Exercise and Sport Sciences Reviews

Volume 19, 1991

EXERCISE AND SPORT SCIENCES REVIEWS

Volume 19, 1991

Editor

JOHN O. HOLLOSZY, M.D.

Professor of Medicine
Department of Internal Medicine
Washington University School of Medicine
St. Louis, Missouri

American College of Sports Medicine Series

 WILLIAMS & WILKINS
BALTIMORE · HONG KONG · LONDON · MUNICH
PHILADELPHIA · SYDNEY · TOKYO

Editor: John P. Butler
Associate Editor: Marjorie Kidd Keating
Copy Editor: Jennifer Conway
Designer: Saturn Graphics
Illustration Planner: Ray Lowman
Production Coordinator: Raymond E. Reter

Printed in the United States of America

Library of Congress Catalog Card Number 72-12187

ISBN 0-683-00048-9

91 92 93 94 95
1 2 3 4 5 6 7 8 9 10

Preface

Exercise and Sport Sciences Reviews is an annual publication sponsored by the American College of Sports Medicine that reviews current research concerning behavioral, biochemical, biomechanical, clinical, physiological, and rehabilitational topics involving exercise science. The Editorial Board for this series currently consists of 15 recognized authorities who have assumed the responsibility for one of the following general topics: athletic medicine, biochemistry, biomechanics, environmental physiology, epidemiology, exercise physiology, gerontology, growth and development, metabolism, molecular biology, motor control, physical fitness, psychology, rehabilitation, and sociology. The organization of the Editorial Board should help foster the commitment of the American College of Sports Medicine to publish timely reviews in broad areas of interest to clinicians, educators, exercise scientists, and students. The goal for this Editorial Board is to provide at least one review in each of these 15 areas for each volume of *Exercise and Sport Sciences Reviews*. Further, the Editor shall select three or four additional topics to be developed into chapters based on current interest, timeliness, and importance to the above audience.

The contributors for each volume are selected by the Editorial Board members and the Editor. Although the majority of these reviews are invited, unsolicited manuscripts of potential chapter topics will be received by the Editor and reviewed by him and/or various members of the Editorial Board for possible inclusion in future volumes. Correspondence should be directed to John O. Holloszy, M.D., Washington University School of Medicine, 2nd Floor, West Building, 4566 Scott Avenue, Campus Box 8113, St. Louis, MO 63110, who assumed the role of Editor of *Exercise and Sport Sciences Reviews* beginning with Volume 19.

John O. Holloszy, M.D.
Editor

Contributors

Kenneth M. Baldwin, Ph.D.
Departments of Physiology and Biophysics
University of California–Irvine
Irvine, California

Jeffrey P. Broker, M.S.
Department of Kinesiology
University of California, Los Angeles
Los Angeles, California

Joseph G. Cannon, Ph.D.
Human Physiology Laboratory
United States Department of Agriculture
Human Nutrition Research Center on Aging
Tufts University
Boston, Massachusetts

Robert C. Cantu, M.D.
Department of Surgery
Chief, Neurosurgical Service
Emerson Hospital
Concord, Massachusetts

Andrew R. Coggan, Ph.D.
Exercise Physiology Laboratory
School of Health, Physical Education, and Recreation
Ohio State University
Columbus, Ohio

Edward F. Coyle, Ph.D.
Human Performance Laboratory
Department of Kinesiology and Health Education
University of Texas at Austin
Austin, Texas

Jerome A. Dempsey, Ph.D.
John Rankin Laboratory of Pulmonary Medicine
Department of Preventive Medicine
University of Wisconsin–Madison Medical School
Madison, Wisconsin

Rod K. Dishman, Ph.D.
Behavioral Fitness Laboratory
University of Georgia
Athens, Georgia

Andrea L. Dunn, Ph.D.
Department of Psychiatry
University of Colorado
Denver, Colorado

V. Reggie Edgerton, Ph.D.
Department of Kinesiology
University of California, Los Angeles
Los Angeles, California

William J. Evans, Ph.D.
Human Physiology Laboratory
United States Department of Agriculture
Human Nutrition Research Center on Aging
Tufts University
Boston, Massachusetts

Martha Flanders, Ph.D.
Department of Physiology
University of Minnesota
Minneapolis, Minnesota

Robert J. Gregor, Ph.D.
Department of Kinesiology
University of California, Los Angeles
Los Angeles, California

Bruce D. Johnson, Ph.D.
John Rankin Laboratory of Pulmonary Medicine
Department of Preventive Medicine
University of Wisconsin–Madison Medical School
Madison, Wisconsin

Abby C. King, Ph.D.
Department of Medicine
Stanford Center for Research in Disease Prevention
Stanford University School of Medicine
Palo Alto, California

Robert Marcus, M.D.
Department of Medicine
Stanford University School of Medicine
Stanford, Connecticut

Frederick O. Mueller, Ph.D.
Department of Physical Education, Exercise, and Sport Science
University of North Carolina at Chapel Hill
Chapel Hill, North Carolina

Roland R. Roy, Ph.D.
Brain Research Institute
University of California, Los Angeles
School of Medicine
Los Angeles, California

Mary Margaret Ryan, M.S.
Department of Kinesiology
University of California, Los Angeles
Los Angeles, California

Douglas R. Seals, Ph.D.
Departments of Exercise and Sport Sciences and Physiology
Arizona Health Science Center
University of Arizona
Tucson, Arizona

Christine Snow-Harter, Ph.D.
Department of Exercise and Sport Science
Oregon State University
Corvallis, Oregon

John F. Soechting, Ph.D.
Department of Physiology
University of Minnesota
Minneapolis, Minnesota

Ronald L. Terjung, Ph.D.
Department of Physiology
State University of New York
Health Science Center Syracuse
Syracuse, New York

James G. Tidball, Ph.D.
Department of Kinesiology and Jerry Lewis Neuromuscular Research
  Center
University of California, Los Angeles
Los Angeles, California

Charles M. Tipton, Ph.D.
Department of Exercise and Sport Sciences
School of Health Related Professions
University of Arizona
Tucson, Arizona

Peter C. Tullson, Ph.D.
Department of Physiology
State University of New York
Health Science Center Syracuse
Syracuse, New York

Ronald G. Victor, M.D.
Department of Medicine, Cardiology Division, and the Harry S. Moss
  Heart Center
University of Texas/Southwestern Medical Center at Dallas
Dallas, Texas

Kevin Young, Ph.D.
Department of Sociology
University of Calgary
Calgary, Alberta, Canada

Contents

1
Carbohydrate Ingestion During Prolonged Exercise: Effects on Metabolism and Performance

ANDREW R. COGGAN, Ph.D.
EDWARD F. COYLE, Ph.D.

INTRODUCTION

The effects of ingesting carbohydrates (CHO) during prolonged exercise have interested physiologists since the early part of the 20th century [25, 27, 46, 47]. This interest arises in large part because CHO ingestion provides a means of rapidly altering CHO availability during exercise and, therefore, represents a useful tool for studying the interrelationships between CHO availability, substrate metabolism, and fatigue. Yet despite this long-standing and widespread interest, detailed studies of the metabolic responses to CHO ingestion during exercise are relatively recent. Similarly, it was only in the last decade that it was conclusively demonstrated that ingesting CHO during prolonged exercise can improve performance [38].

The effects of CHO ingestion during prolonged exercise have been reviewed recently by several authors, mostly from the perspective of determining the optimal fluid replacement beverage during exercise [36, 37, 85, 94]. In this chapter, we focus primarily on the metabolic responses to exercise when fed CHO, and develop a model that we believe is useful in understanding how these metabolic effects may be mechanistically linked to enhanced exercise performance. Because early views of substrate metabolism and the possible causes of fatigue during prolonged exercise have had a major impact on research in this area, we begin with a brief historical overview.

HISTORICAL PERSPECTIVES

At the beginning of this century, studies of exercise metabolism were aimed primarily at defining the fuel(s) used to provide the energy required for muscular activity [6]. These early experiments consisted mainly of determining the respiratory exchange ratio (R) during exercise when CHO availability was increased or decreased by altering a person's

1

chronic diet [26, 79]. In a few studies, however, CHO availability was increased by having subjects ingest CHO during the exercise itself [25, 27, 46, 47]. As early as 1932, for example, Dill et al. [46] reported that feeding one laboratory dog 20 grams (g) of CHO every hour during prolonged exercise maintained blood glucose levels and enabled the animal to run at 124 meters per minute (m/min) up to a 17.6% grade for at least 13 hours without fatiguing. When the dog was supplied with only water to drink during exercise, however, blood glucose concentrations decreased markedly, and he was able to exercise at this intensity for 3 to 6.5 hours (hr) before tiring. In another experiment, the dog ran for 4.25 hr in the fasted state, which resulted in a decline in blood glucose to 2.6 millimole per liter (mmol/L) coincident with fatigue. The animal was then fed 40 g of CHO during an 8-minute (min) rest period, which increased blood glucose to >6 mmol/L and enabled the dog to run for another 1.5 hr, at which time he was still not exhausted. These observations led Dill et al. [46] to conclude that the limiting factor in the performance of prolonged exercise ". . . seems to be merely the quantity of easily available fuel . . ." in the form of blood-borne glucose. Ingestion of CHO during exercise was therefore thought to delay fatigue by maintaining the availability of this important CHO source for oxidation by the exercising musculature.

In contrast to this view, early studies of exercising humans emphasized the ability of CHO ingestion during exercise to supply glucose for use by the central nervous system (CNS) [16, 17, 27, 58, 86]. As early as 1924, for example, Levine et al. [86] noted that some runners competing in the Boston Marathon became hypoglycemic, showing symptoms of neuroglucopenia such as ". . . muscular twitching . . . nervous irritability, and even collapse and unconsciousness." Performance was reportedly improved when these symptoms were prevented by having these same men consume additional CHO on the day before and during the race the following year [58]. Fifteen years later in 1939, Christensen and Hansen [26] observed in three men that consuming a low CHO diet markedly impaired their endurance during moderate-intensity ($\approx$60–65% oxygen uptake peak [$\dot{V}O_2$max]) exercise. This premature fatigue was accompanied by ketosis, a low rate of CHO oxidation, and hypoglycemia severe enough to result in symptoms of neuroglucopenia. In an attempt to distinguish between these three possible causes of fatigue, Christensen and Hansen [27] performed additional experiments in which two of these men were fed 200 g of glucose at almost complete exhaustion. Glucose ingestion resulted in a rapid increase in blood glucose concentration and relief of the neuroglucopenic symptoms, enabling the men to continue exercising for an additional 60 min (Fig. 1.1). The subjects' R values, however, which were much lower than normal owing to the preceding low CHO diet, changed very little either before or after glucose ingestion (Fig. 1.1). Thus, the initial onset of

FIGURE 1.1

*The data of Christensen and Hansen [27]. Blood glucose and respiratory exchange ratio were measured during prolonged exercise in two men who had been consuming a very low CHO diet. At the point of "almost complete exhaustion" the men were fed 200 g of glucose (denoted by "****Feed****"), and they were able to exercise for an additional hour. In subject O.B., R remained relatively constant before and after glucose ingestion. Interestingly, this is the same subject who was studied by Boje in 1940 [17], and who appears to have been unusually susceptible to hypoglycemia during exercise. In subject M.N., R initially fell and then increased again following glucose ingestion. The response of subject M.N. is similar to our observations shown in Figure 1.6. (Modified from Christensen, E.H., and O. Hansen. IV. Hypoglykämie, Arbeitfähigkeit und Ermudung.* Skand. Arch. Physiol. *81:172–179, 1939.)*

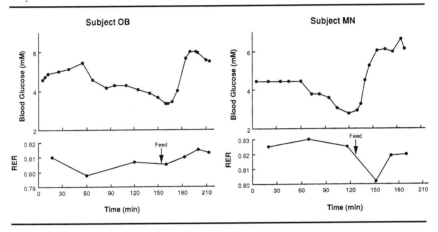

fatigue and its subsequent reversal by CHO ingestion did not appear to be associated with large changes in the rate of CHO oxidation. In another experiment [27], one of these men experienced hypoglycemia and symptoms of neuroglucopenia when exercising 3 hr after ingesting 200 g of glucose, and fatigued prematurely even though R and therefore the estimated rate of CHO oxidation were quite high. Based on these observations, Christensen and Hansen [27] concluded that hypoglycemia must cause fatigue by means of its effects on the CNS, and not by affecting muscle metabolism. A similar conclusion had been reached by Boje in 1936 [16].

With the reintroduction of the muscle biopsy procedure in the 1960s [12], emphasis shifted from blood glucose towards muscle glycogen as the major source of CHO during exercise. Using this technique, muscle glycogen was shown to be depleted after intense exercise performed to fatigue [13, 62]. Dietary manipulations known to affect endurance performance were found to alter preexercise muscle glycogen stores

[14, 57, 75]. In addition, endurance exercise training, which was known to decrease total CHO oxidation and improve exercise performance, was demonstrated to decrease the rate of glycogen utilization [66, 76]. Furthermore, glucose uptake by skeletal muscle during exercise was reported to be minimal [13, 34], and the intravenous infusion of glucose at high rates was found to have little effect on the rate of muscle glycogenolysis [1, 13, 63]. The concept therefore became established that muscle glycogen was the primary CHO source during exercise, and that blood-borne glucose contributed little to the CHO needs of muscle during moderate or intense exercise.

This concept was further reinforced by the notion that CHO ingested during exercise "seems to remain in compartments within an unoxidized glucose pool" [117]. This belief was based on the observation that although carbon-14- (^{14}C) labeled glucose ingested during prolonged exercise at 50–72% $\dot{V}O_2$max rapidly appeared in the circulation, very little of the ^{14}C label was recovered in expired breath as $^{14}CO_2$ [35, 117]. Because blood glucose in general and ingested CHO in particular were thought to contribute little to the CHO needs of muscle during moderate intensity exercise, CHO ingestion during exercise was assumed to benefit only persons suffering from neuroglucopenia [36].

Despite these earlier views, however, substantial evidence exists indicating that blood glucose is an important CHO energy source during exercise [32]. CHO ingestion during prolonged exercise also has been repeatedly demonstrated to enhance performance, even in persons not suffering from neuroglucopenia [28–30, 38, 41]. Indeed, recent evidence indicates that blood glucose becomes the dominant CHO energy source during prolonged (≥ 2 hr) exercise, and that, as originally suggested by Dill et al. [46], CHO ingestion improves performance primarily by maintaining the availability and oxidation of this critical fuel [28–30, 41]. The evidence leading to this interpretation is the subject of the present review.

EFFECTS ON METABOLISM

Rate of Blood Glucose Utilization During Exercise When Fasted

In the fasted state, glucose uptake by resting skeletal muscle is minimal, and most of the glucose produced by the liver is used by the CNS [5]. At the onset of exercise, the arteriovenous difference for glucose across the muscle initially decreases and may actually become negative, indicating net glucose release [34, 74, 78, 123]. This free glucose is presumably derived from the hydrolysis of the α minus 1,6-linkages of glycogen by debranching enzyme, or from the hydrolysis of glucose-6-phosphate by the action of nonspecific phosphatases [34, 123]. After the first few min of exercise, however, this glucose release quickly reverts to glucose uptake [34, 123].

The rate of blood glucose utilization during exercise is curvilinearly related to the exercise intensity [77, 123]. During cycle ergometer exercise, for example, glucose uptake by the legs increases from ≈0.05 g/min at rest to ≈0.2, ≈0.4, and ≈0.7 g/min after 40 min of exercise at approximately 25%, 50%, and 75% of $V_{mO_2}max$, respectively [123]. Most of the glucose taken up at these intensities is probably directly oxidized; blood glucose utilization can therefore account for roughly one-fourth to one-third of total CHO energy production during the early stages of moderate-intensity exercise [32]. Glucose uptake continues to increase with increasing exercise intensity, with rates as high as 1.4 g/min observed during exercise at ≈100% $\dot{V}_{O_2}max$ [77]. During such high-intensity exercise, however, some of the glucose taken up may accumulate within the muscle, owing to inhibition of hexokinase by glucose-6-phosphate produced by rapid glycogenolysis [77].

In addition to increasing with greater exercise intensity, the utilization of blood glucose also increases as the duration of exercise increases. For example, glucose uptake by the legs during cycle ergometer exercise at ≈60% $\dot{V}_{O_2}max$ increases almost 40% between 40 and 90 min of exercise [4]. Rates of blood glucose utilization of over 1.2 g/min have been observed at the end of exercise to fatigue at 67% $\dot{V}_{O_2}max$ [21]. Even very intense, intermittent exercise, which is normally thought to rely primarily on muscle glycogen as a CHO source, eventually results in marked increases in glucose turnover. In two subjects, for example, Hultman [63] observed that splanchnic glucose release increased from 0.4–0.6 g/min early in exercise to 0.9–1.1 g/min at fatigue (≈60 min). In both cases, the arterial blood glucose concentration remained constant, indicating that these high rates of splanchnic glucose production were matched by equally high rates of peripheral glucose utilization.

This increase in blood glucose utilization with time partially compensates for, and may be related to, a steady decrease in the rate of muscle glycogenolysis [32]. Because blood glucose utilization increases over time as muscle glycogen utilization decreases, blood glucose utilization represents a progressively increasing proportion of total CHO oxidation [41]. As indicated above, during the first hour of exercise at ≈60–70% $\dot{V}_{O_2}max$, blood glucose utilization represents only about one-fourth of total CHO oxidation [4, 21, 41, 72]. Late in exercise when muscle glycogen is low, however, blood glucose appears to account for almost all of the CHO being oxidized [21, 28, 41]. However, blood glucose utilization may actually decrease during the later stages of prolonged moderate intensity exercise because of a decrease in blood glucose concentration that results from a decrease in splanchnic glucose production [4, 28, 41].

Blood glucose utilization also increases with time during low-intensity exercise. During prolonged cycle ergometer exercise performed at 30% $\dot{V}_{O_2}max$, glucose uptake by the legs does not plateau until after 90 min of exercise [2]. Nevertheless, fat remains the primary source of energy for skeletal muscle during prolonged, low-intensity exercise [2]. Like moderate-intensity exercise, leg glucose uptake may decrease during the later stages of lower intensity exercise because of a decrease in blood glucose concentration [2].

Substantial data therefore indicate that blood glucose represents a very important source of CHO for exercising skeletal muscle, especially when muscle glycogen stores become depleted during prolonged, moderate-intensity exercise. The contribution of blood glucose to CHO oxidation by muscle may be limited, however, by a decrease in blood glucose concentration late in exercise [2, 4, 28, 41]. This decrease in blood glucose may be prevented by ingesting sufficient amounts of CHO. The effects of such CHO ingestion on blood glucose and muscle and liver glycogen utilization during exercise are considered below.

Rate of Blood Glucose Utilization During Exercise When Fed CHO
During low-intensity exercise (30% $\dot{V}o_2max$), CHO ingestion results in increased blood glucose and insulin concentrations [3]. As a result of this hyperglycemia and hyperinsulinemia, the rate of muscle glucose uptake is up to twofold greater compared to the rate observed during exercise in the fasted state [3]. At the same time, adipose tissue lipolysis is decreased, as indicated by lower plasma free fatty acid (FFA) and glycerol concentrations [3] and a slower rate of plasma FFA turnover [24]. As will be discussed subsequently, muscle glycogen utilization does not appear to be affected by CHO ingestion during exercise. The net result of these metabolic changes is a decreased reliance on adipose tissue (and possibly intramuscular) triglycerides and an increased reliance on blood glucose as the source of energy during exercise, leading to an increase in R [3, 9–11]. Nevertheless, the rate of blood glucose utilization does not exceed that observed during more intense exercise performed in the fasted state [3].

CHO ingestion during moderate intensity exercise (50–75% $\dot{V}o_2max$) tends to produce less marked alterations in substrate metabolism. The insulin response to CHO infusion or ingestion during moderate-intensity exercise is suppressed compared to that observed during low-intensity exercise, probably because of greater sympathetic nervous system inhibition of insulin secretion. Consequently, insulin levels are the same or only slightly higher than those observed during exercise in the fasted state [28–30, 38, 41, 69]. The increases in plasma FFA and glycerol concentrations during exercise are blunted, but not to the same extent as observed following CHO ingestion during low-intensity exercise [38, 41, 69]. Plasma FFA or muscle triglyceride utilization have not been directly determined during moderate-intensity exercise when fed CHO. However, these small differences in plasma FFA and glycerol concentrations, along with little or no difference in R, at least during the first several hours of exercise [38, 41], suggest that the rate of fat oxidation is not greatly affected.

The effects of CHO ingestion on blood glucose metabolism during moderate-intensity exercise also have not been studied directly in humans. As described under "Historical perspectives," early studies that attempted to calculate blood glucose oxidation by feeding subjects ^{14}C-labeled glucose during exercise at 50–72% $\dot{V}O_2$max surmised that very little blood glucose was oxidized under these conditions [35, 117]. This notion was based on the observation that, although up to two-thirds of circulating glucose was derived from the ingested glucose load, <10% of the ^{14}C label was recovered in expired CO_2 during the first hour of exercise following glucose ingestion. However, CO_2 produced by cellular respiration enters the body's bicarbonate pools, which turn over relatively slowly, even during exercise [31, 115, 127]. This limited recovery probably primarily reflects the slow passage of the [14]CO_2 through these pools, not a limited rate of blood glucose oxidation. This interpretation is supported by the observation that, irrespective of the size, timing, or type of ^{14}C-labeled CHO load, the recovery of [14]CO_2 during exercise follows a similar time course [10, 35, 117], which lags well behind the appearance of the label in the blood [35, 117]. Again, considerable data indicate that blood glucose is an important CHO source during moderate-intensity exercise performed in the fasted state. Thus, these studies using ^{14}C-glucose [35, 117] undoubtedly greatly underestimated the extent to which blood glucose is oxidized when CHO are ingested during moderate-intensity exercise.

In contrast, studies that have attempted to measure the oxidation of exogenous CHO by feeding exercising subjects CHO sources that are naturally enriched with carbon-13 (^{13}C) [56, 80, 87, 88, 104–108] have overestimated the rate of oxidation by up to 75% [105]. Because the ^{13}C enrichment of CHO is greater than that of fats [71, 112], an increase in the relative contribution of CHO oxidation to total CO_2 production (i.e., an increase in R) due either to exercise or to CHO ingestion, or both, will result in an increase in [13]CO_2 production from endogenous CHO sources [8, 31, 112, 126]. Indeed, recent data indicate that, when subjects are fed naturally labeled CHO during exercise, up to one-half of the increase in [13]CO_2 production arises from endogenous substrates, not from the ingested CHO load [105]. This increase in endogenous [13]CO_2 production when fed CHO during exercise is not accounted for by measuring the breath [13]CO_2 enrichment at rest prior to exercise, and is only partially accounted for by measuring the [13]CO_2 enrichment in breath during exercise in the absence of CHO ingestion. This may explain why, under otherwise almost identical experimental conditions, the apparent recovery of the label in expired CO_2 during exercise is much greater when subjects ingest CHO sources labeled with [13]C [56, 80, 87, 88, 104–108] rather than [14]C [10, 35, 117]. Similarly, production of $^{13}CO_2$ from endogenous sources may explain why over 50 g of ingested ^{13}C-labeled sucrose are apparently "oxidized" during 4 hr of moderate-intensity exercise, despite the simultaneous ingestion of a potent α-glucosidase inhibitor to block hydrolysis and therefore absorption of the sucrose in the small intestine [56]. Estimates of the rate of exogenous CHO oxidation during exercise obtained using this technique therefore require quantitative reevaluation. Furthermore, these studies have provided no information on the effect of CHO ingestion during exercise on the oxidation of endogenous blood glucose.

The effects of CHO ingestion during moderate-intensity exercise on blood glucose utilization remain uncertain. In the absence of direct data, we attempted to estimate this indirectly by measuring muscle glycogen utilization in subjects fed CHO throughout moderate intensity exercise; any additional CHO oxidized was assumed to represent blood glucose [41]. Because these estimates are indirect, they must be viewed as only a first approximation. Nevertheless, the results of this study suggested that blood glucose utilization initially increased similarly during exercise at 70–75% $\dot{V}O_2$max when fasted or when fed CHO, reaching ≈ 1 g/min after ≈ 2 hr of exercise. After this time, blood glucose utilization appeared to decrease during exercise in the fasted state, owing to a decline in blood glucose concentration. When fed CHO throughout exercise, however, estimated blood glucose utilization continued to increase with time, so that after ≈ 3 hr of exercise, it appeared to account for almost all of the CHO being oxidized. Blood glucose must have been oxidized at ≈ 2 g/min late in exercise to support the observed rate of total CHO oxidation. Most of the blood glucose being oxidized was presumably derived from the ingested CHO load (i.e., ≈ 340 g of maltodextrins during ≈ 4 hr of exercise), because previous studies have demonstrated that up to two-thirds of circulating glucose originates from the exogenous CHO load when much smaller amounts (10–42 g) of CHO are ingested during exercise [35, 117].

These data suggested that when blood glucose concentration is prevented from decreasing during the later stages of moderate-intensity exercise, blood glucose may be oxidized at much higher rates than previously believed possible. To test this hypothesis, we [28] measured whole-body glucose disposal late in exercise using the euglycemic clamp technique [45]. After prolonged exercise that led to muscle glycogen depletion and a decline in blood glucose concentration, glucose was infused intravenously at the rate required to restore and maintain euglycemia while the subjects performed additional exercise. These experiments demonstrated that whole-body glucose disposal averaged 1.13 g/min late in exercise. If completely oxidized, the infused glucose could account for three-quarters of total CHO oxidation under these conditions [28] (Fig. 1.2). It is probable that blood glucose oxidation constituted nearly 100% of total CHO oxidation during glucose infusion,

FIGURE 1.2

Estimated substrate utilization during the final 30 minutes of exercise at ≈70% $\dot{V}_{O_2}$max, when glucose was infused intravenously at the rate required to maintain plasma glucose concentration at ≈5 mmol/L. The relative contributions of fat (55%) and CHO (45%) to total energy expenditure were determined from the mean R value (i.e., 0.84). The rate of total CHO oxidation (i.e., 1.50 g/min) was also determined from R and $\dot{V}_{O_2}$. Exogenous glucose was assumed to be oxidized at the infusion rate required to maintain euglycemia (i.e., 1.13 g/min), and could account for 76% of total CHO oxidation and 34% of total energy expenditure. The rate of oxidation of other CHO sources (i.e., 0.37 g/min) accounted for 24% of total CHO oxidation and 11% of total energy expenditure. This probably reflects primarily the oxidation of endogenous blood glucose, because muscle glycogen concentration did not change during glucose infusion. (Reprinted with permission from Coggan, A.R., and E.F. Coyle. Reversal of fatigue during prolonged exercise by carbohydrate infusion or ingestion. J. Appl. Physiol. *63:2388–2395, 1987.)*

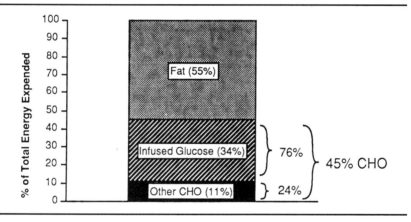

because muscle glycogen concentration did not decrease during this time despite a high rate of total CHO oxidation (i.e., 1.50 g/min). This additional glucose (i.e., 0.37 g/min) would presumably be derived from residual hepatic glycogenolysis or gluconeogenesis, or both, which are not determined by the euglycemic clamp technique [45].

To test this hypothesis further, in a recent pilot experiment we measured plasma glucose turnover and oxidation using a primed, continuous infusion of $[U-^{13}C]$glucose in one well-trained cyclist exercising for 2 hr at 70–75% $\dot{V}_{O_2}$max when fed CHO throughout exercise [A. R. Coggan, D. M. Bier, and J. O. Holloszy, unpublished observations]. By priming the bicarbonate pools with $NaH^{13}CO_3$ and by infusing the $[U-^{13}C]$glucose at a relatively high rate (≈50 μmol/min), it was possible to achieve a plateau in breath $^{13}CO_2$ enrichment during the final 30 min of exercise that was approximately 100 times greater than any potential increase from exercise or CHO ingestion alone [31, 126]. It was therefore possible to accurately quantify glucose oxidation under true steady-state conditions. The results of this experiment indicated that the rate of plasma glucose oxidation during the 90–120 min period of exercise exceeded 1 g/min, which could have accounted for about one-half of the total CHO being oxidized at this time. Although representing only a single subject, these direct measurements of the rate of blood glucose oxidation after 1.5–2 hr of moderate-intensity exercise when fed CHO agree very well with prior indirect estimates derived from the measurement of $\dot{V}O_2$, R, and muscle glycogen concentration [41]. These measurements also agree reasonably well with the rate of whole-body glucose disposal determined after 3 hr of exercise using the euglycemic clamp technique [28].

Obviously, additional experiments will be required to more accurately quantify the rate of blood glucose utilization during moderate-intensity exercise when subjects are fed CHO, especially during exercise of >2 hr duration. In particular, it will important to compare these rates of blood glucose utilization during exercise when fed CHO to rates observed during exercise in the fasted state. More information also is needed on the contribution of ingested CHO to the total glucose pool during exercise. Nevertheless, the available data support the conclusion that blood glucose can be oxidized at very high rates during prolonged, moderate-intensity exercise when fed CHO, and that at least some of this glucose is derived from the ingested CHO load. As developed later in this chapter, it is this ability of CHO ingested during exercise to maintain or increase blood glucose availability and oxidation late in exercise that apparently results in the improvement in exercise performance.

Effect of CHO Ingestion on Muscle Glycogenolysis During Exercise
An important question is whether ingesting CHO during exercise, by maintaining or increasing blood glucose availability and oxidation as previously described, slows the rate of muscle glycogenolysis. This possibility was first raised by the experiments of Hultman and co-workers [1, 13, 63], who reported that the intravenous infusion of glucose at up to 3.5 g/min decreased net glycogen degradation during intermittent exercise by ≈20%. This decrease in glycogen utilization was not statistically significant when only 2 to 6 subjects were studied [1, 63], but did achieve statistical significance (P < 0.001) when a total of 10 men were tested [13]. Similarly, Ehrenstein et al. [49] reported that, although intravenous glucose infusion during 8 hr of intermittent cycle ergometer exercise at 30% $\dot{V}O_2$max did not result in a statistically significant decrease in the amount of muscle glycogen utilized, differences in muscle glycogen utilization between the control and glucose

infusion trials were inversely related to differences in blood glucose concentration ($r = -0.62$; $P < 0.01$). These observations, along with the observation that less muscle glycogen was used when glucose was infused into exercising rats [7], led us to hypothesize that CHO ingestion during exercise improves performance by slowing the rate of muscle glycogen degradation [38, 39]. However, subsequent direct measurements of muscle·glycogen utilization during exercise with and without CHO feedings, both by us [41] and by others [53, 55, 61, 91, 100], have indicated that this hypothesis is incorrect. Nevertheless, some authors have concluded that CHO ingestion during exercise does indeed exert a glycogen-sparing effect [15, 23, 50, 60, 113]. The evidence for and against this hypothesis is considered in detail below.

In apparently the first study to directly examine the effects of CHO ingestion on muscle glycogen use during exercise, Hargreaves et al. [60] reported that feeding subjects 43 g of sucrose every hour during 4 hr of intermittent cycling exercise decreased net glycogen degradation in the vastus lateralis from 126 ± 5 ($X \pm$ S.E.) to 101 ± 10 mmol glucosyl units/kg wet muscle ($P < 0.05$). Interpretation of these results is confounded, however, by the fact that muscle glycogen concentration was significantly higher prior to the placebo trial compared to the CHO feeding trial. In fact, when the data are reanalyzed excluding the four subjects with the largest intertrial difference in pre-exercise glycogen stores (20–63% higher prior to their placebo trial), the difference in glycogen utilization between trials is almost completely eliminated. Thus, the apparent sparing of glycogen in this study appears to be an artifact of the higher pre-exercise glycogen concentration in the placebo trial.

Soon after, Bjorkman et al. [15] measured muscle glycogen concentration and performance time in moderately trained men exercising to fatigue at 68% $\dot{V}o_2$max when fed a placebo, glucose, or fructose throughout exercise. Muscle glycogen concentration decreased similarly in all three trials. However, because the time to fatigue was significantly longer during the glucose feeding trial, the researchers concluded that glucose ingestion decreased the rate of glycogen degradation during exercise. Simard et al. [113] reached a similar conclusion when glycogen degradation was expressed relative to the distance skated during a hockey match. Yet when muscle glycogen is measured in serial biopsies throughout exercise with and without CHO ingestion, no difference in the rate of glycogen utilization is observed [41]. The apparent sparing of muscle glycogen reported by Bjorkman et al. [15] and Simard et al. [113] therefore appears to be due to the greater quantity of exercise made possible by ingesting CHO during exercise, and not to a decrease in the actual rate of glycogenolysis.

Brouns et al. [23] also concluded recently that CHO ingestion during exercise decreases the utilization of muscle glycogen. In these experiments, however, muscle glycogen concentration was measured at rest on one day, and after exercise four days later. In the interim, the subjects (highly trained cyclists) performed two bouts of very strenuous exercise, and ingested extra CHO not only during the exercise itself but also between exercise bouts. It is impossible to determine from this design whether the higher glycogen level observed after exercise when consuming a CHO supplement was caused by a decrease in the rate of glycogen utilization during exercise, or was the result of higher preexercise glycogen levels from an accelerated rate of glycogen resynthesis between exercise bouts.

Definitive evidence of glycogen sparing would require demonstrating that, when preexercise muscle glycogen concentration and the duration of exercise are the same, postexercise muscle glycogen concentration is significantly higher when fed CHO during exercise. To date, in at least seven studies muscle glycogen concentration has been measured before and after exercise of the same duration, performed with and without CHO supplementation during exercise [41, 50, 53, 55, 61, 91, 100]. In six of these studies [41, 53, 55, 61, 91, 100] in which a total of 85 subjects were examined, CHO ingestion had no effect on the decrease in muscle glycogen during exercise. In contrast, Erickson et al. [50] reported that muscle glycogen utilization was significantly reduced when five trained cyclists ingested 70 g of glucose during 90 min of exercise at 65–70% $\dot{V}o_2$max. These results, however, like those of Hargreaves et al. [60], appear to be due to higher preexercise muscle glycogen levels in the control trial, rather than a decrease in the rate of glycogen utilization when fed CHO during exercise.

A review of the literature indicates that CHO ingestion during continuous, moderate-intensity exercise does not reduce the utilization of muscle glycogen. In contrast, some evidence suggests that intravenous glucose infusion during exercise may decrease the rate of muscle glycogenolysis [7, 13, 125]. These studies, however, have generally provided glucose at rates that produced significant hyperglycemia, therefore possibly resulting in a greater impetus to decrease muscle glycogenolysis during exercise.

To address this possibility, we recently measured muscle glycogen utilization in eight men during 2 hr of continuous exercise at 73% $\dot{V}o_2$max, when glucose was infused throughout exercise at a rate which elevated and then maintained blood glucose at 10.8 ± 0.4 mmol/L [42]. This required the infusion of glucose at an average rate of ≈2 g/min. Despite this high rate of glucose infusion and an increase in blood insulin concentrations during the second hour of exercise to 20–25 μU/mL, muscle glycogen degradation was unaffected (glycogen utilization averaged 76 ± 7 mmol glucosyl units/kg wet muscle during the control trial vs. 75 ± 8 mmol glucosyl units/kg wet muscle during the glucose infusion trial). Thus, increasing blood glucose to ≈10 mmol/L during continuous exercise at 70–75% $\dot{V}o_2$max does not reduce utilization of muscle glycogen in humans.

Nevertheless, the decline in muscle glycogen during exercise appears to be attenuated in men when the exercise is intermittent and glucose is infused at higher rates that result in greater hyperglycemia [13]. This may be the result of stimulation of glycogen resynthesis, which may occur either during rest periods between exercise bouts or even during exercise itself [19, 33, 49, 65, 68, 81–83, 118]. However, in glycogen-depleted men fed large amounts of CHO during mild exercise, net glycogen accumulation occurs only in Type II fibers, and not in Type I fibers [82]. Thus, glycogen synthesis during exercise following CHO ingestion appears to occur primarily in resting muscle fibers within the exercising muscle, rather than in exercising muscle fibers themselves. It therefore seems unlikely that CHO ingestion during continuous, moderate-intensity exercise could decrease net muscle glycogen utilization by inducing glycogen synthesis, because most muscle fibers are recruited during this type of exercise [120]. Net glycogen sparing due to glycogen synthesis during exercise may still be a possibility, however, when subjects are fed CHO during low-intensity or intermittent exercise.

Effect of CHO Ingestion on Hepatic Glycogenolysis and Gluconeogenesis During Exercise

In contrast to the lack of effect of CHO ingestion during exercise on muscle glycogen metabolism, hepatic CHO metabolism appears to be affected by CHO supplementation during exercise. Liver glycogenolysis has been shown to be reduced when exercising rats are infused with glucose during mild exercise [7]. Furthermore, the uptake of gluconeogenic precursors by the splanchnic bed has been shown to be greatly reduced when men ingest CHO during low-intensity exercise [3]. These effects are probably mediated by the accompanying hormonal responses of CHO ingestion during low-intensity exercise (i.e., increased insulin and decreased glucagon and epinephrine concentrations [3]).

The effects of CHO ingestion on hepatic glucose metabolism during moderate-intensity exercise are less certain. However, it appears that ingested CHO can at least partially replace the liver as the source of glucose entering the circulation. For example, glucose ingested during exercise at 50–72% $\dot{V}o_2$max has been demonstrated to supply up to two-thirds of the circulating glucose pool [35, 117]. Because the total glucose mass increases only slightly following CHO ingestion during moderate-intensity exercise (as indicated by relatively small increases in blood glucose concentration), these observations suggest that hepatic glycogenolysis or gluconeogenesis, or both, must be reduced. Similarly, glucose infusion during moderate-intensity exercise has been demonstrated to at least partially suppress glucose production in both rats [125] and humans [51, 73]. When hepatic glycogen stores become depleted late in exercise, ingested CHO will represent almost the sole source of blood glucose supply, because the rate of gluconeogenesis in exercising humans seems to be limited to at most 0.2–0.4 g/min [2, 4], and appears to be suppressed by CHO ingestion [3].

EFFECTS OF PERFORMANCE

Early Evidence That CHO Ingestion May Aid Performance
As previously discussed, during the 1970s it was generally believed that CHO ingestion during prolonged exercise would be of little benefit to performance except in persons suffering from neuroglucopenia [36, 117]. This was true despite preliminary attempts to address this question that suggested otherwise [22, 59, 69, 93]. For example, in 1972 Green and Bagley [59] fed subjects either a placebo or a total of 230 g of maltodextrins before and during a ≈2.5 hr canoeing race. CHO ingestion before and during exercise increased blood glucose concentration above preexercise levels, whereas blood glucose decreased moderately (by 1–1.5 mmol/L) during exercise when fed the placebo. CHO ingestion also permitted the athletes to maintain their pace during the final ≈30 min of the race; during the same time in the placebo trial they were forced to reduce their pace by ≈10–15%. The average difference in overall performance time in this study, however, was very small (2%) and not statistically significant.

In a follow-up study, Brooke et al. [22] reported that blood glucose concentration and the rate of CHO oxidation were well maintained during 3 to 4 hr of cycling at 67% $\dot{V}O_2$max when trained cyclists ingested 90 g of CHO in the form of either maltodextrins or rice pudding plus sucrose every 20 minutes during exercise. In contrast, both blood glucose concentration and the rate of CHO oxidation declined when the subjects consumed a low-energy drink or nothing at all during two other trials. These authors reasoned that "... muscle glycogen must be reduced considerably and the only way of maintaining such a high CHO participation is by use of the blood glucose." These observations and this interpretation are generally supported by our more recent findings [28, 41], as discussed below. In addition, Brooke et al. [22] reported that the "work time cut-off" averaged 148 ± 13 min when completely fasted, 180 ± 19 min when fed the low energy drink (P < 0.10 vs. fasted), 200 ± 16 min when fed rice pudding plus sucrose (P < 0.01 vs. fasted), and 214 ± 14 min when fed maltodextrins (P < 0.01 vs. fasted; P < 0.05 vs. the low energy drink). Interpretation of these results is confounded because the subjects' performance time appears to have been defined by a decrease in R or blood glucose, or both, below a certain level, rather than by the inability of the subjects to continue exercising. Furthermore, $\dot{V}O_2$ varied considerably between and within trials, suggesting that the exercise intensity may have been inadequately controlled. Despite these limitations, this study [22] suggested that CHO feedings during prolonged exercise could potentially delay fatigue, and that this was associated with the maintenance of blood glucose concentration and the rate of CHO oxidation.

A further indication that CHO ingestion may improve endurance performance was provided by Ivy et al. [69], who had trained cyclists attempt to maximize their average power production during 2 hr of exercise on a hydraulically braked cycle ergometer. The cyclists ingested ≈13 g of maltodextrins immediately prior to and every 15 min during the first 90 min of exercise during one trial, whereas they ingested a placebo at these time points during another trial. CHO ingestion did not significantly affect the average power produced during the entire 2 hr of exercise. During the last 30 min of exercise, however, when fed CHO the subjects were able to increase their power output during this time period when fed the placebo. It was not specified whether these differences in power output late in exercise were statistically significant.

In contrast, Felig et al. [52] observed only small (+7 to +13 min), insignificant increases in time to fatigue during cycle ergometer exercise at 60–65% $\dot{V}O_2$max when subjects ingested either 10 g or 20 g of glucose instead of a placebo every 15 min during exercise. The subjects in this study, however, were not experienced cyclists and showed great variability in their exercise performances owing to motivation or learning effects. This variability may have obscured any potential improvement in performance as a result of ingesting CHO during exercise.

Studies by the Authors
Green and Bagley [59], Brooke et al. [22], and Ivy et al. [69] suggested, but did not prove, that CHO ingestion may potentially enhance performance during prolonged (≥2 hr) moderate-intensity exercise. To address this question, we had experienced cyclists exercise at ≈74% $\dot{V}O_2$max for as long as possible on two occasions [38]. When the subjects were no longer able to maintain this exercise intensity, they were permitted to reduce their exercise intensity to the highest level they could maintain for at least another 10 min. Fatigue was defined as the time when they were forced to reduce their exercise intensity by 10% of $\dot{V}O_2$max below their initial level (i.e., from ≈74% $\dot{V}O_2$max to ≈64% $\dot{V}O_2$max). Both trials were performed after an overnight fast in order to minimize the acute effects of the last meal on exercise metabolism [40, 92]. During one trial, the subjects ingested 1 g of maltodextrins/kg body weight in a 50% solution after 20 min of exercise, and an additional 0.25 g of maltodextrins/kg body weight in a 6% solution after 60, 90, and 120 min of exercise. During another trial, they received equal volumes of an artificially sweetened and flavored placebo.

CHO ingestion significantly delayed fatigue by 23 min (i.e., from 134

FIGURE 1.3

*Blood glucose concentration and exercise intensity during prolonged exercise by ten cyclists receiving either a placebo or CHO feedings throughout exercise. The seven subjects who became hypoglycemic (blood glucose < 3 mmol/L) during exercise when fasted were able to exercise significantly longer when fed CHO throughout exercise (i.e., 159 ± 6 min CHO vs 126 ± 3 min Placebo; † P < 0.001). Fatigue was not delayed in the three subjects who did not demonstrate a significant decrease in blood glucose concentration during their placebo trial (i.e., 153 ± 14 min CHO vs 150 ± 9 min Placebo). * Blood glucose concentration significantly (P < 0.05) lower than before exercise as well as significantly lower than CHO. § Exercise intensity significantly higher during CHO. (Reprinted with permission from Coyle, E.F., J.M. Hagberg, B.F. Hurley, W.H. Martin, A.A. Ehsani, and J.O. Holloszy. Carbohydrate feedings during prolonged strenuous exercise can delay fatigue. J. Appl. Physiol. 55:230–235, 1983.)*

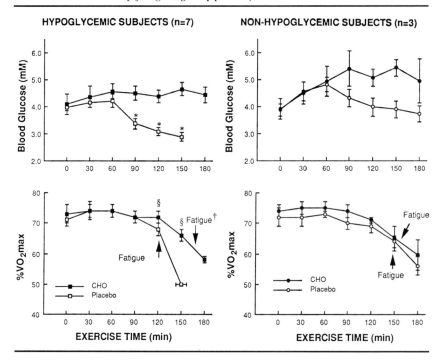

± 6 min to 157 ± 5 min; P < 0.01) for the entire group of 10 subjects. However, as shown in Figure 1.3, this effect was evident only in the seven subjects who experienced a decline in blood glucose concentration to below 3 mmol/L during their placebo trial; in these subjects fatigue was delayed by an average of 33 min (i.e., from 126 ± 3 min to 159 ± 6 min; P < 0.001). This decrease in blood glucose was associated with symptoms of neuroglucopenia in only two of these persons, whereas the other five subjects complained primarily of severe weariness in the exercising muscles as the cause of fatigue. Fatigue was not delayed in the three subjects whose blood glucose concentration did not decline during their placebo trial (Fig. 1.3). To our knowledge, this was the first study to conclusively demonstrate that CHO ingestion during exercise can delay fatigue and improve performance in people not suffering from neuroglucopenia. Furthermore, this effect appeared to be due to prevention of a decline in blood glucose to levels which, although not associated with symptoms of neuroglucopenia in most of the subjects, apparently contributed to local muscular fatigue during the latter stages of prolonged exercise. At the time, however, we incorrectly interpreted these observations to suggest that CHO ingestion during prolonged exercise improves performance by delaying muscle glycogen depletion [38, 39].

To test this hypothesis, we first measured muscle glycogen concentration in the vastus lateralis before and after 105 min of cycling at 71% $\dot{V}o_2$max with and without CHO ingestion throughout exercise. No differences in glycogen utilization were observed [41]. Thinking that CHO feedings may spare muscle glycogen only late in exercise, we next obtained muscle biopsies from another group of cyclists at rest, after 120 min of exercise at 71% $\dot{V}o_2$max, and at fatigue during both a placebo and a CHO ingestion trial [41]. Fatigue occurred after 181 ± 11 min of exercise when fed the placebo, whereas fatigue was delayed (P < 0.01) until 241 ± 20 min when fed CHO throughout exercise (i.e., 1 g of maltodextrins/kg body weight in a 50% solution after 20 minutes of exercise and 0.4 g maltodextrins/kg body weight in a 10% solution every 20 min thereafter). As shown in Figure 1.4C, however, the decline in muscle glycogen concentration during exercise was again similar both with and without CHO ingestion, with the additional 60 ± 16 min of exercise made possible by CHO ingestion accomplished without a further decrease in muscle glycogen.

The rate of total CHO oxidation was also similar during the first 2 hr of exercise in both trials (Fig. 1.4B). However, CHO oxidation began declining during the third hour of the placebo trial, at a time when muscle glycogen was low and blood glucose concentration was also declining (Fig. 1.4C and 1.4A). Blood glucose concentration and the rate of CHO oxidation eventually fell to 2.5 mmol/L and to <1.4 g/min, respectively, at the time of fatigue. Thus, the lowering of blood glucose during the latter stages of prolonged strenuous exercise appeared to play a major role in the development of muscular fatigue. Fatigue under these conditions was clearly preceded by a decline in CHO oxidation, which in turn was preceded by a decline in blood glucose to approximately 2.5–3.0 mmol/L.

In contrast, when blood glucose was maintained at 4–5 mmol/L through CHO ingestion, the high rate of CHO oxidation required by

FIGURE 1.4

Metabolic responses to prolonged cycling at 71% V̇o₂max when fed a placebo or CHO every 20 minutes during exercise. **Panel A:** *Plasma glucose concentration.* **Panel B:** *Total CHO oxidation estimated from V̇o₂ and R.* **Panel C:** *Glycogen concentration in the vastus lateralis muscle, reported both graphically and numerically.* * *Significantly lower (P < 0.05) than CHO. (Reprinted with permission from Coyle, E.F., A.R. Coggan, M.K. Hemmert, and J.L. Ivy. Muscle glycogen utilization during prolonged strenuous exercise when fed carbohydrate.* J. Appl. Physiol. *61:165–172, 1986.)*

exercise at 71% V̇o₂max ($\approx$2 g/min) was also maintained, and the subjects were able to exercise strenuously for an hour longer (Fig. 1.4A & B). As described above, muscle glycogen concentration was already low after 3 hr of exercise and appeared to contribute little to this maintenance of CHO oxidation and exercise tolerance (Fig. 1.4C). It appears that other CHO sources, presumably blood glucose, were able to largely replace muscle glycogen in providing CHO for oxidation during the latter stages of exercise.

We reasoned that, if a decline in plasma glucose during prolonged, glycogen-depleting exercise contributes to fatigue by limiting CHO oxidation, it should be possible to increase CHO oxidation and reverse fatigue late in exercise under these conditions by restoring euglycemia. To test these hypotheses, the study illustrated in Figure 1.5 was performed. On three separate occasions, we had trained cyclists first exercise to fatigue at 70% V̇o₂max after an overnight fast [28]. This required about 170 min and resulted in a reproducible decline in plasma glucose concentration (to 3–3.5 mmol/L) and in R (to 0.81) at fatigue (Exercise Bout 1, Fig. 1.5). In each trial, the subjects attempted to perform further exercise at the same intensity after a 20-minute rest period when one of three treatments was applied (Exercise Bout 2, Fig. 1.5).

In one trial, the subjects ingested a placebo solution at the end of Exercise Bout 1. Although plasma glucose concentration increased slightly during the rest period, plasma glucose decreased again during further exercise, and the subjects were able to tolerate only 10 $\pm$ 1 min of additional exercise (Fig. 1.5). The rate of CHO oxidation, as reflected by R (Fig. 1.5), did not increase from that observed at the end of Exercise Bout 1.

During a second trial, the subjects ingested 3 g of maltodextrins/kg body weight at the end of Exercise Bout 1. This initially increased plasma glucose concentrations and R during Exercise Bout 2 above the levels observed at fatigue in Exercise Bout 1 (Fig. 1.5). Plasma glucose concentration and R were not maintained, however, declining progres-

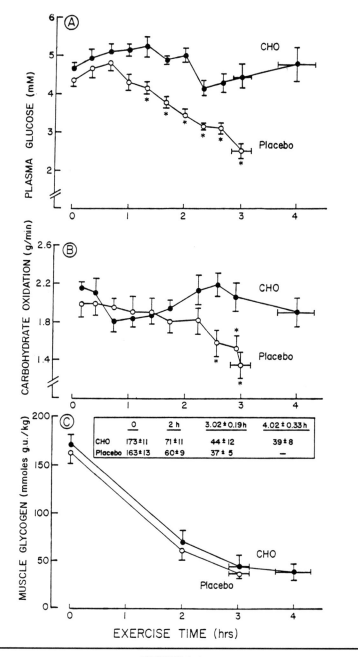

FIGURE 1.4

FIGURE 1.5

Plasma glucose and R during prolonged cycling at 70% V̇o₂max. During three trials, the subjects first exercised to fatigue while drinking only water (Exercise Bout 1). They then attempted to perform additional exercise at this intensity (Exercise Bout 2) after ingesting a placebo and resting 20 minutes (Placebo), after ingesting 200 g of maltodextrins and resting 20 minutes (Feed), or after resting 20 minutes and while glucose was infused intravenously at the rate required to maintain plasma glucose at ≈5 mmol/L (Infusion). The subjects were able to exercise significantly longer when glucose was infused (43 ± 5 min; P < 0.01) or when fed CHO (26 ± 4 min; P < 0.05) in comparison to when fed the placebo (10 ± 1 min). * Significantly lower (P < 0.05) than the initial value during Exercise Bout 1. † Significantly higher (P < 0.05) than the value observed at fatigue of Exercise Bout 1.

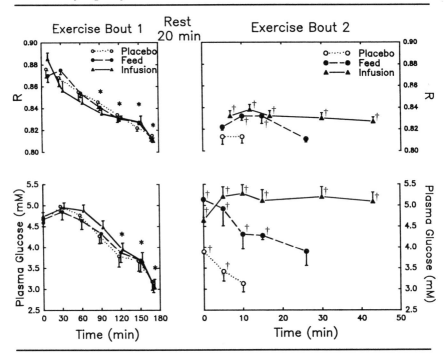

sively until the subjects again fatigued, which occurred after 26 ± 4 min (P < 0.05 vs. placebo) (Fig. 1.5).

During a third trial, glucose was infused intravenously throughout Exercise Bout 2 using a syringe pump. The rate of glucose infusion was adjusted every 5 min during exercise to maintain plasma glucose concentration at ≈5 mmol/L. Restoration and maintenance of euglycemia in this manner increased and maintained R above the levels observed at fatigue during Exercise Bout 1 (i.e., 0.84 vs. 0.81; Fig. 1.5), although R was still lower than observed at the beginning of Exercise Bout 1, when muscle glycogen was probably still high. Infusion of glucose also allowed the subjects to complete an additional 43 ± 5 min of exercise (P < 0.01 vs. both placebo and CHO ingestion at fatigue) (Fig. 1.5). As previously described, glucose had to be infused at over 1 g/min in order to maintain plasma glucose concentrations at ≈5 mmol/L. Because insulin concentrations remained low and muscle glycogen concentration did not change, the infused glucose was probably oxidized at this same high rate.

Finally, in a fourth trial, the subjects were provided with a single large CHO feeding (3 g maltodextrins/kg body weight) during Exercise Bout 1 after 135 min of exercise [30]. This large CHO load reversed the gradual decrease in plasma glucose and R values (Fig. 1.6), similar to glucose infusion or CHO ingestion at fatigue. Unlike ingesting CHO at fatigue, however, ingesting CHO late in exercise was able to maintain plasma glucose and R during additional exercise, thereby delaying fatigue by 36 ± 10 min (P < 0.01).

The above observations form the basis for our model regarding the mechanism by which CHO feedings improve performance during prolonged intense exercise [41]. This model is summarized in Figure 1.7, which depicts the relative contributions of muscle glycogen and blood glucose to energy production during prolonged strenuous exercise when fasted or when ingesting CHO throughout exercise. The percent of total energy derived from CHO oxidation was determined from R. The contribution of muscle glycogen has been estimated using the rate of decline in glycogen measured in the vastus lateralis [41] and by assuming that this reflects the response in a total of 10 kg of muscle. The difference between the rate of total CHO oxidation and muscle glycogen utilization presumably reflects primarily the oxidation of blood glucose. Although the relative contributions of muscle glycogen and blood glucose to total CHO oxidation vary depending on the muscle mass that is used in these calculations, the pattern of response (i.e., steadily decreasing reliance on muscle glycogen and steadily increasing reliance on blood glucose) remains the same.

We interpret Figure 1.7 as follows. During the initial ≈2 hr of exercise at ≈70% $\dot{V}O_2$max, substrate utilization is generally similar both with and without CHO ingestion, although the ingested CHO may partially or completely replace hepatic glycogenolysis or gluconeogenesis as the source of blood glucose [3, 35, 117]. When no CHO is consumed, blood glucose concentration decreases late in exercise, at a time when muscle glycogen is already low. This decline in blood glucose apparently prevents glucose oxidation from increasing sufficiently to offset the reduced contribution of muscle glycogen, resulting in fatigue due to an inadequate rate of CHO oxidation. CHO ingestion, by maintaining blood glucose at 4–5 mmol/L during the latter stages of exercise, allows

FIGURE 1.6

Plasma glucose and R during prolonged cycling at 70% V̇o₂max. The subjects ingested either a placebo or 200 g of maltodextrins after 135 minutes of exercise ("Feed"), which was approximately 30 minutes before the anticipated time of fatigue during the placebo trial. The subjects were able to exercise significantly longer when fed CHO compared to when fed the placebo (205 ± 17 vs 169 ± 12 min; P < 0.01). * Significantly higher (P < 0.05) during Feed. (Reprinted with permission from Coggan, A.R., and E.F. Coyle. Metabolism and performance following carbohydrate ingestion late in exercise. Med. Sci. Sports Exerc. *21:59–65, 1989.)*

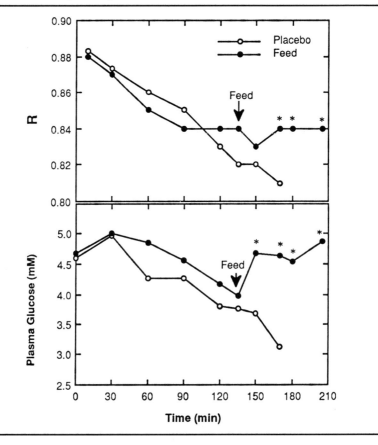

for a progressive increase in blood glucose oxidation to the point where it supplies nearly all of the CHO energy required during exercise. As previously discussed, substantial evidence exists that blood glucose can contribute a major proportion of the CHO energy required during prolonged moderate-intensity exercise. Indeed, when blood glucose

FIGURE 1.7

The authors' model of the percentage of energy and the absolute rate of CHO oxidation derived from various sources during prolonged cycling at 70–75% $\dot{V}O_2$max when fasted or when fed CHO throughout exercise. The rate of muscle glycogen utilization during exercise is the same when fasted or when fed CHO. As the duration of exercise increases, progressively less energy is derived from muscle glycogen and progressively more is derived from blood glucose. During the first 2 hours of exercise, substrate utilization is generally similar when fasted or when fed CHO. However, fatigue occurs after 3 hours of exercise when fasted owing to an insufficient rate of CHO oxidation as a result of a decrease in blood glucose concentration. CHO ingestion prevents this decrease in CHO oxidation by maintaining blood glucose availability and allowing blood glucose oxidation to increase to the point where it accounts for almost all of the CHO being oxidized. Therefore, over the course of 4 hours of exercise when fed CHO, muscle glycogen and blood glucose each contribute approximately one-half of the CHO energy and thus should be considered as equally important substrates. Estimated blood glucose oxidation when fed CHO does not distinguish between endogenous and exogenous sources of glucose. For example, during the first 2 hours of exercise, it is likely that ingested CHO partially replaces endogenous blood glucose. (Reprinted with permission from Coyle, E.F., A.R. Coggan, M.K. Hemmert, and J.L. Ivy. Muscle glycogen utilization during prolonged strenuous exercise when fed carbohydrate. J. Appl. Physiol. *61:165–172, 1986.)*

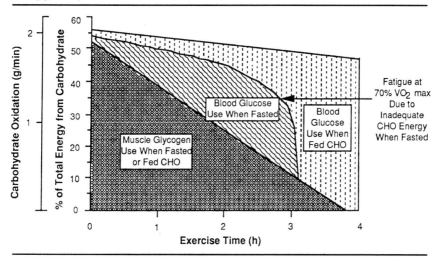

concentration is maintained by CHO ingestion, muscle glycogen and blood glucose each contribute approximately one-half of the CHO energy during prolonged exercise and, therefore, should be considered as equally important substrates. Thus, it appears that CHO ingestion during prolonged exercise improves performance primarily by maintaining blood glucose oxidation at sufficiently high rates late in exercise, as suggested over 50 years ago by Dill et al. [46].

Recent Studies by Others
The model developed above may explain many observations regarding the effects of CHO ingestion on exercise performance. For example, most studies that have reported that CHO ingestion during exercise improves performance have also observed that blood glucose concentration and the rate of total CHO oxidation gradually decrease during exercise performed without CHO supplementation after an overnight fast, but are maintained at higher levels when fed CHO throughout exercise [5, 22, 28–30, 38, 41, 48, 53, 59, 60, 69, 70, 90, 91]. This model may also explain why CHO ingestion during exercise fails to improve performance under certain conditions. CHO ingestion during exercise does not appear to be of benefit to individuals who, in the absence of CHO supplementation, are able to maintain adequate blood glucose concentrations [15, 38, 48]. CHO ingestion during exercise also appears to have less of an effect on performance when the exercise bout is ≤2 hr in duration [69, 89], probably because CHO availability usually does not become limiting during this time. If body CHO stores are reduced prior to the onset of exercise, however, CHO supplementation has improved performance during exercise of shorter duration (i.e., 60 min) [99].

Similarly, CHO ingestion also often has been ineffective in improving exercise performance during prolonged running [100, 110, 111]. This may be because blood glucose concentration does not appear to decrease as readily during prolonged running as it does during prolonged cycling [cf. 32 for discussion]; consequently, there may be less of a need for supplemental CHO. Williams et al. [124] observed, however, that blood glucose concentration decreased to ≈3.5 mmol/L and R fell to 0.86 by the end of a 30 kilometer (km) treadmill run when subjects were provided with only water to drink, whereas glucose ingestion throughout exercise maintained blood glucose at ≈5 mmol/L and R at 0.89–0.90. Consistent with the model developed above, the subjects were able to run significantly faster during the final 5 km when ingesting glucose.

In apparent conflict with this model, several recent studies have reported that CHO ingestion during exercise improves performance even when blood glucose availability and total CHO oxidation do not appear to have been especially limited during the placebo or control trial [43, 44, 90, 91, 95–97]. However, in all of these studies the improvement in exercise performance due to CHO ingestion was associated with a higher blood glucose concentration and a greater rate of total CHO oxidation, as predicted by the model. In addition, performance in these studies was defined as the ability to increase the exercise intensity above the control level, and not as the ability to maintain a given exercise intensity for a longer period of time. Although blood glucose availability and total CHO oxidation may not have been limiting at the exercise intensity that the subjects were able to tolerate in the fasted state, they were apparently insufficient to support exercise at a higher intensity. When fed CHO during exercise, however, the increase in glucose availability and oxidation apparently permitted the subjects to increase their exercise intensity. We interpret these results to indicate that the effects of CHO ingestion during exercise are probably related more to relative changes in CHO availability and oxidation, rather than to some absolute level of blood glucose or CHO oxidation per se.

There appears to be an upper limit, however, to the exercise intensity that can be supported by the oxidation of blood glucose. We have observed that when trained cyclists are fed CHO throughout exercise that alternates every 15 min between 60% and (initially) ≈85% $\dot{V}o_2$max, after 2.5 hr of exercise the subjects were forced to reduce their exercise intensity to ≈75% $\dot{V}o_2$max [29]. This was accompanied by a reduction in total CHO oxidation to ≈2 g/min. Similarly, Davis et al. [43] observed that, even when fed CHO throughout exercise, after ≈2 hr of exercise at ≈75% $\dot{V}o_2$max, subjects are unable to increase their exercise intensity above this level during an additional ≈30 min of exercise. Although blood glucose can apparently be oxidized at much higher rates than previously believed possible, it still does not appear to be able to supply all of the CHO energy required to support very intense, steady-state exercise [29]. When endogenous CHO stores are not depleted, however, increasing the availability of blood glucose by means of CHO ingestion during exercise may still supplement these existing stores sufficiently to increase CHO oxidation [18, 99] and to enhance performance during very high intensity exercise [53, 60, 99].

PRACTICAL APPLICATION

Type of CHO
Studies that have directly determined the effects of ingesting glucose compared to maltodextrins or sucrose during exercise, either alone or in combination, have found little difference among these CHO in their ability to maintain blood glucose concentration and CHO oxidation or to improve performance [22, 88, 97, 103]. Apparent exceptions to this conclusion have been observed in studies in which the amount as well as the type of CHO ingested have been altered [84, 89, 119]. This similarity in response between maltodextrins, sucrose, and glucose is probably related to the fact that all three types of CHO deliver glucose into the circulation at similar rates.

Maltodextrins have become a popular form of CHO for inclusion in sports drinks. The gastric emptying rate of maltodextrins (in g of CHO/min) is generally similar to that of glucose [20, 67, 98, 103], although it has been reported that a 5% solution of maltodextrins may initially empty from the stomach at a slightly faster rate than a similar glucose solution [54]. Because maltodextrins are rapidly hydrolyzed in the small intestine and absorbed as glucose, it is not surprising that the metabolic responses to maltodextrin ingestion are similar to that of glucose. However, the osmolality of a maltodextrin solution is only approximately one-fifth that of an equally concentrated glucose solution, so that the ingestion of maltodextrins results in somewhat smaller gastric secretion and volume [54, 103]. Probably the major difference is that maltodextrins are not very sweet tasting; solutions containing ≥10% CHO are therefore more palatable for most people. In support of this, Rehrer et al. [109] have observed that cyclists expending 20 MJ of energy per day voluntarily ingest enough of a supplemental maltodextrin solution to maintain energy and nitrogen balance, but do not ingest enough of a 50% fructose solution. It seems likely that the cyclists became prematurely satiated when consuming the 50% fructose supplement because of the excessively sweet taste.

In contrast to these other sugars, the ingestion of fructose during prolonged exercise apparently does not improve performance [15, 97]. This may be a result of its slower rate of absorption from the gut and subsequent conversion to glucose in the liver. Fructose tends to result in lower blood glucose and insulin concentrations and lower rates of CHO oxidation in comparison to other types of sugars [15, 87, 88, 97]. Alternatively, the failure of fructose ingestion to improve performance may be due to the gastrointestinal distress that often accompanies the ingestion of large amounts of fructose [97].

Liquid Versus Solid CHO
Although at least two studies have compared the metabolic and performance effects of ingesting water plus CHO in solid form (i.e., candy bars) versus those of an artificially sweetened placebo drink during prolonged, intermittent exercise [53, 60], no direct comparisons between solid and liquid forms of CHO appear to have been performed. Because ingested CHO will be in a liquid or semiliquid state when leaving the stomach, however, and because an additional purpose of feeding during exercise is to supply the water needed to maintain hydration, there appears to be little reason to anticipate any physiological advantage to solid forms of CHO. Solid forms of CHO may be preferred by some exercising individuals, however, for reasons of satiety.

Timing of CHO Ingestion
In addition to using different types and forms of CHO, researchers also have employed a wide variety of CHO supplementation schedules

in studies in which the influence of CHO ingestion during exercise has been examined. The performance criteria as well as the training status of the subjects have also varied greatly from study to study. Direct comparisons among these various studies regarding the optimal timing of CHO ingestion during exercise are therefore difficult to make. However, as previously described, we have used four different means of supplying supplemental CHO during exercise to fatigue at 70–75% $\dot{V}O_2$max [28, 30, 41]. The subjects in all of these studies were well-trained cyclists, and, in many cases, a single subject has been studied using three or even four of these treatments. Summarized in Table 1.1 are our observations of the additional length of time (in min) that exercise could be tolerated by each subject (1) when CHO was ingested throughout exercise, (2) when CHO was ingested 30 minutes prior to the anticipated time of fatigue, (3) when glucose was infused intrave-

TABLE 1.1

Comparison of the Length of Time (in min) that Fatigue is Delayed During Exercise at 70–75% $\dot{V}O_2$max by Various Means of CHO Supplementation

	Treatment			
Subject Number	CHO Ingestion Throughout Exercise[a]	CHO Ingestion 30 min Before Fatigue[b]	Intravenous Glucose Infusion at Fatigue[c]	CHO Ingestion at Fatigue[d]
1			33	27
2		41	60	29
3		43	53	44
4		52	30	29
5		50	27	21
6		−13	50	21
7	**149**	46	47	11
8	63			
9	60			
10	47			
11	40			
12	36			
12	21			
X ± S.E. of all	60 ± 16	37 ± 9	43 ± 5	26 ± 4*
X ± S.E. without data shown in bold	45 ± 6	46 ± 2	43 ± 5	26 ± 4*

* Significantly less than all other treatments.
[a] Data from Coyle et al. [41]. Subjects ingested 1 g CHO/kg body weight after 20 minutes of exercise and 0.4 g CHO/kg body weight every 20 minutes thereafter.
[b] Data from Coggan and Coyle [30]. Subjects ingested 3 g CHO/kg body weight 30 minutes before the anticipated time of fatigue.
[c] Data from Coggan and Coyle [28]. After the subjects exercised to fatigue and then rested for 20 minutes, they resumed exercising while glucose was infused intravenously at the rate required to maintain plasma glucose at ≈5 mmol/L.
[d] Data from Coggan and Coyle [28]. After the subjects exercised to fatigue, they ingested 3 g CHO/kg body weight, rested for 20 minutes, then resumed exercising.

nously after fatigue had already occurred, or (4) when CHO was ingested after fatigue had already occurred. On average, little difference existed in the time that fatigue was delayed when the subjects were supplemented with CHO using the first three approaches. In fact, when two seemingly spurious individual responses in Table 1.1 are eliminated, all three methods of CHO supplementation appear to be able to delay fatigue by ≈45 min. Because fatigue is delayed just as much when CHO supplementation is withheld until late in exercise as when CHO is ingested throughout exercise, these observations support the concept that fatigue is delayed as a result of maintaining blood glucose availability and oxidation late in exercise, when muscle glycogen is low, and is not caused by a sparing of muscle glycogen throughout exercise.

Nevertheless, as illustrated in Table 1.1 and Figures 1.5 and 1.8, CHO feeding at fatigue is usually not effective in restoring and maintaining blood glucose concentration or exercise tolerance [28, 116]. Individual subjects differed widely, however, in the extent to which CHO ingestion at fatigue was able to restore and maintain plasma glucose concentration and exercise tolerance. Several of the subjects were able to maintain euglycemia and a high rate of CHO oxidation for an additional 30 to 45 min of exercise after the large CHO feeding and 20 min of rest, whereas plasma glucose concentration and the rate of CHO oxidation decreased progressively during exercise in others (Fig. 1.8). On the other hand, CHO ingestion and 20 min of rest did little to raise plasma glucose concentration in some fatigued persons, the response of one of whom is shown in Figure 1.8. These results suggest that CHO ingested after fatigue has occurred may not be absorbed into the blood rapidly enough to match the rate at which glucose is removed from the circulation (i.e., at ≈1 g/min; see below).

Although it is possible to postpone CHO supplementation until later in exercise, and still delay fatigue, it is also possible to delay CHO ingestion too long, and fail to enhance performance. It is also important to keep in mind that these results apply to continuous exercise performed at 70–75% $\dot{V}O_2$max. As previously discussed, it is theoretically possible that CHO supplementation at high rates throughout intermittent or low-intensity exercise may potentially promote glycogen resynthesis in resting muscle fibers [33, 49, 65, 82]. Under these conditions, CHO ingestion throughout exercise may prove more beneficial to performance than ingesting CHO only late in exercise. This has yet to be demonstrated experimentally, however.

Rate of CHO Ingestion
Based on the rate of intravenous glucose infusion required to restore and maintain blood glucose availability and CHO oxidation late in

FIGURE 1.8

Plasma glucose concentration in individual subjects during Exercise Bout 2. As shown in Figure 1.5, the subjects first exercised to fatigue at ≈70% V̇O₂max (Exercise Bout 1), then ingested 200 g of maltodextrins and rested 20 minutes before performing Exercise Bout 2. Note the variation between subjects in their ability to maintain plasma glucose concentration during Exercise Bout 2 as well as differences in their time to fatigue. (Reprinted with permission from Coggan, A.R., and E.F. Coyle. Reversal of fatigue during prolonged exercise by carbohydrate infusion or ingestion. J. Appl. Physiol. *63:2388–2395, 1987.)*

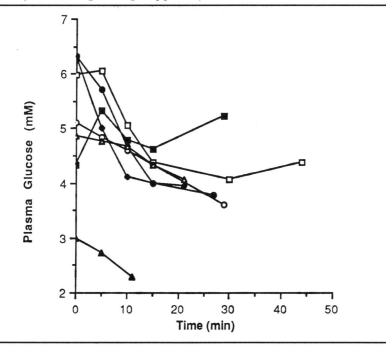

exercise [28], trained cyclists need to ingest sufficient supplemental CHO to supply the blood with exogenous glucose at approximately 1 g/min late in exercise, at least during continuous exercise at 70–75% V̇O₂max. Because fatigue is delayed by ≈45 min, this amounts to a total of ≈45–60 g of glucose. As discussed above, it does not appear to be critical whether this demand is met by ingesting small amounts of CHO throughout exercise or by ingesting larger amounts late in exercise. To ensure that 45–60 g of exogenous glucose are readily available late in exercise, however, it seems that large amounts of CHO must be ingested.

It is clear that the two most important factors determining the rate at which a CHO solution is emptied from the stomach are the CHO concentration and the volume of solution ingested [20, 54, 67, 90, 109].

FIGURE 1.9

The average rate of emptying of CHO from the stomach during 2 hours of exercise when ingesting 600 mL/h of solutions containing 6, 12, and 18 g of CHO/100 mL (g%). (Reprinted with permission from Mitchell, J.B., D.L. Costill, J.A. Houmard, W.J. Fink, R.A. Robergs, and J.A. Davis. Gastric emptying: influence of prolonged exercise and carbohydrate concentration. Med. Sci. Sports Exerc. 21:269–274, 1989.)

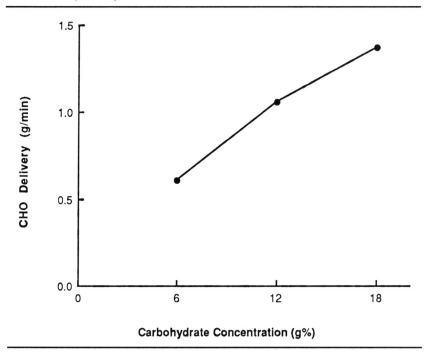

Carbohydrate Concentration (g%)

Mitchell et al. [90] have clearly demonstrated that when 600 mL of solution are ingested per hour, the rate of CHO delivery to the small intestine during exercise increases in proportion to the CHO concentration (Fig. 1.9). Figure 1.9 also indicates that it is possible to empty CHO from the stomach at ≥1 g/min when solutions containing ≥12% CHO are consumed. This agrees with our observations that by ingesting 400 mL of a 50% maltodextrin solution approximately 30 min before the time of fatigue when fasted, subjects were able to exercise an additional ≈45 min (i.e., ≈75 min beyond the time of ingestion) [30]. Presumably the presence of this large volume of concentrated CHO was able to provide CHO to the intestines at ≥1 g/min late in exercise. Therefore, if CHO supplementation is withheld until late in exercise, it appears that sufficient volumes (≥400 mL/h) of relatively concentrated (10–50% CHO) solutions should be ingested.

In the majority of studies in which CHO ingestion throughout exercise was shown to improve performance, subjects were provided with 25–60 g of CHO/h [15, 29, 38, 41, 60, 69, 70, 95–97, 124]. Although the extent to which this ingested CHO replaces endogenous blood glucose oxidation, is stored, or remains unabsorbed is not known, it does appear that these rates of supplementation have been sufficient to provide the additional 45–60 g of CHO required to maintain blood glucose oxidation late in exercise. Neither the minimal nor the optimal rate of CHO ingestion throughout exercise needed to improve performance has been systematically determined. It is likely that these rates will differ depending on the criteria used to assess performance. It should also be recognized that there are substantial intraindividual differences in the quantity of CHO required to maintain blood glucose availability and oxidation during prolonged exercise. As indicated previously, some subjects are apparently able to exercise for prolonged periods without evidence of a decrease in blood glucose concentration [15, 38, 48], whereas other individuals appear to rely on blood glucose to a greater extent during exercise [31] and are therefore particularly susceptible to a decline in blood glucose concentration.

UNANSWERED QUESTIONS

Although the model developed in this chapter appears to explain the mechanism by which CHO ingestion during exercise enhances performance, a number of unanswered questions remain. For example, the model we have presented predicts that, during prolonged exercise in the fasted state, the ability of the exercising muscles to resynthesize adenosine triphosphate (ATP) becomes insufficient when CHO availability decreases late in exercise. There is evidence to support this hypothesis [21, 64, 101, 102]. Presumably, CHO ingestion throughout or late in exercise enhances performance by maintaining or restoring the rate of ATP production. However, this latter hypothesis has yet to be verified experimentally.

It is also not certain whether CHO ingestion during exercise enhances blood glucose utilization only during the later stages of exercise, by merely maintaining blood glucose concentration, or whether CHO ingestion increases blood glucose utilization throughout exercise. It is theoretically possible, for example, that the small differences in insulin and FFA concentrations that result from CHO ingestion during moderate-intensity exercise cause an increase in glucose oxidation throughout exercise, which contributes to the enhancement in exercise capacity. An argument in favor of this possibility is the fact that fructose ingestion throughout exercise, which maintains blood glucose concentration but has less of an effect on insulin or FFA levels than does the ingestion of glucose, maltodextrins, or sucrose, fails to improve performance [15, 97]. An argument against this hypothesis is that CHO ingestion throughout exercise at 70–75% $\dot{V}o_2$max appears to have very little effect on substrate utilization during the first 2 to 2.5 hr of exercise, when blood glucose concentrations are similar to those observed in the fasted state, even though insulin and FFA concentrations differ [38, 41]. Furthermore, subjects who do not show a decrease in blood glucose concentration during prolonged exercise at 70–75% $\dot{V}o_2$max performed in the fasted state do not appear to benefit from CHO feedings [15, 38, 48, 110, 111]. This is true even though changes in insulin and FFA in response to CHO ingestion in these subjects are similar to those in men who do benefit from CHO ingestion [38]. Finally, CHO ingestion or infusion late in exercise increases blood glucose concentration and total CHO oxidation and enhances performance without measurably altering insulin or FFA concentrations [28, 30]. Nevertheless, the possibility remains that very small but physiologically significant changes in insulin and FFA may contribute to the maintenance of CHO oxidation and the enhancement of performance as a result of CHO ingestion during exercise.

Perhaps the most important remaining question concerns the cause of fatigue during exercise when blood glucose concentration is maintained by feeding CHO during exercise. Based on R values, although the estimated rate of CHO oxidation is low, it does not appear to decrease prior to fatigue when receiving CHO supplementation (Fig. 1.7). This could be interpreted to suggest that, because CHO availability is not limiting, other causes of fatigue have emerged. Many possibilities exist, including depletion of muscle potassium [114], a decrease in force-generating capacity at the myofibrillar level [122], or fatigue of neural origin [121]. Alternatively, Figure 1.7 raises the possibility that, although relative contribution of muscle glycogen to energy production is small during the hours prior to fatigue, fatigue during exercise when fed CHO occurs at the same general time that this contribution becomes zero. It is therefore possible that, although blood glucose appears to be able to supply almost all of the CHO required during moderate intensity exercise, some small but critical requirement for muscle glycogen exists. If so, CHO availability may indeed eventually become limiting even when fed CHO throughout exercise, even though this limitation is too small to be manifested by changes in R.

Further experimentation will obviously be required to answer these questions. The point of such speculation, however, is to emphasize that this experimental model could be helpful in designing future studies of the causes of fatigue during prolonged exercise. CHO ingestion during exercise, by providing a means of altering CHO availability, will continue to be a useful tool in attempting to answer these questions.

SUMMARY

It is well recognized that energy from CHO oxidation is required to perform prolonged strenuous (>60% $\dot{V}O_2$max) exercise. During the past 25 years, the concept has developed that muscle glycogen is the predominant source of CHO energy for strenuous exercise; as a result, the potential energy contribution of blood glucose has been somewhat overlooked. Although during the first hour of exercise at 70–75% $\dot{V}O_2$max, most of the CHO energy is derived from muscle glycogen, it is clear that the contribution of muscle glycogen decreases over time as muscle glycogen stores become depleted, and that blood glucose uptake and oxidation increase progressively to maintain CHO oxidation (Fig. 1.7).

We theorize that over the course of several hours of strenous exercise (i.e., 3–4 h), blood glucose and muscle glycogen contribute equal amounts of CHO energy, making blood glucose at least as important as muscle glycogen as a CHO source. During the latter stages of exercise, blood glucose can potentially provide all of the CHO energy needed to support exercise at 70–75% $\dot{V}O_2$max if blood glucose availability is maintained. During prolonged exercise in the fasted state, however, blood glucose concentration often decreases owing to depletion of liver glycogen stores. This relative hypoglycemia, although only occasionally severe enough to result in fatigue from neuroglucopenia, causes fatigue by limiting blood glucose (and therefore total CHO) oxidation.

The primary purpose of CHO ingestion during continuous strenuous exercise is to maintain blood glucose concentration and thus CHO oxidation and exercise tolerance during the latter stages of prolonged exercise. CHO feeding throughout continuous exercise does not alter muscle glycogen use. It appears that blood glucose must be supplemented at a rate of ≈ 1 g/min late in exercise. Feeding sufficient amounts of CHO 30 minutes before fatigue is as effective as ingesting CHO throughout exercise in maintaining blood glucose availability and CHO oxidation late in exercise. Most persons should not wait, however, until they are fatigued before ingesting CHO, because it appears that glucose entry into the blood does not occur rapidly enough at this time. It also may be advantageous to ingest CHO throughout intermittent or low-intensity exercise rather than toward the end of exercise because of the potential for glycogen synthesis in resting muscle fibers. Finally, CHO ingestion during prolonged strenuous exercise delays by approximately 45 minutes but does not prevent fatigue, suggesting that factors other than CHO availability eventually cause fatigue.

ACKNOWLEDGEMENTS

The authors' research has been supported by grants from Ross Laboratories, The United States Olympic Committee Sports Medicine Council, The Quaker Oats Company, and the National Institutes of Health. We sincerely thank Lisa Mendenhall and Greg Wimer for their assistance in preparing this manuscript.

REFERENCES

1. Ahlborg, B., J. Bergström, L.-G. Eklund, and E. Hultman. Muscle glycogen and muscle electrolytes during prolonged physical exercise. *Acta Physiol. Scand.* 70:129–142, 1967.
2. Ahlborg, G., P. Felig, L. Hagenfeldt, R. Hendler, and J. Wahren. Substrate turnover during prolonged exercise in man. *J. Clin. Invest.* 53:1080–1090, 1974.
3. Ahlborg, G., and P. Felig. Influence of glucose ingestion on the fuel-hormone response during prolonged exercise. *J. Appl. Physiol.* 41:683–688, 1976.
4. Ahlborg, G., and P. Felig. Lactate and glucose exchange across the forearm, legs, and splanchnic bed during and after prolonged leg exercise. *J. Clin. Invest.* 69:45–54, 1982.
5. Andres, R., G. Cader, and K.L. Zierler. The quantitatively minor role of carbohydrat in oxidative metabolism by skeletal muscle in intact man in the basal state. Measurements of O_2 and glucose uptake and CO_2 and lactate production in the forearm. *J. Clin. Invest.* 35:671–682, 1956.
6. Asmussen, E. Muscle metabolism during exercise. A historical survey. B. Pernow and B. Saltin (eds). *Advances in Experimental Medicine and Biology, Vol. 11: Muscle Metabolism during Exercise.* New York: Plenum Press, 1971, pp. 1–12.
7. Bagby, G.J., H.J. Green, S. Katsuta, and P.D. Gollnick. Glycogen depletion in exercising rats infused with glucose, lactate, or pyruvate. *J. Appl. Physiol.* 45:425–429, 1978.
8. Barstow, T.J., D.M. Cooper, S. Epstein, and K. Wasserman. Changes in breath $^{13}CO_2/^{12}CO_2$ consequent to exercise and hypoxia. *J. Appl. Physiol.* 66:936–942, 1989.
9. Benadé, A.J.S., C.H. Wyndham, N.B. Strydom, and G.G. Rogers. The physiological effects of a mid-shift feed of sucrose. *S. Afr. Med. J.* 45:711–718, 1971.
10. Benadé, A.J.S., C.R. Jansen, G.G. Rogers, C.H. Wyndham, and N.B. Strydom. The significance of an increased RQ after sucrose ingestion during prolonged exercise. *Pflügers Arch.* 342:199–206, 1973.
11. Benadé, A.J.S., C.H. Wyndham, C.R. Jansen, G.G. Rogers, and E.J.P. de Bruin. Plasma insulin and carbohydrate metabolism after sucrose ingestion during rest and prolonged aerobic exercise. *Pflügers Arch.* 342:207–218, 1973.
12. Bergström, J., and E. Hultman. The effect of exercise on muscle glycogen and electrolytes in normals. *Scand. J. Clin. Lab. Invest.* 18:16–20, 1966.
13. Bergström, J., and E. Hultman. A study of the glycogen metabolism during exercise in man. *Scand. J. Clin. Lab. Invest.* 19:218–228, 1967.
14. Bergström, J., L. Hermansen, E. Hultman, and B. Saltin. Diet, muscle glycogen, and physical performance. *Acta Physiol. Scand.* 71:140–150, 1967.
15. Björkman, O., K. Sahlin, L. Hagenfeldt, and J. Wahren. Influence of glucose and fructose ingestion on the capacity for long-term exercise. *Clin. Physiol.* 4:483–494, 1984.
16. Boje, O. Der Blutsucker während und nach körperlicher Arbeit. *Skand. Arch. Physiol.* 74(*Suppl.* 10):1–46, 1936.
17. Boje, O. Arbeitshypoglykämie nach Glukoseeingabe (Vorläufige Mitteilung). *Skand. Arch. Physiol.* 83:308–312, 1940.
18. Bonen, A., S.A. Malcolm, R.D. Kilgour, K.P. MacIntyre, and A.N. Belcastro. Glucose ingestion before and during intense exercise. *J. Appl. Physiol.* 50:766–771, 1981.
19. Bonen, A., G.W. Ness, A.N. Belcastro, and R.L. Kirby. Mild exercise impedes glycogen repletion in muscle. *J. Appl. Physiol.* 58:1622–1629, 1985.

20. Brenner, W., T.R. Hendrix, and P.R. McHugh. Regulation of the gastric emptying of carbohydrates. *Gastroenterology* 85:76–82, 1983.

21. Broberg, S., and K. Sahlin. Adenine nucleotide degradation in human skeletal muscle during prolonged exercise. *J. Appl. Physiol.* 67:116–122, 1989.

22. Brooke, J.D., G.J. Davies, and L.F. Green. The effects of normal and glucose syrup work diets on the performance of racing cyclists. *J. Sports Med.* 15:257–265, 1975.

23. Brouns, F., W.H.M. Saris, E. Beckers, et al. Metabolic changes induced by sustained exhaustive cycling and diet manipulations. *Int. J. Sports Med.* 10(*Suppl.* 1):S49–S62, 1989.

24. Carlson, L.A., R.J. Havel, L.-G. Ekelund, and A. Holmgren. Effect of nicotinic acid on the turnover rate and oxidation of the free fatty acids of plasma in man during exercise. *Metabolism* 12:837–845, 1963.

25. Carpenter, T.M., and E.L. Fox. The effect of muscular work upon the respiratory exchange of man after the ingestion of glucose and fructose. II. Heat production, efficiency, oxygen debt, excess respiratory quotient, and metabolism of carbohydrates. *Arbeitsphysiol.* 4:568–599, 1931.

26. Christensen, E.H., and O. Hansen. III. Arbeitsfähigkeit und Ernährung. *Skand. Arch. Physiol.* 81:161–171, 1939.

27. Christensen, E.H., and O. Hansen. IV. Hypoglykamie, Arbeitfähigkeit und Ermudung. *Skand. Arch. Physiol.* 81:172–179, 1939.

28. Coggan, A.R., and E.F. Coyle. Reversal of fatigue during prolonged exercise by carbohydrate infusion or ingestion. *J. Appl. Physiol.* 63:2388–2395, 1987.

29. Coggan, A.R., and E.F. Coyle. Effect of carbohydrate feedings during high-intensity exercise. *J. Appl. Physiol.* 65:1703–1709, 1988.

30. Coggan, A.R., and E.F. Coyle. Metabolism and performance following carbohydrate ingestion late in exercise. *Med. Sci. Sports Exerc.* 21:59–65, 1989.

31. Coggan, A.R., W.M. Kohrt, R.J. Spina, D.M. Bier, and J.O. Holloszy. Endurance training decreases plasma glucose turnover and oxidation during moderate intensity exercise in men. *J. Appl. Physiol.* 68:990–996, 1990.

32. Coggan, A.R. Plasma glucose metabolism during exercise in humans. *Sports Med.* 11:102–124, 1991.

33. Constable, S.H., J.C. Young, M. Higuchi, and J.O. Holloszy. Glycogen resynthesis in leg muscles of rats during exercise. *Am. J. Physiol.* 247:R880–R883, 1984.

34. Corsi, A., M. Midrio, and A.L. Granata. In situ utilization of glycogen and blood glucose by skeletal muscle during tetanus. *Am. J. Physiol.* 216:1534–1541, 1969.

35. Costill, D.L., A. Bennett, G. Branam, and D. Eddy. Glucose ingestion at rest and during prolonged exercise. *J. Appl. Physiol.* 34:764–769, 1973.

36. Costill, D.L., and J.M. Miller. Nutrition for endurance sport: carbohydrate and fluid balance. *Int. J. Sports Med.* 1:2–14, 1980.

37. Costill, D.L. Carbohydrates for exercise: dietary demands for optimal performance. *Int. J. Sports Med.* 9:1–18, 1988.

38. Coyle, E.F., J.M. Hagberg, B.F. Hurley, W.H. Martin, A.A. Ehsani, and J.O. Holloszy. Carbohydrate feedings during prolonged strenuous exercise can delay fatigue. *J. Appl. Physiol.* 55:230–235, 1983.

39. Coyle, E.F., and A.R. Coggan. Effectiveness of carbohydrate feeding in delaying fatigure during prolonged exercise. *Sports Med.* 1:446–458, 1984.

40. Coyle, E.F., A.R. Coggan, M.K. Hemmert, R.C. Lowe, and T.J. Walters. Substrate usage during prolonged exercise following a preexercise meal. *J. Appl. Physiol.* 59:429–433, 1985.

41. Coyle, E.F., A.R. Coggan, M.K. Hemmert, and J.L. Ivy. Muscle glycogen utilization during prolonged strenuous exercise when fed carbohydrate. *J. Appl. Physiol.* 61:165–172, 1986.

42. Coyle, E.F., M.T. Hamilton, J.G. Alonso, S.J. Montain, and J.L. Ivy. Carbohydrate metabolism during intense exercise when hyperglycemic. *J. Appl. Physiol.* (in press).

43. Davis, J.M., D.R. Lamb, R.R. Pate, C.A. Slentz, W.A. Burgess, and W.P. Bartoli. Carbohydrate-electrolyte drinks: effects on endurance cycling in the heat. *Am. J. Clin. Nutr.* 48:1023–1030, 1988.

44. Davis, J.M., W.A. Burgess, C.A. Slentz, W.P. Bartoli, and R.R. Pate. Effects of ingesting 6% and 12% glucose/electrolyte beverages during prolonged intermittent cycling in the heat. *Eur. J. Appl. Physiol.* 57:563–569, 1988.

45. DeFronzo, R.A., J.D. Tobin, and R. Andres. Glucose clamp technique: a method for quantifying insulin secretion and resistance. *Am. J. Physiol.* 237:E214–E223, 1979.

46. Dill, D.B., H.T. Edwards, and J.H. Talbott. Studies in muscular activity. VII. Factors limiting the capacity for work. *J. Physiol. (Lond.)* 77:49–62, 1932.

47. Edwards, H.T., R. Margaria, and D.B. Dill. Metabolic rate, blood sugar, and the utilization of carbohydrate. *Am. J. Physiol.* 58:203–209, 1934.

48. Edwards, T.L., D. Santeusanio, and K.B. Wheeler. Endurance of cyclists given carbohydrate solutions during moderate-intensity rides. *Texas Med.* 83:29–31, 1986.

49. Ehrenstein, W., C. Emans, and W. Müller-Limroth. Der Glycogenabbau im arbeitenden Muskel während 8stündiger Ergometerarbeit und seine Hemmung durche mässige Blutzuckerspiegeleröhung. *Pflügers Arch.* 320:233–246, 1970.

50. Erickson, M.A., R.J. Schwarzkopf, and R.D. Mckenzie. Effects of caffeine, fructose, and glucose ingestion on muscle glycogen utilization during exercise. *Med. Sci. Sports Exerc.* 19:579–583, 1987.

51. Felig, P., and J. Wahren. Role of insulin and glucagon in the regulation of hepatic glucose production during exercise. *Diabetes* 28(*Suppl.* 1):71–75, 1979.

52. Felig, P., A. Cherif, A. Minagawa, and J. Wahren. Hypoglycemia during prolonged exercise in normal men. *New. Eng. J. Med.* 306:895–900, 1982.

53. Fielding, R.A., D.L. Costill, W.J. Fink, D.S. King, M. Hargreaves, and J.E. Kovaleski. Effect of carbohydrate feeding frequency and dosage on muscle glycogen use during exercise. *Med. Sci. Sports Exerc.* 17:472–476, 1985.

54. Foster, C., D.L. Costill, and W.J. Fink. Gastric emptying characteristics of glucose and glucose polymer solutions. *Res. Quart. Exerc. Sport.* 51:299–305, 1980.

55. Flynn, M.G., D.L. Costill, J.A. Hawley, et al. Influence of selected carbohydrate drinks on cycling performance and glycogen use. *Med. Sci. Sports Exerc.* 19:37–40, 1987.

56. Gerard, J., B. Jandrain, F. Pirnay, et al. Utilization of oral sucrose load during exercise in humans. Effect of the α-glucosidase inhibitor Acarbose. *Diabetes* 35:1294–1301, 1986.

57. Gollnick, P.D., K. Piehl, C.W. Saubert, R.B. Armstrong, and B. Saltin. Diet, exercise, and glycogen changes in human muscle fibers. *J. Appl. Physiol.* 33:421–425, 1972.

58. Gordon, B., L.A. Kohn, S.A. Levine, M. Matton, W. de M. Scriver, and W.B. Whiting. Sugar content of the blood in runners following a marathon race. With especial reference to the prevention of hypoglycemia: further observations. *J. A. M. A.* 85:508–509, 1925.

59. Green, L.F., and R. Bagley. Ingestion of a glucose syrup drink during long distance canoeing. *Br. J. Sports Med.* 6:125–128, 1972.

60. Hargreaves, M., D.L. Costill, A.R. Coggan, W.J. Fink, and I. Nishibata. Effect of carbohydrate feedings on muscle glycogen utilization and exercise performance. *Med. Sci. Sports Exerc.* 16:219–222, 1984.

61. Hargreaves, M., and C.A. Briggs. Effect of carbohydrate ingestion on exercise metabolism. *J. Appl. Physiol.* 65:1553–1555, 1988.

62. Hermansen, L., E. Hultman, and B. Saltin. Muscle glycogen during prolonged severe exercise. *Acta Physiol. Scand.* 71:129–139, 1971.

63. Hultman, E. Physiological role of muscle glycogen in man, with special reference to exercise. *Circ. Res.* 20–21(*Suppl.* 1):I99–I114, 1967.

64. Hultman, E., J. Bergström, and N. McLennan-Anderson. Breakdown and resynthesis

of phosphorylcreatine and adenosine triphosphate in connection with muscular work in man. *Scand. J. Clin. Lab. Invest.* 19:56–66, 1967.

65. Hultman, E., J. Bergström, and A.E. Roch-Norlund. Glycogen storage in human skeletal muscle. B. Pernow and B. Saltin (eds). *Advances in Experimental Medicine and Biology, Vol. 11: Muscle Metabolism During Exercise.* New York: Plenum Press, 1971, pp. 273–288.

66. Hultman, E., and J. Bergström. Local energy-supplying substrates as limiting factors in different types of leg muscle work in normal man. J. Keul (ed). *Limiting Factors of Physical Performance.* Stuttgart: Thieme, 1973, pp. 113–125.

67. Hunt, J.N., J.L. Smith, and C.L. Jiang. Effect of meal volume and energy density on the gastric emptying of carbohydrates. *Gastroenterology* 89:1326–1330, 1985.

68. Hutber, C.A., and A. Bonen. Glycogenesis in muscle and liver during exercise. *J. Appl. Physiol.* 66:2811–2817, 1989.

69. Ivy, J.L., D.L. Costill, W.J. Fink, and R.W. Lower. Influence of caffeine and carbohydrate feedings on endurance performance. *Med. Sci. Sports* 11:6–11, 1979.

70. Ivy, J.L., W. Miller, V. Dover, L.G. Goodyear, W.M. Sherman, S. Farrel, and H. Williams. Endurance improved by ingestion of a glucose polymer supplement. *Med. Sci. Sports Exerc.* 15:466–471, 1983.

71. Jacobsen, B.S., B.N. Smith, S. Epstein, and G.G. Laties. The prevalence of carbon-13 in respiratory carbon dioxide as an indicator of the type of endogenous substrate. *J. Gen. Physiol.* 55:1–17, 1970.

72. Janssen, E., and L. Kaijser. Substrate utilization and enzymes in extremely endurance-trained men. *J. Appl. Physiol.* 62:999–1005, 1987.

73. Jenkins, A.B., D.J. Chisholm, D.E. James, K.Y. Ho, and E.W. Kraegen. Exercise-induced hepatic glucose output is precisely sensitive to the rate of systemic glucose supply. *Metabolism* 34:431–436, 1985.

74. Jorfeldt, J., and J. Wahren. Human forearm muscle metabolism during exercise. IV. Quantitative aspects of glucose uptake and lactate production during exercise. *Scand. J. Clin. Lab. Invest.* 26:73–81, 1970.

75. Karlsson, J., and B. Saltin. Diet, muscle glycogen, and endurance performance. *J. Appl. Physiol.* 31:203–206, 1971.

76. Karlsson, J., L.-O. Nordesjö, and B. Saltin. Muscle glycogen utilization during exercise after training. *Acta Physiol. Scand.* 90:210–217, 1974.

77. Katz, A., S. Broberg, K. Sahlin, and J. Wahren. Leg glucose uptake during maximal dynamic exercise in humans. *Am. J. Physiol.* 251 (*Endocrinol. Metab.* 14):E65–E70, 1986.

78. Klassen, G.A., G.M. Andrew, and M.R. Becklake. Effect of training on total and regional blood flow and metabolism in paddlers. *J. Appl. Physiol.* 28:397–406, 1970.

79. Krogh, A., and J. Lindhard. Relative value of fat and carbohydrate as a source of muscular energy. With appendices on the correlation between standard metabolism and the respiratory quotient during rest and work. *Biochem. J.* 14:290–298, 1920.

80. Krzentowski, G., B. Jandrain, F. Pirnay, et al. Availability of glucose given orally during exercise. *J. Appl. Physiol.* 56:315–320, 1984.

81. Kuipers, H., D.L. Costill, D.A. Porter, W.J. Fink, and W.M. Morris. Glucose feeding in trained rats: mechanisms for glycogen sparing. *J. Appl. Physiol.* 61:859–863, 1986.

82. Kuipers, H., H.A. Keizer, F. Brouns, and W.H.M. Saris. Carbohydrate feeding and glycogen synthesis during exercise in man. *Pflügers Arch.* 410:652–656, 1987.

83. Kuipers, H., W.H.M. Saris, F. Brouns, H.A. Keizer, and C. ten Bosch. Glycogen synthesis during exercise and rest with carbohydrate feeding in males and females. *Int. J. Sports Med.* 10(*Suppl.* 1):S63–S67, 1989.

84. Kujula, U., Heinonen, O.J., M. Kvist, O.P. Kärkkäinen, J. Marniemi, K. Niittymäki, and E. Havas. Orienteering performance and ingestion of glucose and glucose polymer. *Br. J. Sports Med.* 23:105–108, 1989.

85. Lamb, D.R., and G.R. Brodowicz. Optimal use of fluids of varying formulations to minimise exercise-induced disturbances in homeostasis. *Sports Med.* 3:247–274, 1986.

86. Levine, S.B., T.A. Schultz, D.K. Westbie, J.E. Gerich, and J.D. Wallin. Some changes in the chemical constituents of the blood following a marathon race. With special reference to the development of hypoglycemia. *J. A. M. A.* 82:1778–1779, 1924.

87. Massicotte, D., F. Peronnet, C. Allah, C. Hillaire-Marcel, M. Ledoux, and G. Brisson. Metabolic response to [^{13}C]glucose and [^{13}C] fructose ingestion during exercise. *J. Appl. Physiol.* 61:1180–1184, 1986.

88. Massicotte, D., F. Peronnet, G. Brisson, K. Bakkouch, and C. Hilliare-Marcel. Oxidation of a glucose polymer during exercise: comparison of glucose and fructose. *J. Appl. Physiol.* 66:179–183, 1989.

89. Maughn, R.J., C.E. Fenn, and L.B. Leiper. Effects of fluid, electrolyte and substrate ingestion on endurance capacity. *Eur. J. Appl. Physiol.* 58:481–486, 1989.

90. Mitchell, J.B., D.L. Costill, J.A. Houmard, W.J. Fink, R.A. Roberts, and J.A. Davis. Gastric emptying: influence of prolonged exercise and carbohydrate concentration. *Med. Sci. Sports Exerc.* 21:269–274, 1989.

91. Mitchell, J.B., D.L. Costill, J.A. Houmard, W.J. Fink, D.D. Pascoe, and D.R. Pearson. Influence of carbohydrate dosage on exercise performance and glycogen metabolism. *J. Appl. Physiol.* 67:1843–1849, 1989.

92. Montain, S.J., M.K. Hopper, A.R. Coggan, and E.F. Coyle. Exercise metabolism at different time intervals following a meal. *J. Appl. Physiol.* (in press).

93. Muckle, D.S. Glucose syrup ingestion and team performance in soccer. *Br. J. Sports Med.* 7:340–343, 1973.

94. Murray, R. The effects of consuming carbohydrate-electrolyte beverages on gastric emptying and fluid absorption during and following exercise. *Sports Med.* 4:322–351, 1987.

95. Murray, R., D.E. Eddy, T.W. Murrary, J.G. Seifert, G.L. Paul, and G.A. Halaby. The effect of fluid and carbohydrate feedings during intermittent cycling exercise. *Med. Sci. Sports Exerc.* 19:597–604, 1987.

96. Murray, R., J.G. Siefert, D.E. Eddy, G.L. Paul, and G.A. Halaby. Carbohydrate feeding and exercise: effect of beverage carbohydrate content. *Eur. J. Appl. Physiol.* 59:152–158, 1989.

97. Murray, R., G.L. Paul, J.G. Siefert, D.E. Eddy, and G.A. Halaby. The effects of glucose, fructose, and sucrose ingestion during exercise. *Med. Sci. Sports Exerc.* 21:275–282, 1989.

98. Neufer, P.D., D.L. Costill, W.J. Fink, J.P. Kirwan, R.A. Fielding, and M.G. Flynn. Effects of exercise and carbohydrate composition on gastric emptying. *Med. Sci. Sports Exerc.* 18:658–662, 1986.

99. Neufer, P.D., D.L. Costill, M.G. Flynn, J.P. Kirwan, J.B. Mitchell, and J. Houmard. Improvements in exercise performance: effects of carbohydrate feedings and diet. *J. Appl. Physiol.* 62:983–988, 1987.

100. Noakes, T.F., E.V. Lambert, M.I. Lambert, P.S. McArthur, K.H. Myburgh, and A.J.S. Benadé. Carbohydrate ingestion and muscle glycogen depletion during marathon and ultramarathon racing. *Eur. J. Appl. Physiol.* 57:482–489, 1988.

101. Norman, B., A. Sollevi, L. Kaijser, and E. Jannson. ATP breakdown products in human skeletal muscle during prolonged exercise to exhaustion. *Clin. Physiol.* 7:503–509, 1987.

102. Norman, B., A. Sollevi, and E. Jannson. Increased IMP content in glycogen-depleted muscle fibres during submaximal exercise in man. *Acta Physiol. Scand.* 133:97–100, 1988.

103. Owen, M.D., K.C. Kregel, P.T. Wall, and C.V. Gisolfi. Effects of ingesting carbohydrate beverages during exercise in the heat. *Med. Sci. Sports Exerc.* 18:568–575, 1986.

104. Pallikarakis, N., B. Jandrain, F. Pirnay, et al. Remarkable metabolic availability of

oral glucose during long duration exercise in humans. *J. Appl. Physiol.* 60:1035–1042, 1986.

105. Peronnet, F., D. Massicotte, C. Hillaire-Marcel, and G. Brisson. Use of carbon-13 (^{13}C) labeled glucose during exercise: effect of changes in background $^{13}CO_2$ production. *Med. Sci. Sports Exerc.* 22:S52, 1990 (Abstract).
106. Pirnay, F., M. Lacroix, M. Mosora, F. Lucykx, and P. Lefebvre. Glucose oxidation during prolonged exercise evaluated with naturally labeled [^{13}C]glucose. *J. Appl. Physiol.* 31:416–422, 1977.
107. Pirnay, F., M. Lacroix, M. Mosora, F. Lucykx, and P. Lefebvre. Effect of glucose ingestion on energy substrate utilization during prolonged muscular exercise. *Eur. J. Appl. Physiol.* 36:247–254, 1977.
108. Pirnay, F., J.M. Crielaard, N. Pallikarakis, et al. Fate of exogenous glucose during exercise of different intensities in humans. *J. Appl. Physiol.* 53:1620–1624, 1982.
109. Rehrer, N.J., E. Beckers, F. Brouns, F. Ten Hoor, and W.H.M. Saris. Exercise and training effects on gastric emptying of carbohydrate beverages. *Med. Sci. Sports Exerc.* 21:540–549, 1989.
110. Riley, M.L., R.G. Israel, D. Holbert, E.B. Tapscott, and G.L. Dohm. Effect of carbohydrate ingestion on exercise endurance and metabolism after a 1-day fast. *Int. J. Sports Med.* 9:320–324, 1988.
111. Sasaki, H., I. Takaoka, and T. Ishiko. Effects of sucrose or caffeine ingestion on running performance and biochemical responses to endurance running. *Int. J. Sports Med.* 8:203–207, 1987.
112. Schoeller, D.A., C. Brown, K. Nakamura, et al. Influence of metabolic fuel on the $^{13}C/^{12}C$ ratio of breath CO_2. *Biomed. Mass. Spectrom.* 11:557–561, 1984.
113. Simard, C., A. Tremblay, and M. Jobin. Effects of carbohydrate intake before and during an ice hockey match on blood and muscle energy substrates. *Res. Q. Exerc. Sport* 59:144–147, 1988.
114. Sjoggard, G. Water and electrolyte fluxes during exercise and their relation to muscle fatigue. *Acta Physiol. Scand.* 128 (*Suppl.* 556):129–136, 1986.
115. Slanger, B.H., N. Kusubov, and H.S. Winchell. Effect of exercise on human CO_2–HCO^{3-} kinetics. *J. Nucl. Med.* 11:716–718, 1970.
116. Tabata, I., Y. Atomi, and M. Miyashita. Blood glucose concentration dependent ACTH and cortisol responses to prolonged exercise. *Clin. Physiol.* 4:299–307, 1984.
117. Van Handel, P.J., W.J. Fink, G. Branam, and D.L. Costill. Fate of ^{14}C glucose ingested during prolonged exercise. *Int. J. Sports Med.* 1:127–131, 1980.
118. Villa Maruzzi, E., E. Bergamini, and Z. Gori Bergamini. Glycogen metabolism and the function of fast and slow muscles of the rat. *Pflügers Arch.* 391:338–342, 1981.
119. Viinamäki, O.J. Heinonen, U.M. Kujala, and M. Alén. Glucose polymer syrup attenuates prolonged endurance exercise-induced vasopressin release. *Acta Physiol. Scand.* 136:69–73, 1989.
120. Vollestäd, N.K., and P.C.S. Blom. Effect of varying exercise intensity on glycogen depletion in human muscle fibers. *Acta Physiol. Scand.* 125:395–405, 1985.
121. Vollestäd, N.K., O.M. Sejersted, R. Bahr, J.J. Woods, and B. Bigland-Ritchie. Motor drive and metabolic responses during repeated submaximal contractions in humans. *J. Appl. Physiol.* 64:1421–1427, 1988.
122. Vollestäd, N.K., J. Wesche, and O.M. Sejersted. Gradual increase in leg oxygen uptake during repeated submaximal contractions in humans. *J. Appl. Physiol.* 68:1150–1156, 1990.
123. Wahren, J. Glucose metabolism during leg exercise in man. *J. Clin. Invest.* 50:2715–2725, 1971.
124. Williams, C., M.G. Nute, L. Broadbank, and S. Vinall. Influence of fluid intake on endurance running performance. A comparison between water, glucose, and fructose solutions. *Eur. J. Appl. Physiol.* 60:112–119, 1990.

125. Winder, W.W., J. Arogyasami, H.T. Yang, et al. Effects of glucose infusion in exercising rats. *J. Appl. Physiol.* 64:2300–2305, 1988.
126. Wolfe, R.R., J.H.F. Shaw, E.R. Nadel, and M.H. Wolfe. Effect of substrate intake and physiological state on background $^{13}CO_2$ enrichment. *J. Appl. Physiol.* 56:230–234, 1984.
127. Wolfe, R.R., M.H. Wolfe, E.R. Nadel, and J.H.F. Shaw. Isotopic determination of amino acid-urea interactions in exercise in humans. *J. Appl. Physiol.* 56:221–229, 1984.

2
Exercise and the Neurobiology of Depression

ANDREA L. DUNN, Ph.D.
ROD K. DISHMAN, Ph.D.

As too much and violent exercise offends on the one side, so doth an idle life on the other . . . Opposite to Exercise is Idleness or want of exercise, the bane of body and minde, . . . the chiefe author of all mischiefe, one of the seven deadly sinnes, and a sole cause of Melancholy.

BURTON, 1632

INTRODUCTION

Since the time of Herodicus and Hippocrates, physicians have recognized the potential efficacy of exercise for the prevention and treatment of melancholia or depression [31]. Medical interest in the use of exercise as an adjunct for mental hygiene waned in the middle of this century [36], while psychopharmacology and neurobiology developed clinically effective drugs for depression and while psychotherapy was adopted by psychiatrists and clinical psychologists. The reemerging role of behavior in the prevention of disease and the promotion of health [235] has refocused attention on the role of exercise in the etiology and treatment of some types of depression.

This attention has culminated in a recent controversy over interpreting the scientific evidence linking exercise with moderate depression. Since 1980, numerous reviews of the literature have concluded that exercise is associated with reduced depression [66, 83, 157, 188, 230], which also was the consensus of the Workshop on Exercise and Mental Health sponsored by the National Institute of Mental Health in 1984 [159]. Moreover, a recent meta-analysis of 80 studies concluded that exercise is accompanied by a decrease in depression approximating one-half standard deviation [166]. Despite these interpretations of the literature, other reviews have concluded that exercise does not reduce depression [115, 242]. The U.S. Preventive Services Task Force of the U.S. Office of Disease Prevention and Health Promotion concluded that the quality of the available evidence was poor and stated that the

41

relationship between exercise and depression was poorly understood [106].

It is our view that no progress toward reconciling the controversy will be made until major strides are taken in improving the internal and external validity of exercise studies of depression. Past reviews have either ignored the importance of epidemiological traditions and evidence, have not adequately addressed definitions and measures of depression and physical activity, or have given only perfunctory attention to the neurobiological aspects of depressive disorders [149]. The independent efficacy, generalizability, and population effectiveness of exercise for decreasing depression cannot be described without redressing these shortfalls of past reviews and most of the research studies they have interpreted. In particular, biologically plausible mechanisms that might explain the previously documented association between exercise and reduced depression must be clarified for future research. Herein we briefly review past studies on exercise and depression from the perspective of epidemiology, but our focus is on neurobiological models of depression that can guide future research. Although cognitive models of depression [17] represent important approaches for understanding the role of exercise, we agree with prior reviews [157, 166, 188] that endorse a preeminent role for neurobiology. Exercise and sport scientists interested in the effect of exercise on depression must become conversant with contemporary models of depression derived from the traditions of psychobiology and neuropharmacology. Likewise, study of the neurobiological aspects of exercise may add to a more complete understanding of the etiology and treatment of depression.

We include (1) a brief overview of the epidemiology of depression; definitions of (2) depression and (3) exercise; (4) evidence for the efficacy of exercise as a treatment for depression; (5) the present state of knowledge about the neurobiological mechanisms underlying depressive symptoms and antidepressant drugs; (6) the current evidence from human and animal studies that describe changes in monoamines after acute and chronic exercise; (7) speculations about exercise effects on the hypothalamic-pituitary-adrenal (HPA) axis that appear relevant for depression; (8) new directions for animal models of exercise and depression; and (9) questions and recommendations for future research.

EPIDEMIOLOGY OF DEPRESSION

The National Institute of Mental Health conducted the Epidemiologic Catchment Area study which sampled more than 20,000 adults from five diverse U.S. communities. The six-month prevalence rate of persons suffering from affective disorders (Major Depression, Bipolar Disorder, or Dysthymia) was 5.8%; the lifetime prevalence rate was 8.3% [247,

251]. These rates are similar to those found in other industrialized countries. In studies conducted in England, Denmark, Sweden and the U.S., the point prevalence rate for nonbipolar depression was between 1.8 to 3.2 cases per 100 for men and 2.0 to 9.3 cases per 100 for women [74, 107, 250].

The finding that rates of depression are approximately twice as high for women compared to men is consistent in most studies conducted in the U.S. and other developed nations [249]. These ratios do not seem to be due a higher rate of help-seeking behavior or symptom-reporting by females [170, 249]. Whether the higher rate in females is due to genetic factors, endocrine differences, or learning consequent to social roles is unknown [6]. More recently, evidence indicates that the difference in relative risk for depression between females and males is diminishing. This appears less the result of lowered incidence of depression among females than the result of rising incidence of depression among young men [162, 248]. Hagnell and colleagues [104] found the risk of depression to be ten times higher for young adults from 1957 through 1972 as compared with the period from 1947 to 1957.

High or rising rates for depression are alarming because approximately 15% of patients suffering from severe primary depressive disorder for at least one month commit suicide. Within the U.S. population, suicide ranks tenth as a cause of death in all ages, and it is the leading cause of death in young adults [3, 252]. The total cost of suicide due to depression has been estimated at $4.2 billion per year [223]. The estimated cost for the single affective disorder of major depression has been estimated at $16.3 billion dollars per year in the U.S. Of this total, $2.1 billion has been spent directly on inpatient and outpatient treatment. The remaining $14.2 billion is indirectly expended by lost productivity through morbidity and mortality and expenses for family care [223]. These economic costs and the human suffering that underlies them could be curtailed if more of those suffering from depression entered effective treatment programs. It is estimated that only one of three persons suffering from depression seeks treatment from a medical doctor or a specialist in mental health [209]. Furthermore, there is evidence that those who do seek help are either undertreated, inappropriately treated, or the symptoms of depression are not recognized [123]. Consensus estimates indicate that 80–90% of those suffering from major depression can be treated successfully [191]. Self-help behaviors including regular exercise may offer useful adjuncts to primary and secondary prevention [58, 235], and there is some population evidence that physical inactivity may be one risk factor for depression [77, 220].

Established risk factors for nonbipolar depression include: (1) female gender, especially for ages 35 to 45 years; (2) a family history of depression or alcoholism; (3) a negative home environment; (4) recent negative life events, particularly those involving loss; (5) a lack of a confiding relationship, and; (6) parturition in the last six months [248]. Risk factors for depression in youth have not been established but are thought to include factors such as increased geographic mobility and loss of social attachments, social anomie, and changing roles in the family structure [126]. Although these risk factors are not directly rooted in neurobiology, all involve stress emotions linked by neurobiological processes [183].

Disruptions of neurotransmitter and hormone systems, and their interaction, represent the most widely studied area in the search for the underlying neurobiological mechanisms of depression [110]. It has been proposed that exercise may re-regulate neurobiological systems involved in stress emotions [159, 188], but specific hypotheses about antidepressant effects of exercise that are biologically plausible have not yet been advanced. This is largely explained by an incomplete consideration in past exercise research and review articles of 1) the etiological and nosological complexity of the depression disorders and 2) neurobiological models of depression. The efficacy of exercise for reducing depression, and the potential neurobiological mechanisms for exercise effects, could differ across diagnostic categories.

DEFINITION OF DEPRESSION

The etiology of depression is not fully understood. This in part is due to heterogeneity of symptoms. For example, depression can present either an increase or decrease in appetite and either insomnia or hypersomnia. Refinements in diagnosis have lead to the establishment of specific criteria for the varieties of depression. Research Diagnostic Criteria (RDC) [219] were developed to facilitate the uniformity of patient diagnosis for depression research. Only a handful of exercise studies have conformed to RDC definitions of depression [101, 124, 143, 144, 146, 147]. The Diagnostic and Statistical Manual of Mental Disorders, third edition, revised (DSM-III-R) [5] provides the most used standard for treatment and research on depression [191]. Although designed for use in the United States, DSM-III-R is widely employed in international research and has been translated into Chinese, Dutch, Danish, Finnish, French, German, Greek, Italian, Japanese, Norwegian, Portuguese, Spanish and Swedish. Many DSM-III-R criteria will be included in the tenth revision of the International Classification of Diseases (ICD-10) which is expected to be available in 1992 [5]. Although we recognize their theoretical limitations [76] and alternative classification systems [183], herein we utilize DSM-III-R definitions.

Depressive disorders are defined within the classification of Mood Disorders. Mood Disorders are broadly divided into Bipolar Disorders which include Bipolar Disorder, and Cyclothymia and Depressive Disorders which include Major Depression and Dysthymia. Bipolar Disorder requires the presence of one or more manic or hypomanic episodes intermixed or alternating with at least one full day of Major Depression; a history of major depressive symptoms is typical. Major Depression does not include episodes of mania or hypomania. A manic episode is described as a period of elevated, expansive, or irritable mood usually accompanied by impairment in occupational and social functioning. Symptoms of a manic episode include elevated self-esteem, decreased need for sleep, increased involvement in goal-directed activity, psychomotor agitation, and a high degree of involvement in pleasurable activities that may cause the person harm. In hypomania these symptoms are not severe enough to impair social or occupational functioning [5].

In Cyclothymia the essential diagnostic criteria is a chronic mood disturbance lasting at least two years (one year in children and adolescents) with alternating episodes of depression and hypomania. The depression must not be severe enough to meet the criteria for Major Depression and the hypomania must not be severe enough to be considered manic.

Major Depressive Episode is defined as a change of mood that has been present at least two weeks and is marked by symptoms of depressed mood or a loss of pleasure or interest. Symptoms that can be attributed to physical illness are excluded from the differential diagnosis; depression is the primary, not secondary, disorder. Also, at least five of the following associated symptoms should be present: (1) depressed mood (irritability in children or adolescents) which lasts most of the day; (2) a diminished interest or no pleasure in all or almost all activities; (3) weight loss or weight gain of not more than 5% per month or a decrease or increase in appetite nearly every day; (4) insomnia or hypersomnia for most of this two-week period; (5) psychomotor agitation or retardation; (6) fatigue or loss of energy even when no physical work has been performed; (7) feelings of worthlessness or guilt; (8) an inability to think or concentrate; and (9) recurrent thoughts of suicide or death [5].

DSM-III-R also subdivides Major Depression into a number of subtypes. Among these are Melancholia which is a severe form of a Major Depressive Episode that responds well to somatic therapy including tricyclic antidepressants and monoamine oxidase (MAO) inhibitors. In addition to Major Depression, a second major type of depression is Dysthymia, in which the person has suffered from depressed mood for the majority of days over the last two years but symptoms were not severe enough to be classified as major depression [5].

In this review we primarily address Major Depression and its subtype, Melancholia. However, our use of the term depression will refer to diagnosed depressive disorders of varying severity in humans and to signs and behaviors in animals that are consistent with depression in humans. We will exclude Bipolar Disorder or Cyclothymia, except when discussing studies that have assessed metabolites of monoamines in bipolar patients following acute physical activity.

DEFINITION OF EXERCISE

It is also important to define exercise for this review. The American College of Sports Medicine (ACSM) classifies exercise into three types: (1) cardiorespiratory or aerobic endurance, (2) muscular strength and endurance, and (3) flexibility. The majority of studies of exercise and depression have examined supervised programmatic exercise consistent with ACSM guidelines [4]. Most studies have used aerobic exercise such as running, swimming, or bicycling. A few have investigated anaerobic exercise, which is defined as weight training or vigorous sports [146, 166]. No studies have utilized flexibility training as an intervention. For our purposes the term exercise will indicate programmatic aerobic exercise unless otherwise specified. Epidemiological definitions of exercise [39] measured by global estimates of energy expenditure or the frequency, intensity, and duration of free-living activity, regardless of type, must also be considered if the population effectiveness of exercise as an antidepressant behavior is to be established. Descriptive epidemiological methods will not, however, permit the direct study of neurobiological explanations for the efficacy of exercise.

THE EFFICACY OF EXERCISE IN THE TREATMENT OF DEPRESSION

Most studies have examined the effects of exercise on depression by comparison with no-treatment controls or other treatments for depression such as psychotherapy, or both. In the first experimental study by Greist and colleagues at the University of Wisconsin [101], running was found to be comparable to either time-limited or time-unlimited group therapy in relieving symptoms of minor depression. This finding was replicated with a larger sample of volunteers diagnosed according to RDC criteria for unipolar, minor depression [124]; similar decreases in the depression scale of the Symptom Checklist-90 were observed for running, medication, and group therapy.

Since these early studies, a number of correlational quasi-experimental and experimental studies have examined the efficacy of exercise for reducing depression. Reviews of these studies have generally concluded that aerobic exercise is associated with a reduction in symptoms of mild and moderate depression [66, 83, 157, 188, 230]. However, others have not reached the same conclusions [115, 241]. Many of the studies reviewed had serious design and methodological flaws. Typically, depression was not assessed by uniform measures or standard diagnostic criteria and exercise was not adequately quantified.

Subsequent reviews by Martinsen [143, 144] were limited to experimental studies of clinically depressed patients meeting RDC or DSM-III-R diagnostic category of nonbipolar depression of mild to moderate severity who participated in aerobic forms of exercise. It was concluded that aerobic exercise was as effective as group psychotherapy, individual psychotherapy, and meditative relaxation. Furthermore, exercise was more effective than no treatment or a placebo treatment [144].

These narrative conclusions by Martinsen have been recently supported by a quantitative meta-analysis of exercise and depression conducted by North et al. [166]. A mean effect size (ES) of $-0.53 \pm$ .85 was obtained, indicating that depression scores were decreased by about one-half of one standard deviation in exercise groups compared to leisure activity, psychotherapy, and nonexercising control groups. The meta-analysis indicated an effect for 1) all forms of depression reported, including major and minor depressive disorders, primary and secondary types of depression, and self-rated depressive mood in nonpatients who scored in the normal range on questionnaires; 2) cardiorespiratory or aerobic endurance and muscular strength and endurance, as defined by ACSM; and 3) exercise programs of varying length ranging from less than 4 weeks to more than 24 weeks.

A number of shortcomings of meta-analysis limit the confidence that can be placed in the conclusion that exercise reduces depression. It is instructive to place these shortcomings in the perspective of epidemiological principles of 1) independence, 2) dose-response, 3) and biological plausibility for demonstrating a cause-effect relationship between exposure and disease [149]. First, only a handful of randomized trials with clinically depressed subjects have been reported, none of which shows an independent effect of exercise on depression. Collectively, studies show exercise effects that parallel those shown for psychotherapy or other minimally effective interventions such as meditation or recreation. Furthermore, the finding that exercise combined with psychotherapy produces an effect ($+.81 \pm .57$) that exceeds the effects of exercise alone ($-.53 \pm .84$) or psychotherapy alone ($-.19 \pm .71$) is difficult to interpret because of the unusually low psychotherapy effect reported in exercise studies. Meta-analysis of the large literature on psychotherapy and depression [212] has shown an independent effect size of .93 for psychotherapy compared to control conditions and an effect size approximating .20 for minimally effective or placebo interventions [69]. This suggests that the psychotherapy conditions contrasted in exercise studies have been ineffectively presented, poorly evaluated, or they involved persons who were not clinically depressed. In addition, the use of a true no-treatment control group in studies of depression is rare owing to ethical concerns over withholding treatment. However, it is known that episodes of moderate depression can remit spontaneously within several weeks or a few months, and this period falls within the duration of a number of prospective studies of exercise and depression. When all treatment groups respond favorably with a reduction in depression symptoms within this period, it is difficult to discount that results are due to spontaneous remission or to nonspecific effects of the experimental or clinical setting rather than to specific therapeutic components of the interventions. The North et al. [166] observation that the reduction in depression was correlated with length of the exercise program is consistent with a spontaneous remission of symptoms when exercise effects do not differ from other minimally effective interventions such as meditation or relaxation.

A dose-response relationship of exercise volume or increased fitness with decreased depression would present a more convincing case for an independent effect of physical activity on depression. Although many studies have followed ACSM guidelines for type, intensity, duration, and frequency known to increase fitness, several studies have shown no change in depression. Other studies show decreased depression with types and amounts of activity unlikely to influence fitness, whereas most studies have not assessed fitness with standardized measures. We have located only one prospective report linking increased fitness with decreased depression [144]. This report used submaximal exercise heart rate to estimate fitness, and the changes seen could have resulted from autonomic nervous system changes accompanying the abatement of depression. Moreover, the relationship between increased fitness and decreased depression was not replicated in a later study by the same investigators using a more direct measure of peak oxygen consumption [146].

Contrary to the assumptions of meta-analysis [166], the methodological problems of past research cannot be resolved by any type of review of the existing human literature on exercise and depression. They collectively place an even greater burden on exercise research to demonstrate cognitive and neurobiological mechanisms that offer plausible mechanisms for explaining the associations previously seen between physical activity and depression.

A number of findings from the North et al. [166] meta-analysis are, however, relevant to the discussion of neurobiological mechanisms common to exercise and depression. First, a significant effect size was found for single exercise sessions (-0.31 ± 0.44), for exercise programs of greater length ($-0.59 \pm .89$), and for follow-up periods up to nine months ($-0.50 \pm .80$). This appears inconsistent with findings of other studies [156, 238] indicating that antidepressant effects of exercise do not occur after acute bouts of exercise. It is difficult to explain this discrepancy in terms of pharmacological and neurobiological pathways that exercise might share with other somatic treatments such as the tricyclic antidepressants. For example, tricyclic antidepressant drugs block the reuptake systems for norepinephrine and serotonin as soon as they are applied, but clinical responses are typically not observed for two to three weeks following administration [12, 13]. When viewed in this context of the clinical time course for typical antidepressant therapy, the discrepancy between exercise studies reporting similar results for acute and chronic protocols illustrates that any postulated neurobiological explanation for antidepressant effects of exercise should account for both acute and chronic responses to exercise.

One explanation for the discrepancy between the North et al. [166] meta-analysis and other narrative reviews is nonuniformity in the definitions of depression. The meta-analysis incorporated all measures and forms of depression. It is likely that some studies have included subjects suffering from depression with a primary anxiety component. This inference is based on epidemiological findings that 33–91% of patients who meet the DSM-II-R criteria for agoraphobia with panic attacks are currently suffering from depression or have a history of depression [133]. Acute bouts of exercise can lower state anxiety for a period of 2 to 4 hours following exercise [11, 137, 187]. It is possible that reduced state anxiety results in an acute improvement in mood which could also lead to lower depression scores. Indeed, most exercise studies assessing state anxiety have employed Form X of the State-Trait Anxiety Inventory [217] which is known to be confounded by depression [218]. Careful clinical trials need to be conducted to examine the effects of acute and chronic exercise in patients suffering from depression and anxiety compared to those suffering from depression without anxiety [147].

Another finding of the meta-analysis with implications for neurobiological mechanisms of depression was the effectiveness of both aerobic and anaerobic exercise as antidepressants. The effect size of the weight training group was $-1.78 \pm .82$, compared to other types of aerobic training for which effect sizes ranged from -0.67 ± 1.22 to -0.48 ± 0.38. The effect size of the weight training group was based on only two studies, compared to 64 studies which utilized aerobic training. Because of the small number of studies utilizing anaerobic exercise programs, more needs to be done with greater numbers of depressed patients before confidence can be placed in these findings [160].

A recent well-controlled study supports the efficacy of anaerobic exercise, however. Martinsen and his colleagues [146] sampled a large subject pool of depressed patients and compared aerobic versus anaerobic training programs. They found that both groups had similar improvements in depression that were not dependent on an improvement in oxygen uptake peak ($\dot{V}O_2$ peak), and it was concluded that increased aerobic fitness was not necessary for an antidepressant effect of exercise. It has been argued that increased physical work capacity, i.e. an increase in $\dot{V}O_2$ peak, is indirect evidence for biochemical hypotheses of exercise on depression because it would be consistent with a biological dose-response adaptation to exercise training. This conclusion seems premature, however. We have not located studies that show either a correlational or cause-effect relationship between increased $\dot{V}O_2$ peak and adaptations in central nervous system neurotransmitters or neuromodulaters following aerobic or anaerobic exercise in either humans or animals.

In summary, studies of the efficacy of exercise on depression indicate that both aerobic and anaerobic exercise can alleviate symptoms of depression. Two questions are raised by these studies, however. First, do antidepressant effects occur after an acute bout of exercise, or are these effects only seen following a chronic exercise treatment; is the symptom abatement similar to that found for antidepressant drugs, e.g. a clinical response is not observed for two to three weeks? Second, are increases in fitness necessary for a decrease in symptoms of depression; is there a dose response between exercise and depression that is independent of fitness change?

Carefully controlled clinical trials addressing epidemiological issues of independence, time course, dose response, and population effectiveness will provide a better understanding of the neurobiology of exercise in depression. It is necessary, however, to directly examine neurobiological models of depression and changes in neurotransmitter and neuroendocrine systems following acute and chronic exercise that are relevant for these models.

NEUROBIOLOGICAL FACTORS INVOLVED IN DEPRESSION

Etiology and Genetics

A genetic vulnerability to depressive disorders has been established as a contributing factor to the onset of depression [3, 94, 252]. This is particularly true for recurrent affective disorders such as bipolar disorder and major depressive disorder [110]. The greatest evidence for the heritability of depression comes from twin studies in which concordance rates for major affective disorder are 65–75% in monozygotic twins compared to 14–19% in dizygotic twins [168, 231]. Arguably, the effect of a shared environment is difficult to determine when separating genotypic and cultural origins of phenotypic expression. It is possible that monozygotic twins are treated more alike than are dizygotic twins. Adoption studies indicate less genetic involvement in the etiology of depression. A recent adoption study found that affective disorders were diagnosed in 5.2% of biological relatives suffering from affective disorders, compared to 2.3% in the biological relative of unaffected adoptees [240].

Molecular biology research has suggested an X-linked gene for manic depressive illness [15, 152], but early findings have not been replicated [20]. In addition, bipolar depression was linked to a dominant gene on chromosome 11 in an Amish pedigree [71]; however, these results also have not been replicated [122]. Similar studies are being conducted on other affective disorders, but results are inconclusive [168, 180].

Nonetheless, it is likely that genetic influence on depression involves multiple genes. If so, part of the variability seen in affective disorders [180] would be explained. Siever [210] has suggested that individuals inherit a susceptibility to depressive illness, and that stress-related factors interacting with genetic influences potentiate a depressive episode. Because 20% of the variability in physical activity patterns are apparently explained by genetically transmissible variation [178], descriptive epidemiological research on the effects of exercise on depression [77, 197, 200] must ultimately discount an association due to correlated or common genotypes.

Dysregulation of monoaminergic neurotransmitter systems and the hypothalamic-pituitary-adrenal axis are prominent models of depression. Because each is responsive to pharmacological interventions believed to function through physiological systems that adapt to acute and chronic exercise, monoamine, and HPA responses are of particular interest for our review.

Dysregulation of Noradrenergic/Serotonergic Systems in Depression
The most widely studied biological hypotheses of affective disorders have involved the biogenic amines, norepinephrine (NE), dopamine (DA), and serotonin (5-HT) [53, 205]. Other putative neurotransmitters have also been implicated in depression, e.g. acetylcholine (ACh) and gamma-aminobutyric acid (GABA) [110, 116]. Because the bulk of exercise studies have examined NE and 5-HT, we will focus on these neurotransmitters.

SYNTHESIS AND METABOLISM OF NE AND 5-HT TRANSMITTERS. The monoamine neurotransmitters are located in neurons primarily in the brain stem reticular formation. The catecholamine neurotransmitters, which include dopamine, norepinephrine, and epinephrine, are synthesized from tyrosine. The rate of synthesis of NE varies with the degree of sympathetic nerve activity and its associated changes in tyrosine hydroxylase activity [233]. Tyrosine hydroxylase is the rate limiting enzyme in NE synthesis. If NE is not taken back up into the presynaptic neuron and bound in storage vesicles, it is metabolized by the enzymes MAO and catechol-o-methyl transferase (COMT). The synthesis and metabolism of NE is shown in Figure 2.1.

The indoleamine transmitter, serotonin (5-hydroxytryptamine or 5-HT) is synthesized from the amino acid tryptophan. The rate of synthesis of serotonin is more complex than NE. The rate-limiting enzyme, tryptophan hydroxylase, is not fully saturated under normal physiological conditions, and its activity depends on the amount of available L-tryptophan which, in turn, is controlled by a variety of factors, including its concentration in plasma and its rate of uptake into the brain and presynaptic terminals. Like NE, unbound 5-HT is converted to inactive metabolites by MAO. The synthesis and metabolism of 5-HT is shown in Figure 2.2 [52].

The function of monoaminergic systems in the CNS. Norepinephrine cell bodies represent two groups which innervate both rostral and dorsal structures. The major noradrenergic nucleus is the locus coeruleus (LC) which contains approximately half of all NE neurons in the brain. (See Figure 2.3). The LC is located in the caudal pontine central gray. Fibers from the LC form five major tracts which are mostly ipsilateral. Three of the tracts are ascending and innervate the periaqueductal gray, superior, and inferior colliculi, thalamic nuclei, amygdala, hippocampus, and all of the frontal cortex. One other ascending tract innervates the cerebellum. The remaining descending tract innervates the mesencephalon and spinal cord [52, 234, 239].

A large number of NE neurons also lie outside the LC and are located throughout the lateral ventral tegmental fields. Fibers from these neurons intermingle with the LC neurons, all of which contribute to the innervation of the mesencephalon and spinal cord as well as forebrain and diencephalon [52].

Norepinephrine is mediated by two types of adrenergic receptors, α-receptors and β-receptors, which have been further subdivided into α-1 and α-2 and β-1 and β-2. When α-1 receptors are stimulated, the second messenger, phosphoinositide cascade, is activated. Alpha-2 receptor stimulation is associated with an inhibition of noradrenergic activity. Presynaptic α-2 autoreceptors have been found to decrease presynaptic neuron activity and the amount of NE released. When β-1 receptors are excited there is a stimulation of adenylate cyclase by the stimulatory G protein (Gs) and a subsequent rise in the level of intracellular cyclic adenosine monophosphate (AMP) which acts as a second messenger for neural transmission. In the brain, β-2 receptors are primarily associated with glial cells [54].

Unlike the neurons of the noradrenergic system, the 5-HT neurons are distributed to all areas of the central nervous system (CNS). However, several discrete areas of serotonergic neurons have been identified [84, 176] (see Figure 2.4). Nine serotonin nuclei are near the midline raphe regions in the pons, medulla, and mesencephalon. Other

FIGURE 2.1

(1) *Tyrosine is converted to dihydroxyphenylalanine (DOPA) by tyrosine hydroxylase, the rate-limiting enzyme in the synthesis to NE. This reaction requires molecular O_2, Fe^{++}, and tetrahydropteridine cofactor.* **(2)** *DOPA is converted to dopamine by L-aromatic amino acid decarboxylase. It requires pyroxidal phosphate (vitamin B_6) as a cofactor.* **(3)** *Dopamine is converted to norepinephrine by dopamine β-hydroxylase. It requires ascorbic acid and molecular O_2 as cofactors. Dopamine β-hydroxylase contains cupric ion and is believed to be localized in the amine storage granules.* **(4)** *Reserpine interferes with the storage and uptake mechanism of the amine granules, which causes irreversible damage.* **(5)** *Presynaptic α-2 adrenergic receptors inhibits the release of NE.* **(6)** *Tricyclic drugs inhibit reuptake of NE, whose action is terminated by return to the presynaptic neuron.* **(7)** *NE that is not taken back up into storage vesicles is degraded by MAO.* **(8)** *NE remaining in the cleft is inactivated by COMT. Normetanephrine (NM) is further metabolized by MAO.* **(9)** *Following chronic antidepressant treatment, there is a reduction in β-adrenergic receptors.* **(10)** *Increased affinity for and sensitivity to $α_1$-adrenergic after chronic treatment with tricyclic antidepressants.* **(11)** *Downregulation of postsynaptic (and presynaptic) $α_2$-adrenergic receptors with chronic antidepressant treatment.*

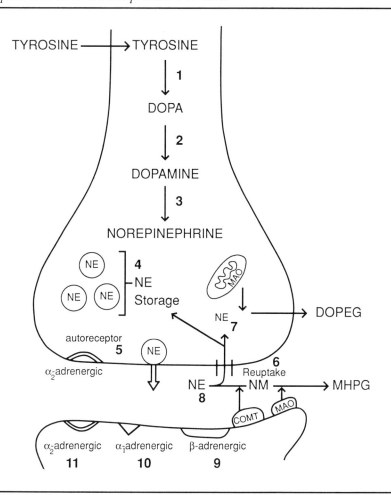

FIGURE 2.2

(1) *Tryptophan is converted to 5-hydroxytryptophan (5-HTP) by trytophan hydroxylase, the rate limiting enzyme in the synthesis of 5-HT. This reaction requires molecular O_2, tetrahydropteridine, and a sulfhydryl-stabilizing substance, e.g., mercaptoethanol.* **(2)** *5-HTP is converted to 5-HT by 5-HTP decarboxylase. It requires pyroxidal phosphate (vitamin B_6) as a co-factor.* **(3)** *Reserpine interferes with the storage and uptake mechanism of the amine granules which causes irreversible damage.* **(4)** *5-HT$_{1A}$ is the autoreceptor for 5-HT. Agonists such as 8-hydroxydiproplaminotetraline (8-OH-DPAT) selectively bind to 5-HT$_{1A}$ receptors, which inhibit the activity of serotonergic neurons in the midbrain raphe neurons.* **(5)** *Tricyclic drugs inhibit reuptake of 5-HT whose action is terminated by return to the presynaptic neuron.* **(6)** *5-HT that is not taken back up into storage vesicles is degraded by MAO and aldehyde dehydrogenase to 5-hydroxyindole acetic acid (5-HIAA).* **(7)** *Chronic administration of tricyclic antidepressants causes increased sensitivity to 5-HT. At this time their effect on 5-HT receptors is uncertain.*

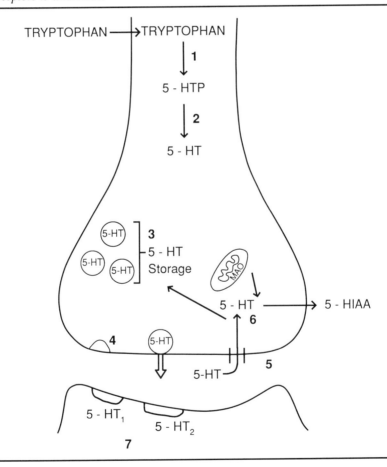

FIGURE 2.3

Diagram of the projections of the locus coeruleus viewed in the sagittal plane. See text for description. Abbreviations: AON, anterior olfactory nucleus; AP-VAB, ansa peduncularis-ventral amygdaloid bundle system; BS, brainstem nuclei; C, cingulum; CC, corpus callosum; CER, cerebellum; CTT, central tegmental tract; CTX, cerebral neocortex; DPS, dorsal periventricular system; DTB, dorsal catecholamine bundle; EC, external capsule; F, fornix; FR, fasciculus retroflexus; H, hypothalamus; HF, hippocampal formation; LC, locus coeruleus; ML, medial lemniscus; MT, mammillothalamic tract; OB, olfactory bulb; PC, posterior commissure; PT, pretectal area; RF, reticular formation; S, septal area; SC, spinal cord; SM, stria terminalis; T, tectum; TH, thalamus. (From observations of Lindvall, O., and A. Björklund. The organization of the ascending catecholamine neuron systems in the rat brain as revealed by the glyoxylic acid fluorescence method. Acta Physiol Scand. Suppl. *412:1–48, 1974. Jones, M.T., R.Y. Moore, and F.E. Bloom. Central catecholamine neuron systems: anatomy and physiology of the norepinephrine and epinephrine systems.* Ann. Rev. Neurosci. *2:113–168, 1979. Moore, R.Y., and F.E. Bloom. Central catecholamine neuron systems: anatomy and physiology of norepinephrine and epinephrine systems.* Annual Review of Neuroscience, Vol. 2. *Palo Alto, CA: Annual Reviews, Inc. 1979, pp. 129–165.)*

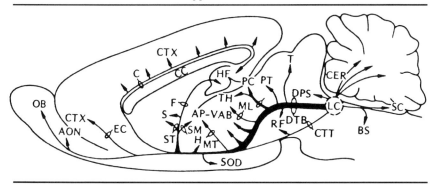

serotonergic nuclei have been detected in the caudal LC, the area postrema, and the interpendicular nucleus. Rostral serotonergic nuclei are thought to innervate the diencephalon and telencephalon which include many of the same structures innervated by noradrenergic fibers, including the thalamus, hypothalamus, amygdala, hippocampus, and frontal cortex. A dorsal serotonergic pathway also innervates the periaqueductal gray and posterior hypothalamus. There is also a minor innervation of the cerebellum, pons, medullary reticular formation, and spinal cord [52, 81, 239].

Sertonergic receptors have not been as widely studied as have noradrenergic receptors, but binding studies have distinguished two

FIGURE 2.4

Schematic representation of serotonin-containing pathways in brain as demonstrated by administration of 5,6-DHT or 5,7-DHT. (Modified from Björklund, A., A. Nobin, and U. Stenevi. The use of neurotoxic dihydroxytryptamine on nerve terminal serotonin and serotonin uptake in the rat brain. Brain Res. *50:214–220, 1973. Fuxe, K., and G. Johnson. Further mapping of central 5-hydroxytryptamine neurons: studies with neurotoxic dihydroxytryptamines. E. Costa, B.L. Gessa, M. Sandler (eds.).* Advances in Biochemical Psychopharmacology, Volume 10. *New York: Raven Press, 1974, pp. 1–12.*

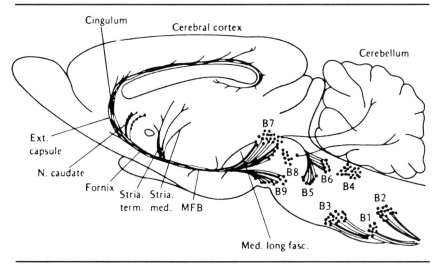

types of serotonergic receptors, 5-HT$_1$ and 5-HT$_2$ receptors. These receptors also appear coupled with adenylate cyclase and mediate inhibitory and excitatory effects [177]. 5-HT$_1$ receptors have been further subdivided into 5-HT$_{1A}$ and 5-HT$_{1B}$. Autoreceptors seem to be of the 5-HT$_{1A}$ type [52].

The consensus view holds that monoaminergic neurons modulate a wide range of functions in the CNS. Noradrenergic neurons are implicated in hormonal release [86], cardiovascular function [72], sleep [88], and analgesic responses [192]. Serotonergic activity is associated with pain, fatigue, appetitive behavior, periodicity of sleep, and corticosteroid activity [52]. Both NE and 5-HT have been implicated in the regulation of emotion by virtue of their action in the limbic system and the frontal cortex.

History and Evidence for the Monoaminergic Hypotheses of Depression. The first hypothesis concerning central amines in depression was the catecholamine hypothesis [29, 205], which posited that depression resulted from a deficiency of NE at central adrenergic receptors and that mania resulted from excess catecholamines. The indoleamine hypothesis of depression postulated a deficiency of 5-HT [53, 132]. These hypotheses arose from serendipitous observations of two different clinical populations. In the 1950s treatment of hypertension with reserpine led to depletion of NE and to symptoms of depression in approximately 15% of the patients treated. It was found that reserpine inactivates the storage granules containing NE and 5-HT and depleted these neurotransmitters intracellularly. The loss of intracellular vesicles also prevents the reuptake of NE or 5-HT into the presynaptic neuron, thus increasing the likelihood of their degradation by MAO [75].

Next it was observed that depressed tuberculosis patients treated for tuberculosis with iproniazid experienced elevated mood. It was later found that iproniazid inhibits MAO and thus reduces the metabolism of NE and 5-HT [13].

Each observation led to the inference that depression was precipitated by low monoamine levels and abated with increased levels. Considerable support has been generated for both monoamine hypotheses of depression. Evidence for involvement of central noradrenergic and serotonergic systems comes primarily from two sources. First, pharmacological studies have examined the actions and effects of antidepressant drugs which are known to raise the levels of amines in the synapse. Tricyclic antidepressants such as imipramine hydrochloride and desipramine hydrochloride prevent NE from being taken back up into the presynaptic neuron, thus enabling NE to remain in the synaptic cleft longer to bind with receptors. Another class of antidepressants, monoamine oxidase inhibitors such as phenelzine sulfate, prevents oxidative deamination which also increases availability of NE at postsynaptic receptor sites. A new atypical drug, fluoxetine hydrochloride, selectively blocks the reuptake of serotonin. The efficacy of these antidepressant treatments is between 65–80%; the placebo response rate is between 20–40% [12, 191].

A second line of evidence more directly examines the role of monoaminergic systems in depressed patients by sampling metabolites of NE and 5-HT in cerebrospinal fluid (CSF) or urine. It is assumed that excretion of metabolites such as 3-methoxy-4-hydroxyphenylethylene glycol (MHPG) from NE and 5-hydroxyindolacetic acid (5-HIAA) from 5-HT reflects the activity of noradrenergic and serotonergic systems. In general the results of these studies demonstrate that in bipolar depression there are reduced levels of MHPG during depressive episodes and higher than normal levels during mania [18, 204]. Reduced urinary MHPG also has been reported in schizoaffective depression and in subgroups suffering from unipolar depression [18, 206].

5-HIAA in urine also has been found to be below normal in depressed patients [53]. The same has been found to be true when examining 5-HIAA in CSF. Hirschfeld and Goodwin [110] suggest however, that, these low levels may be more strongly correlated with suicidal tendencies than with depression. Lower than normal MHPG levels in CSF have not been substantiated [110]. The circadian rhythm of urinary MHPG excretion may explain this discrepancy. Urinary MHPG is generally collected over a 24-hour sampling period, while the lumbar puncture is acute. Therefore, samples of MHPG from CSF could exhibit a great deal of variability depending on the time of sampling [241].

On the surface there seems to be good support for monoaminergic hypotheses of depression. Closer examination, however, of the pharmacological and metabolite studies reveals issues that are not easily resolved by a deficiency of NE or 5-HT. First, pharmacological data reveal that both tricyclic antidepressants and monoamine oxidase inhibitors increase the availability of NE and 5-HT to the receptors. If depression is the result of low NE or 5-HT, then raising the levels should alleviate symptoms of depression in a matter of hours. Yet clinical responses from antidepressant drugs generally are not observed for two to three weeks. In addition, some of the atypical antidepressants such as iprindole neither block the reuptake of NE nor alter the metabolism of NE or 5-HT [12, 225]. Iprindole also lacks the ability to suppress the firing of NE cells in the LC, which is a common response to the tricyclic antidepressants [169]. These discrepancies indicate that the site of action of a drug is not tantamount to the mechanisms responsible for its therapeutic action.

Baldessarini [12] has recently discussed consensus effects of antidepressants on NE and 5-HT systems. Firstline acute effects block the reuptake of monoamines. In general the reuptake of NE is blocked to a greater extent than is 5-HT, except in cases where an atypical antidepressant is used such as fluoxetine which selectively blocks the reuptake of 5-HT. A second acute effect is a reduction of firing rates for NE and 5-HT neurons in the brainstem. Third, the synthesis and turnover of NE and 5-HT is temporarily reduced. Fourth, receptors of the monoaminergic systems are blocked. Alpha-1 adrenergic receptors have a higher affinity for tricyclic antidepressants, whereas β receptors have the lowest affinity. The affinity of tricyclic antidepressants for the α-2 receptor is also low [12].

Chronic effects of tricyclic antidepressants include (1) continued blockade of reuptake; (2) a temporary and reversible down-regulation of presynaptic and postsynaptic α-2 receptors; (3) a normalization of firing rates and turnover which can lead to levels of monoamines that are above normal; (4) increased release of NE; (5) a down-regulation of β receptors; (6) an increased affinity and sensitivity to α-1 agonists that may increase the number of α-1 receptors, and; (7) a possible increase in the sensitivity to 5-HT, although the effects on 5-HT receptors are uncertain at this time [12].

The chronic changes seen with antidepressant drugs present some problems for both of the original monoaminergic hypotheses. Also, the MHPG data are not entirely consistent with the prediction of central NE depletion. In some patients with unipolar depression, normal or higher than normal levels of MHPG have been detected. Schildkraut et al. [206] subsequently proposed that the differences in MHPG can discriminate three subtypes of unipolar depression. Subtype I presents low levels of urinary MHPG prior to treatment. This low NE output may be due to a decrease in NE synthesis or to decreased release from the NE neurons. Subtype II presents intermediate levels of MHPG. These patients may have normal NE metabolism but other neurochemical systems may be abnormal. Subtype III presents high MHPG prior to treatment possibly because of less responsive noradrenergic receptors or increased cholinergic activity, or both [206]. Maas [140] has proposed that two subgroups of depression exist: one presenting low MHPG and normal 5-HIAA and the other presenting normal MHPG but low 5-HIAA. Although initial data from aggregated trials were consistent with these subtypes, recent cohort findings [59] have not supported this view.

Although these revised models are compatible with the catecholamine hypotheses, each assumes that all of the MHPG in CSF, plasma, or urine is derived from the brain. Maas and his colleagues [141] have estimated that 60% of MHPG is derived from brain, whereas Blomberry et al. [22] have derived a much lower estimate of 20%. MHPG can be assayed as a free molecule in plasma and as total free and conjugated MHPG in urine. In peripheral tissue, phenolsulfotransferase conjugates MHPG sulfate and glucuronosyltransferase conjugates MHPG glucuronide. In brain, only MHPG sulfate is conjugated. Although peripheral MHPG can be weakly or highly correlated with central MHPG, recent consensus holds that urinary MHPG sulfate is a more reliable estimate of brain NE metabolism [179]. In human plasma, total MHPG comprises about 30% free, 35% sulfate, and 35% glucuronide conjugates. In human urine less than 10% of total MHPG is free, with 40% sulfoconjugated and 50% in the glucuronide conjugate form. Based on these distributions, MHPG sulfate, rather than total MHPG or the glucuronide conjugate, appears to be the metabolite of choice for estimating central noradrenergic activity by assays of peripheral tissues [179].

Because of these problems, several revised hypotheses have been proposed that more fully consider the chronic effects of antidepressant drugs on monoaminergic neurons [3, 140,210]. There is consensus that monoamines are involved in depression. Examination of metabolic pathways for the monoamines suggests, however, a structural and functional relationship between the noradrenergic and serotonergic systems, revealing a number of places where homeostatic mechanisms could lose their self-regulatory ability (see Figures 2.1 and 2.2). Also, neurotransmitter systems not only influence each other, but they also are intimately linked to the HPA axis. Growing evidence indicates a role for the HPA axis in depression.

The HPA Axis and Depression

The symptomatology of typical Major Depression, including weight loss and early morning awakening, implicates the neuroendocrine system in the etiology and psychopathology of depression. For example, hypothalamic nuclei such as the preoptic area have been found to be crucial in the regulation of eating and body temperature. The supra-chiasmatic nucleus plays a role in the circadian secretion of various hormones; the ventromedial nucleus is the source of growth hormone-releasing factor and is critical in controlling visceral responses. An abnormality in the ventromedial nucleus can lead to hyperphagia, irritability, and decreased spontaneous activity [38, 151].

It is likely that multiple hormonal systems are disrupted in depressive illness. Although it is beyond our scope to review all of them, detailed reviews of the dysregulation of other hormonal systems in depression can be found [37, 145, 192]. We will focus only on the HPA axis. Our purpose will be to (1) understand how regulation of this system implicates neuroendocrine strategies for testing monoaminergic theories of depression, and (2) speculate how exercise might readjust these mechanisms in depression.

HPA ANATOMY AND REGULATION. The HPA axis refers to the paraventricular nucleus of the hypothalamus which releases corticotro-pin-releasing hormone (CRH) into the median eminence and the blood vessels of the anterior pituitary (see Figure 2.5). The anterior pituitary then releases adrenocorticotropin hormone (ACTH) and β-endorphin from the precursor molecule proopiomelanocortin (POMC). ACTH causes increased synthesis and secretion of cortisol or corticosterone from the adrenal cortex. These glucocorticoid hormones, in turn, inhibit CRH production and release at the level of the hypothalamus. They also can inhibit gene transcription of POMC and ACTH/β-endorphin secretion at the level of the pituitary. Inhibition of ACTH secretion occurs more rapidly than inhibition of POMC gene transcription [57, 118, 151, 239]. Dallman and Yates [57] have termed the former regulatory mechanism fast feedback. Its function is to precisely control ACTH during basal and acute stress states. Inhibition of POMC gene transcription has been termed delayed feedback and maintains the overall set point for the regulation of the transcription of the POMC gene. Fast feedback can only adjust levels of ACTH within the limits established by the amount of POMC messenger ribonucleac acid avail-able for transcription [118].

Young, Watson, and Akil [253] also suggest that because β-endorphin is coreleased with ACTH, it, too, may play a role in moderating the release of corticotropin-releasing factor (CRF), although this remains

FIGURE 2.5

Schematic illustration of neuroendocrine and neurotransmitter influences on the HPA axis. In response to stress, signals from multiple pathways are relayed to the paraventricular nucleus (PVN) of the hypothalamus which then releases CRH into the portal vessels through the infundibular stalk to the anterior pituitary. CRF causes POMC to be expressed. ACTH, β-endorphin, and other neuropeptides are cleaved from the POMC molecule. ACTH causes increased synthesis and secretion of cortisol or corticosterone from the adrenal cortex. These glucocorticoids then influence subsequent responses through a number of negative feedback mechanisms at pituitary, hypothalamus, and higher centers.

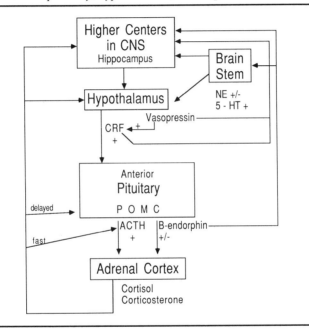

unclear. Preliminary studies indicate that β-endorphin may be both inhibitory or excitatory depending on its affinity with receptor subtypes [253]. Stubbs et al. [224] found an inhibition of ACTH and cortisol release with a *m*-opiate receptor selective enkephalin analog, Sandoz FK-33824. Conversely, DeSouza and Van Loon [63] found an initial stimulation and then a subsequent inhibition of ACTH and cortisol with an opioid peptide that has been found to prefer the *d*-opiate receptor, [D-Ala^2]-Met-enkephalin.

Neurotransmitters such as DA, NE, and 5-HT can also modulate the secretion of hypothalamic-releasing hormones [181, 201, 232]. Catecholamines and arginine vasopressin (AVP) have both been found to potentiate CRH-induced ACTH secretion [10, 236]. Because of these multiple regulatory strategies at the various levels of the HPA axis and the modulating influences from higher centers, it is possible that numerous interactions could differentially affect feedback in order to maintain homeostasis; these may become disrupted in depression.

EVIDENCE FOR HPA DISRUPTION IN DEPRESSION. At rest, the secretion of cortisol follows a well-defined circadian rhythm. ACTH and cortisol levels peak during the early morning hours, then decline during the day, with the lowest levels occurring during the first few hours of sleep. The early morning cortisol surge is the result of the episodic secretions of ACTH and cortisol six to eleven times throughout the day [89, 129]; the majority of these surges are in the morning. As the frequency of surges increases, the amplitude of cortisol secretion increases because cortisol has a longer half-life than ACTH [96]. The evidence for disruption of the HPA axis in depression comes primarily from clinical studies in which hypercortisolism was found in approximately 50% of patients suffering from primary major depression and melancholia. This has been demonstrated by measures of (1) 24-hour urinary-free cortisol, (2) plasma cortisol concentrations, (3) circadian secretion of cortisol, (4) cortisol concentrations in CSF, and (5) the dexamethasone suppression test [38, 151].

Studies examining the circadian rhythm of cortisol production show that it follows the same pattern for depressed patients and normal control patients [105]. Although the pattern is similar, however, about one-half of depressed patients have higher cortisol levels during the afternoon and evening [37, 198, 199]. This pattern is similar to the hypersecretion in Cushing's disease, and many persons who suffer from Cushing's disease also suffer from depression [93, 97]. This hypersecretion of cortisol is typically resistant to feedback by dexamethasone, a synthetic corticosteroid.

A series of studies conducted by Sachar and colleagues [198, 199] found that depressed patients have a greater than expected number of secretory episodes of cortisol at higher levels, that total cortisol is particularly increased at certain periods during the day, i.e., late evening and early morning, and that increases in cortisol secretion are not dependent on external stressors. These responses return to normal as the patient recovers [9, 49]. Because the hypercortisolism documented in depression is also present with other disorders such as anorexia nervosa [90] and alcoholism [221], it is not viewed as a causal factor in depression.

Although the origin and mechanisms of hypercortisolism in depression remain unclear, infusion of cortisol, synthetic steroids such as dexamethasone, or CRF followed by sensitive radioimmunoassay has characterized the disruption of these regulatory mechanisms in acute and chronic stress in animals and to a lesser extent in humans. Results from these strategies provide direction for developing neurobiological models of antidepressant effects of exercise.

HPA Mechanisms in Acute and Chronic Stress and their Relationship to Depression

There is controversy and uncertainty over the regulatory mechanisms of the HPA axis in acute and chronic stress. In this section we briefly review areas of clear relevance for exercise. More detail on the regulatory mechanisms of the HPA axis during stress is available elsewhere [8, 10, 118].

In acute experimental stress, i.e., the injection of synthetic ovine CRF (oCRF) in rats, there is an immediate increase in plasma ACTH. This response is dose-dependent and can be blocked by CRF antibodies. Vasopressin also causes the release of ACTH in a dose-dependent manner in the rat, and this can be blocked by vasopressin antagonists [194].

However, when stress is chronic or repeated, HPA responses are more complex and can be confounded by the types of stress and the timing of the stress [118]. DeSouza and Van Loon [64] found an attenuation of the adrenocortical response using restraint stress with an interval of less than two hours. This attenuation has also been demonstrated with ether stress [120]. Conversely, a potentiation of the ACTH response can occur subsequent to footshock or laparotomy [56]. Jones and Gillham [118] have suggested that potentiation occurs after neurogenic stresses, such as restraint and laparotomy, but that inhibition occurs after systemic stresses such as hypoglycemia or hypotension. They hypothesize that this is because of the ratios of ACTH secretagogues released into the systemic circulation; the response of the pituitary is likely to be different depending on the ratios of vasopressin, oxytocin, and CRF released.

For the study of chronic stress, Akil et al. [2] have developed an in vitro pituitary model in which animals are given footshock for 30 min/day for 14 days and either a 24-hour recovery period or an acute shock prior to decapitation. Results indicate an increased response to CRF, with an increase in the content of POMC peptides and a decrease in glucocorticoid negative feedback. The responses seen in this chronic stress model resemble those seen in Cushing's disease, which has provided the primary human model for studies of HPA axis disruption [253].

A characteristic sign of Cushing's disease is the failure to suppress pituitary ACTH in response to endogenous glucocorticoids or exogenous steroids like the synthetic dexamethasone (DEX). DEX challenge provides information about the delayed feedback regulatory mechanism defined earlier (see Figure 2.5). On the other hand, the infusion of cortisol or CRF stimulation provides an evaluation of fast feedback mechanisms. Reader et al. [190] and Fehm et al. [80] administered cortisol in order to observe the fall in ACTH with rising cortisol and found that nearly twice the concentration of plasma cortisol was required to stimulate the decrease in ACTH in patients with Cushing's disease. This inability to suppress plasma ACTH with cortisol infusion indicates a loss of sensitivity in steroid-negative feedback mechanisms. Furthermore, studies that have examined ACTH responses as a result of CRF stimulation have found a hyperresponsiveness of ACTH in Cushing's patients compared to normal controls [161, 172, 173].

In summary, the pattern of HPA responsivity in Cushing's disease is very similar to the chronic stress model developed by Akil et al. [2]. There is (1) an overall increase in ACTH, (2) a loss of sensitivity in steroid-negative feedback, and (3) an increased sensitivity to all doses of CRF [253].

HIGHER CENTER CONTROL OF THE HPA AXIS IN DEPRESSION. Numerous studies conducted by Gold and his colleagues [95, 96] as well as by Holsboer et al. [112] report a decreased ACTH response to CRF stimulation in depressed patients. This blunted response suggests that, unlike the case for Cushing's patients, the pituitary corticotroph cell functions normally in depressed patients. Thus, Gold et al. [94, 95] have hypothesized that the hypercortisolism in depression is due to a defect at the level of the hypothalamus or higher.

There are several lines of evidence to support this hypothesis. First, it has been found that a continuous infusion of oCRF in normal volunteers demonstrates the same circadian pattern and amplitudes of hypercortisolism seen in depression [207]. Second, the level of CSF CRF has been found to be elevated in depression [164]. Third, neurotransmitters such as NE, ACh, and GABA can modulate the effects of the secretion of CRH [33, 34, 35]. Norepinephrine injected into the posterior hypothalamus increases corticosteroid secretion, whereas CRF applied locally to neurons in the LC increases their NE activity [95]. Fourth, experimental studies have demonstrated that hypercortisolism can damage or destroy hippocampal cells containing glucocorticoid receptors that mediate the suppression of the CRF neuron [201, 202]. Because depressed patients have higher free cortisol levels than normal patients, even though ACTH release is small during CRH stimulation, the adrenal cortex has apparently become hyperresponsive to ACTH. Chronic elevations or exaggerated episodic pulses of cortisol could lead to neuron damage to the hippocampus or to a downregulation of hippocampal glucocorticoid receptors [94, 95, 203].

In summary, hypersecretion of cortisol in humans and corticosterone in rats may be explained by disruption at any of several sites in the HPA axis: hypersensitivity of the adrenals to ACTH, hyposensitivity of the pituitary to glucocorticoid feedback, hypersensitivity of the pituitary to secretagogues, hypersecretion of secretagogues by the hypothalamus, and resistance to neural feedback [201]. In depression, ACTH secretion following CRF challenge is blunted. This could result from competition for pituitary responsiveness to CRF coming from feedback signals of elevated glucocorticoids. Because evidence indicates, however, that in depression the pituitary is less sensitive to glucocorticoid feedback, it appears the pituitary becomes less responsive to CRF possibly because of prolonged exposure to high CRF and subsequent downregulation of CRF receptor density. It is argued [95, 201] that elevated ACTH, despite diminished response by the pituitary to CRF, indicates increased hypothalamic secretagogue activity. A similar pattern also has been suggested for AVP [95, 201].

Although the hypothalamus mediates HPA feedback, it appears subordinate to higher command. For example, deafferentation of the hypothalamus leads to resistance to dexamethasone suppression of ACTH. Sopolsky and Plotsky [201] argue that the hippocampus exerts an inhibitory central command on the hypothalamus and that damage or disruption of hippocampal activity can explain part of the hypercortisolism of depression. Lesioning the hippocampus or severing its neural connection to the hypothalamus leads to hypersecretion of glucocorticoids, ACTH, CRF, AVP, and oxytocin (OT) during basal and stressful conditions. Because the primate hippocampus has corticosteroid receptor densities similar to those in rats, and because stimulation of rat hippocampus [68] and the human hippocampus during neurosurgery [142] is followed by reduced glucocorticoid secretion and inhibition of CRF and AVP neurons projecting to the median eminance [200], there is evidence that the hippocampus downregulates the HPA axis in both rats and primates.

Sopolsky et al. [202, 203] show that sustained exposure to stressors also is associated with decreased receptor density in hippocampus. In addition to CRF, arginine vasopressin, oxytocin, catecholamines, and angiotensin stimulate ACTH directly or in synergy with CRF. The pattern of secretagogues appears stereotyped for different stressors [8]. It, therefore, will be important to determine if exercise and depression share common secretagogue patterns while examining the plausibility that either acute or chronic exercise might influence HPA regulation by influencing hippocampal activity or regulation.

Integration of Monoamine and HPA Systems
Collectively, the evidence [95] is consistent with the hypothesis that the CRH and LC-NE systems reinforce one another's activity. In melancholic depression the glucocorticoids or the LC-NE system, or both, may fail to provide the appropriate regulation or restraint on the HPA axis. This system then becomes excessively activated. The resulting model of prolonged or excessive activation of the HPA stress response provides a useful heuristic for understanding the neurobiology of depression.

Moreover, an HPA model of depression does not directly challenge monoaminergic theories of depression. Excess NE could stimulate the overproduction of CRF. Another view is that the central action of NE on the HPA is inhibitory thus reducing CRH and ACTH secretion. Central administration of catecholamine synthesis inhibitors such as reserpine and α-methyl-p-tyrosine leads to increased plasma corticosterone and ACTH [226].

Conclusions over the stimulatory or inhibitory effects of NE on the HPA remain equivocal because NE apparently exerts differential effects on ACTH at different levels of the HPA axis. In addition, NE actions are paradoxical at presynaptic and postsynaptic receptors. It has been hypothesized that NE reduces CRH and ACTH secretion through α-one receptors and enhanced somatostatin release, whereas NE stimulation of α-two receptors increases ACTH release [181, 232].

Other monoamines also have demonstrated effects on CRF-ACTH secretion. For example, 5-HT generally has been found to have stimulatory effects on resting and stress-induced ACTH-corticosteroid secretion [1, 130, 196].

We have reviewed the major neurobiological models of depression. The historically preeminent models are the monoamine theories which include the catecholamine and indoleamine hypotheses that depression is the result of a deficit of these neurotransmitters. Recent studies have emphasized the disruption of the HPA axis and hypothesize that depression is the result of loss of regulatory mechanisms at the level of the hypothalamus or the hippocampus which restrain the secretion of corticosteroids. This lack of restraint is thought to lead to overactivation of the CRH/LC-NE systems. The HPA model of overactivation of the CRH/LC-NE systems does not discredit the monoamine theories, however. Models of monoamine and HPA dysregulation can be integrated. Sachar et al. [198] have proposed that depletion of NE in the hypothalamus causes a loss of inhibition to the CRH neuron which then stimulates the secretion of ACTH; this may eventually lead to the hypercortisolism seen in depression.

Other integrations of the monoamine and HPA models of depression have been proposed. Siever and Davis [210] argue that depression is the result of dysregulation in one or more neurotransmitter systems, and that these systems should be evaluated in terms of their circadian and ultradian periodicities [211]. The neurobiological systems models proposed by Gold et al. [95] and Siever and Davis [210] more fully describe depression as a heterogeneous illness with many paradoxical signs and symptoms, e.g., high or low urinary MHPG and hypersomnia or insomnia. In this way, integrated models are more easily reconciled with clinical diagnosis for human patients.

Each of the preceding perspectives provides directions for examining how exercise might cause adaptations to restore homeostasis in depressed patients. Monoaminergic theories have been explored by describing changes in neurotransmitters such as NE and 5-HT with acute and chronic training in rats. They also have been investigated by observing changes in urinary MHPG in acute and chronic exercise in depressed and nondepressed humans. In the next sections we review the effects of exercise in humans and rats in relation to the neurobiological aspects of depression.

EXERCISE AND MONOAMINE STUDIES IN HUMANS

If exercise has independent antidepressant effects, then it is reasonable to expect that its biological mechanisms of action could be similar to those believed to be affected by pharmacological treatments for depression. Of the plausible neurobiological responses common to pharmacological interventions and exercise, only changes in the monoamines have received sustained study.

In humans, changes in monoamines have been assessed by measuring MHPG in urine, plasma or CSF; it has been assumed that increased MHPG would reflect increased central noradrenergic activity. Studies examining the effects of acute physical activity on MHPG have been summarized elsewhere [158]. Acute studies which measured urinary MHPG found either increased MHPG excretion [18, 163, 184] or no change [61, 226, 229].

There are some methodological problems with these studies. First, sample sizes were small, and different types of depression were present in the same treatment group. For example, both unipolar and bipolar patients were assigned to the exercise condition. Also, exercise levels were not quantified or very low levels of exercise were used.

Studies of acute activity and MHPG in nondepressed subjects have typically quantified the exercise and some have relativized exercise intensity to work capacity. Again, the findings are mixed. Typically, plasma MHPG is increased, but urinary MHPG remains unchanged [98, 114]. Other studies have found increases in glucuronide and sulphated subfractions of MHPG [179, 213, 228]. Continued debate, however, over the central or peripheral origins of plasma and urinary MHPG and their meaning for NE metabolism in the brain hinders interpretations of the exercise studies for models of depression. In plasma or urine, MHPG sulfate appears more reflective of NE activity in the brain than total MHPG or the glucuronide conjugate [179]. Because free MHPG originating in brain can be sulfoconjugated in the blood, however, the relevance for monoamine models of depression of exercise studies showing increased MHPG sulfate in plasma following acute exercise [228] remains unclear. To determine the origin of the MHPG, a recent study [82] used ethanol to block the metabolism of

MHPG to vanillylmandelic acid in the liver. The findings were consistent with a central origin for MHPG sulfate, and showed similar excretion rates for MHPG subfractions in depressed patients and normal controls following high intensity exercise.

We have located no chronic exercise studies that have examined MHPG response. Cross-sectional studies of nondepressed subjects have, however, compared MHPG levels between fitness groups based on $\dot{V}o_2$max and have found no differences [214, 215, 216]. An inverse relationship between $\dot{V}o_2$ peak and self-rated depression has been reported [135], as have multivariate relationships among fitness and urinary NE metabolites with depression and anxiety for normal males following resting and occupational conditions [215, 216].

Although these studies provide a base for the study of exercise and depression from the neurobiological perspective, they collectively yield no clear conclusions owing to the absence of prospective controlled studies, a lack of uniformity in diagnosis and quantification of exercise in the patient studies, the unclear relevance for depression of exercise studies with nonpatients, and the inherent limitations of peripheral metabolites of NE for understanding central noradrenergic activity.

Despite these shortcomings, the measurement of plasma or urinary MHPG remains an important clinical tool in depression research. It is likely that it could also be used effectively in understanding noradrenergic adaptations with exercise in depressed patients with more tightly controlled studies. Future studies should ensure a more homogenous diagnosis of depression and establish that baseline MHPG excretion patterns are similar in patient groups [206]. Prospective studies employing repeated measures are needed to assess changes over both days and weeks due to the disruption of circadian and ultradian rhythms common in Major Depression [211]. It also is important to strictly quantify exercise intensity and to examine both aerobic and anaerobic modes of exercise. Peripheral monoamines and β-endorphin are acutely increased by prolonged exercise (e.g., 20 min to 1 hr) at intensities above 80% of $\dot{V}o_2$ peak, and a dependent or correlated response in the CNS remains a plausible explanation for an antidepressant effect of exercise [27, 99, 208].

Change in monoaminergic systems also can be assessed by receptorology. We are unaware of studies that have examined changes in α or β receptors following exercise in depressed patients. Lymphocyte β-adrenoreceptor density is reported to decrease with training, however [32]. Conversely, $α_2$-adrenergic receptors on platelets appear to increase with training [136]. The mechanism of these changes in receptor density is unknown. Furthermore, it is not certain that changes in peripheral noradrenergic receptors parallel those in the CNS. The development of imaging methods such as positron emission tomography (PET) and the future development of suitable positron-emitting ligands for noradrenergic and serotonergic receptors will enable researchers to study changes in monoaminergic receptors in depressed persons using more specific, dynamic methods [54].

EXERCISE AND MONOAMINE STUDIES IN ANIMALS

We have located no studies on the chronic effects of exercise using an animal model of depression such as learned helplessness or other behavioral deficit models. We did find reports of increased LC activity [242] and increased NE and MHPG [246] following acute bouts of swimming stress. Both studies employed the Porsolt [182] test as an index of motivational deficit. Because fitness or training/habituation was not controlled in these studies, their results are unclear for salutary models of exercise and depression.

A number of studies have examined brain NE, 5-HT, and 5-HIAA with acute and chronic training protocols which are detailed in Tables 2.1 and 2.2 For example, decreases in whole brain NE have been found with acute exercise [14, 50, 99, 148, 153, 154, 222]. Conversely, chronic exercise studies have found elevation in brain NE levels [26, 27, 28, 274, 219]. Acute exercise causes a rise in NE in the periphery if intensity is over 30% of $\dot{V}o_2$ peak. Chronic training causes an adaptation in the peripheral noradrenergic system in a one to three week period [87]. The mechanism of this adaptation is unknown. As noted, however, it is plausible that there may be a downregulation of β-adrenergic receptors and an upregulation of α_2-adrenergic receptors that are correlated with changes in fitness [32, 136].

Acute exercise studies have found increased [14, 195] or no change [50] in 5-HT levels. Two acute exercise studies that have measured both 5-HT and 5-HIAA, commonly used to estimate turnover, found increased turnover [43, 48]. On the other hand, chronic wheel-running decreased 5-HT turnover in the midbrain, cortex, hippocampus, and posterior hypothalamus but increased turnover in the pons-medulla [113]. Chaouloff et al. [47] also found decreased turnover with chronic treadmill training.

It is not possible to determine from these studies how exercise affects noradrenergic or serotonergic activity because the lack of uniformity in their methods prevents direct comparisons of results. First, early studies measured only concentration levels using fluorometry. The measure of a concentration of a neurotransmitter is not a good indicator of its activity because many types of stress are likely to alter levels of NE in both brain and periphery depending on factors such as severity [10, 62]. Turnover, estimated by the neurotransmitter and major metabolites, provides a more accurate estimate of activity of the neurotransmitter of interest. Yet there are some potential problems with

TABLE 2.1
Summary—Acute Exercise and Changes in NE, 5-HT, and Metabolites

Study (Author, Subjects)	Exercise Protocol	Other Stressors	Method of Measurement	Brain Area
Barchas and Freedman (1962) [14] (More than 50 rats in each experimental condition)	Swim to exhaustion in 15°C & 23°C water, treadwheel for 3 hours at 6 rpm.		Fluorometry	Whole brain
Moore and Lariviere (1964) [154] (7 groups, 12 female Sprague-Dawley rats in each group)	Forced swim for 4 hours. One group in 23°C, the other in 37°C.	Other groups: tail shock, restraint, sound, grid shock D-amphetamine to all groups to deplete catecholamines	Fluorometry	Whole brain
Gordon, Spector, Sjoerdsma, and Udenfriend (1966) [99] (4 groups, female Sprague-Dawley rats, total = 46)	Rotating drum at 7 kpm for 3 hours and 5 hours Rotating drum at 7 kpm for 1 hour	α-metyl tyrosine in two groups, one with exercise, one with no exercise tyrosine-C^{14} to all groups	Fluorometry	Brain stem
Moore (1968) [153] (8 male albino mice)	Spontaneous activity wheel measured for 10 minutes	Diet with 0, 0.3, or 1% α-methyl tyrosine	Fluorometry	Whole brain
Stone (1973) [222] Adult male Sprague-Dawley rats. 10 in control (c); 4 to 8 rats in running groups. Some also injected with reserpine and α-methyl tyrosine (AMT).	3 hours on motor-driven activity wheel 330–475 m/h	Injection of [^{3}H]NE under light anesthesia 10 or 30 minutes after running	Radioactive labelling	Hypothalamus brain stem
Romanowski and Grabiec (1974) [195] (2 groups, 10 each, male Wistar rats)	Treadmill 24 m/min for 90 minutes		Spectrofluorometric	Whole brain
Lukaszyk, Buczko and Wisniewski (1983) (5 male Wistar rats; no controls [138])	Treadmill—20 min at 30 m/min	Shock used to facilitate treadmill running: Dopamine receptor agonists: DL-amphetamine sulfate, apomorphine hydrochloride; antagonists: haloperidol; and trasylol, aproteolytic enzyme inhibitor, given IP.	Flourometry	Striatum, hypothalamus, hippocampus, midbrain, frontal cortex, cerebellum

NE	MHPG	5-HT	5-HIAA	*Conclusions*
Decreased in exercise conditions		Increased in exercise conditions		Physiological significance of changes is unclear. Changes in brain amines did correlate with changes in behavioral state e.g. sporadic uncoordinated activity after cold swim. 5-HT levels approached normal after 2 hours, NE by 6 hours.
Decreased in exercise more than in control conditions				No difference in catecholamine levels in rats swimming at 23°C & 37°C.
				Only grid-shock and swim rats had lower brain NE than controls.
				Appears both chemical and physical stimuli can deplete brain stores of NE.
Slight depletion of NE in exercise alone; lowered more with α-methyl tyrosine. Increased radioactivity in NE due to tyrosine-C^{14} in exercise (increased synthesis).				Both exercise and cold with little effect by themselves, produced marked depletion of NE when synthesis was blocked.
				Increased radioactivity after injection with tyrosine-C^{14} must be the result of increased synthesis.
				Increased synthesis probably is not due to increased substrate because tyrosine levels do not change.
				Release of catecholamines may free tyrosine hydroxylase from end-product inhibition.
				Increased tyrosine hydroxylase activity may result from interaction with hormones of the pituitary-adrenal axis.
				Mechanism for increased tyrosine hydroxylase activity may involve increased synthesis of the enzyme.
Decreased in dose dependent manner w/α-methyl tyrosine but not with exercise				NE and locomotor activity both decreased in a dose dependent manner w α-methyl tyrosine.
				Locomotor activity continued to diminish with administration of the drug until 10 days after which there was no further reduction in activity. The tolerance developed to α-methyl tyrosine may be due to increased sensitivity of adrenergic receptors.
Decreased in exercise. Reserpine treated lost 95% NE. AMT reduced NE 41%	Exercise increased MHPG. Reserpine treated increased MHPG. AMT slightly reduced MHPG.			Running stress did not affect the storage of NE as determined by no change in accumulation of [H^3]NE injected at various intervals.
				Stores of NE depleted by stress are replenished from newly synthesized stores, not by reuptake.
				Prior stress (i.e., running), which resulted in increased MHPG, might be reflective of NE released by nerve activity.
		Increased		5-HT was nearly doubled in exercise rats compared to controls.
Increased in striatum, frontal cortex, and hippocampus; decreased in hypothalamus; unchanged in cerebellum and midbrain. Exercise effects less than trasylol condition.		Decreased in striatum, frontal cortex and midbrain.		Acute exercise enhanced the action of dopamine receptor antagonists. Trasylol facilitated the action of dopaminomimetic drugs and increased NE; exercise normalized this effect.

(continued)

TABLE 2.1 *(continued)*

Study (Author, Subjects)	Exercise Protocol	Other Stressors	Method of Measurement	Brain Area
Chaouloff, Elghozi, Guezennec, and Laude (1985) [48] (4 groups, 6 per group, fasted and fed, exercise and control male Wistar)	Treadmill—4 or 5 adaptation sessions. Day of experiment 1 hour at 20 m/min or 2 hours at 20 m/min.	Shock during adaptations. Two groups food deprived.	Liquid chromatography with ultraviolet and amperometric detection.	Whole brain minus cerebellum
Cicardo, Carbone, De-Rondina and Mastronardi (1986) [50] (10 groups, 6 male Wistar rats in each group)	Swim to exhaustion in 23°C water	Injections of mianserin or moclobemide acutely and chronically	Spectrofluorometric	Whole brain
Chaouloff, Kennett, Serrurrier, Merino, and Curzon (1986) [43] (4 resting control, 5 brain, 6 CSF male Wistar rats)	Treadmill—4 or 5 adaptation sessions. Last session all rats ran 20 m/min for 1 hour.	Shock during adaptations	Liquid chromatography	Whole brain & CSF
Heyes, Garnett and Coates (1988) [109] (25 male Sprague-Dawley rats split into performance groups: exhaustion and control groups and early (5.9 min), mid (10.9 min), and late (16.6 min) stages of the endurance test)	Motor driven treadmill-run to exhaustion (19.6 ± 0.6 min) at 37 m/min.	Shock used to facilitate treadmill running	Liquid chromatography	Striatum, brain stem and hypothalamus

this. Turnover is an index of the functional state of the neurons and is defined as the rate in which amine stores are replaced. This is not always the same as biosynthesis. Turnover can be measured directly by isotope methods and use of inhibitors, or indirectly through measurement of metabolites in CSF and plasma. These methods make a number of assumptions which may lead to errors in the estimation of turnover. One assumption is that NE is contained in one homologous pool. This is erroneous as demonstrated by neuroanatomical studies which have mapped NE in the brain [24, 155]. Another assumption is that labelled

NE	MHPG	5-HT	5-HIAA	Conclusions
		Increased with exercise	Increased with exercise	Brain 5-HT turnover is indirectly increased during running as a consequence of accelerated fat catabolism (running did not diminish brain tryptophan uptake as much as food deprivation).
				Valine injected before exercise prevented tryptophan increases. This raises questions about stress during running. When animals are trained, stress induced variations in metabolism may be minimized.
				Desipramine, an antidepressant, affected only peripheral tryptophan in runners. Both plasma free and total were increased. Desipramine increased ratio of brain tryptophan to plasma free tryptophan. Brain 5-HT and 5-HIAA were increased in desipramine treated controls and runners.
				Results suggest running accelerates lipolysis, increases brain tryptophan and 5-HT turnover.
Decreased in exercise more than control		No change		Mianserin, a tetracyclic antidepressent which does not inhibit presynaptic reuptake of NE, did not modify the decrease in NE when administered acutely or chronically in rats forced to swim.
				Moclobemide, a MAO inhibitor, did not inhibit the decrease in NE when administered acutely in rats forced to swim. It did inhibit the decrease when administered chronically.
		Increased brain & CSF tryptophan (5-HT substrate)	Increased brain & CSF	Running increased 5-HT turnover as indicated by increased tryptophan and 5-HIAA. Lvels of tryptophan and 5-HIAA returned to prerunning values in 1 hour.
Decreased in hypothalamus and brain stem		No change in striatum, brain stem, and hypothalamus	Increased in striatum	Although dopamine concentration and estimated turnover were increased in striatum and brain stem, concentrations of 5-HT were unchanged in all brain regions. NE concentration increased in brain stem and hypothalamus but not striatum.

NE is taken up only in NE neurons. NE also can be taken up by dopamine-containing neurons. Use of inhibitors potentially has other pharmacological effects which may affect the rates of the depletion, or the rates of depletion itself may influence control processes abnormally. Problems with indirect turnover measures already have been discussed [52].

Second, measurement of a single neurotransmitter concentration does not provide much information on relationships between neurotransmitters. More sensitive methods such as high performance liquid

TABLE 2.2
Summary—Chronic Exercise and Changes in NE, 5-HT, and Metabolites

Study (Author, Subjects)	Exercise Protocol	Other Stressors	Method of Measurement	Brain Area	NE
Brown and Van Huss (1973) [27] 80, Male Sprague-Dawley ÷ Exercise and Control (6 conditions × 2 groups = 12)	Specially developed electronically controlled runner wheel	Shock	Fluorometric	Whole brain	Average concentration is higher in exercised groups, independent of brain weight.
Ostman and Nyback (1976) [174] 24, Male Sprague-Dawley rats ÷ into swimming and control	Swimming in 35°C ± 1° water 1 hr → 2.5 hr/day for 17 weeks	Injection 2 or 6 hours prior to decapitation	Radioactive labelling	Whole brain	26% higher in exercise than control. NE also higher.
Brown, Payne, Kim, Moore, Krebs, and Martin (1979) [28] 40 adult female rats ÷ Exercise (E) and Control (2 conditions × 2 groups F = high fat N = normal)	30 min/day, 1.5 feet/ second, 5 days/week	High fat diet	Fluorometric	Cerebral cortex, cerebellum, midbrain	NE in cerebral cortex higher among E-N vs. sedentary E-N and E-F higher in midbrain and whole brain but not from each other.
Hellhammer, Hingten, Wade, Shea, and Aprison (1983) [108] 20 male Wistar rats—3 groups Activity wheel, food limited (AWF) Activity wheel (AW), ad libatum Sedentary, food limited (SED)	Spontaneous	1 hr feeding period	HPLC-electrochemical detection	Pons-Medulla Midbrain Thalamus Posterior Hypothalamus Septum Striatum Hippocampus Cortex	
Rea and Hellhammer (1984) [189] (21 Wistar rats—3 groups Activity wheel, food limited (AWF) Sedentary, food limited (FC) Sedentary, unlimited food (UC))	Spontaneous	1 hr feeding period	HPLC-EC	Pons-Medulla Midbrain Thalamus Hypothalamus Septum Striatum Hippocampus Neocortex Cerebellum	NS FC ↑ UC NS AWF ↑ FC NS AWF ↑ UC AWF ↓ Controls NS NS
deCastro and Duncan (1985) [60] 18 male Long-Evans hooded rats—2 groups, AW vs. control (yoked, allowed to run but not reinforced)	Variable reinforcement food schedule for wheel running 5 days/week for 8 weeks	None	Radioenzymatic	½ of brain	NS

MHPG	5-HT	5-HIAA	Fitness	Conclusions
			Larger heart weight in trained rats	Increased NE in trained vs. sedentary may indicate a higher level of maintained sympathetic output.
				Exercise and/or shock did not significantly lower NE.
				LSD tests showed that exercise and/or shock can augment NE brain depletion in trained rats.
				Brain catecholamines are altered in a differential fashion depending on conditions imposed.
			Cardiac hypertrophy in exercised rats	Some adrenergic neurons in the brain react to chronic increases in their impulse flow by increasing their stores of transmitter, like noradrenergic neurons in heart and chromaffin cells of adrenal medulla.
				Chronically exercised animals display marked adaptive changes in the functioning of peripheral sympathetic neurons. Little if any sympathetic activity in the heart and spleen during rest.
				There is an inverse relationship between changes in activity in central compared with peripheral noradrenergic neurons as a result of adaptation to chronic exercise.
	Concentration in exercise fat higher sed. fat in cerebellum. E-F and E-N higher, lower respectively in cerebral cortex. In mid-E-N higher than both sedentary.		Not measured	Midbrain and whole brain levels of NE and 5-HT were highly related.
	AW ↑ Sed.	AW ↑ Sed.	Not measured	AWF ↓ 5-HT and 5-HIAA levels in midbrain, cortex, hippocampus and posterior hypothalamus. Decreases in both might reflect reduced metabolism. Might indicate a negative feedback mechanism regulated at post-synaptic receptor sites.
	AWF ↓ AW and Sed.	NS		
	NS	NS		
	AWF ↓ Sed.	AWF ↓ Sed.		
	AWF ↑ Sed.	NS		Pons/Medulla changes in the opposite direction. May indicate a general increase in 5-HT metabolism to stress.
	AWF ↓ AW and Sed.	NS		Contains vagal complex which contain parasympathetic preganglionic cells of vagus. Suggest 5-HT may influence cholinergic outflow of X cranial nerve.
	AW ↑ Sed. AWF ↓ Sed.	AWF ↓ Sed.		
	AWF ↓ AW	NS		
AWF ↑ Controls			Not measured	One possible explanation for 25% decrease of NE in hippocampus is that dorsal hippocampus projections become depleted with prolonged stress.
AWF ↑ Controls				
AWF ↑ Controls				
AWF ↑ Controls				
—				
NS				
NS				
AWF ↑ Controls				
AWF ↑ Controls				
			Not measured	Reason for no difference in NE may be that yoked animals were not sedentary. Reinforced group ran almost twice as much.

(continued)

TABLE 2.2 (*continued*)

Study (Author, Subjects)	Exercise Protocol	Other Stressors	Method of Measurement	Brain Area	NE
Elam, Svensson, and Thoren (1987) [73] 25, Male Wistar ÷ into spontaneous running and control groups (half of spontaneous group sacrificed immediately after exercise, others sacrificed 24 hours after)	Spontaneous running stabilized after 4 weeks at 5 km/12 hr Animals ran for 7 days after this period	Injection 30 minutes prior to decapitation	Chromatography-spectro-photo-fluorimetry	Limbic forebrain, corpus striatum, remaining hemispheric parts, brain stem, spinal cord	
Chaouloff, Laude, Serrurier, Merino, Guezennec, and Elghozi (1987) [47]	Treadmill 4 or 5 days adaptation 8 weeks, 5 days/week, 20 m/min or last week or 8-week period 20 m/min	Shock during adaptation	Liquid chromatography with amperometric and ultra-violet detection	Whole brain minus cerebellum	
Broocks, Liu, and Pirke (1990) [26] (168 male Wistar groups divided into 5 groups. Food deprived and nondeprived in running and sedentary groups)	Spontaneous running for 10 days	Food deprivation	HPLC-EC	Mediobasal hypothalami (MBH) preoptic areas (POA)	Increased in both running groups (i.e. food deprived vs. ac lib) in MBH. Increased in both running groups in POA

chromatography are now available which allow sensitive measurement of multiple neurotransmitters and metabolites within the same sample.

Third, most exercise studies have used other stressors in addition to exercise. Swim protocols can be confounded by fear and cold [103, 175]. Shock has commonly been used during treadmill exercise. It is possible that shock could differentially affect neurotransmitter systems. As deCastro and Duncan [60] point out, the use of shock may confound comparative animal models of neurobiology extended to exercise training programs with humans. The added stress of shock is not present in human exercise programs. Humans also are allowed to adjust the intensity and duration of exercise, which is not permitted by treadmill training protocols with animals.

Further, few studies have assessed fitness and the relationship between oxidative metabolism and fitness. This might be particularly important because oxygen is an important co-factor in the synthesis of both NE and 5-HT. At the present time, it is not known whether cardiorespiratory fitness induced by training or physical activity is necessary for changes in neurotransmitters to occur.

Fourth, these studies have not assessed the same brain regions. In

MHPG	5-HT	5-HIAA	Fitness	Conclusions
	No differences between groups		Not measured	Immediately after heavy spontaneous exercise, DOPA accumulation was decreased in dopamine-brain rich regions, i.e., limbic forebrain and corpus striatum, indicating a decreased rate of synthesis.
				DOPA accumulation was increased in the noradrenaline predominated region of brain stem, indicating increased synthesis of noradrenaline.
				Alterations in monoamine metabolism were normalized in exercising animals analyzed 24 hours post-exercise.
	Unchanged in short-term trained rats	Increased in short-term trained	Soleus glycogen content decreased more in short-term than long-term after running.	In short-term trained rats, running increased 5-HT which remains stable under normal conditions.
	Decreased in long-term trained rats	Increased in long-term trained		In long-term trained rats, running decreased 5-HT content. This cannot be explained by synthesis because tryptophan and 5-HIAA are increased by long-term running. Running may have a disruptive effect on 5-HT storage, similar to reserpine.
Increased in both running groups in MBH. Increased in food deprived in POA and decreased in ad lib in POA.			Not measured	In starved and ad lib episodes, running activity corresponded with maximal MHPG concentration, indicating a causal role of activity on hypothalamic and preoptic NE turnover.
				Activity stress might alter transport kinetic at the blood-brain barrier, increasing precursor influx into the brain.

fact, some have commonly examined whole brain and others have examined brain areas which have not been linked to depression. As seen in Figures 2.1 and 2.2, the various neurotransmitters are differentially associated with specific brain regions. According to a number of studies [26, 44, 108, 189], turnover is likely to vary from one brain region to another. It is important to examine localized brain regions which are known to be associated with the specific behaviors of interest, e.g., NE and 5-HT in the pons-medulla for the study of depression.

Finally, the studies are not comparable because different rat strains and genders were studied. For example, Wistar rats have higher circulating levels of corticosterone than Sprague-Dawley rats [131]. Because of the reciprocal nature of glucocorticoids and catecholamines, one might expect varied responses and adaptations to stress in these species. Moreover, estrogen levels can differentially affect functioning of monoamine neurons [85].

As the studies in Tables 2.1 and 2.2 demonstrate, a number of questions are raised by past studies of monoamine levels following exercise. A second line of studies is needed to examine specific aspects of synthesis and metabolism of these neurotransmitters. For example,

Stone [222] found that running stress did not adversely alter storage of NE, and that NE depleted by running was probably derived from newly synthesized NE and not from reuptake mechanisms. This study was done by comparing running stress to rats injected with either reserpine or α-methyltyrosine, all of which were later injected with radioactively labelled NE and observed for accumulation. Chaouloff and colleagues [41, 44, 45] have reported a series of studies that examine the effects of running on the synthesis and metabolism of 5-HT in various brain regions. An inhibitor of aromatic amino acid decarboxylase was injected into a resting control group. The effects of a tryptophan (TRP) load were then compared in running and resting groups as measured by levels of TRP and 5-hydroxytryptophan (5-HTP). Tryptophan was increased equally in the hippocampus, midbrain, and striatum for the running group, but 5-HTP accumulation was increased in the midbrain, was unchanged in the striatum, and decreased in the hippocampus. A follow-up study examined the effects of a TRP load on 5-HT and 5-HIAA. Running differentially affected TRP utilization in the 5-HT pathway, with no change in the cell bodies (i.e., midbrain), and reduced turnover in the nerve terminals (i.e., hippocampus and striatum).

Other studies have begun to examine the interactions with other neurotransmitters [42, 46] on synthesis and metabolism during exercise. For example, injection of amphetamine and α-methyl-p-tyrosine has been found that catecholaminergic activity influences the availability of tryptophan during exercise [46].

Future studies also need to examine changes in receptor distribution because single neurotransmitters can have both inhibitory and excitatory effects. This can be done in animal models of exercise by labeling receptors with radioligands using autoradiography.

It is also important to find plausible biological hypotheses that explain why monoamine systems might be stimulated by exercise. A number of candidates exist but are essentially unstudied. First, there may be direct innervation between brain motor regions and limbic structures. Because the locus coeruleus innervates the cerebellum and the corpus striatum as well as the hippocampus, frontal cortex, and spine, neural effects are structurally possible. Acute swimming stress is associated with increased LC activity [246]. Other NE neurons in the brain stem project to the ventral tegmentum region, a major reward center. Because GABAergic, serotonergic, and endorphin receptors are located on the brain stem and may be responsive to exercise, there may be exercise effects on hedonic responses as well. It is also plausible that Type II, III, and IV sensory afferents from muscle could stimulate higher limbic centers through the thalamus. We have located no studies that bear directly on these speculations for exercise, but we believe they deserve further investigation.

Another plausible alternative [165] proposes that increases in the plasma ratios of tryptophan to branched-chain amino acids could promote brain entry of tryptophan and subsequently increase 5-HT synthesis and storage. Increased use of branched-chain amino acids by muscle during prolonged exercise could also decrease their plasma levels and increase tryptophan ratios. Finally, increased free fatty acid with prolonged exercise could increase the concentration of free tryptophan which appears to limit the rate of tryptophan uptake in the brain [24]. Human [23] and rat [43] studies are consistent with this hypothesis and justify its consideration for exercise studies of depression that address the monoamine hypotheses.

EXERCISE STUDIES RELEVANT FOR THE HPA AXIS IN DEPRESSION

In humans, postexercise changes in the regulation of the HPA system and its interaction with the sympathetic nervous system have not been studied by methods directly relevant for understanding their effects on depression. Acute effects at the HPA axis during exercise regulate cardiovascular, thermoregulatory, fluid, electrolyte, and fuel needs of increased metabolism [87]. Aside from increases in NE and epinephrine that can range from eight- to twelvefold for intense, prolonged exercise [87], several hormonal changes accompany exercise that may bear on HPA disruption in depression. Prolactin and growth hormone can increase two- to threefold during acute exercise, whereas increases in ACTH, cortisol, and β-endorphin are similar in rate and magnitude during prolonged exercise at intensities approximating 80% $\dot{V}o_2$ peak [227]. Some evidence from naltrexone blockade [78, 79] suggests that endogenous opioid peptides, including perhaps β-endorphin, can inhibit secretion of growth hormone, cortisol, and catecholamines during acute exercise. Because all of these hormones have been implicated as potential secretagogues acting on the pituitary, hypothalamus, hippocampus, and locus coeruleus, research is needed to determine their patterns of release and action during exercise in relationship to patterns observed with other stressors studied in HPA models of depression.

Owing to past unavailability of assay techniques sensitive to the small resting levels found in plasma, the effects of chronic exercise on tonic levels of monoamines and HPA hormones are poorly understood. Changes in response to DEX and oCRF infusion may provide useful information regarding parallel regulatory responses of the HPA axis that occur with depression and with exercise. A recent study [139] reported a decreased resting ACTH and cortisol response to oCRH among highly trained runners compared with sedentary and moderately trained runners. This response was interpreted as consistent with sustained hypercortisolism in the highly trained group, despite comparable increases in ACTH and cortisol during exercise that were proportional to relative exercise intensity for all groups. The cross-sectional design of this study precludes inferences about training status over other intrinsic HPA differences related to higher centers. Another recent cross-sectional comparison between highly trained endurance athletes and sedentary individuals showed no differences in plasma catecholamine responses to non-exertional stressors including a reaction-time shock avoidance task and the cold pressor test [51]. Because a prior meta-analysis [55] concluded that an association exists between various estimates of aerobic fitness and neuroendocrine and sympathetic nervous system responses to nonexertional stressors, well-controlled prospective studies of HPA adaptations to nonexertional stress following acute and chronic exercise training are needed. This need is further evidenced by reports of lower plasma cortisol, ACTH, growth hormone, and prolactin response to insulin-induced hypoglycemia. These responses returned to normal after a four-week rest [17]. Elevated salivary cortisol concomitant with elevated total mood disturbance has also been found following overtraining in endurance athletes [171].

Related to the HPA axis hypercortisolism in Major Depression is the disruption of circadian rhythms. Perturbation of these rhythms is seen in the pattern of cortisol secretion in depression as well as in abnormalities of sleep. For example, a shortened rapid eye movement (REM) latency, the period between sleep onset and the first period of dreaming, is consistently seen in Major Depression. Other sleep abnormalities also have been noted in depression, such as an absence of slow-wave sleep (SWS) (stages 3 and 4) and an increased number of spontaneous awakenings [193].

Quasi-experimental studies of normal subjects have shown that acute exercise of submaximal and exhaustive intensities is followed by increased SWS during the evening of the exercise [67]. High intensity (50–70% $\dot{V}o_2$max) exercise to exhaustion leads to increased SWS early in the sleep period concomitant with a decrease in REM sleep [67]. Cross-sectional comparisons of fit and unfit subjects indicate that sleep differences are not dependent on daily exercise [67]. Although this implies that a training effect is necessary for sleep effects, selection bias is an equally compelling explanation, and convincing prospective studies of initially low fit persons have not been reported. Regional changes in brain blood flow and thermal effects have been proposed as plausible mechanisms for promoting sleep because of their established association with altered activity in both noradrenergic and serotonergic activity under resting conditions in rats. Porcine data indicate that during acute exercise only blood flow to the cerebellum is increased following acute exercise [167]. In humans, body temperature during exercise has been linked with changes in SWS in highly fit females who were normal sleepers [113], but we have not located prospective evidence that sleep is altered among patients with sleep disorders. No studies have been conducted with depressed patients to see if exercise might cause REM latency to lengthen or whether SWS might increase in depressed patients.

NEW DIRECTIONS FOR ANIMAL MODELS OF EXERCISE AND DEPRESSION

It is our view that an understanding of the relationship between exercise and depression can be advanced by the prudent, careful use of animal models. We next integrate selected interpretations of the rat literature on the neurobiology of depression that appear most consistent with plausible mechanisms by which exercise might exert antidepressant effects. Two issues are addressed: (1) the similarity between the monoamine and HPA axis disruption found in depression and in anxiety and the clinical importance of this similarity for exercise studies, and (2) the limitations of monoamine and HPA models of depression for fully explaining the anhedonia that is uniquely characteristic of Major Depression.

Depression and Anxiety

Recent human evidence supports that the anxiety accompanying Major Depression is a principal clinical feature linked with HPA axis disruption measured by a dexamethasone suppression test (DST) [150]. This clinical finding is consistent with animal research using behavioral deficit models for depression such as learned helplessness to uncontrollable shock, the Porsolt swim test, or open-field behavior [244]. Weiss and colleagues [243] have proposed that deficits in motivated behavior are the result of depleted NE in the LC, so that the normal inhibition of LC by its α-2 autoreceptors for NE is removed, leading to augmented release of NE from LC neurons projecting to other receptor fields in the limbic system and the spine. This view is in contrast to the serotonin hypothesis that behavioral deficits are due to a decreased release of 5-HT [80]. However, Weiss and Simson [244] argue that the release of NE decreases 5-HT release. Alpha-2 agonists, clonidine, and NE decrease LC activity concomitant with increases in swimming and open-field ambulation, whereas the α-2 antagonist yohimbine increases LC activity concomitant with behavioral deficit. Similarly, stimulation of α-1 receptors by phenylephrine and β receptors by isoproterenol has led to a behavioral deficit when infused proximal to the lateral ventricle, but it has led to increased activity when infused in the region of the brain stem or spine. This specificity of response is particularly relevant for exercise studies because of the likelihood of afferent stimulation of the spine and thalamus from Type II, III, and IV sensory nerves.

It is believed that the LC fires in pulsatile bursts, followed by a period of autoinhibition, and that α-2 autoinhibition modulates the response of LC neurons to excitatory stimuli. In addition to α-2 autoreceptor-mediated inhibition, it has been proposed that membrane changes in ion conductance lead to hyperpolarization of LC neurons because of a calcium-dependent influx of potassium [7]. Because evidence for other ion conductance models for depression have some clinical support [3, 111, 252], exercise studies of LC activity should consider mechanisms complementary to α-2 autoreceptors.

Gray [100] has argued that the LC-NE depletion model of Weiss and colleagues [244] conceptualizes the role of the dorsal ascending nor-adrenergic bundle for the regulation of depression in a way similar to its established role in inhibiting behavior under conditions of threat that is characteristic of anxiety. In this way, Gray argues that the prevailing animal models of anxiety and neurotic depression share similar neurobiological pathways consistent with their shared clinical symptoms of agitation, hypervigilance, decreased motor activity under threat, and HPA axis disruption. For this reason, exercise studies using an animal model of depression must employ behavioral or pharmacological methods to assess both anxiolytic and antidepressant components of exercise effects.

A further parallel comes from the paradoxical phenomenon of "toughening up", in which chronic exposure (approximating two weeks) to the same uncontrollable stress that leads to a behavioral deficit (lasting 24 to 72 hours) under acute exposure eliminates the behavioral deficit [243]. The simple interpretation of this paradox is depletion or insufficient release of NE from LC following acute uncontrollable stress but increased synthesis of NE as an adaptive accommodation to chronic exposure [100]. The similarity between the concept of "toughening up" with chronic monoamine or HPA adaptations to graduated exercise conditioning is appealing and deserves direct study. It is plausible that acute episodes of both controllable and uncontrollable exercise stress could lead to increased metabolism and synthesis of monoamines as well as an inoculation against central depletion or motivational deficits, or both, following acute uncontrollable stress.

Anhedonia

The effects of uncontrollable shock in the rat correspond directly with all DSM-III-R symptoms required for the diagnosis of Major Depression in humans, except self-reports of hopelessness, worthlessness, and recurrent thoughts of suicide or death [244]. For this reason, it is important that exercise studies of depression using a behavioral deficit model also address other models that may better explain the dysphoric mood which is the defining characteristic unique to human depression.

We believe the most compelling case for an animal model complementary to the uncontrollable stress model is offered by anhedonia [127]. Major Depressive Episode is distinguished by dysphoric mood and the loss of interest or pleasure in all or almost all usual activities. Melancholia places even more emphasis on loss of pleasure in activities and the absence of reactivity to usually pleasurable events [127]. Anhedonia in the rat is typically modeled after intracranial electrical self-stimulation (ICSS), by which animals are operantly conditioned for reward-motivated behavior using ICSS as the reinforcer. The brain region associated with the highest rates of responding for the lowest stimulus are in the mid-brain hypothalamic region circumscribing the medial forebrain bundle and the ventral tegmentum. A lower response slope for ICSS also can be found in the area of the LC and its dorsal projection to the forebrain and in major dopamine projections of the mesolimbic and nigrostriatal systems. Although NE has been implicated in ICSS owing to LC responses, most evidence favors dopamine as the main neurotransmitter. Specific dopamine receptor blockers attenuate ICSS at low doses, whereas typically therapeutic doses of NE reuptake blockers like imipramine do not alter ICSS. Stimulation of raphe nuclei appears to support ICSS; inhibition of tryptophan hydroxylase attenuates it. More evidence implicates cholinergic effects on ICSS. Hypothalamic ICSS is reduced by central but not peripheral cholinesterase inhibition. Furthermore, evidence supports a muscarinic inhibition but nicotinic facilitation of ICSS [127].

Recent study has shown that inescapable shock in mice leads to reduced ICSS in the nucleus accumbens, medial forebrain bundle, and ventral tegmentum, but not the substantia nigra [254]; chronic administration of desmethylimipramine (10 days) mitigates the ICSS reduction. Because ICSS can condition increased running behavior in rats [30], it will be important to determine if acute or chronic exercise can support or influence ICSS in a behavioral deficit model of animal depression.

QUESTIONS AND RECOMMENDATIONS

To address current controversy over the existence of an antidepressant effect with exercise, we examined available evidence from the perspective of biological plausibility. We restricted our view to programmatic exercise and Major Depression including Melancholia. We briefly summarized the epidemiology of depression and the prominent neurobiological models that characterize Major Depression. Because depression has been linked to chronic stress through dysregulation of brain monoamines and the HPA axis, exercise could play a role in the prevention and treatment of depression by promoting regulatory adaptation of brain monoamines and HPA systems.

We conclude that the efficacy of exercise in the treatment or prevention of depression cannot be determined from the available data and the prevailing research strategies used in exercise studies. Important clinical questions relevant to the neurobiological plausibility of exercise remain. These include the antidepressant effects of single exercise sessions compared to long-term exercise programs and the comparability of exercise responses with effective antidepressant drugs. Additional issues include the effects of aerobic versus anaerobic exercise, the existence or importance of a dose-response relationship between increased exercise or fitness and decreased depression, the independence of exercise effects compared to minimally effective interventions, the role of anxiolytic responses to exercise in the antidepressant effect, gender differences, and what monoamine or HPA mechanisms in depression might be responsive to various types and amounts of exercise.

Exercise studies of monoaminergic brain activity in humans have relied on peripheral metabolites as CNS estimates. No clear conclusion can be drawn from these studies. Although urinary or plasma changes in MHPG following exercise deserve continued study using repeated measures designs with depressed patients, investigators using the sulfated subfraction of MHPG as an indicator of CNS activity must consider that MHPG can be sulfoconjugated in plasma during exercise. More studies are needed to determine the origin of increased central and peripheral sulfated MHPG with physical activity.

Receptorology presents a necessary approach for future studies of the effects of exercise in depressed patients. We did not locate studies examining changes in monoaminergic receptors in depressed patients following exercise, but exercise studies inferring central changes from peripheral measures will encounter method problems similar to those described for peripheral metabolites as estimates of brain monoamine activity. The use of PET or other dynamic imaging technology for measuring receptor changes, regional brain blood flow, and glucose uptake will help resolve the measurement uncertainty of the available literature.

Effects of exercise on HPA axis in depressed patients can be assessed by neuroendocrine challenge tests. Changes in markers of circadian and ultradian rhythms with exercise should also be studied. Changes in the daily pattern of resting cortisol represent one approach. Studies that examine sleep architecture after acute or chronic exercise in depressed patients represent another approach.

We also recommend that comparative studies be conducted with a variety of animal models of depression, although limitations of animal models must be recognized. Animal models cannot totally replicate depression; instead they are most appropriately used to examine its specific aspects. They can control depression-inducing conditions in specific ways or to isolate specific behavior patterns linked with depression [128]. For example, rats exposed to clomipramine (CLI) neonatally exhibit many of the same symptoms as seen with endogenous depression, e.g. decreased sexual, aggressive, and intracranial self-stimulation activities as well as REM sleep abnormalities [237]. Primate and rodent separation models, in which either mothers and infants or peers are isolated from one another also lead to abnormalities in eating, drinking, activity, and sleep seen in human depression [128]. Thus, developmental models may use social or pharmacological interventions to induce depression, and the putative role of exercise may differ for these models despite common signs and symptoms that result from each induction approach.

Another purpose of animal models is to evaluate treatments and mechanisms underlying treatment. Exercise researchers should therefore adopt a model most suited to questions asked. Learned helplessness, defined as an inability to learn subsequent escape procedures, is induced by exposing an animal to an uncontrollable stress. This helplessness is accompanied by changes in neurotransmitters such as NE, DA, and ACh and is reversed by antidepressant drugs.

The use of uncontrollable stress would be unsuitable for studying the effects of chronic exercise on symptoms of depression in rats, because most of the depressive symptoms induced (e.g., decreased food and water intake, sleep reduction with early morning awakening) last only 48 to 72 hours. A better model for the study of chronic exercise might include developmental models such as CLI in which symptoms are longer lasting. Uncontrollable stress models, however, do appear suited for addressing the prevention of depression with chronic exercise. For this purpose, animals first would be chronically conditioned with exercise to determine if increased exercise or fitness exerts a protective effect.

Many human and animal studies are needed to confirm and explain an antidepressant effect with exercise. Clinical and descriptive epidemiological studies can address the population effectiveness of exercise. Moreover, social and cognitive-behavioral models of depression present alternatives to those we have discussed. We have attempted in this review to integrate the exercise and depression literatures in a way that will lead to biologically plausible hypotheses about why exercise may help prevent and treat Major Depression. We have limited this review to the most widely recognized neurobiological theories of depression. Other neurobiological models of depression, including sodium-potassium transport mechanisms [111], should be considered for exercise studies. Understanding the role that exercise may play in reregulating monoaminergic and HPA mechanisms is indicated, however, by the growing evidence that dysregulation of these systems contributes in a causal manner to Major Depression and by the plausibility that exercise could induce adaptations in these systems in ways that may help prevent or treat depression.

ACKNOWLEDGMENTS

Thanks go to Donna Smith and Melinda Brewer for their help in preparing this manuscript.

REFERENCES

1. Abe, K., and T. Hiroshige. Changes in plasma corticosterone and hypothalamic CRF levels following intraventricular injection drug induced changes of brain biogenic amines in the rat. *Neuroendocrinology*, 14:195–211, 1974.
2. Akil, H., H. Shiomi, and J. Matthews. Induction of the intermediate pituitary by stress: synthesis and release of a nonopioid form of beta-endorphin. *Science* 227:424–427, 1985.
3. Akiskal, H.S., and W.T. McKinney, Jr. Overview of recent research in depression. Integration of ten conceptual models into a comprehensive clinical frame. *Arch. Gen. Psychiatry* 32:285–305, 1975.
4. American College of Sports Medicine. Position statement on the recommended quantity and quality of exercise for developing and maintaining fitness in health adults. *Med. Sci. Sports Exerc.* 22:3, 1990.
5. American Psychiatric Association. *Diagnostic and Statistical Manual of Mental Disorders (3rd ed. rev.) (DSM-III-R)*. Washington, D.C.: American Psychiatric Association, 1987.
6. American Psychological Association. *Developing a National Agenda to Address Women's Mental Health Needs*. Washington, D.C.: American Psychological Association, 1985.
7. Andrade, R., and G.K. Aghajanian. Locus coeruleus activity in vitro: intrinsic regulation by a calcium-dependent potassium conductance but not alpha-2 adrenoreceptors. *J. Neurosc.* 4:161–170, 1984.
8. Antoni, F.A. Hypothalamic control of adrenocorticotropin secretion: advances since the discovery of 41-residue corticotropin releasing factor. *Endocrine Rev.* 7:351–378, 1986.
9. Asnis, G.M., U. Halbreich, E.J. Sachar, et al. The relationship of dexamethasone (2 mg) and plasma cortisol secretion in depressive illness: clinical and neuroendocrine parameters. *Psychopharm. Bull.* 18:122–126, 1982.
10. Axelrod, J., and T.D. Resine. Stress hormones: their interaction and regulation. *Science* 224:452–459, 1984.
11. Bahrke, M.S., and W.P. Morgan. Anxiety reduction following exercise and meditation. *Cognit. Ther. Res.* 2:323–333, 1978.
12. Baldessarini, R.J. Current status of antidepressants: clinical pharmacology and therapy. *J. Clin. Psychiatry* 50:117–126, 1989.
13. Baldessarini, R.J. Drugs and the treatment of psychiatric disorders. A.G. Goodman, L.S. Goodman, T.W. Rall, F. Murad (eds.). *Goodman and Gilman's The Pharmacological Basis of Therapeutics* (7th ed.). New York: Macmillan Publishing Company, 1985, pp. 387–445.
14. Barchas, J.D., and D.X. Friedman. Brain amines: responses to physiological stress. *Biochem. Pharmacol.* 12:1232–1235, 1962.
15. Baron, M., N. Risch, R. Hamburger, et al. Genetic linkage between X-chromosome markers and bipolar affective illness. *Nature* 326:289–292, 1987.
16. Barron, J.L., T.D. Noakes, W. Levy, C. Smith, and R.P. Millar. Hypothalamic dysfunction in overtrained athletes. *J. Clin. Endocrinol. and Metab.* 60:803–806, 1985.
17. Beck, A.T., A.J. Rush, B.F. Shaw, and G. Emery. *Cognitive Therapy of Depression*. New York: Guilford Press, 1979.
18. Beckmann, H., and F.K. Goodwin. Urinary MHPG in subgroups of depressed patients and normal controls. *Neuropsychobiology* 6:91–100, 1980.

19. Beckmann, H., M.H. Ebert, R.M. Post, et al. Effect of moderate exercise on urinary MHPG in depressed patients. *Pharmacopsychiatria* 12:351–356, 1979.

20. Berrettini, W.H., L.R. Goldin, J. Gelernter, P.V. Gejman, E.S. Gershon, and S. Detera-Wadleigh. X-chromosome markers and manic-depressive illness: rejection of linkage to Xq28 in nine bipolar pedigrees. *Arch. Gen. Psychiatry* 47:336–373, 1990.

21. Björklund, A., A. Nobin, and U. Stenevi. The use of neurotoxic dihydroxytryptamine on nerve terminal serotonin and serotonin uptake in the rat brain. *Brain Res.* 50:214–220, 1973.

22. Blomberry, P.A., I.J. Kopin, E.K. Gordon, S.P. Markey, and M.H. Ebert. Conversion of MHPG to vanillylmandelic acid. *Arch. Gen. Psychiatry* 37:1095–1098, 1980.

23. Blomstrand, E., F. Celsing, and E.A. Newsholme. Changes in plasma concentrations of aromatic and branched chain amino acids during sustained exercise in man and their possible role in fatigue. *Acta Physiol. Scand.* 133:115–121, 1988.

24. Bloxham, P.L., M.D. Tricklebank, A.J. Patel, and G. Curzon. Effects of albumin, amino acids and clofibrate on the uptake of tryptophan by the rat brain. *J. Neurochem.* 34:43–49, 1980.

25. Breese, G.R. Chemical and immunochemical lesions by specific neurotoxic substances and antisera. L.L. Iverson, S.D. Iverson, and S.H. Snyder (eds.). *Handbook of Psychopharmacology: Volume 1 Biochemical Principles and Techniques in Neuropharmacology.* New York: Plenum Press, 1975, pp. 137–189.

26. Broocks, A., J. Liu, and K.M. Pirke. Semistarvation-induced hyperactivity compensates for decreased norepinephrine and dopamine turnover in the mediobasal hypothalamus of the rat. *J. Neural Transm.* 79:113–124, 1990.

27. Brown, B.S., and W. Van Huss. Exercise and rat brain catecholamines. *J. Appl. Physiol.* 34:664–669, 1973.

28. Brown, B.S., T. Payne, C. Kim, G. Moore, P. Krebs, and W. Martin. Chronic response to rat brain norepinephrine and serotonin levels to endurance training. *J. Appl. Physiol.* 34:664–669, 1973.

29. Bunney, W.E., Jr., and J.M. Davis. Norepinephrine in depressive reactions: a review. *Arch. Gen. Psychiatry* 13:483–494, 1965.

30. Burgess, M.L., J.M. Davis, and J. Buggy. Physiological responses to exercise for brain reward versus electric shock in rats. *Med. Sci. Sports Ex.* 22:S31, 1990.

31. Burton, R. *The Anatomy of Melancholy.* Oxford: Printed by Ion Lichfield for Henry Cripps, 1632.

32. Butler, J., M. O'Brien, K. O'Malley, and J.G. Kelly. Relationship of B-adrenoceptor density to fitness in athletes. *Nature* 298:60–62, 1982.

33. Calogero, A.E., W.T. Gallucci, G.P. Chrousos, and P.W. Gold. Catecholamine effects upon rat hypothalamic corticotropin releasing hormone secretion in vitro. *J. Clin. Invest.* 82:839–846, 1988.

34. Calogero, A.E., W.T. Gallucci, R. Bernardini, C. Saoutis, P.W. Gold, and G.P. Chrousos. Effect of cholinergic agonists and antagonists on rat hypothalamic corticotropin releasing hormone secretion in vitro. *Neuroendocrinology* 47:303–308, 1988.

35. Calogero, A.E., W.T. Gallucci, G.P. Chrousos, and P.W. Gold. Multiple feedback regulatory loops upon rat hypothalamic corticotropin releasing hormone secretion. *J. Clin. Invest.* 82:767–777, 1988.

36. Campbell, D.D., and J.E. Davis. Report of research and experimentation in exercise and recreational therapy. *Am. J. Psychiatry* 96:915–933, 1939–1940.

37. Carpenter, W.T., and W.E. Bunney. Adrenal cortical activity in depressive illness. *Am. J. Psychiatry* 128:65–71, 1971.

38. Carroll, B.J., and J. Mendels. Neuroendocrine regulation in affective disorders. E.J. Sachar (ed.). *Hormones Behavior and Psychopathology.* New York: Raven Press, 1976, pp. 193–224.

39. Caspersen, C.J., K.E. Powell, and G.M. Christenson. Physical activity, exercise, and

physical fitness: definitions and distinctions for health-related research. *Pub. Health Rep.* 100:126–130, 1985.

40. Chodakowsa, J., B. Wocial, B. Skorka, K. Nazar, and J. Chwalbinska-Moneta. Plasma and urinary catecholamines and metabolites during physical exercise in essential hypertension. *Acta Physiol. Pol.* 31:623–630, 1980.

41. Chaouloff, F. Physical exercise and brain monoamines: a review. *Acta Physiol. Scand.* 137:1–13, 1989.

42. Chaouloff, F., J. Danguir, and J.L. Elghozi. Dextrafenfluramine, but not 8-OH-DPAT affects the decrease in food consumed by rats submitted to physical exercise. *Pharmacol. Biochem. Behav.* 32:573–576, 1989.

43. Chaouloff, F., G.A. Kennett, B. Serrurrier, D. Merino, and G. Curzon. Amino acid analysis demonstrates that increased plasma free tryptophan causes the increase of brain tryptophan during exercise in the rat. *J. Neurochem.* 46:1647–1650, 1986.

44. Chaouloff, F., D. Laude, and J.L. Elghozi. Physical exercise: evidence for differential consequences of tryptophan on 5-HT synthesis and metabolism in central serotonergic cell bodies and terminals. *J. Neural Transm.* 78:121–130, 1989.

45. Chaouloff, F., D. Laude, Y. Guezennec, and J.L. Elghozi. Motor activity increases tryptophan, 5-hydroxyindoleacetic acid, and homovanillic acid in ventricular cerebrospinal fluid of the conscious rat. *J. Neurochem.* 46:1313–1316, 1986.

46. Chaouloff, F., D. Laude, D. Merino, B. Surrurrier, Y. Guesennec, and J.L. Elghozi. Amphetamine and α-methyl-*p*-tyrosine affect the exercise-induced imbalance between the availability of tryptophan and synthesis of serotonin in the brain of the rat. Neuropharmacology 26:1099–1106, 1987.

47. Chaouloff, F., D. Laude, B. Serrurrier, D. Merino, Y. Guezennec, and J. Elghozi. Brain serotonin response to exercise in the rat: the influence of training duration. *Biogenic Amines* 4:99–106, 1987.

48. Chaouloff, R., J.L. Elghozi, Y. Guezenncec, and D. Laude. Effects of conditioned running on plasma, liver and brain tryptophan and on brain 5-hydroxytryptamine metabolism of the rat. *Br. J. Pharmacol.* 86:33–41, 1985.

49. Christensen, L., C.B. Kristensen, L.F. Gram, P. Christensen, D.L. Pedersen, and P.K. Sorensen. Afternoon plasma cortisol in depressed patients: a measure of diagnosis or severity. *Life Sci.* 32:617–623, 1983.

50. Cicardo, V.H., S.E. Carbone, D.C. De Rondina, and I.O. Mastronardi. Stress by forced swimming in the rat. Effects of misanserin and moclobemide on GABAergic and monoaminergic systems in the brain. *Comp. Biochem. Physiol.* 83:133–135, 1986.

51. Claytor, R.P., R.H. Cox, E.T. Howley, K.A. Lawler, and J.E. Lawler. Aerobic power and cardiovascular response to stress. *J. Appl. Physiol.* 65:1416–1423, 1988.

52. Cooper, J.R., F.E. Bloom, and R.H. Roth. *The Biochemical Basis of Neuropharmacology (5th ed.)* New York: Oxford University Press, 1986.

53. Coppen, A. Depressed states and indolealkylamines. *Advances in Pharmacology Volume 6.* New York: Academic Press, 1968, pp. 283–291.

54. Coyle, J.T. Neuroscience and psychiatry. J.A. Talbott, R.E. Hales, S.C. Yudofsky (eds.). *The American Psychiatric Press Textbook of Psychiatry.* Washington, D.C.: The American Psychiatric Press, Inc., 1988, pp. 3–31.

55. Crews, D.J., and D.M. Landers. A meta-analytic review of aerobic fitness and reactivity to psychosocial stressors. *Med. Sci. Sports Exerc.* 19(suppl):S114–S120, 1987.

56. Dallman, M.F., and M.T. Jones. Corticosteroid feedback control of ACTH secretion: effect of stress-induced corticosterone secretion on a subsequent stress response in the rat. *Endocrinology* 92:1367–1375, 1973.

57. Dallman, J.F., and F.E. Yates. Dynamic asymmetries in the corticosteroid feedback pathway and distribution binding and metabolism elements of the adrenocortical system. *Ann. N.Y. Acad. Sci.* 156:696–721, 1969.

58. Daniels, M.L., L.S. Linn, N. Ward, and B. Leake. A study of physician preferences

in the management of depression in the general medical setting. *Gen. Hosp. Psychiatry* 8:229–235, 1986.

59. Davis, J.M., S.H. Koslow, R.D. Gibbons, et al. Cerebrospinal fluid and urinary biogenic amines in depressed patients and health controls. *Arch. Gen. Psychiatry* 45:705–717, 1988.

60. deCastro, J.M., and G. Duncan. Operantly conditioned running effects on brain catecholamine concentrations and receptor densities in the rat. *Pharmacol. Biochem. and Behav.* 23:495–500, 1985.

61. DeLeon-Jones, F., J.W. Maas, H. Dekirmenjian, and J. Sanchez. Diagnostic subgroups of affective disorders and their urinary excretion of catecholamine metabolites. *Am. J. Psychiatry* 132:1141–1148, 1975.

62. DePocas, F., and W.A. Behrens. Effects of handling, decapitation, anesthesia, and surgery on plasma noradrenaline levels in the white rat. *Can. J. Physiol. Pharmacol.* 55:212–219, 1977.

63. DeSouza, E., and G. Van Loon. D-Ala-2-met-enkephalinamide, a potent opioid peptide, alters pituitary-adrenocortical secretion in rats. *Endocrinology* 111:1483–1490, 1982.

64. DeSouza, E., and G. Van Loon. Stress-induced inhibition of the plasma corticosterone response to a subsequent stress in rats: a noradrenocorticotropin mediated mechanism. *Endocrinology* 110:23–33, 1982.

65. Detera-Wadleigh, S.D., W.H. Berretini, L.R. Goldin, D. Boorman, S. Anderson, and E.S. Gershon. Close linkage of c-Harvey-ras-1 and the insulin gene to affective disorder is ruled out in three North American pedigress. *Nature* 325:806–808, 1987.

66. Dishman, R.K. Medical psychology in exercise and sport. *Med. Clin. N. Am.* 69:123–143, 1985.

67. Dishman, R.K. Mental health. V. Seefeldt (ed.). *Physical Activity and Well Being*, Reston, VA: American Alliance for Health, Physical Education, Recreation and Dance, 1986, pp. 303–341.

68. Dunn, J., and S. Orr. Differential plasma corticosterone responses to hippocampal stimulation. *Exp. Brain Res.* 54:1–9, 1984.

69. Dush, D.M. The placebo in psychosocial outcome evaluations. *Evaluation and the Health Professions* 9:421–438, 1986.

70. Ebert, M.H., R.M. Post, and F.K. Goodwin. Effects of physical activity on urinary MHPG excretion in normal subjects. *Lancet* 11:766, 1972.

71. Egeland, J.A., D.S. Gerhard, D.L. Pauls, et al. Bipolar affective disorders linked to DNA markers on chromosome 11. *Nature* 325:783–787, 1987.

72. Elam, M., T.H. Svensson, and P. Thoren. Brain monoamine metabolism is altered in rats following spontaneous, long-distance running. *Acta Physiol. Scand.* 130:313–316, 1987.

73. Elam, M., H.S. Torngy, and P. Thoren. Differentiated cardiovascular afferent regulation of locus coeruleus neurons and sympathetic nerves. *Brain Res.* 358:77–84, 1985.

74. Essen-Moller, E., and O. Hagnell. The frequency and risk of depression within a rural population group in Scandia. *Acta Psychiat. Scand.* 162:81–90, 1961.

75. Everett, G.M., and J.E.P. Toman. Mode of action of Rauwolfia alkaloids and motor activity. J.H. Masserman (ed.). *Biological Psychiatry*. New York: Grune & Stratton, 1959, pp. 75–81.

76. Eysenck, H.J., J.A. Wakefield, and A.F. Friedman. Diagnosis and clinical assessment: The DSM-III. *Ann. Rev. Psychol.* 34:167–193, 1983.

77. Farmer, M.E., B.Z. Locke, E.K. Moscicki, A.L. Dannenberg, D.B. Larson, and L.S. Radloff. Physical activity and depressive symptoms: the Njanes I epidemiologic follow-up study. *Am. J. Epidem.* 128:1340–1351, 1988.

78. Farrell, P.A., A.B. Gustafson, T.L. Garthewaite, R.K. Kalkhoff, A.W. Cowley, and

W.P. Morgan. Influence of endogenous opioids on the response of selected hormones to exercise in man. *J. Appl. Physiol.* 61:1051–1057, 1987.

79. Farrell, P.A., A.B. Gustafson, W.P. Morgan, and C.B. Pert. Enkephalins, catecholamines, and psychological mood alterations: effects of prolonged exercise. *Med. Sci. Sports Exer.* 19:347–353, 1987.

80. Fehm, H.L., K.H. Voigt, R. Lang, K.E. Beinert, K.E. Kummer, and E.F. Pfeiffer. Paradoxical ACTH response to glucocorticoids in Cushing's disease. *N. Engl. J. Med.* 297:904–907, 1977.

81. Felten, D.L., and J.R. Sladek, Jr. Monoamine distribution in primate brain. V. Monoaminergic nuclei: anatomy, pathways and local organization. *Brain Res. Bull* 10:171–284, 1983.

82. Filser, J.G., J. Spira, M. Fischer, et al. The evaluation of 4-hydroxy-3-methoxyphenylglycol sulfate as a possible marker of central norepinephrine turnover: Studies in health volunteers and depressed patients. *J. Psychiat. Res.* 22:171–181, 1988.

83. Folkins, C.H., and W.E. Sime. Physical fitness training and mental health. *Am. Psychol.* 36:373–389, 1981.

84. Fuxe, K., and G. Jonsson. Further mapping of central 5-hydroxytryptamine neurons: studies with neurotoxic dihydroxytryptamines. E. Costa, G.L. Gessa, M. Sandler (eds.). *Advances in Biochemical Psychopharmacology, Volume 10.* New York: Raven Press, 1974, pp. 1–12.

85. Fuxe, K., A. Cintra, L.F. Agnati, et al. Studies on the cellular localization and distribution of glucocorticoid receptor and estrogen receptor immunoreactivity in the central nervous system of the rat and their relationship to the monoaminergic and peptidergic neurons of the brain. *J. Steroid Biochem.* 27:159–170, 1987.

86. Fuxe, K., T. Hokfelt, K. Andersson, et al. The transmitters of the hypothalamus. B. Cox, I.D. Morris, and A.H. Weston (eds.). *Pharmacology of the Hypothalamus.* Baltimore: University Park Press, 1978, pp. 63–104.

87. Galbo, H., M. Kjaer, M. Mikines, et al. Discussion: hormonal adaptation to physical activity. C. Bouchard, R.J. Shephard, T. Stephens, J.R. Sutton, and B.D. McPherson (eds.). *Exercise, Fitness and Health: A Consensus of Current Knowledge.* Champaign, IL: Human Kinetics Publishers, 1990, pp. 259–263.

88. Gaillard, J.M. Involvement of noradrenaline in wakefulness and paradoxical sleep. A. Wauguier, J.M. Gaillard, J.M. Monti, and M. Radulovacki (eds.). *Sleep Neurotransmitters and Neuromodulators.* New York: Raven Press, 1985, pp. 57–68.

89. Gallagher, T.F., K. Yoshida, H.D. Roffwarg, D.K. Fukushima, E.D. Weitzman, and L. Hellman. ACTH and cortisol secretory patterns in man. *J. Clin. Endocrinology Metab.* 36:1058–1073, 1973.

90. Gerner, R.H., and H.E. Gwirtsman. Abnormalities of dexamethasone suppression test and urinary MHPG in anorexia nervosa. *Am. J. Psychiatry* 138:650–653, 1981.

91. Gerner, R.H., R.M. Post, and W.E. Bunney, Jr. A dopaminergic mechanism in mania. *Am. J. Psychiatry* 133:1177–1180, 1976.

92. Gold, P.W. Stress-responsive neuromodulators. *Biol. Psychiatry* 24:371–374, 1988.

93. Gold, P.W., G. Chrousos, C. Kellner, et al. Psychiatric implications of basic and clinical studies with corticotropin-releasing factor. *Am. J. Psychiatry* 141:619–627, 1984.

94. Gold, P.W., F.K. Goodwin, and G.P. Chrousos. Clinical and biochemical manifestations of depression, relation to the neurobiology of stress (first of two parts). *N. Engl. J. Med.* 319:348–353, 1988.

95. Gold, P.W., F.K. Goodwin, and G.P. Chrousos. Clinical and biochemical manifestations of depression, related to the neurobiology of stress (second of two parts). *N. Engl. J. Med.* 319:413–420, 1988.

96. Gold, P.W., M.A. Kling, M.A. Demitrack, H. Whitfield, D.L. Loriaux, and G.P. Chrousos. Clinical studies with corticotropin releasing hormone. Implications for hypothalamic-pituitary-adrenal dysfunction in depression and related disorders. D.

Ganten and D. Pfaff (eds.). *Current Topics in Neuroendocrinology Volume 8.* Berlin: Springer-Verlag. 1988, pp. 55–77.

97. Gold, P.W., D.L. Loriaus, A. Roy, et al. Responses to corticotropin-releasing hormone in the hypercortisolism of depression and Cushing's disease: pathophysiologic and diagnostic implications. *N. Engl. J. Med.* 314:1329–1335, 1986.

98. Goode, D.J., H. Dekirmenjian, H.Y. Meltzer, and J.W. Maas. Relation of exercise to MHPG excretion in normal subjects. *Arch. Gen. Psychiatry* 29:391–396, 1973.

99. Gordon, R., S. Spector, A. Sjoerdsma, and S. Udenfriend. Increased synthesis of norepinephrine and epinephrine in the intact rat during exercise and exposure to cold. *J. Pharmacol. Exper. Ther.* 153:440–447, 1966.

100. Gray, J.A. Issues in the neuropsychology of anxiety. A.H. Tuma and J.D. Masser (eds.). *Anxiety and the Anxiety Disorders.* Hillsdale, N.J., Lawrence Erlbaum Associates, Inc., 1985, pp. 5–26.

101. Greist, J.H., M.H. Klein, and R.R. Eischens, J.W. Faris, A.S. Gurman, and W.P. Morgan. Running through your mind. *J. Psychosom. Res.*, 22:259, 1978.

102. Grossman, A.P., P. Bouloux, P. Price, et al. The role of opioid peptides in the hormonal responses to acute exercise in man. *Clin. Sci.* 67:483–491, 1984.

103. Haari, M., and P. Kuusela. Is swimming exercise or cold exposure for rats? *Acta Physiol. Scand.* 126:189–197, 1986.

104. Hagnell, O., J. Lanke, B. Rorsman, et al. Are we entering an age of melancholy? Depressive illness in a prospective epidemiological study over 25 years: the Lundby Study, Sweden. *Psychol. Med.* 12:279–289, 1982.

105. Halbreich, U., B. Zumoff, J. Kream, and D.K. Fukushima. The mean 1300–1600 h plasma cortisol concentrations as a diagnostic test for hypercortisolism. *J. Clin. Endocrinology Metab.* 54:1262–1264, 1982.

106. Harris, S.S., C.J. Caspersen, G.H. DeFriese, and E.H. Estes, Jr. Physical activity counseling for healthy adults as a primary preventive intervention in the clinical setting. *J.A.M.A.* 261:3590–3598, 1989.

107. Helgason, T. Frequency of depressive states within geographically delimited population groups: the frequency of depressive states in Iceland as compared with other Scandinavian countries. *Acta Psychiatr. Scand.* 162:81–90, 1961.

108. Hellhammer, D.H., J. Hingten, S.E. Wade, P. Shea, and M.A. Aprison. Serotonergic changes in specific areas of rat brain associated with activity stress gastric lesions. *Psychosom. Med.* 45:115–122, 1983.

109. Heyes, M.P., E.S. Garnett, G. Coates. Nigrostriatal dopaminergic activity is increased during exhaustive exercise stress in rats. *Life Sci.* 42:1537–1542, 1988.

110. Hirschfeld, R.M.A., and F.K. Goodwin. Mood disorders. J.A. Talbott, R.E. Hales, S.C. Yodofsky, (eds.). *The American Psychiatric Press Textbook of Psychiatry.* Washington, D.C.: American Psychiatric Press, Inc., 1988, pp. 403–441.

111. Hokin-Neaverson, M., and J.W. Jefferson. Erythrocyte sodium pump activity in bipolar affective disorder and other psychiatric disorders. *Neuropsychobiology* 22:1–7, 1989.

112. Holsboer, F., U. Bardeleben, A., Gerken, G.K. Stalla, and O.A. Muller. Blunted corticotropin and normal cortisol response to human corticotropin releasing factor in depression. *N. Engl. J. Med.* 311:1127, 1984.

113. Horne, J.A. The effects of exercise upon sleep: a critical review. *Biological Psychol.* 12:241–290, 1981.

114. Howlett, D.R., and F.A. Jenner. Studies relating to the clinical significance of urinary 3-methoxy-4-hydroxyphenylethylene glycol. *Br. J. Psychiatry* 132:49–54, 1978.

115. Hughes, J.R. Psychological effects of habitual aerobic exercise. A critical review. *Preventive Medicine* 13:66–78, 1984.

116. Janowsky, D.S., K. El-Yousef, M. Davis, and H.J. Sekerke. A cholinergic-adrenergic hypothesis of mania and depression. *Lancet* 2:632:635, 1972.

117. Jones, B.E., and R.Y. Moore. Ascending projections of the locus coeruleus in the rat. II. *Brain Res.* 127:25–53, 1977.

118. Jones, M.T., and B. Gillham. Factors involved in the regulation of adrenocorticotropic hormone/ʙ-lipotropic hormone. *Physiol. Rev.* 68:743–818, 1988.

119. Jones, M.T., B. Gillham, B.D. Greenstein, U. Beckford, and M.C. Holmes. Feedback actions of adrenal steroid hormone. D. Ganten and D. Pfaff (eds.). *Current Topics in Endocrinology.* Heidelberg, FRG: Springer-Verlag, 1982, pp. 46–68.

120. Jones, M.T., and M.A. Stockham. The effect of previous stimulation of the adrenal cortex by adrenocorticotropin on the function of the pituitary-adrenal axis in response to stress. *J. Physiol.* 184:741–750, 1966.

121. Moore, R.Y., and F.E. Bloom. Central catecholamine neuron systems: anatomy and physiology of the norepinephrine and epinephrine systems. *Ann. Rev. Neurosci.* 2:113–168, 1979.

122. Kelsoe, J.R., E.I. Ginns, J.A. Egeland, et al. Re-evaluation of linkage relationship between chromosome 11p loci and the gene for bipolar affective disorder in the old order Amish. *Nature* 342:238–243, 1989.

123. Kessler, L.G., B.J. Burns, S. Shapiro, et al. Psychiatric diagnoses of medical service users: evidence from the epidemiologic catchment area program. *Am. J. Public Health* 77:18–24, 1987.

124. Klein, M.H., J.H. Greist, R.A. Gurman, et al. A comparative outcome study of group psychotherapy vs. exercise treatments for depression. *Int. J. Ment. Health* 13:148–177, 1985.

125. Klerman, G.L. Depressive disorders. *Arch. Gen. Psychiatry* 46:856–858, 1989.

126. Klerman, G.L., and M.M. Weissman. Increasing rates of depression. *J.A.M.A.* 261:2229–2235, 1989.

127. Koob, G.F. Anhedonia as an animal model of depression. G.F. Koob, C.L. Ehlers, and D.J. Kupfer (eds.). *Animal Models of Depression.* Boston: Birkhauser, 1989, pp. 162–183.

128. Koob, G.F., C.L. Ehlers, and D.J. Kupfer (eds.). *Animal Models of Depression.* Boston: Birkhauser, 1989.

129. Krieger, D.T., Rhythms in CRF, ACTH, and corticosteroids. D.T. Krieger (ed.). *Endocrine Rhythms.* New York: Raven Press, 1979, pp. 123–142.

130. Krieger, H.P. and D.T. Krieger. Chemical stimulation of the brain. Effect on adrenal corticoid release. *Am. J. Physiol.* 218:1632–1641, 1970.

131. Kuhn, E.R., K. Bellon, L. Huybrechts, and W. Heyns. Endocrine differences between the Wistar and Sprague-Dawley laboratory rat: influence of cold adaptation. *Horm. Metabol. Res.* 15:491–498, 1983.

132. Lapin, I., and G. Oxenkrug. Intensification of the central serotonergic process as a possible determinant of thymoleptic effect. *Lancet* 1:132–136, 1969.

133. Leckman, J.F., M. Weissman, K.R. Merikangask, et al. Panic disorder and major depression: increased risk of depression, alcoholism, panic and phobic disorders in families or depressed probands with panic disorders. *Arch. Gen. Psychiatry* 40:1055–1060, 1983.

134. Lindvall, O., and A. Björklund. The organization of the ascending catecholamine neuron systems in the rat brain as revealed by the glyoxylic acid fluorescence method. *Acta Physiol. Scand. Suppl.* 412:1–48, 1974.

135. Lobstein, D.D., B.J. Mosbacher, and A.H. Ismail. Depression as a powerful discriminator between physically active and sedentary middle-aged men. *J. Psychosom. Res.* 27:69–76, 1983.

136. Lockette, W., R. McCurdy, S. Smith, and O. Carretero. Endurance training and α_2-adrenergic receptors on platelets. *Med. Sci. Sports Exer.* 19:7–10, 1987.

137. Luborsky, L.P., P. Crits-Christoph, J.P. Brady, et al. Behavioral versus pharmacological treatments for essential hypertension—a needed comparison. *Psychosom. Med.* 44:203–213, 1982.

138. Lukaszyk, A., W. Buczko, K. Wisniewski. The effect of strenuous exercise on the reactivity of the central dopaminergic system in the rat. *Pol. J. Pharmacol. Pharm.* 35:29–30, 1983.

139. Luger, A., P.A. Deuster, S.B. Kyle, et al. Acute hypothalamic-pituitary-adrenal responses to the stress of treadmill exercise: physiological adaptations to physical training. *New Eng. J. Med.* 316:1309–1315, 1987.

140. Maas, J.W. Neurotransmitters and depression: too much, too little, or too unstable? *Trends in the Neurosciences* 2:306–308, 1979.

141. Maas, J.W., and J.F. Leckman. Relationships between central nervous system noradrenergic function and plasma and urinary MHPG and other norepinephrine metabolites. J.W. Maas (ed.). *MHPG: Basic Mechanisms and Psychopathology.* New York: Academic Press, 1983, pp. 33–43.

142. Mandell, A., L. Chapman, and R. Rand. Plasma corticosteroids: changes in concentration after stimulation of hippocampus and amygdala. *Science.* 139:1212–1215, 1963.

143. Martinsen, E.W. Benefits of exercise for the treatment of depression. *Sports Med.* 9:380–389, 1990.

144. Martinsen, E.W. The role of aerobic exercise in the treatment of depression. *Stress Med.* 3:93–100, 1987.

145. Martinsen, E.W., A. Medhus, and L. Sandirk. Effects of aerobic exercise on depression: a controlled study. *Br. Med J.* 291:109–110, 1985.

146. Martinsen, E.W., A. Hoffart, and O. Solberg. Comparing aerobic with nonaerobic forms of exercise in the treatment of clinical depression: a randomized trial. *Compr. Psychiat.* 30:324–331, 1989.

147. Martinsen, E.W., J. Strand, G. Paulsson, and J. Kaggestad. Physical fitness level in patients with anxiety and depressive disorders. *Int. J. Sports Med.* 10:58–61, 1989.

148. Matlina, E. Effects of physical activity and other types of stress on catecholamine metabolism in various animal species. *J. Neural Tran.* 60:11–18, 1984.

149. Mausner, J.S., and A.K. Bahn. *Epidemiology: An Introductory Text.* Philadelphia: W.B. Saunders, 1974.

150. Meador-Woodruff, J.H., J.F. Greden, L. Grunhaus, and R.F. Haskett. Severity of depression and hypothalamic-pituitary-adrenal axis dysregulation: identification of contributing factors. *Acta. Psychiatr. Scand.* 81:364–371, 1990.

151. Meltzer, H.Y., and M.T. Lowy. Neuroendocrine function in psychiatric disorders and behavior. S. Arieti (ed.). *American Handbook of Psychiatry (2nd ed.) Volume 8.* P.A. Berger and H.K.H. Brodie (eds.). *Biological Psychiatry.* New York: Basic Books, 1986, pp. 111–150.

152. Mendlewicz, J., P. Simon, S. Sevy, et al. Polymorphic DNA marker on X chromosome and manic depression. *Lancet* 1:1230–1232, 1987.

153. Moore, K.E. Development of tolerance to the behavioural depressant effects of α-methyltyrosine. *J. Pharm. Pharmac.* 20:805–806, 1968.

154. Moore, K.E., and E.W. Lariviere. Effects of stress and d-amphetamine on rat brain catecholamines. *Biochem. Pharmacol.* 13:1098–1100, 1964.

155. Moore, R.Y., and F.E. Bloom. Central catecholamine neuron systems: anatomy and physiology of norepinephrine and epinephrine systems. *Annual Review of Neuroscience, Vol. 2.* Palo Alto, CA: Annual Reviews, Inc., 1979, pp. 129–165.

156. Morgan, W.P. A pilot investigation of physical working capacity in depressed and non-depressed males. *Res. Q.* 40:859–861, 1969.

157. Morgan, W.P. Affective beneficence of vigorous physical activity. *Med. Sci. Sports Exer.* 17:94–100, 1985.

158. Morgan, W.P., and P.J. O'Connor. Exercise and Mental Health. R.K. Dishman (ed.). *Exercise Adherence: It's Impact on Public Health.* Champaign, IL: Human Kinetics Books, 1988, pp. 91–121.

159. Morgan, W.P., and S.E. Goldston (eds.). *Exercise and Mental Health.* Washington Hemisphere Publishing Corporation, 1987.

160. Morgan, W.P., J.A. Roberts, and A.D. Feinerman. Psychological effect of physical activity. *Arch. Phys. Med. Rehabil.* 52:422–425, 1971.

161. Muller, O., H.G. Dorr, B. Hagen, G.K. Stalla, and K. Von Werder. Corticotropin releasing factor (CRF)-stimulation test in normal controls and patients with disturbances of the hypothalamopituitary-adrenal axis. *Klin. Wchnschr.* 60:1485–1491, 1982.

162. Murphy, J., A.M. Sobol, R.K. Neff, D.C. Olivier, and A.H. Leighton. Stability of prevalence: depression and anxiety disorders. *Arch. Gen. Psychiatry* 41:990–997, 1984.

163. Muscettola, G., W.Z. Potter, D. Pickor, and F.K. Goodwin. Urinary 3-methoxy-4-hydroxyphenylglycol and major affective disorders. *Arch. Gen. Psychiatry* 41:337–342, 1984.

164. Nemeroff, C.B., E. Widerlov, G. Bissette, et al. Elevated immunoreactive corticotropin releasing hormone in depressed patients. *Science* 224:1342–1344.

165. Newsholme, E.A. Effects of exercise on aspects of carbohydrate, fat, and amino acid metabolism. C. Bouchard, R.J. Shephard, T. Stephens, J.R. Sutton, and B.D. McPherson (eds). *Exercise, Fitness, and Health: A Consensus of Current Knowledge.* Champaign, IL: Human Kinetics Publishers, 1990, pp. 293–308.

166. North, T.C., P. McCullagh, and Z. Vu Tran. Effect of exercise on depression. *Ex. Sport Sci. Rev.* 18:379–415, 1990.

167. Norton, K.I., M.T. Delp, M.T. Jones, C. Duan, D.R. Dengel, and R.B. Armstrong. Distribution of blood flow during exercise following blood volume expansion in swine. *J. Appl. Physiol.* (in press).

168. Nurnberger, Jr., J.I., and E.S. Gershon. Genetics of affective disorder. R.M. Post and J.C. Ballenger (eds.). *Neurobiology of Mood Disorders.* Baltimore: Williams and Wilkins, 1984, pp. 76–101.

169. Nyback, H.V., J.V. Walters, G.K. Aghajanian, and R.H. Roth. Tricyclic antidepressants. Effects on the firing rate of brain noradrenergic neurons. *Eur. J. Pharmacol.* 32:302–312, 1975.

170. Oakes, R. Sex patterns in DSM-III: bias or basis for theory development. *Am. Psychol.*, 39:1320–1322, 1984.

171. O'Connor, P.J., W.P. Morgan, J.S. Raglin, C.N. Barksdale, and N.H. Kalin. Mood state and salivary cortisol levels following overtraining in female swimmers. *Psychoneuroendocrinology* 14:303–310, 1989.

172. Orth, D.N., C.R. DeBold, G.S. DeCherney, et al. Pituitary microadenomas causing Cushing's disease response to corticotropin-releasing factor. *J. Clin. Endocrinol. Metab.* 55:1017–1019, 1982.

173. Orth, D.N., R.V. Jackson, G.S. DeCherney, et al. Effect of synthetic ovine corticotropin-releasing factor: dose response of plasma adrenocorticotropin and cortisol. *J. Clin. Invest.* 71:587–595, 1983.

174. Ostman, I., and H. Nyback. Adaptive changes in central and peripheral noradrenergic neurons in rats following chronic exercise. *Neuroscience* 1:41–47, 1976.

175. Ostman, I., and N.O. Sjostrand. Reduced urinary noradrenaline excretion during rest, exercise and cold stress in trained rats. A comparison between physically-trained rats, cold-acclimated rats and warm-acclimated rats. *Acta Physiol. Scand.* 95:209–218, 1975.

176. Palkovits, M., M. Brownstein, J.S. Kizer, J.M. Saavedra, and I.J. Kopin. Effect of stress on serotonin and tyrosine hydroxylase activity of brain nuclei. E. Usdin, R. Kvetnansky, and I.J. Kopin (eds.). *Catecholamines and Stress.* Oxford: Pergamon Press, 1976, pp. 51–59.

177. Peroutka, S.J., R.M. Lebovitz, and S.H. Snyder. Two distinct central serotonin receptors with different physiological functions. *Science* 212:827–829, 1981.

178. Perusse, L., A. Tremblay, C. Leblanc, and C. Bouchard. Genetic and familial

environmental influences on level of habitual physical activity. *Am. J. Epid.* 129:1012–1022, 1989.

179. Peyrin, L. Urinary MHPG sulfate as a marker of central norepinephrine metabolism: a commentary. *J. Neural Transm.* 80:51–65, 1990.

180. Plomin, R. The role of inheritance in behavior. *Science* 248:183–188, 1990.

181. Plotsky, P.M., E.T. Cunningham, Jr., and E.P. Widmaier. Catecholaminergic modulation of corticotropin-releasing factor and adrenocorticotropin secretion. *Endocrine Rev.* 10:437–458, 1989.

182. Porsolt, R.D., M. LePichon, and M. Jalfre. Depression: A new animal model sensitive to antidepressant treatments. *Nature. London.* 226:730–732, 1977.

183. Post, R.M., and J.C. Ballenger (eds.). *Neurobiology of Mood Disorders.* Baltimore: Williams & Wilkins, 1984.

184. Post, R.M., J. Kotin, and F.K. Goodwin. Psychomotor activity and cerebrospinal fluid amine metabolites in affective illness. *Am. J. Psychiatry* 130:67–72, 1973.

185. Price, L.H., D.S. Charney, P.L. Delgado, and G.R. Heninger. Lithium and serotonin function: implications for the serotonin hypothesis of depression. *Psychopharmacology* 100:3–12, 1990.

186. Raglin, J.S. Exercise and mental health: Beneficial and detrimental effects. *Sports Med.* 9:323–329, 1990.

187. Raglin, J.S., and W.P. Morgan. Influence of exercise and quiet rest on state anxiety and blood pressure. *Med. Sci. Sports Exerc.* 19:456–463, 1987.

188. Ransford, C.P. A role for amines in the antidepressant effects of exercise: a review. *Med. Sci. Sports Exer.* 14:1–10, 1982.

189. Rea, M.A., and D.H. Hellhammer. Activity wheel stress changes in brain norepinephrine turnover and the occurrence of gastric lesions. *Psychother Psychosom.* 42:218–223, 1984.

190. Reader, S.C.J., W.R. Robertson, J. Alaghband-Zadeh, and J.R. Daly. Negative effects on adrenocorticotropin secretion by cortisol in Cushing's syndrome. *J. Endocrinol.* 87:60–61, 1980.

191. Regier, D.A., R.M.A. Hirschfeld, F.K. Goodwin, J.D. Burke, J.B. Lazar, and L.L. Judd. The NIMH depression awareness, recognition, and treatment program: structure, aims, and scientific basis. *Am. J. Psychiatry* 145:1351–1357, 1988.

192. Reigle, T.G. Increased brain norepinephrine metabolism correlated with analgesia produced by the periaqueductal gray injection of opiates. *Brain Res.* 338:155–159, 1985.

193. Reynolds, C.F. III, L.S. Taska, D.B. Jarrett, P.A. Coble, and D.J. Kupfer. REM latency in depression: Is there one best definition? *Biol. Psychiatry* 18:849–863, 1983.

194. Rivier, C., and W. Vale. Modulation of stress-induced ACTH release by corticotropin releasing factor, catecholamines and vasopressin. *Nature* 305:325–327, 1983.

195. Romanowski, W., and S. Grabiec. The role of serotonin in the mechanism of central fatigue. *Acta Physiol. Pol.* 25:127–134, 1974.

196. Rose, J.C., and W.F. Gannong. Neurotransmitter regulation of pituitary gland. W.F. Essman and L. Valzelli (eds.). *Current Developments in Psychopharmacology.* New York: Spectrum, 1976, pp. 87–123.

197. Ross, C.E., and D. Hayes. Exercise and psychologic well-being in the community. *Am. J. Epid.* 127:762–771, 1988.

198. Sachar, E.J., G. Asnis, U. Halbreich, R.S. Nathan, and F. Halpern. Recent studies in the neuroendocrinology of major depressive disorders. *Psychiatr. Clin. North Am.* 3:3113–3126, 1980.

199. Sachar, E.J., L. Hellman, D.K. Fukushima, T.F. Gallagher. Cortisol production in depressive illness: a clinical and biochemical classification. *Arch. Gen. Psychiatry* 23:289–298, 1970.

200. Saphier, D., and S. Feldman. Effects of septal and hippocampal stimuli on paraventricular neurons. *Neuroscience.* 20:749–755, 1987.

201. Sapolsky, R.M., and P.M. Plotsky. Hypercortisolism and its possible neural bases. *Biol. Psychiatry* 27:937–952, 1990.
202. Sapolsky, R.M., L.C. Krey, and B.S. McEwen. Glucocorticoid-sensitive hippocampal neurons are involved in terminating the adrenocortical stress response. *Proc. Natl. Acad. Sci.* 81:6174–6177, 1984.
203. Sapolsksy, R.M., L.C. Krey, and B.S. McEwen. Stress down-regulates corticosterone receptors in a site-specific manner in the brain. *Endocrinology* 114:287–292, 1984.
204. Schildkraut, J.J. Catecholamine metabolism and affective disorders: studies of MHPG excretion. E. Usdin and S. Snyder (eds.). *Frontiers in Catecholamine Research.* New York: Pergamon Press, 1975, pp. 1165–1171.
205. Schildkraut, J.J. The catecholamine hypothesis of affective disorders: a review of supporting evidence. *Am. J. Psychiatry* 122:509–522, 1965.
206. Schildkraut, J.J., P.J. Orsulak, A.F. Schatzberg, and A.H. Rosenbaum. Relationship between psychiatric diagnostic groups of depressive disorders and MHPG. J.W. Maas (ed.). *MHPG: Basic Mechanisms and Psychopathology.* New York: Academic Press, 1983, pp. 129–144.
207. Schulte, H.M., G.P. Chrousos, P.W. Gold, et al. Continuous infusion of CRF in normal volunteers. Physiological and pathophysiological implications. *J. Clin. Invest.* 75:1781–1785.
208. Sforzo, G.A., T.F. Seeger, C.B. Pert, A. Pert, and C.O. Dotson. In vivo opioid receptor occupation in the rat brain following exercise. *Med. Sci. Sports Ex.* 18:380–384, 1986.
209. Shapiro, S., E.A. Skinner, L.G. Kessler, et al. Utilization of health and mental services. *Arch. Gen. Psych.* 41:971–978, 1984.
210. Siever, L.J., and K.L. Davis. Overview toward a dysregulation hypothesis of depression. *Am. J. Psychiatry* 142:1017–1031, 1985.
211. Siever, L.J., E.F. Coccaro, and K.L. Davis. Chronobiologic instability of the noradrenergic system in depression. A. Halaris (ed.). *Chronobiology and Psychiatric Disorders.* New York: Elsevier, 1987, pp. 2–21.
212. Smith, M.L., G.V. Glass, and T.E. Miller. *The Benefits of Psychotherapy.* Baltimore: Johns Hopkins University Press, 1980.
213. Sothmann, M.S., J. Blaney, T. Woulfe, et al. Plasma free and sulfoconjugated catecholamines during sustained exercise. *J. Appl. Physiol.* 68:452–456, 1990.
214. Sothmann, M.S., and A.H. Ismail. Factor analytic derivation of the MHPG/NM ration. Implications for studying the link between physical fitness and depression. *Biol. Psychiatry* 20:570–583, 1985.
215. Sothmann, M.S., and A.H. Ismail. Relationships between urinary catecholamine metabolites, particularly MHPG, and selected personality and physical fitness characteristics in normal subjects. *Psychosom. Med.* 46:523–533, 1984.
216. Sothmann, M.S., A.H. Ismail, and W. Chodepki-Zajiko. Influence of catecholamine activity on the hierarchical relationships among physical fitness condition and selected personality characteristics. *J. Clin. Psychol.* 40:1308–1317, 1984.
217. Spielberger, C.D., R.L. Gorsuch, and R. Lushene. *Manual for the State-Trait Anxiety Inventory (Self-Evaluation Questionnaire).* Palo Alto, CA: Consulting Psychologists Press, 1970.
218. Spielberger, C.D., R.L. Gorsuch, R. Lushene, P.R. Vagg, and G.A. Jacobs. *Manual for the State-Trait Anxiety Inventory (STAI) Form Y.* Palo Alto, CA: Consulting Psychologists Press, Inc., 1983.
219. Spitzer, R.L., J. Endicott, and E. Robins. Research diagnostic criteria rationale and reliability. *Arch. Gen. Psychiatry* 35:773–783, 1978.
220. Stephens, T. Physical activity and mental health in the United States and Canada: Evidence from four population surveys. *Prev. Med.* 17:35–47, 1988.
221. Stokes, P.E., P.M. Stoll, S.H. Koslow, et al. Pretreatment DST and hypothalamic-

pituitary-adrenocortical function in depresed patients and comparison groups. *Arch. Gen. Psychiatry* 41:257–267, 1984.

222. Stone, E.A. Accumulation and metabolism of NE in rat hypothalamus after exhaustive stress. *J. Neurochem.* 21:589–601, 1973.

223. Stoudemire, A., R. Frank, N. Hedemark, M. Kamlet, and D. Blazer. The economic burden of depression. *Gen. Hosp. Psychiatry* 8:387–394, 1986.

224. Stubbs, W.A., A. Jones, C.R.W. Edwards, et al. Hormonal and metabolic responses to an enkephalin analogue in normal man. *Lancet* December 9:1225–1227, 1978.

225. Sulser, F., J. Ventulani, and P. Mobley. Mode of action of antidepressant drugs. *Biochem. Pharmacol.* 27:257–261, 1978.

226. Sweeney, D.R., J.W. Maas, and G.R. Heninger. State anxiety, physical activity and urinary 3-methoxy-4-hydroxyphenylglycol excretion. *Arch. Gen. Psychiatry* 35:1418–1425, 1978.

227. Sutton, J.R., P.A. Farrell, and V.J. Harber. Hormonal adaptations to physical activity. C. Bouchard, R.J. Shephard, T. Stephens, J.R. Sutton, and B.D. McPherson (eds.). *Exercise, Fitness and Health: A Consensus of Current Knowledge.* Champaign, IL: Human Kinetics Publishers, 1990, pp. 17–257.

228. Tang, S.W., H.C. Stancer, S. Takahashi, R.J. Shephard, and J.J. Warsh. Controlled exercise elevates plasma but not urinary MHPG and VMA. *Psychiat. Res.* 4:13–20, 1981.

229. Taube, S.L., L.S. Kirstein, D.R. Sweeney, G.R. Heninger, and J.W. Maas. Urinary 3-methoxy-4-hydroxyphenylglycol and psychiatric diagnosis. *Am. J. Psychiatry* 135:78–81, 1978.

230. Taylor, C.B., J.F. Sallis, and R. Needle. The relation of physical activity and exercise to mental health. *Pub. Health Rep.* 100:195–202, 1985.

231. Torgersen, S. Genetic factors in moderately severe and mild affective disorders. *Arch. Gen. Psychiatry* 43:222–226, 1986.

232. Tuomisto, J., and P. Mannisto. Neurotransmitter regulation of anterior pituitary hormones. *Pharmacol. Rev.*, 37:249–332, 1985.

233. Udenfriend, S., and W. Dairman. Regulation of norepinephrine synthesis. G. Weber (ed.). *Advances in Enzyme Regulation Volume 9.* Oxford: Pergamon Press, 1971, pp. 145–165.

234. Ungerstedt, U. Stereotaxic mapping of the monoamine pathways in the rat brain. *Acta Physiol. Scand.* 367:1–48, 1971.

235. U.S. Department of Health and Human Services. *Promoting Health/Preventing Disease: Year 2000 Objectives for the Nation.* Washington, D.C.: U.S. Government Printing Office, 1990.

236. Vale, W., J. Vaughan, M. Smith, G. Yamomoto, J. Rivier, and C. Rivier. Effects of synthetic ovine corticotropin-releasing factor, glucocorticoids, catecholamines, neurohypophysial peptides and other substances on cultured corticotropic cells. *Endocrinology* 113:1121–1131, 1983.

237. Vogel, G., D. Neill, M. Hagler, and D. Kors. A new animal model of endogenous depression: a summary of present findings. *Neurosci. Behav. Rev.* 14:85–91, 1990.

238. Walker, J.M., T.C. Floyd, G. Fein, C. Cavness, R. Lualhati, and I. Feinberg. Effects of exercise on sleep. *J. Appl. Physiol.* 44:945–951, 1978.

239. Watson, S.J., H. Khachaturian, M.E. Lewis, and H. Akil. Chemical neuroanatomy as a basis for biological psychiatry. S. Arieti (ed.). *American Handbook of Psychiatry (2nd ed.) Volume 8.* P.A. Berger and H.K.H. Brodie (eds.) *Biological Psychiatry.* New York: Basic Books, 1986, pp. 4–33.

240. Wender, P.H., S.S. Kety, D. Rosenthal, et al. Psychiatric disorders in the biological and adoptive families of adopted individuals with affective disorders. *Arch. Gen. Psychiatry* 43:923–929, 1986.

241. Wehr, T.A., and F.K. Goodwin. Biological rhythms and psychiatry. S. Arieti and

H.K.H. Brodie (eds.). *American Handbook of Psychiatry* (vol. 7, 2nd ed.), 1981, pp. 344–378.

242. Weinstein, W.S., and A.W. Meyers. Running as a treatment for depression: is it worth it? *J. Sport Psychol.* 5:288–301, 1983.

243. Weiss, J.M., H.I. Glazer, L.A. Pohorecky. Coping behavior and neurochemical changes: an alternative explanation for the "learned helplessness" experiments. G. Serban and A. King (eds.). *Animal Models in Human Psychobiology*. New York: Plenum, 1976, pp. 141–173.

244. Weiss, J.M., and P.E. Simson. Electrophysiology of the locus coeruleus: implications for stress-induced depression. G.F. Koob, C.L. Ehlers, and D.J. Kupfer (eds.). *Animal Models of Depression*. Boston: Birkhauser, 1989, pp. 111–134.

245. Weiss, J.M., and P.G. Simson. Neurochemical mechanisms underlying stress-induced depression. T. Field and N. Schneiderman, (eds.). *Stress and Coping, Vol. 1*. Hillsdale, N.J.: Lawrence-Erlbaum, 1988.

246. Weiss, J.M., P.G. Simson, L.J. Hoffman, M.J. Ambrose, S. Cooper, and A. Webster. Infusion of adrenergic receptor agonists and antagonists into the locus coeruleus and ventricular system of the brain: effects on swim-motivated and spontaneous motor activity. *Neuropharmacology* 25:367–384, 1986.

247. Weissman, M.M. Advances in psychiatric epidemiology: rates and risks for major depression. *Am. J. Public Health* 77:445–451, 1987.

248. Weissman, M.M., and J.H. Boyd. The epidemiology of affective disorders. R.M. Post and Ballenger (eds.). *Neurobiology of Mood Disorders*. Baltimore: Williams and Wilkins, 1984, pp. 60–75.

249. Weissman, M.M., and G.L. Klerman. Sex differences and the epidemiology of depression. *Arch. Gen. Psychiatry* 34:98–111, 1977.

250. Weissman, M.M., and G.L. Klerman. Epidemiology of mental disorders: emerging trends in the U.S. *Arch. Gen. Psychiatry* 35:705–712, 1978.

251. Weissman, M.M., P.J. Leaf, G.L. Tischler, et al. Affective disorders in 5 U.S. communities. *Psychol. Med.* 18:141–153, 1988.

252. Whybrow, P.C., H.S. Akiskal, and W.T. McKinney, Jr. *Mood Disorders Toward a New Psychobiology*. New York: Plenum Press, 1984.

253. Young, E.A., S.J. Watson, and H. Akil. Pituitary regulation in endogenous depression. *Prog. Brain Res.* 65:153–166, 1986.

254. Zacharko, R.M., W.J. Bowers, L. Kokkinidis, and H. Anisman. Region-specific reductions of intracranial self-stimulation after uncontrollable stress: possible effects on reward processes. *Behav. Brain Res.* 9:129–141, 1983.

3
The Metabolic Effects of Exercise-Induced Muscle Damage

WILLIAM J. EVANS, Ph.D.
JOSEPH G. CANNON, Ph.D.

INTRODUCTION

The responses to damaging exercise often do not manifest themselves during the exercise. Pain does not develop for several hours; membrane damage or protein breakdown may take days or weeks to become evident (Figure 3.1). In this review we focus on the delayed nature of exercise-induced muscle damage and discuss mechanisms that may be involved. Eccentric exercise is often used to induce experimental muscle damage and, therefore, is a major topic of this review, but damage resulting from other forms of exercise is also discussed. The review is organized in the following manner:

ECCENTRIC EXERCISE AS A PARADIGM OF MUSCLE DAMAGE
    Oxygen Consumption
    Integrated Electromyography
    Muscle Weakness
MYOCELLULAR ENZYME RELEASE
    Type and Intensity of Exercise
    Training
    Mechanisms of Enzyme Release
THE ACUTE PHASE RESPONSE
    Complement
    Neutrophils
    Monocytes
    Cytokines and Acute Phase Proteins
    Trace Metals
ULTRASTRUCTURAL DAMAGE
PROTEIN METABOLISM
    Hydrolytic Enzymes
    Calcium Ion (Ca^{2+})
    Cytokines
    Anti-inflammatory Drugs
    Hypertrophy
SUMMARY

FIGURE 3.1

Delayed responses to eccentric exercise. Density of shading in each bar corresponds to the intensity of the response at the time indicated on the horizontal axis. This figure was compiled from the results of several studies [18, 39, 92, 97].

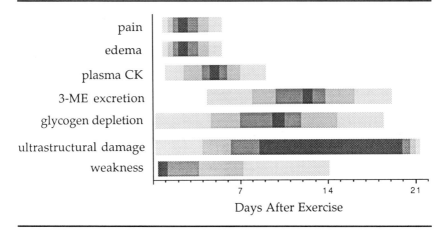

ECCENTRIC EXERCISE AS A PARADIGM OF MUSCLE DAMAGE

All physical activity consists of some combination of concentric, isometric, and eccentric muscle contractions. When a weight is lifted, muscles contract and shorten to produce sufficient force. When the same weight is lowered, the same muscle groups are used; however, force is generated by the muscles as they lengthen. Although the same amount of force is generated to lift and lower the weight, lowering it seems easier, just as walking up stairs is more difficult and requires more oxygen to perform than walking down stairs. Erling Asmussen [7, p. 364] compared the effort of climbing up and down a rope and remarked that the fact that it is easier to climb down was

"astonishing, as the force necessary to keep the body in constant movement upwards must be the same as the force necessary to keep the body moving at the same speed in the downward direction, since the force in both cases equals the weight of the body. If the muscular movements in the two cases are exactly reversed, the tensions produced by the active muscles must be exactly equal at corresponding phases of the two movements, the only difference being that in climbing the rope the active muscles are shortening during the movement while they are being forcibly lengthened during the descent."

FIGURE 3.2

Oxygen cost of eccentric and concentric exercise on a cycle ergometer (n = 6 subjects) [unpublished data].

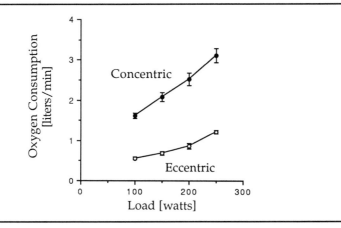

Oxygen Consumption

By having his subjects ride a bicycle with pedals linked directly to the rear wheels on an inclined, motor-driven treadmill, uphill for concentric and downhill for eccentric contractions, Asmussen [7] found that the ratio of the oxygen uptake, or the cost of positive work (2.08 liters per minute [L/min]), to the cost of negative work (0.28 L/min) was 7.4:1. He also demonstrated that eccentric exercise resulted in delayed onset muscle soreness (24 to 48 hours later) [8]. Figure 3.2 shows data from our laboratory [unpublished observations] comparing the oxygen cost of concentric and eccentric cycle ergometry at varying intensities. The relative difference in $\dot{V}O_2$ becomes more pronounced as the intensity of the exercise increases.

Integrated Electromyography

The integrated electromyographic (IEMG) analyses of concentric and eccentric contractions that produce similar amounts of force are quite different [9]. Not only is the IEMG of eccentric exercise smaller, but unlike concentric exercise in which the IEMG increases directly in proportion to the intensity, the IEMG of eccentric muscle contractions does not go up with increasing force production. Komi and Buskirk [71] examined the effects of seven weeks of conditioning the forearm flexors in groups of young men. One group used only concentric muscle contractions, another only eccentric contractions, while a third (control) group remained sedentary. They measured maximal force production as well as the IEMG during eccentric, isometric, and concentric contractions. During the first week of conditioning, the eccentric group complained of muscle soreness; by the second week, however, the eccentric contractions produced no soreness. When compared to the control group, only the eccentrically conditioned group showed a significant increase in the IEMG, with a linear increase during the first three weeks of conditioning. Both the eccentric and concentric groups showed increases in force production, but the subjects in the eccentric group showed the greatest increase in maximal force production during eccentric muscle contractions. Moreover, compared to the control group, only the upper arm girth of the eccentric group increased in size as a result of the conditioning.

The IEMG was also measured by Newham et al. [93] during chair-stepping exercise, with one leg raising the body (concentric exercise) and the contralateral leg lowering the body (eccentric exercise). They found that fewer motor units were recruited during eccentric exercise and that, unlike the concentric leg, the IEMG rose progressively during the eccentric exercise. They concluded that "the fact that greater tension per muscle fiber is generated under eccentric contraction conditions provides a situation where relatively few fibres are recruited and are producing relatively large forces" [93, p. 384].

The IEMG has also been shown [31] to increase progressively during a bout of prolonged submaximal exercise (downhill running, 40 min, 3.83 m $\cdot$ sec^{-1}, 44% of $\dot{V}o_2$max), but it remains unchanged during level running at the same speed. The authors concluded that this increased recruitment of motor units during eccentric exercise caused the upward drift in $\dot{V}o_2$ seen by them and other investigators [68]. Armstrong [4] suggested that the increase in IEMG during a bout of eccentric exercise indicates that injury to initially recruited motor units may have necessitated recruitment of additional units to produce the required forces. The fact that this upward drift in $\dot{V}o_2$ during prolonged eccentric exercise is eliminated by eccentric exercise training [69] lends credence to Armstrong's suggestion. Because eccentric exercise training greatly reduces the amount of muscle damage caused by the exercise, the initial injury to the fibers would not occur, obviating the need for increased recruitment of motor units.

Muscle Weakness
Davies and White [29] measured the separate effects of eccentric and concentric exercise (chair stepping at a rate of 20 lifts of the body/min for 1 hour) on stimulated and voluntary isometric contraction of triceps surae. The maximal twitch and tetanic tensions in the eccentric leg at 10, 20, 50, and 100 hertz (Hz) were substantially reduced for a prolonged period, whereas the contralateral concentric leg was unaffected. In addition, the eccentric leg was more fatiguable than the concentric leg. Although these investigators did not examine morphological changes

in the muscles affected by the exercise, they ascribed these long-lasting changes in twitch characteristics to prolonged muscle damage caused by the eccentric exercise. They also noted that their subjects experienced muscle soreness for 5 to 7 days after the exercise only in the eccentric leg. Newham and co-workers [93], using a similar exercise (chair stepping, 15 lifts/min for 15 to 20 minutes), found that maximal voluntary force and electrically stimulated force were decreased for 24 hours after the stepping in the eccentric leg, but not in the concentric leg.

MYOCELLULAR ENZYME RELEASE

The appearance of myocellular enzymes in the circulation is generally taken as an indication of "muscle damage." Following myocardial ischemia, the plasma concentrations of individual enzymes have been correlated to infarct size [117]. In addition, the relative release of different enzymes during shock have been correlated to the inverse of the molecular radius of each enzyme, supporting the concept that the enzyme efflux is a diffusional process through holes introduced into the plasma membrane [72]. Holes of sufficient size to allow passage of macromolecules ranging in size up to several hundred kilodaltons would seem incompatible with continued cell viability, but the release of enzymes does not appear to correlate with ultrastructural damage or loss of function. The extent of the postexercise rise in circulating skeletal muscle enzymes appears to be most closely related to the type and intensity of the exercise and the previous activity of the subjects.

Type and Intensity of Exercise

Friden et al. [456] examined serum muscle enzyme activities (glutamic oxaloacetic transaminase [SGOT], lactic dehydrogenase [LDH], and creatine kinase [CK]) in young subjects performing eccentric, concentric, or isometric exercise of the lower-leg anterior compartment. The SGOT and circulating CK activities increased significantly 48 hours after the eccentric exercise only. Serum LDH levels were not affected by any of the exercise interventions. The increases in serum enzyme activities were relatively small for this study (36% and 17% for CK and SGOT, respectively, probably because of the low intensity of the exercise (15% of the subject's maximal torque) and the small mass of muscle used during the exercise. Much larger increases in circulating CK have been seen following other eccentric exercise protocols. A 351% increase in circulating CK activity was seen following downhill running (45 min, 57% $\dot{V}o_2$max, -10% incline) but no change was seen following running on the level [116]. Newham et al. [93] examined circulating CK after stepping exercise and found a remarkably variable response: some subjects showed only a small two- to threefold increase 24 hours after the exercise, whereas others displayed a 70- to 100-fold increase peaking up to 6 days following the exercise. They found no relationship between peak-circulating CK and body weight, but neither the aerobic capacity or the activity patterns of the subjects were described.

Training

Hunter et al. [56] demonstrated that a single maximal exercise test elicited increases in circulating CK, SGOT, and LDH activities in previously sedentary men. After 10 weeks of endurance training, however, the exercise-induced changes in these enzymes were attenuated. This same training phenomenon has been seen in rats. Schwane and Armstrong [115] showed that training by downhill running or level running greatly reduced or eliminated the postexercise rise in circulating CK activity, but that uphill training did not effect the increase. Byrnes et al. [19] found that a single bout of downhill running (heart rate of 170 beats/min, 30 min, −10% incline) diminished or eliminated the amount of delayed onset muscle soreness and circulating CK activity following subsequent bouts of downhill running up to 6 weeks later. Evans et al. [39] found that in previously sedentary men, 45 minutes of eccentric exercise (250W) caused an average 33-fold increase in circulating CK activity which did not return to preexercise levels for 10 days. In the same study, a group of endurance athletes performing the same exercise had a mild twofold increase that was only significant 24 hours after the exercise. The endurance athletes in this study also had higher resting circulating CK activity than did the sedentary men.

The large intersubject variability reported by many investigators [25, 26, 39, 93] in the rise in circulating CK activity following exercise is an indication that CK is not an accurate predictor of skeletal muscle damage. Clarkson and Ebbeling [26, 260] have pointed out that the increase in circulating CK is "unrelated to either the development of muscle soreness, the amount of strength loss after exercise, fitness level of the subject, or lean body weight." We have seen no difference in circulating CK response following high-intensity eccentric exercise that produced very different amounts of skeletal muscle damage as assessed by electron and light microscopy of muscle biopsies [83]. It is likely that the postexercise rise in circulating CK activity is a manifestation of skeletal muscle damage but not a direct indicator of it. Clearly, the magnitude of the rise in circulating CK is a net result of release of the protein from skeletal muscle and its clearance by the liver.

Mechanisms of Enzyme Release

Is the release of myocellular enzymes following severe exercise analogous to myocardial infarction? Armstrong et al. [5] have postulated that the enzyme efflux following an initial exposure to high-intensity eccentric exercise does in fact indicate irreversible destruction of muscle fibers. Based on this hypothesis, Newham et al. [92] proposed that the "training effect" (the dramatically reduced enzyme efflux in response to a second exposure to eccentric exercise) is attributable to the elimination of weak or susceptible fibers by the first exposure.

One possible mechanism of cellular destruction could be physical shearing of membranes or filaments by excessive loads experienced during exercise. Eccentric exercise can easily expose muscles to excessive loads, which may explain why it is particularly damaging. Figure 3.2 shows the differences in oxygen consumption at equivalent loads in concentric versus eccentric modes of cycle ergometry. During concentric exercise, aerobic capacity may limit the length of time a person can develop forces sufficiently high to cause damage. In contrast, the external forces imposed on a person's muscles during eccentric exercise are not strictly limited by aerobic capacity, thus increasing the risk of overload.

Cellular destruction could also stem from transient ischemia caused by compression of vasculature during force development. Again, eccentric exercise accentuates this potential mechanism for damage. Friden et al. [44] determined that eccentric contractions caused 50% higher intramuscular pressures than concentric contractions at the same loads. Nielsen et al. [95] have shown, however, that muscle blood flow, measured by ^{133}Xe clearance, is not different between the two modes of exercise. The mass of muscle tissue likely to become ischemic is therefore probably small, which is in line with the focal damage observed immediately after exercise [43]. In most tissues, ischemia and subsequent reperfusion cause a conversion of xanthine dehydrogenase to xanthine oxidase, leading to the production of superoxide and hydrogen peroxide [84]. This conversion does not occur in skeletal muscle, but neutrophils that localize in muscle after ischemia are an abundant source of oxygen radicals [119]. Alternatively, heavy exercise may disrupt mitochondrial respiratory control, releasing oxygen free radicals that cause lipid peroxidation [100]. In a perfused heart model, Gauduel et al. [47] observed an association between lipid peroxidation products and creatine kinase leakage. Kanter et al. [63] related CK and LDH to lipid peroxidation following an 80 km run.

Other investigators [32, 60, 137] have suggested that enzyme leakage is a consequence of disturbances in cell volume or in energy state, or both. One possibility is that a reduced metabolic state inhibits sarcolemmal Na-K-ATPase, resulting in swelling from intracellular accumulation of sodium and water [79, 106]. The swelling then leads to stretching and ultimate rupture of the membrane, allowing intracellular enzymes to escape. Enzyme efflux was not affected, however, in rats treated with ouabain [85]. Jones et al. [60] also found an association between adenosine 5'-triphosphate (ATP) depletion by muscle and the efflux of enzymes. Although they offered no mechanistic interpretation of the delayed efflux, the reseachers did observe that it was qualitatively different from the rapid enzyme efflux caused by membrane disruption with detergents. Edema and swelling following exercise-induced muscle damage has been seen by a number of investigators. The evidence for this swelling has ranged from increased circumference of exercised muscle 24 to 48 hours after exercise [25], to ultrastructural evidence of postexercise muscle edema [133], to direct measurement of intramuscular resting pressure. Friden, et al. [44] used a slit catheter placed in the leg anterior compartments to measure pressure during and following eccentric exercise in one leg and concentric exercise in the other. Average peak muscle pressure was greater during eccentric than concentric exercise and resting pressure was elevated for a prolonged period in the eccentrically, but not the concentrically, exercised leg. Friden et al. [46] also have seen an increase in the water content of muscles following eccentric exercise. This increase in intramuscular pressure is thought to occur as a result of increased amounts of small protein or peptide fragments and the release of protein-bound ions in damaged muscle cells. The release of intracellular proteins into the circulation likely results from an increase in intracellular pressure.

Diederichs et al. [32] examined release of LDH following manipulations that caused swelling of isolated rat peroneus longus. By introducing the muscle to varying concentrations of hypotonic media in the presence or absence of dinitrophenol (to poison ATP-producing systems), they found that the greater the amount of swelling, the greater the release of LDH. Actual swelling deviated, however, from the theoretical swelling curve; the deviation was associated with increased LDH release and was ATP-dependent. Zierler [137] observed increased aldolase efflux from isolated skeletal muscle treated with metabolic inhibitors of glycolysis, oxidative phosphorylation, and mitochondrial electron transport. Based on these data, he proposed a dynamic membrane structure containing metabolically regulated pores capable of allowing transient macromolecule passage. Notably, the release rate of intracellular proteins into the circulation is closely correlated with their molecular weight [72]. It is likely that varying amounts of muscle cell edema produce varying amounts of stretch and membrane permeability. Skeletal muscle CK activity is found in the soluble fraction, sarcoplasmic reticulum, and mitochondria, and is an integral element in the M-line structure of myofibrils [129, 131, 132]. It therefore seems likely that the prolonged release of skeletal muscle CK into the circulation represents both the soluble CK fraction initially released as well as the CK protein released as a result of muscle protein degradation (specifically, actomyosin protein) [39].

The postexercise elevation in circulating CK activity appears to be different between men and women. At the same level of exercise, men showed a significant postexercise rise in circulating CK, whereas women did not [12, 118]. The postmarathon rise in circulating CK is much greater in men than in women, even after accounting for differences in body size [3]. This postmarathon rise in circulating CK was not related to age or finishing time. Moreover, the resting circulating CK levels of pregnant women with very high estrogen levels are lower than that of menstruating women with normal estrogen levels and much lower than in premenarchal and postmenopausal women with low estrogen levels [128]. The presence of estrogen can markedly reduce the release of intracellular protein from the erythrocytes of women but not men [128]. Amelink and Bar [2] found that after two hours of treadmill running, circulating CK activity was elevated by 335% in male rats but unchanged in female rats. Amelink and Bar also ran female rats that had been ovariectomized at different stages of sexual maturity (early, 22 days old, 6 weeks before the exercise; late, 45 days old, 2 weeks before exercise), and both ovariectomized groups showed a greater rise than control female rats. The rats ovariectomized before reaching sexual maturity showed a greater postexercise rise in circulating CK activity than those ovariectomized after reaching sexual maturity. These data and those of Thomson and Smith [128] indicate that estrogen may directly affect the cell membrane to reduce the efflux of intracellular proteins.

If changes in muscle membrane permeability are truly brought about by host factors, do the changes represent some kind of adaptive response? Cannon et al. [22] recently observed that CK release was more pronounced in young persons, who are usually considered to be more resilient to physical stress, than in older persons. This calls into question the assumption that the efflux of myocellular enzymes represents undesirable "damage" to muscle membranes. The CK release may indicate turnover of proteins rendered dysfunctional by physical or oxidative stresses. Salminen and Vihko [113] put forward a similar hypothesis after finding that the acid proteolytic capacity of young mice increased to a greater extent than in older mice following prolonged exercise.

Exercise that results in muscle damage also initiates a well-orchestrated response that ultimately results in the repair of the damaged tissue. Indeed, exercise that may result in a great deal of muscle damage, such as lifting and lowering a heavy weight, also has the capability of producing skeletal muscle hypertrophy, which ultimately decreases the risk of future muscle damage from that particular exercise.

THE ACUTE PHASE RESPONSE

Tissue damage and infection initiate a stereotyped sequence of host defense reactions, known as the acute phase response [62]. Although the acute phase response generally is recognized for its antibacterial and antiviral actions, it also promotes clearance of damaged tissue and sets the stage for repair and growth [104]. These latter activities may be a teleological explanation for why an acute phase response is initiated by exercise. The generation of an acute phase response depends on the duration, and possibly to a lesser extent, the intensity of exercise. Running a 42 kilometer (km) marathon is an adequate stimulus of an acute phase response [57], but as the duration decreases, acute phase reactions are less clear [70]. Experimental complications arise because the facets of the acute phase response are transient and sequential. Some are very rapid in onset (within minutes) because the elements are preformed (complement, neutrophils). Others require hours or days to become maximal owing to time-dependent transport processes (trace metals) or protein synthesis (acute phase proteins). Reports indicating no changes in acute phase reactants following exercise can sometimes be attributed to sampling that was done too early, measuring trace metals immediately after short-duration exercise [6], or too late, sampling for circulating neutrophils 24 hours after exercise [17]. The following overview will focus on the aspects of the acute phase response that are associated with tissue damage and repair, and present the evidence that these occur following exercise. Figure 3.3 shows the temporal development of the acute phase response following exercise.

Complement
The complement system consists of 20 plasma proteins that circulate as inactive precursors [89]. Activation of the system by proteolytic cleavage

FIGURE 3.3
Temporal development of an acute phase response following exercise. Note logarithmic time scale on the horizontal axis. This figure was compiled from the results of several studies [21, 22, 36, 61, 77, 127].

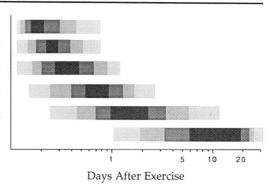

of certain complement components results in several active fragments: some catalyze cleavage of other complement components, some catalyze assembly of components. The result is a fast-acting, self-amplifying process analogous to the blood-clotting cascade. The end products of this cascade include membrane-attack complexes that disrupt the membranes of nonself cells; anaphylatoxins (C3a, C4a and C5a) that are activators of mast cells, neutrophils, and monocytes; and opsonins (C3b) that coat foreign particles, aiding phagocytosis. The complement system can be activated by antigen-antibody complexes (the "classical pathway") or by foreign pathogens and damaged host cells (the "alternative pathway") [126].

An early manifestation of the acute phase response after exercise is activation of complement (Figure 3.3). Dufaux and Order [36] observed a twofold increase in plasma C3a and C4a immediately after a 2.5 hour running protocol. Exercise of this magnitude may have caused damage to contractile or connective elements, releasing fragments that activate complement through the alternate pathway. In addition, Dufaux et al. [35] found an approximately 10% increase in circulating immune complexes 1 hour after a similar running protocol, raising the possibility that complement may be activated by the classical pathway following exercise as well.

Neutrophils
Within hours of injury or infection, the number of circulating neutrophils can increase several fold. This rapid increase is possible because only about half of the mature neutrophils released from the bone marrow usually circulate, the other half adhere to vessel walls ("marginated") [30]. Neutrophil half-life in the circulation is usually <10 hours, and is reduced during inflammation as the cells migrate to the site of injury, drawn by chemoattractants including C5a. The life span of the neutrophil within tissue is thought to be only one or two days [11]. Neutrophils phagocytize pathogens and tissue debris, and release an array of cytotoxic factors, including elastase, lysozyme, and oxygen radicals [10]. These factors affect intact host tissue with adaptive and maladaptive consequences. For example, elastase, collagenase, and oxygen radicals increase vascular permeability by breaking down basement membranes of the microvasculature near a site of injury, thus promoting migration of leukocytes [88]. If released in an uncontrolled manner, however, these agents also can break down healthy surrounding tissue and are the basis of several inflammatory diseases [82].

The number of circulating neutrophils increases during exercise [123] and can continue to increase for several hours afterwards [22], depending on the duration and intensity of exercise. The mechanism responsible for the increase in circulating neutrophils is not settled. Administration of epinephrine can cause similar increases [124], but β-blockers do not significantly attenuate the postexercise rise in circulating neutrophils [42, 107]. It has been proposed that the increased blood flow during exercise shears marginated neutrophils free of vessel walls [42], but it is not clear how this mechanism can account for the continued increase in circulating neutrophils for several hours after extended periods of exercise. Administration of the cytokines interleukin-1 (IL-1), tumor necrosis factor (TNF), or interleukin-6 (IL-6) will cause an increase in circulating neutrophils in laboratory animals; perhaps the modest increases in circulating cytokine levels observed for several hours after exercise [21, 37, 96] contribute to postexercise leukocytosis.

Greater neutrophil increases have been observed after eccentric exercise than after concentric exercise in the same subjects at similar levels of oxygen consumption [120]. These data raise the possibility that other factors, possibly tissue damage, may contribute to the increase in circulating neutrophils. It should be pointed out, however, that the subjects in this investigation had higher heart rates during the eccentric exercise, raising the possibility that hemodynamic shear forces may have been different in the two forms of exercise.

High intramuscular pressures, especially during eccentric exercise [44], may cause transient, localized interruptions of blood flow. On a whole-muscle scale, experimental ischemia and subsequent reperfusion result in reduced function, increased histological evidence of cellular damage, and increased release of CK and other cytoplasmic enzymes [67]. During reperfusion, an increase in tissue neutrophil content has been observed [119]. In isolated, perfused organ systems, reperfusion after ischemia with neutrophil-containing buffer caused more histological and functional damage than buffer alone, indicating a causal association [78]. Neutrophils have been observed in muscle tissue following a marathon [55], but have not been mentioned in reports of leukocytic infiltration following eccentric exercise [61, 110]. It is possible that the timing of the muscle biopsies is responsible for these discrepancies, with earlier sampling times (within 24 hours) more likely to find neutrophils than later times (beyond 4 days).

Several lines of evidence suggest that neutrophils are activated following exercise. Degranulation of neutrophils apparently occurs, based on increased plasma concentrations of lactoferrin (100% increase immediately after a triathalon) [127] and elastase (50% increase immediately after a 10 km run) [70]. In addition, postexercise plasma lysozyme concentrations increases with concurrent decreases in neutrophil lysozyme content [87].

Monocytes

Monocytes circulate with a half-life of about 3 days, and their life span is thought to be on the order of months after egress into tissue [59]. Within tissue, monocytes undergo morphological and functional differentiation, becoming macrophages. During inflammation, monocytes accumulate at the site of injury by chemotaxis. Like neutrophils, monocytes and macrophages are capable of phagocytosis and secretion of cytotoxic factors [1], but in addition, these cells are prime sources of cytokines that mediate most of the physiological and inflammatory reactions accompanying injury and infection [33]. Cytokines, especially IL-1 and TNF, influence leukocytes and organ function throughout the body.

Substantial numbers of mononuclear cells were found in muscle interstitium 24 hours after completion of a marathon [55], and in the muscle of rats 24 hours after eccentrically biased exercise [5]. In some studies of eccentric exercise in humans, 4 to 7 days elapsed before significant accumulations of mononuclear cells were observed [61, 110]. These cells bring with them not only phagocytic and clearance capabilities, but also the capacity to promote repair. Carlson and Faulkner [23, p. 190] have stressed the importance of the macrophage in no uncertain terms: "Unless the damaged muscle fiber becomes invaded by macrophages, it remains arrested in the stage of intrinsic degeneration, and the activation of satellite cells and regeneration proceed no further." Macrophages secrete fibronectin and proteoglycans that help stabilize the extracellular matrix, promote cell adhesion [90], and stimulate fibroblast proliferation [114] and collagen synthesis [73] by means of IL-1. Immunohistochemical evidence of IL-1 has been observed in muscle up to 5 days following eccentric exercise [20].

Kelso et al. [65] have found that pentose phosphate pathway enzyme activity attributable to macrophages and fibroblasts was increased sevenfold by 7 days, and remained for at least 21 days, following muscle overload by removal of synergists. This elevated pentose phosphate activity in damaged or overloaded muscle may contribute to the prolonged state of glycogen depletion observed after eccentric exercise [97].

Cytokines and Acute Phase Proteins
Although exceedingly diverse, cytokine-mediated reactions are functionally related. At the site of injury, cytokines potentiate cytotoxic and inflammatory mechanisms. For example, TNF induces production of oxygen radicals and release of proteolytic enzymes from neutrophils. Both IL-1 and TNF alter endothelial permeability, leading to leukocyte infiltration and edema [88]. Systemically, cytokines promote adaptations that protect the organism as a whole. Injection of IL-1 or TNF into laboratory animals causes liberation of branched-chain amino acids from skeletal muscle [91]. This proteolysis is thought to provide a pool of free amino acids needed to support cytokine-accelerated rates of hepatic protein synthesis. The action on the liver is selective: plasma concentrations of some proteins, such as C-reactive protein (CRP), can

increase 1000-fold in severe injury [75], while albumin synthesis declines. One of the functions of CRP appears to be opsonization of pathogens, and in a model of muscle injury CRP has been shown to localize in the affected tissue, possibly serving as an opsonin for damaged cells [105]. Other plasma proteins that increase as a result of cytokine-stimulated hepatic protein synthesis include antioxidant enzymes (such as ceruloplasmin) and antiproteases (including $a_1$antitrypsin) that neutralize oxygen radicals and proteases distal to the site of injury. Increased intracellular concentrations of antioxidant enzymes such as catalase, superoxide dismutase [135], and metallothionein [64] are also promoted by IL-1.

The first evidence linking exercise to the acute phase response comes from the studies of Haralambie et al. [51, 52], Poortmans and Haralambie [103], and Rocker et al. [108], who compared chronic levels of acute-phase proteins in trained versus untrained subjects, and from Liesen et al. [77], who documented transient changes in acute phase reactants following a 3-hour run. Acute phase plasma protein concentrations are sometimes elevated immediately after unusually long-duration exercise, such as an 100 km run [103], but normally these concentrations are not significantly increased until approximately 24 hours after exercise. The investigations cited above, along with more recent investigations [57, 127], have shown that CRP, $a_1$antitrypsin, $a_2$macroglobulin, ceruloplasmin, and transferrin concentrations all increase significantly following long-duration ($\geqslant 2$ hours) exercise, whereas albumin concentrations decrease [122].

The primary mediators of acute phase protein synthesis are IL-1, IL-6, and TNF. Cannon and Kluger [21] demonstrated that 1 hour of concentric cycling at 60% of aerobic capacity resulted in increased IL-1 activity in the circulation about 3 hours later. Furthermore, monocytes isolated after exercise exhibited enhanced release of IL-1 activity in that study and others involving human subjects [76] and animals [81]. IL-1 activity increased following eccentric exercise in plasma from untrained subjects [39]. In contrast, the trained subjects in the same investigation exhibited elevated plasma IL-1 activity in resting samples, which is in line with the observations that acute-phase protein concentrations are elevated in trained persons. There also is recent evidence that plasma TNF increased after a 2.5-hour run [37], with a time course similar to IL-1, and that plasma IL-6 activity was increased twofold after a marathon [96].

Trace Metals

Inflammation, or systemic administration of IL-1 or TNF, causes a redistribution of trace metals within the body: plasma iron and zinc concentrations fall and plasma copper concentrations rise [62]. The ability to sequester iron in intracellular depots during infection reduces the availability of this nutrient to bacteria that require it for growth and replication [134]. The adaptive value of the redistribution of the other metals is not understood at present.

Physical training is associated with reductions in hematocrit, blood hemoglobin concentration, and plasma iron concentration [50]. These changes have sometimes been mistaken for an iron deficiency and termed "runner's anemia." In fact, hematocrit and hemoglobin concentrations are lower because of the increases in plasma volume that are a part of the training response. Magnusson and co-workers [80] have demonstrated that total red cell numbers and hemoglobin mass in the circulation are usually increased, and erythropoiesis is normal in highly trained individuals. The chronically lower plasma iron concentration in trained subjects is accompanied by lower plasma zinc [16] and higher plasma copper concentrations [51], and is most likely another manifestation of the acute phase response [6]. Furthermore, acute changes in plasma iron [127], zinc [99], and copper [52] have been observed after long-duration exercise. These changes in plasma iron concentrations may have adaptive value in reducing oxidative stress. Iron catalyzes the production of highly reactive oxygen radicals and converts lipid peroxides to cytotoxic aldehydes [6]. As exercise is associated with increases in oxygen radical-induced lipid peroxidation [100], lowering plasma iron and subsequent formation of deleterious oxygen radicals may reduce damage to tissues during exercise. In addition, most of the copper in the circulation is complexed with the antioxidant ceruloplasmin [49]. Thus, increased plasma copper concentrations may be an indirect indication of another adaptation aimed at preventing oxidative damage.

ULTRASTRUCTURAL DAMAGE

Exercise causes a number of immediate and delayed ultrastructural and histochemical changes in skeletal muscle. Highman and Altland [54] demonstrated that long-duration endurance exercise produced a marked number of necrotic muscle cells. They also found that tissue necrosis was not present in the postexercise muscle of endurance-trained rats (20 consecutive days of 6 hours of walking). The necrotic or partially necrotic muscle fibers were infiltrated with macrophages or large mononuclear cells. Jones and co-workers [61] examined muscle biopsies from eccentrically exercised muscles immediately after the exercise and in at least one subject up to 20 days later. Using histochemical techniques, they found minimal evidence of damage immediately after and up to 7 days after the exercise. However, later biopsies contained many fibers and endo- and perimysial areas infiltrated with mononuclear cells, with maximal infiltration seen at 12 days following the exercise. Long-distance running events such as the marathon also cause extensive skeletal muscle damage. Warhol and co-workers [133] examined the ultrastructure of biopsies taken from the gastrocnemius muscle of runners immediately after and up to 12 weeks after a marathon. They showed a characteristic pattern of muscle damage, with tearing of sarcomeres at the Z-band level followed by movement of fluid into the muscle cells. Mitochondrial and myofibrillar damage showed progressive repair by 3 to 4 weeks after the marathon. Late biopsies (8 to 12 weeks after the race) showed central nuclei and satellite cells characteristic of a regenerative response. Biopsies taken from veteran marathon runners displayed intracellular collagen deposition suggestive of a fibrotic response to repetitive injury [133]. The damage seen by these and other investigators [55] is similar to the damage resulting from eccentric exercise.

Friden et al. [43] examined ultrastructural changes in human skeletal muscle after high-tension eccentric exercise. The sore muscles showed disturbances of the cross-striated band pattern, with disorganized myofibrillar material making up $\frac{1}{3}$, $\frac{1}{2}$, and $\frac{1}{10}$ of the total amount of tissue analyzed 1 hour, 3 and 6 days after exercise, respectively. These lesions were localized in the Z-band, indicating that the Z-band may be the weak link in the chain of contractile units. He also found that eccentric exercise training reduced the risk for muscle soreness and myofibrillar lesions and improved strength. Biopsies taken 10 days after eccentric exercise [97] reveal necrotic fibers that can be characterized by loss of myofibrillar organization, mitochondrial alterations, incomplete glycogen repletion, and inflammatory cell infiltration.

Like Friden, Newham et al. [94] found that the eccentrically exercised leg in their stepping protocol exhibited some immediate damage, but biopsies taken 24 to 48 hours after the exercise had more marked damage and involved a greater number of muscle fibers. No damage was seen in any of the biopsies from the muscles exercised concentrically.

PROTEIN METABOLISM

Hydrolytic Enzymes

The fact that eccentric exercise causes more extensive delayed damage, rather than immediate damage, indicates that there is continued active myofibrillar protein degradation. Vihko et al. [130] found muscle fiber necrosis and a marked increase in the activities of a number of acid hydrolases 5 days after exhaustive exercise in untrained but not trained mice. They, like Friden et al. [43], found that exercise training caused an apparent resistance to the damaging effects of exercise. They concluded that this increased hydrolase activity reflects an increase in muscle protein turnover. Salminen et al. [111] found that the lysosomal response to prolonged running was age-related, but only after exercise that caused necrotic and inflammatory changes in muscle.

Calcium Ion (Ca^{2+})

One possible stimulator of skeletal muscle protein turnover is an increase in intracellular [Ca^{2+}]. A postexercise elevation in intramuscular [Ca^{2+}] could result from damage from the sarcoplasmic reticulum (SR), failure of the SR to take up Ca^{2+} following activation, or diffusion of extracellular Ca^{2+} through the exercise-damaged sarcolemma. Extracellular [Ca^{2+}] is 10^3–10^4 greater than that inside cells and, when cell membranes are damaged, [Ca^{2+}] enters the cells along a steep concentration gradient [40]. Bupivacaine has been used to produce muscle injury experimentally [15]. When incubated with bupivacaine, intact isolated skeletal muscles demonstrate a large efflux of CK into the incubation media. If the culture medium is free of Ca^{2+}, however, the bupivacaine-induced CK release is greatly reduced during the first hour of incubation [125]. Calcium has been shown to increase muscle protein turnover [13], perhaps by increasing prostaglandin E_2 (PGE_2) production [14], a proposed stimulator of skeletal muscle breakdown [109]. Duan and co-workers [34] found a significant inverse relationship (r = -0.91, P < 0.05) between mitochondrial [Ca^{2+}] (a good indicator of sarcoplasmic [Ca^{2+}]) and intact muscle fibers 2 days after downhill treadmill walking. They also found that attenuating the rise in mitochondrial [Ca^{2+}], by blocking the entry of extracellular Ca^{2+} with verapamil, or chelating Ca^{2+} with EDTA and EGTA, significantly increased the number of intact, noninjured fibers. These data suggest that Ca^{2+} is an important stimulator of skeletal muscle protein breakdown.

Cytokines

Several studies have linked cytokines to the muscle breakdown associated with trauma and sepsis. A 4 kD protein isolated from the plasma of septic patients caused muscle proteolysis in vitro [28]. When natural, monocyte-derived IL-1 was found to induce the same effect, the plasma factor was thought to be a fragment of IL-1 [14]. Injection of natural IL-1 into laboratory animals caused increases in tyrosine oxidation and urinary 3-methylhistidine excretion [136], but intact recombinant IL-1 (17 kD) does not produce proteolysis consistently [86]. Clowes et al. [27] reported that fragments of recombinant IL-1 do induce proteolysis in vitro, but these data conflict with a recent report by Goldberg et al. [48]. Likewise, conflicting data have been reported regarding the ability of recombinant TNF to induce proteolysis [102, 66]. In addition, Moldawer et al. [86] report that recombinant IL-1 and TNF will induce PGE_2 in muscle tissue, but Goldberg et al. [48] claim they do not. Generally speaking, evidence from in vivo experiments indicates that IL-1 and TNF are involved in muscle protein catabolism, but in vitro experiments often do not support this concept. It is possible that these cytokines require a cofactor or processing (i.e., cleavage to 4 kDa), or they are intermediaries that induce another factor that acts on the muscle itself.

Anti-inflammatory Drugs

The hypothesis that muscle proteolysis requires the induction of PGE_2 which then stimulates lysosomal release of proteases has been tested by several investigators using cyclooxygenase inhibitors. Some researchers have been unable to reduce proteolysis associated with IL-1 infusion [121], sepsis [53], or muscle damaged by burns [98], calcium ionophore or dinitrophenol [58], or following eccentric exercise [74]. On the other hand, lipoxygenase inhibitors reduced creatine kinase efflux following calcium ionophore or dinitrophenol-induced muscle injury [58], but not protein degradation rates after full-thickness burn injury [98]. Perhaps the severity of the injury accounts for this discrepancy. The burn-induced proteolysis was reduced by high doses of indomethacin which the author contended was due to reduced lysosomal protease activity through a noncyclooxygenase pathway. Salminen and Kihlström [112] also found that indomethacin would block the lysosomal protease activity and ultrastructural muscle damage induced in mice by prolonged exercise. Thus, although pharmacological evidence argues against PGE_2 as the mediator of proteolysis, a mechanism involving lipoxygenase products or other arachidonic acid metabolites that stimulate lysosomal proteases remains tenable. It should be kept in mind, however, that indomethacin is not a specific inhibitor of cyclooxygenase, but affects several enzymes involved in arachidonic acid metabolism, as well as cyclic nucleotide and pyrimidine metabolism [38].

Hypertrophy

Whether the stimulus for altered rates of protein turnover is increased intramuscular $[Ca^{2+}]$, an immunological factor (summarized in Figure 3.4), or a combination of several factors, exercise-induced muscle damage leads to a long-term increase in protein breakdown and synthesis [39, 41]. These studies suggest that exercise of sufficient intensity to cause some skeletal muscle damage will cause long-term changes in muscle protein metabolism.

Few studies have compared the longitudinal effects of high-intensity eccentric and concentric exercise training. Most progressive resistance-training devices and free weights have substantial concentric and eccentric components. The study by Komi and Buskirk [71] described earlier showed that arm circumference increased only in the arm trained eccentrically. Ciriello et al. [24] examined the effects of 4 months of high-intensity strength training on a Cybex isokinetic dynamometer which has little or no eccentric component. Although the strength of

FIGURE 3.4

Proposed roles of acute phase reactants in delayed muscle damage. Muscle tissue fragments resulting from physical overload or ischemia activate complement (1). C3a, C5a and tissue fragments serve as chemoattractants and activators of neutrophils (2). Neutrophils (and later, monocytes and macrophages) phagocytize damaged tissue (3). Neutrophils (and monocytes) release oxygen radicals, degradative enzymes that further break down muscle (4) as well as increase vascular permeability (5). Monocytes further enhance neutrophil activation by means of secretion of TNF (6), and stimulate hepatic acute phase protein synthesis by means of IL-1, TNF, and IL-6 (7). Some acute phase proteins, such as ceruloplasmin and a₁antitrypsin, neutralize cytotoxic products that stray away from the site of injury (8); others, such as CRP, opsonize damaged tissue (9). Cytokines promote transendothelial transit of leukocytes (10), muscle proteolysis (11), and production of growth factors (12).

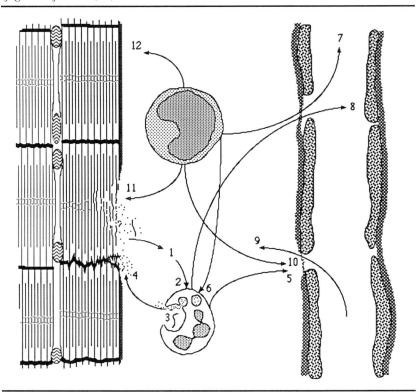

the subjects increased significantly, there was no evidence of hypertrophy of Type I or Type II muscle fibers. Pierson and Costill [101] examined the effects of a progressive resistance weight-training protocol (with eccentric and concentric components) on one leg and isokinetic training (with no eccentric component) on the contralateral leg. Only the leg trained with a significant eccentric component increased in size because of the training. These studies certainly suggest that eccentric exercise-induced skeletal muscle damage and its subsequent repair are important for increasing muscle fiber size in response to strength training.

SUMMARY

Exercise-induced skeletal muscle damage results in a remarkable number of localized and systemic changes, including release of intracellular proteins, delayed onset muscle soreness, the acute-phase response, and an increase in skeletal muscle protein turnover. These exercise-induced adaptations appear to be integral to the repair of the damaged muscle and may be essential for hypertrophy. Chronic exercise produces adaptations in skeletal muscle, resulting in increased capacity of oxidative metabolism; the repair of damaged muscle resulting in hypertrophy may be an important mechanism for protection against further exercise-induced damage. Although the release of CK from skeletal muscle following damage is a commonly observed phenomenon, circulating CK activity is not a quantitative and, in some cases, even a qualitative indicator of skeletal muscle damage. Eccentric exercise-induced skeletal muscle damage offers an opportunity to investigate the signals and modulators of the repair of muscle damage, a process that may be central to the adaptations in muscle as a result of chronic activity.

ACKNOWLEDGEMENTS

This project has been funded in part by federal grants from the U.S. Department of Agriculture, Agricultural Research Service under contract number 53-3K06-5-10 and by National Institutes of Health grant number AR 39595. The contents of this chapter do not necessarily reflect the views or policies of either agency, nor does mention of trade names, commercial products, or organizations imply endorsement by the U.S. government.

REFERENCES

1. Adams, D.O., and T.A. Hamilton. Phagocytic cells: cytotoxic activities of macrophages. J.I. Gallin, I.M. Goldstein and R. Snyderman (eds.). *Inflammation: Basic Principles and Clinical Correlates.* New York: Raven Press, 1988, pp. 471–492.

2. Amelink, G.J., and P.R. Bär. Exercise-induced muscle protein leakage in the rat. *J. Neurol. Sci.* 76:61–68, 1986.

3. Apple, F.S., and M. Rhodes. Enzymatic estimation of skeletal muscle damage by analysis of changes in serum creatine kinase. *J. Appl. Physiol.* 65:2598–2600, 1988.

4. Armstrong, R.B. Mechanisms of exercise-induced delayed onset muscular soreness: a brief review. *Med. Sci. Sports. Exerc.* 16:529–538, 1984.

5. Armstrong, R.B., R.W. Ogilvie, and J.A. Schwane. Eccentric exercise-induced injury to rat skeletal muscle. *J. Appl. Physiol.* 54:80–93, 1983.

6. Aruoma, O.I., T. Reilly, D. MacLaren, and B. Halliwell. Iron, copper, and zinc concentrations in human sweat and plasma; the effect of exercise. *Clin Chim Acta.* 177:81–88, 1988.

7. Asmussen, E. Positive and negative muscular work. *Acta Physiol. Scand.* 28:364–382, 1953.

8. Asmussen, E. Observations on experimental muscular soreness. *Acta Rhum. Scand.* 2:109–116, 1956.

9. Aura, O., and P.V. Komi. Mechanical efficiency of pure positive and pure negative work with special reference to the work intensity. *Int. J. Sports Med.* 7:44–49, 1986.

10. Babior, B.M., R.S. Kipnes, and J.T. Curnutte. The production by leukocytes of superoxide, a potential bactericidal agent. *J. Clin. Invest.* 52:741–744, 1973.

11. Bainton, D.F. Phagocytic cells: development biology of neutrophils and eosinophils. J.I. Gallin, I.M. Goldstein, and R. Snyderman (eds.). *Inflammation: Basic Principles and Clinical Correlates.* New York: Raven Press, 1988, pp. 265–280.

12. Bär, P.R., M.F. Driessen, B. Rikken, and F.G.I. Jennekens. Muscle protein leakage after strenuous exercise: sex and chronological differences. *Neurosci. Lett.* Suppl. 22:288, 1985.

13. Baracos, V., R.E. Greenburg, and A.L. Goldberg. Influence of calcium and other divalent cations on protein turnover in rat skeletal muscle. *Am. J. Physiol.* 250:E702–E710, 1986.

14. Baracos, V., H.P. Rodemann, C.A. Dinarello, and A.L. Goldberg. Stimulation of muscle protein degradation and prostaglandin E2 release by leukocytic pyrogen (Interleukin-1). *N. Engl. J. Med.* 308:553–558, 1983.

15. Benoit, P.W., and W.D. Belt. Destruction and regeneration of skeletal muscle after treatment with a local anaesthetic, Bupivacaine (Marcaine). *J. Anat. (Lond.).* 107:547–556, 1970.

16. Berg, A., F. Kieffer, and J. Keul. Acute and chronic effects of endurance exercise on serum zinc levels. G. Benzi, L. Packer and N. Siliprandi (eds.). *Biochemical aspects of physical exercise.* Amsterdam: Elsevier, 1986, pp. 201–217.

17. Bobbert, M.F., A.P. Hollander, and P.A. Huijing. Factors in delayed onset muscular soreness. *Med. Sci. Sports Exerc.* 18:75–81, 1986.

18. Brendstrup, P. Late edema after muscular exercise. *Arch. Phys. Med. Rehab.* 401–405, 1962.

19. Byrnes, W.C., P.M. Clarkson, J.S. White, S.S. Hsieh, P.N. Frykman, and R.J. Maughan. Delayed onset muscle soreness following repeated bouts of downhill running. *J. Appl. Physiol.* 59:710–715, 1985.

20. Cannon, J.G., R.A. Fielding, M.A. Fiatarone, S.F. Orencole, C.A. Dinarello, and W.J. Evans. Interleukin-1β in human skeletal muscle following exercise. *Am. J. Physiol.* 257:R451–R455, 1989.

21. Cannon, J.G., and M.J. Kluger. Endogenous pyrogen activity in human plasma after exercise. *Science* 220:617–619, 1983.

22. Cannon, J.G., S.F. Orencole, R.A. Fielding, et al. The acute phase response in exercise. The interaction of age and vitamin E on neutrophils and muscle enzyme release. *Am. J. Physiol.* in press.

23. Carlson, B.M., and J.A. Faulkner. The regeneration of skeletal muscle fibers following injury: a review. *Med. Sci. Sports Exerc.* 15:187–198, 1983.

24. Ciriello, V.M., W.L. Holden, and W.J. Evans. The effects of two isokinetic training regimens on muscle strength and fiber composition. H.G. Knuttgen, J.A. Vogel, and J. Poortmans (eds.). *Biochemistry of Exercise.* Champaign, IL: Human Kinetics Publishers, Inc., 1983, pp. 787–793.

25. Clarkson, P.M., W.C. Byrnes, K.M. McCormic, and P. Triffletti. Muscle soreness and serum creatine kinase activity following isometric eccentric and concentric exercise. *Int. J. Sports Med.* 7:51–56, 1986.

26. Clarkson, P.M., and C. Ebbling. Investigation of serum creatine kinase variability after muscle damaging exercise. *Clin. Sci.* 75:257–261, 1988.

27. Clowes, G.H.A., B.C. George, S. Bosari, and W. Love. Induction of muscle protein degradation by recombinant interleukin-1 and its spontaneously occurring fragments. *J. Leukocyte Biol.* 42:547–548, 1987.

28. Clowes, G.H.A., B.C. George, C.A. Villee Jr., and C.A. Saravis. Muscle proteolysis induced by a circulating peptide in patients with sepsis or trauma. *N. Engl. J. Med.* 380:545–552, 1983.

29. Davies, C.T.M., and M.J. White. Muscle weakness following eccentric work in man. *Pflügers Arch.* 392:168–171, 1981.

30. Davis, J.M., and J.I. Gallin. The neutrophil. J.J. Oppenheim, D.L. Rosenstreich, and M. Potter (eds.). *Cellular Functions in Immunity and Inflammation.* New York: Elsevier North Holland, 1981, pp. 77–102.

31. Dick, R.W., and P.R. Cavanaugh. An explanation of the upward drift in oxygen uptake during prolonged sub-maximal downhill running. *Med. Sci. Sports Exerc.* 19:310–317, 1987.

32. Diederichs, F., K. Mühlhaus, I. Trautschold, and R. Friedel. On the mechanism of lactate dehydrogenase release from skeletal muscle in relation to the control of cell volume. *Enzyme* 24:404–415, 1979.

33. Dinarello, C.A., J.G. Cannon, and S.M. Wolff. New concepts in the pathogenesis of fever. *Rev. Infect. Diseases* 10:16189, 1988.

34. Duan, C., M.D. Delp, D.A. Hayes, P.D. Delp, and R.B. Armstrong. Rat skeletal muscle mitochondrial $[Ca^{2+}]$ and injury from downhill walking. *J. Appl. Physiol.* 68:1241–1251, 1990.

35. Dufaux, B., R. Muller, and W. Hollmann. Assessment of circulating immune complexes by a solid-phase C_{1q}-binding assay during the first hours and days after prolonged exercise. *Clin. Chim. Acta* 145:313–317, 1985.

36. Dufaux, B., and U. Order. Complement activation after prolonged exercise. *Clin. Chim. Acta* 179:45–50, 1989.

37. Dufaux, B., and U. Order. Plasma elastase-α1-antitrypsin, neopterin, tumor necrosis factor, and soluble interleukin-2 receptor after prolonged exercise. *Int. J. Sports Med.* 10:1–5, 1989.

38. Dunn, M.J., and V.L. Hood. Prostaglandins and the kidney. *Am. J. Physiol.* 233:F169–F184, 1977.

39. Evans, W.J., C.N. Meredith, J.G. Cannon, et al. Metabolic changes following eccentric exercise in trained and untrained men. *J. Appl. Physiol.* 61:1864–1868, 1986.

40. Farber, J.L. The role of calcium in cell death. *Life Sci.* 29:1289–1295, 1981.

41. Fielding, R.A., C.A. Meredith, K.P. O'Reilly, W.R. Frontera, J.G. Cannon, and W.J. Evans. Enhanced protein breakdown following eccentric exercise in young and old men. *J. Appl. Physiol.* in press, 1991.

42. Foster, N.K., J.B. Martyn, R.E. Rangno, J.C. Hogg, and R.L. Pardy. Leukocytosis of exercise: role of cardiac output and catecholamines. *J. Appl. Physiol.* 61:2218–2223, 1986.

43. Friden, J., J. Seger, M. Sjostrom, and B. Ekblom. Adaptive response in human skeletal muscle subjected to prolonged eccentric training. *Int. J. Sports Med.* 4:177–183, 1983.

44. Friden, J., P.N. Sfakianos, and A.R. Hargens. Muscle soreness and intramuscular

fluid pressure: comparison between eccentric and concentric load. *J. Appl. Physiol.* 61:2175–2179, 1986.

45. Friden, J., P.N. Sfakianos, and A.R. Hargens. Blood indices of muscle injury associated with eccentric muscle contractions. *J. Orth. Res.* 7:142–145, 1989.

46. Friden, J., P.N. Sfakianos, A.R. Hargens, and W.H. Akeson. Residual muscular swelling after repetitive eccentric contractions. *J. Orth. Res.* 6:493–498, 1988.

47. Gauduel, Y., P. Menasche, and M. Duvelleroy. Enzyme release and mitochondrial activity in reoxygenated cardiac muscle: relationship with oxygen-induced lipid peroxidation. *Gen. Physiol. Biophys.* 8:327–340, 1989.

48. Goldberg, A.L., I.C. Kettelhut, K. Furuno, J.M. Fagan, and V. Baracos. Activation of protein breakdown and prostaglandin E_2 production in rat skeletal muscle in fever is signaled by a macrophage product distinct from interleukin-1 or other known monokines. *J. Clin. Invest.* 81:1378–1383, 1988.

49. Gutteridge, J.M.C., and J. Stocks. Ceruloplasmin: physiological and pathological perspectives. *CRC Crit. Rev. Clin. Lab. Sci.* 14:257–329, 1981.

50. Hallberg, L., and B. Magnusson. The etiology of "sports anemia." *Acta Med. Scand.* 216:145–148, 1984.

51. Haralambie, G., and J. Keul. Serum glycoprotein levels in athletes in training. *Experentia* 26:959–960, 1970.

52. Haralambie, G., J. Keul, and F. Theumert. Protein, eisen, und kupfer veranderungen im serum bei schwimmern vor und nach hohentraining. *Eur. J. Appl. Physiol.* 35:21–31, 1976.

53. Hasselgren, P., P. Pedersen, H.C. Sax, B.W. Warner, and J.E. Fischer. Current concepts of protein turnover and amino acid transport in liver and skeletal muscle during sepsis. *Arch. Surg.* 123:992–999, 1988.

54. Highman, B., and P.D. Altland. Effects of exercise and training on serum enzyme and tissue changes in rats. *Am. J. Physiol.* 205:162–166, 1963.

55. Hikida, R.S., R.S. Staron, F.C. Hagerman, W.M. Sherman, and D.L. Costill. Muscle fiber necrosis associated with human marathon runners. *J. Neuro. Sci.* 59:185–203, 1983.

56. Hunter, J.B., and J.B. Critz. Effect of training on plasma enzyme levels in man. *J. Appl. Physiol.* 31:20–23, 1971.

57. Irving, R.A., T.D. Noakes, G.A. Irving, and R.V. Zyl-Smit. The immediate and delayed effects of marathon running on renal function. *J. Urol.* 136:1176–1180, 1986.

58. Jackson, M.J., A.J.M. Wagenmakers, and R.H.T. Edwards. Effect of inhibitors of arachidonic acid metabolism on efflux of intracellular enzymes from skeletal muscle following experimental damage. *Biochem. J.* 241:403–407, 1987.

59. Johnston, R.B. Monocytes and macrophages. *N. Engl. J. Med.* 318:747–752, 1988.

60. Jones, D.A., M.J. Jackson, and R.H.T. Edwards. Release of intracellular enzymes from an isolated mammalian skeletal muscle preparation. *Clin. Sci.* 65:193–201, 1983.

61. Jones, D.A., D.J. Newham, J.M. Round, and S.E.J. Tolfree. Experimental human muscle damage: morphological changes in relation to other indices of damage. *J. Physiol. (London)* 375:435–448, 1986.

62. Kampschmidt, R. Leukocytic endogenous mediator/endogenous pyrogen. P.G.C.M.C. Powanda (ed.). *The Physiologic and Metabolic Responses of the Host.* Amsterdam: Elsevier/North Holland, 1981, pp. 55–74.

63. Kanter, M.M., G.R. Lesmes, L.A. Kaminsky, J. La-Ham-Saeger, and N.D. Nequin. Serum creatine kinase and lactate dehydrogenase changes following an eighty kilometer race. Relationship to lipid peroxidation. *Eur. J. Appl. Physiol.* 57:60–63, 1988.

64. Karin, M., R.J. Imbra, A. Heguy, and G. Wong. Interleukin-1 regulates human metallothionein gene expression. *Molec. Cell. Biol.* 5:2866–2869, 1985.

65. Kelso, T.B., C.R. Shear, and S.R. Max. Enzymes of glutamine metabolism in inflammation associated with skeletal muscle hypertrophy. *Am. J. Physiol.* 257:E885–E894, 1989.

66. Kettlehut, I.C., and A.L. Goldberg. Tumor necrosis factor can induce fever in rats without activating protein breakdown in muscle or lipolysis in adipose tissue. *J. Clin. Invest.* 81:1384–1389, 1988.

67. Kihlström, M., H. Kainulainen, and A. Salminen. Enzymatic and nonenzymatic lipid peroxidation capacities and antioxidants in hypoxic and reoxygenated rat myocardium. *Exper. Mol. Pathol.* 50:230–238, 1989.

68. Klausen, K., and H. Knuttgen. Effect of training on oxygen consumption in negative muscular work. *Acta Physiol. Scand.* 83:319–323, 1971.

69. Knuttgen, H.G., E.R. Nadel, K.B. Pandolf, and J.F. Patton. Effects of training with eccentric muscle contractions on exercise performance, energy expenditure, and body temperature. *Int. J. Sports Med.* 3:13–17, 1982.

70. Kokot, K., R.M. Schaefer, M. Teschner, U. Gilge, R. Plass, and A. Heidland. Activation of leukocytes during prolonged physical exercise. *Adv. Exp. Med. Biol.* 240:57–63, 1988.

71. Komi, P.V., and E.B. Buskirk. Effect of eccentric and concentric muscle conditioning on tension and electrical activity of human muscle. *Ergonomics* 15:417–434, 1972.

72. Kopprasch, S., H. Orlik, and D.W. Scheuch. Kinetic aspects of enzyme activity changes in blood plasma during canine hemorrhagic shock. *Enzyme* 34:122–128, 1985.

73. Krane, S.M., J.M. Dayer, L.S. Simon, and S. Byrne. Mononuclear cell conditioned medium containing mononuclear cell factor, homologous with interleukin-1, stimulates collagen and fibronectin synthesis by adherent rheumatoid synovial cells: effects of prostaglandin E_2 and indomethacin. *Collagen Rel.* 5:99–117, 1985.

74. Kuipers, H., H.A. Keizer, F.T.J. Verstappen, and D.L. Costill. Influence of a prostaglandin-inducing drug on muscle soreness after eccentric work. *Int. J. Sports Med.* 6:336–339, 1985.

75. Kushner, I. The phenomenon of the acute phase response. I. J. Kushner, E. Volanakis, and H. Gewurz (eds.). *C-Reactive Protein and the Plasma Protein Response to Tissue Injury.* New York: Annals of the New York Academy of Sciences, 1982, pp. 39–48.

76. Lewicki, R., H. Tchorzewski, E. Majewska, Z. Nowak, and Z. Baj. Effect of maximal physical exercise on T-lymphocyte subpopulations and on interleukin-1 (IL-1) and interleukin-2 (IL-2) production in vitro. *Int. J. Sports Med.* 9:114–117, 1988.

77. Liesen, H., B. Dufaux, and W. Hollman. Modifications of serum glycoproteins the days following a prolonged physical exercise and the influence of physical training. *Eur. J. Appl. Physiol.* 37:243–254, 1977.

78. Linas, S.L., P.F. Shanley, D. Whittenburg, E. Berger, and J.E. Repine. Neutrophils accentuate ischemia-reperfusion injury in isolated perfused rat kidney. *Am. J. Physiol.* 255:F728–F735, 1988.

79. Macknight, A.D.C., and A. Leaf. Regulation of cellular volume. *Physiol. Rev.* 57:510–573, 1977.

80. Magnusson, B., L. Hallberg, L. Rossander, and B. Swolin. Iron metabolism and "sports anemia": a hematological comparison of elite runners and control subjects. *Acta Ned. Scand.* 216:157–164, 1984.

81. Mahan, M.P., and M.R. Young. Immune parameters of untrained of exercise-trained rats after exhaustive exercise. *J. Appl. Physiol.* 66:282–287, 1989.

82. Malech, H.L., and J.I. Gallin. Neutrophils in human diseases. *N. Engl. J. Med.* 317:687–694, 1987.

83. Manfredi, T.G., R.A. Fielding, K.P. O'Reilly, C.N. Meredith, H.Y. Lee, and W.J. Evans. Serum creatine kinase activity and exercise-induced muscle damage in older men. *Med. Sci. Sports Exerc.* (in press), 1991.

84. McCord, J.M. Oxygen-derived free radicals in postischemic tissue injury. *N. Engl. J. Med.* 312:159–163, 1985.
85. Meltzer, H.Y. Lack of effect of ouabain on creatine phosphokinase efflux from skeletal muscle. *Biochem. Pharm.* 24:419–421, 1975.
86. Moldawer, L.L., G. Svaninger, J. Gelin, and K.G. Lundholm. Interleukin-1 and tumor necrosis factor do not regulate protein balance in skeletal muscle. *Am. J. Physiol.* 253:C766–C773, 1987.
87. Morozov, V.I., S.A. Priatkin, and I.B. Nazarov. Secretion of lysozyme by blood neutrophils during physical exertion. *Fiziol. Zh. SSSR* 75:334–337, 1989.
88. Movat, H.Z., M.I. Cybulsky, I.G. Colditz, M.K.W. Chan, and C.A. Dinarello. Acute inflammation in gram-negative infection: endotoxin, interleukin-1, tumor necrosis factor and neutrophils. *Fed. Proc.* 46:97–104, 1987.
89. Muller-Eberhard, H.J. Complement: chemistry and pathways. J.I. Gallin, I.M. Goldstein, and R. Snyderman (eds.). *Inflammation: Basic Principles and Clinical Correlates*. New York: Raven Press, 1988, pp. 21–53.
90. Nathan, C.F. Secretory products of macrophages. *J. Clin. Invest.* 79:319–326, 1987.
91. Nawabi, M.D., K.P. Block, M.C. Chakrabarti, and M.G. Buse. Administration of endotoxin, tumor necrosis factor, or interleukin-1 to rats activates skeletal muscle branched-chain α-keto acid dehydrogenase. *J. Clin. Invest.* 85:256–263, 1990.
92. Newham, D.J., D.A. Jones, and P.M. Clarkson. Repeated high-force eccentric exercise: effects on muscle pain and damage. *J. Appl. Physiol.* 63:1381–1386, 1987.
93. Newham, D.J., D.A. Jones, and R.H.T. Edwards. Large delayed plasma creatine kinase changes after stepping exercise. *Muscle Nerve* 6:380–385, 1983.
94. Newham, D.J., G. McPhail, K.R. Mills, and R.H.T. Edwards. Ultrastructural changes after concentric and eccentric contractions of human muscle. *J. Neur. Sci.* 61:109–122, 1983.
95. Nielsen, B., S.L. Nielsen, and F.B. Petersen. Thermoregulation during positive and negative work at different environmental temperatures. *Acta Physiol. Scand.* 85:249–257, 1972.
96. Northoff, H., W. Flegel, D. Mannel, and A. Berg. Increased levels of interleukin-6 in sera from long-distance runners. *Cytokine.* 1:140 (abstract), 1989.
97. O'Reilly, K.P., M.J. Warhol, R.A. Fielding, W.R. Frontera, C.N. Meredith, and W.J. Evans. Eccentric exercise-induced muscle damage impairs muscle glycogen repletion. *J. Appl. Physiol.* 63:252–256, 1987.
98. Odessey, R. Effect of inhibitors of proteolysis and arachidonic acid metabolism on burn-induced protein breakdown. *Metabolism* 34:616–620, 1985.
99. Oh, S.H., J.T. Deagen, P.D. Whanger, and P.H. Weswig. Biological function of metallothionein. V. Its induction in rats by various stresses. *Am. J. Physiol.* 3:E282–E285, 1978.
100. Packer, L. Vitamin E, physical exercise and tissue damage in animals. *Med. Biol.* 62:105–109, 1984.
101. Pearson, D.R., and D.L. Costill. The effects of constant external resistance exercise and isokinetic exercise training on work-induced hypertrophy. *J. Appl. Sport Sci. Res.* 2:39–41, 1988.
102. Pomposelli, J.J., E.A. Flores, B.R. Bistrian, S. Zeisel, C.A. Dinarello, M. Drabik, and G.L. Blackburn. Dose response of recombinant mediators in the acute phase response. *Clin. Res.* 35:514A, 1987.
103. Poortmans, J.R., and G. Haralambie. Biochemical changes in a 100 km run: proteins in serum and urine. *Eur. J. Appl. Physiol.* 40:245–254, 1979.
104. Powanda, M.C., and E.D. Moyer. Plasma proteins and wound healing. *Surg. Gyn. Obstet.* 153:749–755, 1981.
105. Rees, R.F., H. Gewurz, J.N. Siegel, J. Coon, and L.A. Potempa. Expression of a C-reactive protein neoantigen (neo-CRP) in inflamed rabbit liver and muscle. *Clin. Immunol. Immunopath.* 48:95–107, 1988.

106. Robinson, J.D. Regulating ion pumps to control cell volume. *J. Theoret. Biol.* 19:90–96, 1968.

107. Rocker, L., and I.-W. Franz. Effect of chronic β-adrenergic blockade on exercise-induced leukocytosis. *Klin. Wochenschr.* 64:270–273, 1986.

108. Rocker, L., K.A. Kirsch, and H. Stoboy. Plasma volume, albumin and globulin concentrations and their intravascular masses. A comparative study in endurance athletes and sedentary subjects. *Eur. J. Appl. Physiol.* 36:57–64, 1976.

109. Rodemann, H.P., and A.L. Goldberg. Arachidonic acid, prostaglandin E_2 and F_2 alpha influence rates of protein turnover in rat skeletal muscle. *J. Biol. Chem.* 257:1632–1638, 1982.

110. Round, J.M., D.A. Jones, and G. Cambridge. Cellular infiltrates in human skeletal muscle: exercise-induced damage as a model for inflammatory muscle disease? *J. Neuro. Sci.* 82:1–11, 1987.

111. Salminen, A., H. Kainulainen, and V. Vihko. Lysosomal changes related to ageing and physical exercise in mouse cardiac and skeletal muscles. *Experientia* 38:781–782, 1982.

112. Salminen, A., and M. Kihlstrom. Protective effects of indomethacin against exercise-induced injuries in mouse skeletal muscle fibers. *Int. J. Sports Med.* 8:46–49, 1987.

113. Salminen, A., and V. Vihko. Effects of age and prolonged running on proteolytic capacity in mouse cardiac and skeletal muscles. *Acta Physiol. Scand.* 112:89–95, 1981.

114. Schmidt, J.A., S.B. Mizel, D. Cohen, and I. Green. Interleukin-1, a potential regulator of fibroblast proliferation. *J. Immunol.* 128:2177–2182, 1982.

115. Schwane, J.A., and R.B. Armstrong. Effect of training on skeletal muscle injury from downhill running in rats. *J. Appl. Physiol.* 55:969–975, 1983.

116. Schwane, J.A., S.R. Johnson, and C.B. Vandenakker. Delayed onset muscular soreness and plasma CPK and LDH activities after downhill running. *Med. Sci. Sports Exerc.* 15:51–56, 1983.

117. Shell, W.E., J.K. Kjekshus, and B.E. Sobel. Quantitative assessment of the extent of myocardial infarction in the conscious dog by means of analysis of serial changes in serum creatine phosphokinase activity. *J. Clin. Invest.* 50:2614–2625, 1971.

118. Shumate, J.B., M.H. Brooke, J.E. Carroll, and J.E. Davis. Increased serum creatine kinase after exercise: A sex-linked phenomenon. *Neurology* 29:902–904, 1979.

119. Smith, J.K., M.B. Grisham, D.N. Granger, and R.J. Korthuis. Free radical defense mechanisms and neutrophil infiltration in postischemic skeletal muscle. *Am. J. Physiol.* 256:H789–H793, 1989.

120. Smith, L.L., M. McCammon, S. Smith, M. Chamness, R.G. Israel, and K.F. O'Brien. White blood cell response to uphill walking and downhill jogging at similar metabolic loads. *Eur. J. Appl. Physiol.* 58:833–837, 1989.

121. Sobrado, J., L.L. Moldawer, B.R. Bistrian, C.A. Dinarello, and G.L. Blackburn. Effect of ibuprofen on fever and metabolic changes induced by continuous infusion of leukocytic pyrogen (interleukin-1) or endotoxin. *Infect. Immunol.* 42:997–1005, 1983.

122. Soeder, G., S.W. Golf, V. Graef, H. Temme, A. Brüstle, L. Róka, F. Bertschat, and K. Ibe. Enzyme catalytic concentrations in human plasma after a marathon. *Clin. Biochem.* 22:155–159, 1989.

123. Steel, C.M., J. Evans, and M.A. Smith. Physiological variation in circulating B cell: T cell ratio in man. *Nature* 247:387–388, 1974.

124. Steel, C.M., E.B. French, and W.R.C. Aitchison. Studies on adrenaline-induced leukocytosis in normal man. *Br. J. Haematol.* 21:413–421, 1971.

125. Steer, J.H., F.L. Mastaglia, J.M. Papadimitriou, and I. Van Bruggen. Bupivacaine-induced muscle injury, the role of extracellular calcium. *J. Neurol. Sci.* 73:205–217, 1986.

126. Storrs, S.B., W.P. Kolb, and M.S. Olson. C1q binding and C1 activation by various isolated cellular membranes. *J. Immunol.* 131:416–422, 1983.

127. Taylor, C., G. Rogers, C. Goodman, et al. Hematologic, iron-related, and acute-phase protein responses to sustained strenuous exercise. *J. Appl. Physiol.* 62:464–469, 1987.
128. Thomson, W.H.S., and I. Smith. Effects of oestrogens on erythrocyte enzyme efflux in normal men and women. *Clin. Chim. Acta.* 103:203–208, 1980.
129. Turner, D.C., and H.M. Eppenberger. Developmental changes in creatine kinase and aldolase isoenzymes and their possible function in association with contractile elements. *Enzyme* 15:224–238, 1973.
130. Vihko, V., A. Salminen, and J. Rantamaki. Exhaustive exercise, endurance training, and acid hydrolase activity in skeletal muscle. *J. Appl. Physiol.* 47:43–50, 1979.
131. Wallimann, T., G. Pelloni, D.C. Turner, and H.M. Eppenberger. Monovalent antibodies against MM-creatine kinase remove the M line from myofibrils. *Proc. Natl. Acad. Sci.* 75:4296–4300, 1978.
132. Wallimann, T., D.C. Turner, and H.M. Eppenberger. Localization of creatine kinase isoenzymes in myofibrils. *J. Cell Biology* 75:297–317, 1977.
133. Warhol, M.J., A.J. Siegel, W.J. Evans, and L.M. Silverman. Skeletal muscle injury and repair in marathon runners after competition. *Am. J. Pathol.* 118:331–339, 1985.
134. Weinberg, E.D. Iron withholding: a defense against infection and neoplasia. *Phys. Rev.* 64:65–75, 1984.
135. White, C.W., P. Ghezzi, S. McMahon, C.A. Dinarello, and J.E. Repine. Cytokines increase rat lung antioxidant enzymes during exposure to hyperoxia. *J. Appl. Physiol.* 66:1003–1007, 1989.
136. Yang, R.D., L.L. Moldawer, A. Sakamoto, et al. Leukocyte endogenous mediator alters protein dynamics in rats. *Metabolism* 32:654–660, 1983.
137. Zierler, K.L. Increased muscle permeability to aldolase produced by depolarization and by metabolic inhibitors. *Am. J. Physiol* 193:534–538, 1958.

4
The Biomechanics of Cycling

ROBERT J. GREGOR, Ph.D.
JEFFREY P. BROKER, M.S.
MARY MARGARET RYAN, M.S.

The rhythmic alternating movements of the legs during cycling are important for exercise, rehabilitation, studies in neural control, and mechanics of lower extremity function. The rider's interface with the bicycle also is related to human factors engineering in which the man and machine must work together to reach a certain objective. Because cycling is ubiquitous in many disciplines and related research is found in a variety of journals—both popular and scientific—our review will focus on the biomechanics of cycling, with only selected references to related fields.

Because the general objective of cycling is to reach an end point as effectively as possible, understanding environmental demands is critical. These demands take the form of wind resistance, rolling resistance, gravitational acceleration on altered terrain, and friction within the machinery of the bicycle. The major form of resistance to the rider, of course, is wind. In this review, we briefly discuss the environmental demands imposed on the rider and bicycle, but refer the reader to Kyle [68, 69, 70] for a more in-depth review.

Interfaces between the rider and bicycle include the seat, handlebars, and pedals. Although the interaction at the pedals has received the greatest scientific attention, the impact of seat and handlebar geometry and loading on the performance of the rider-bicycle system cannot be ignored. In the second section of this chapter, we review how loads are imparted to the bicycle at the seat, handlebars, and pedals, provide historical account of the development of pedal force measurement devices, and describe popular methods of representing pedal force application patterns and subsequent motive effectiveness.

Kinematic features of cycling (i.e., displacements, velocities, and accelerations) are principally affected by cadence (pedalling rate), rider-bicycle geometry, hip motion, and ankling pattern. The effects of these operational and configurational variables on cycling performance are of great interest, and are reserved for a discussion of "optimal" cycling systems. The focus of the kinematics section is, therefore, limited to the frontal plane with a discussion of muscle length and velocity changes during cycling.

127

Kinetic features of cycling are reviewed, with particular emphasis placed on joint moment patterns and associated effects of load, cadence, and seat height. We also briefly review joint reaction and varus and valgus loads on the lower extremity in an effort to understand, for example, cycling as a rehabilitative tool for knee patients.

Muscle activation patterns (electromyography–EMG) have been employed extensively to define both function and dysfunction associated with the cycling motion. Literature on EMG in cycling is reviewed in an effort to understand the magnitude of information available and its relevance to performance both in an exercise and in a clinical setting. As an appropriate follow-up to the joint kinetic and EMG sections, a novel experiment is discussed which used direct measurement of muscle forces in conjunction with EMG and muscle length changes to explore, in greater detail, the musculoskeletal mechanics of cycling.

With these data as background, both physiological and mechanical aspects of the cycling task are integrated in a discussion of an "optimal" rider-bicycle representation. We explore experimental and analytical derivations of the "optimal" cycling system, addressing a spectrum of topics from perceived exertion to muscle-stress-based cost functions.

Recent advances in on-line data acquisition systems permit the use of real-time kinematic or kinetic feedback to modify cycling technique. The utility of such feedback environments in the enhancement of cycling performance and the optimization of therapeutic rehabilitation is becoming obvious. In a final section of this chapter the integration of the biomechanics of cycling with questions of neural control, learning, and biofeedback are discussed.

EXTERNAL RESISTIVE FORCES

Aside from factors such as humidity, temperature, and varying terrain, two major categories of resistive or retarding forces affect the rider. The first of these forces is rolling resistance which is inversely proportional to the wheel diameter [117]. Rolling resistance depends on the type of tire as well as the tire pressure. The larger the cross section, the larger the rolling resistance. Dill et al. [27] found that a 71.1×5.4 cm ($28 \times 2\frac{1}{8}$ inch) tire required an oxygen consumption equivalent to 0.19 liters per minute more than when the same rider under the same conditions used a 68.6×3.2 cm (27 inch $\times 1\frac{1}{4}$ inch) tire. A second and much smaller type of friction is found in the internal machinery of the bicycle. This friction accounts for less than 5% of the total resistive forces [36], and gearing has been reported to be 98–99% efficient [118]. Certainly the largest source of drag cyclists must overcome involves aerodynamic loading. The equation for aerodynamic drag is:

$$F = 0.5 \, C_d A \rho v^2 \qquad [1]$$

where F is the drag force, C_d the drag force coefficient, A the area exposed, ρ the density of the air, and v the relative air velocity.

The major way in which aerodynamic drag can be reduced is to decrease the frontal area; for example, crouch down over the handlebars and assume a streamline racing position. In this manner, an average size male cyclist can reduce his frontal area from approximately 0.5 m^2 for touring posture, to approximately 0.35 m^2 in a fully crouched racing position, resulting in an overall 30% reduction in frontal area [36]. As discussed later, going from an upright position to a racing position not only affects the wind resistance but has potential implications for rider-bicycle interface and the ability to transmit power to the bike.

Clothing also is a factor, because a rider wearing smooth, tight-fitting racing clothes can reduce drag by up to 30% compared to the same rider wearing loose-fitting pants with a jacket. Greater detail about different body positions and the effect these positions and clothing have on wind resistance are presented by Brooks and Hibbs [10], and Faria and Cavanagh [36]. Information about the reduction of frontal area and subsequent reductions in aerodynamic drag also ventures into the science of human-powered vehicles which employ aerodynamic farings around either a land-based bicycle or one used for human-powered flight. Although these applications of cycling science are interesting, they are not discussed in this chapter.

Recent experiments by Kyle [70] performed in wind tunnels provide data on the aerodynamics of various bicycle wheels. The following general conclusions were made:

1. Air resistance of a three-spoke, composite, aerodynamic wheel is equal to or better than that of the best disc wheels.
2. Disc wheels or three-spoke, composite, aerodynamic wheels were better than any of the steel-spoked wheels tested, including a wheel with 16 aero-bladed spokes, aero-rims, and narrow 18 mm tires.
3. In a mild crosswind, the drag of disc wheels or the three-spoke wheels actually decreased because of aerodynamic lift in the direction of motion generated by the airfoil shape.

Interestingly, the aerodynamic advantages of these types of wheels was presented by Sharp in 1896 [107] (Fig. 4.1).

An equation used to calculate total environmental drag has been presented by Kyle [69] and takes the form:

$$D = W (Crr_1Crr_2V) + A_3V^2 \qquad [2]$$

where D is the drag force, W is the rider plus bicycle mass, Crr_1 is a static rolling resistance coefficient, Crr_2 is a dynamic rolling resistance

FIGURE 4.1

Solid disc and four-spoked wheel designs developed in the late 1800s. (Reprinted with permission from Sharp, A. Bicycles and Tricycles. *Cambridge: MIT Press, 1977, p. 352, Fig. 356.)*

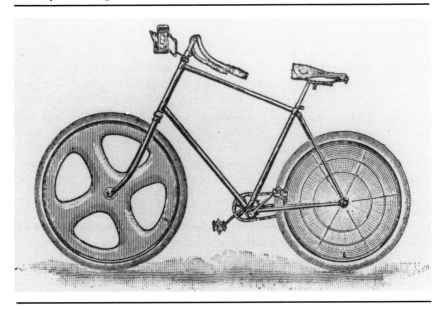

coefficient (which includes wheel bearing losses and dynamic tire losses), V is the speed, and A_3 is a combined aerodynamic drag factor. A_3 may be calculated from:

$$A_3 = 1/2 \, \rho \, C_d A \qquad [3]$$

where ρ is the air density, C_d is the aerodynamic drag coefficient (about .7 to .9 for bicycles), and A is the projected frontal area. For high-quality racing tires, Crr_1 is between 0.0022 and 0.0025; for touring tires, it is between 0.0030 and 0.0035. Crr_2 is about 0.0000344.

In addition to the work done on wheels, Kyle recently reviewed the results from tests on the aerodynamics of helmets and handlebars [69]. Certainly the newer handlebars and teardrop helmets have enhanced rider performance by decreasing aerodynamic drag, and the different types of handlebars employed in road racing, track racing, and triathlon competition have generated renewed interest in efficient rider position. Generally it is known that, (a) aero-helmets have lower drag than no helmet at all (aero-helmets smooth the flow over the head and lower the drag by approximately 1.0 N [neuton] at 48 km/hr [30 mph]); (b) blunt, blocky helmets, commonly used in racing today, can increase air resistance from 1.0 to 1.76 N over that calculated for a good aero model (riders who wear standard helmets may lose more than 1.6 sec per kilometer to a rider wearing an aero-helmet); and (c) there is an optimal head position for each helmet in which drag will be minimized (in general, the bottom of the helmet should be held parallel to the upper back).

Kyle [70] conducted additional studies of elbow rest handlebars, elbow position on handlebars, bar adjustment, and the combined effect on aerodynamic drag of wheels and helmets. Previous wind tunnel tests indicated that clip-on handlebars and other models such as Scott triathlon bars can reduce a rider's drag at 48 km/hr (30 mph) by over 4.45 N (1.0 lb) when compared to a rider using normal "cow-horn" time trial bars. Elbow position on the handlebars also was found to be critical—an elbow-in position can reduce aerodynamic drag up to 8% relative to a normal elbow position. Kyle noted that drag was lowest when the hands and forearms were either level or tilted upward about 30°.

With the interest generated by the success of Greg LeMond in the 1989 Tour de France, Kyle [69] reported the results of a simulation using the equipment and riding positions of LeMond and Fignon. Results indicated that Fignon's standard bike, unzipped jersey, no helmet, ponytail, dangling pendants, and standard cow-horn time trial bars, resulted in over 4.45 N (1.0 lb) higher drag at 48 km/hr (30 mph) when compared to LeMond. In the final 24 km (15 mile) time trial, this would have placed him about 1 minute and 30 seconds behind LeMond. Although this exaggerates the actual 58 seconds that LeMond gained, his bike had a low tech, 32-spoke front wheel which would narrow the predicted advantage. In general, rider position and aerodynamic clothing were likely related to LeMond's success.

The challenge in cycling does not end with testing of equipment aerodynamics, but with the usage of this equipment and subsequent positions assumed by each person on the bicycle and the effect of the equipment and positions on one's ability to transmit power to the bike. With these ideas in mind, we now proceed to the human side of the machine and discuss the biomechanics of the rider-bicycle interface.

INTERACTIVE AND PROPULSIVE FORCES

SEAT AND HANDLEBAR FORCES. To understand completely the rider-bicycle interface, reaction forces at the handlebars, seat, and pedals must be determined. Many authors present information related to pedal forces, but few present data on forces generated at the handlebars and seat. Among those few are two recent studies by Soden and Adeyefa

[110] and by Bolourchi and Hull [4]. Soden and Adeyefa were interested in assessing the strength and performance of bicycle frames and made estimates of forces at the handlebars, seat, and pedals during starting, climbing, and steady-level cycling. Using measurements of rider positions taken from 8 mm film, these authors reported a net pull applied to the handlebars of 0.64 BW (bodyweight) during starting, with a maximum pull of 1.08 BW with one arm and a push of 0.44 BW with the other. These asymmetric forces offset the asymmetric loads applied to the pedals in an effort to begin forward movement of the bicycle. During climbing, a pulling force of 0.36 BW and a pushing force of 0.27 BW are reported, whereas during steady-level cycling, they reported a pull of only 0.11 BW and a push of 0.17 BW. These force estimates were verified in the laboratory using specially constructed pedals, with the difference between the theoretical values and the measured values typically less than 20%.

In the only report in which all load components at both the seat and handlebars were presented, Bolourchi and Hull [4] measured the effect of pedalling rate on rider-induced loads. Varying cadence from 63 to 100 rpm at a constant workload, these authors reported handlebar and seat-load profiles that were independent of subject and cadence; e.g., both load profiles went through two complete periods for each crank cycle (Fig. 4.2). Handlebar forces peaked at 140° of the pedalling cycle, and average horizontal seat forces were significantly related to cadence. Although reactive to pedal loads, other load components at the handlebar and seat were not significantly related to cadence.

PEDAL FORCE DETERMINATION. Although interactive forces at the handlebars and seat are significant, the forces applied to the pedals represent the most important input by the rider to the bicycle. The earliest account of instrumentation employed to measure pedal reaction forces was presented by Sharp [107] (Fig. 4.3A), who described a specially designed pedal employing springs mounted between two surfaces to measure a pedal reaction force component orthogonal to the pedal surface. His data showed orthogonal force components similar to those presented today. Hill's [53] interest in muscle physiology and the relationship between muscle force and contraction velocity stimulated Dickinson [26] to use the bicycle to study mechanics of lower extremity muscles. Fenn [37] studied cycling efficiency and movement speed and presented comparisons between the kinetics of cycling and running. He estimated pedal loads and examined changes in potential and kinetic energy of the leg segments. Similarly to Dickinson, Fenn matched velocity and load to estimate individual muscle forces and velocities.

These early accounts illustrated the potential for studying rider-induced loads, but it is only recently that advancements in instrumented bicycle pedals and their applications have emerged. Hoes et al. [54]

FIGURE 4.2

Loading patterns for the seat and handlebars at three different rpm. (Reprinted with permission from Bolourchi, F., and M. Hull. Measurement of rider-induced loads during stimulated bicycling. Int. J. Sports Biomech. *1:308–329, 1985.)*

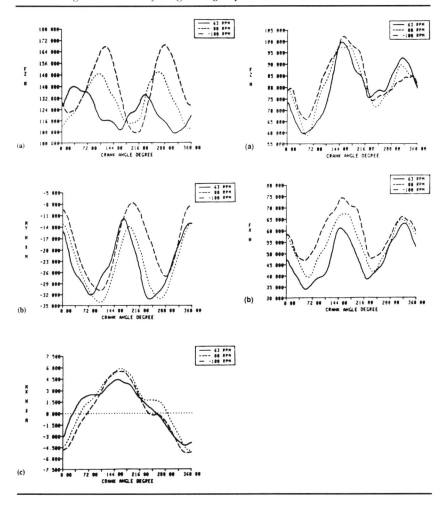

measured the orthogonal component of the pedal reaction force and crank torque on an instrumented bicycle ergometer. Although earlier reports focused on force measurements and estimates of forces at the pedals, Hoes et al. were among the first to evaluate systematically forces at the pedal and crank. Using a pedalling speed of 60 rpm with no toeclips, they report that maximal force at the pedal and crank occurred at approximately 90° of the pedalling cycle. The propulsive leg also assisted the recovery leg, but this assistance decreased as load increased.

FIGURE 4.3

Four exemplar pedal designs reported in the literature between 1896 and 1990. Each design reflects a significant advancement in measurement capability: (**A**) *is the spring design reported by Sharp (reprinted with permission from Sharp, A.* Bicycles and Tricycles. *Cambridge: MIT Press, 1977, p. 269, Fig. 232);* (**B**) *is the strain-gauged design developed at the Biomechanics Laboratory, Pennsylvania State University (reprinted with permission from Cavanagh, P.R., and D.J. Sanderson. The biomechanics of cycling: studies of the pedalling mechanics of elite pursuit riders. E.R. Burke (ed.).* Science of Cycling. *Champaign, IL: Human Kinetics Pub., 1986, p. 98, Fig. 5);* (**C**) *is the design presented by Hull and Davis (reprinted with permission from Hull, M.L., and R.R. Davis. Measurement of pedal loading in bicycling—I. Instrumentation.* J. Biomech. *14:843–855, 1981);* (**D**) *is the design presented by Broker and Gregor (reprinted with permission from Broker, J.P., and R.J. Gregor. A dual piezoelectric force pedal for kinetic analysis of cycling.* Int. J. Sports Biomech. *6:394–403, 1990).*

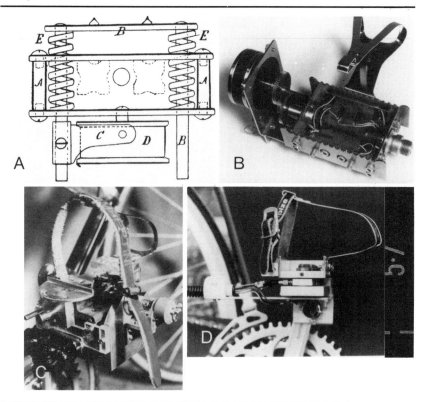

The question addressed by these authors was that of a force-time relation and the varying force production observed at the foot-pedal interface and at the crank during the pedalling cycle. Sargeant and Davies [103] and Sargeant et al. [104], using similar equipment, studied single- and two-legged cycling (50 rpm). Daly and Cavanagh [21] used similar instrumentation to study questions related to cycling asymmetry, and their data supported earlier reports [26, 107] that considerable asymmetry exists at the crank during standard cycling ergometry.

Identifying the need to study more completely the pedal reaction forces, Dal Monte et al. [20] developed transducers to measure pedal reaction force components orthogonal and tangential to the pedal surface. Their technical advancement permitted the analysis of varying foot positions and exploration of the best technique riders should employ to impart forces to the bicycle. They presented data at cadences ranging from 60 to 120 rpm in both the seated and standing positions. Gregor [43] used similar instrumented pedals to study lower extremity kinetics during cycling at four different loads in a group of five experienced cyclists (Fig. 4.3B). Two components of the pedalling reaction force and joint moments were calculated for five subjects riding at 50, 65, and 80% of their maximum aerobic capacity, as well as at a constant load for all subjects representing between 40% and 68% of their maximum aerobic capacity. Asymmetry between right and left limbs was evident, maximum pedal forces occurred at approximately 105° of the pedalling cycle, and substantial differences emerged between subjects regarding their power generation techniques. Similar instrumentation employed in the study of cycling kinetics also has been reported by Miller and Seireg [82] in the evaluation of rider-induced loads in conjunction with lower extremity muscle activity patterns (EMG), and by Soden and Adeyefa [110] in their validation of rider-bicycle interactive forces. Similar to Gregor [43], Soden and Adeyefa reported both normal and tangential components of the pedal reaction forces. They also reported forces orthogonal to the pedal surface of approximately 0.8 BW (90 rpm at 434 Watts [W]) for a seated position. In the seated position, as load increased the force orthogonal to the pedal surface approached bodyweight (120 rpm at 772 W), during standing (83 rpm at 370 W) orthogonal loads approached 1.6 BW, and at the start, up an incline with the rider out of the saddle, orthogonal pedal forces approached 3.1 BW.

A significant advancement in pedal instrumentation was introduced by Hull and Davis [23, 56] in which triaxial, strain-gauged force pedals were used to measured loads in three directions and the three respective moments (Fig. 4.3C). Previous studies relied on planar analyses (two components of the pedal reaction force), but Davis and Hull [23] reported significant medial-lateral forces and moments about the vertical, medial-lateral, and anterior-posterior pedal axes. Peak forces directed normally and tangentially to the surface of the pedal occurred simultaneously at about 100° of the pedalling cycle. These authors confirmed previous reports by Gregor [43] that pedal loads increased with workload and that efficiency was not related to cycling experience.

Other studies by Bolourchi and Hull [4] indicate that cadence had a significant effect on pedal reaction forces. As cadence increased, the load orthogonal to the pedal surface decreased during the power phase and increased during recovery. Pedal force components in both the anterior-posterior and medial-lateral shear also were affected by cadence, with significant changes observed during recovery. Peak pedal load was recorded between 90 and 110° of the pedalling cycle, but cadence appeared to have no effect on the temporal aspects of the load profiles.

Although the triaxial force pedal developed by Hull and Davis [23, 56] contributes significantly to our understanding of pedalling mechanics, the six-element strain-gauge design exhibits significant cross sensitivity. Uniaxial loading and applied pure moments introduce gauge deformations in out-of-plane axes. Consequently, the use of this pedal may be restricted to laboratories equipped with the elaborate calibration equipment and procedures necessary to develop the 6 × 6 coefficient sensitivity matrix employed in the derivation of the applied moments and loads. In 1988, Newmiller et al. [86] addressed the cross-sensitivity problem and presented information on a mechanically decoupled force pedal. Because this pedal measures only normal and anterior-posterior tangential components of the applied load, its application is limited to a planar analysis. Musculoskeletal models and evaluation of cycling performance, however, are typically formulated within the single plane.

Use of multidirectional piezoelectric transducers within the pedal body provides an alternative to mechanical decoupling of the loading axis. Ericson and colleagues [30] used a single piezoelectric element mounted between two surfaces. This pedal offered high-frequency response and employed commercially available components to measure uniaxial loads without the need for cross-sensitivity correction. Ericson et al. [30, 31, 33, 34] reported varus and valgus loads at the knee, forces at the ankle joint, and moments at the hip and knee using a standard bicycle ergometer with six subjects at various workloads and pedalling. Mean ankle joint compressive forces approached 1.4 BW; mean Achilles tendon forces approached 1.1 BW. The mean compressive force varied with workload and rider foot position on the pedal.

Extending the Ericson design, Broker and Gregor [8] reported the use of dual piezoelectric load washers (Kistler Type 9251A) mounted between two surfaces with the capability of measuring three components of the pedal reaction force, a moment about the vertical axis through the center of the pedal, and the point of force application (medial-lateral) during the pedalling cycle (Fig. 4.3D). Exemplar data from the various pedal designs, illustrated in Figure 4.3A-D, are displayed in Figure 4.4a-d. Similarities in force patterns are apparent. Moreover, the UCLA pedals have recently been modified to interface effectively with clipless cycling shoes (Fig. 4.5).

PEDALLING "EFFECTIVENESS." The "effectiveness" of forces produced at the pedal has been evaluated by resolving the resultant pedal load into two components: one orthogonal to the crank (F_E–effective force) and another component along the crank (F_I or F_u–ineffective or unused force) [15, 36, 56, 71, 72]. These vector components calculated from the pedal reaction force components (F_N and F_T) and pedal and crank position ($Ø_1$ and $Ø_4$) yield an index of effectiveness (IE), representing the percentage of the applied linear impulse used to generate the angular impulse during the pedalling cycle (Fig. 4.6). These studies show considerable variability in force effectiveness, both within subjects across cycles and between subjects. Recent data from our laboratory [unpublished observations] nevertheless illustrate limitations of this variable, and suggest that it should not be used exclusively to document "effectiveness" of cycling technique. For example, preliminary measurements indicate that as saddle height increases, force effectiveness increases. Force effectiveness was greatest at the highest saddle position tested (i.e., 115% pubic symphysis height)—one that would never be chosen by cyclists. Force effectiveness should therefore be used with caution and may not be a useful indicator of riding efficiency.

KINEMATICS

Kinematic parameters of the lower extremities, i.e., displacements, velocities, and accelerations, are principally affected by the cadence, hip and ankle motion, and bicycle geometry (e.g., seat height, crank length, and foot position) chosen by the rider. The complex interactions between these operational and geometric variables and the kinetics of the bicycle-rider system have been the subject of the majority of studies on cycling. To understand how one might "optimally" impart energy to the bicycle, many authors have chosen to vary systematically rider-bicycle kinematics by changing either rider-bicycle configurations or pedalling cadence, or both. In this review, the effects that rider-bicycle configurational manipulations and changes in cadence have on rider-bicycle performance, as well as issues concerning hip motion and constancy of crank angular velocity, will be reserved for a discussion focused on cycling optimization. We refer the reader to Faria and Cavanagh [36] and Pons and Vaughan [93] for information concerning general cycling kinematics and the effect that different seat positions have on ranges of motion at the hip and knee.

Although much of the research on cycling has examined sagittal

FIGURE 4.4

Pedal reaction force patterns reported using the pedals described in Figure 4.3. **(A)** *are the force patterns orthogonal to the pedal surface reported by A. Sharp (reprinted with permission from Sharp, A.* Bicycles and Tricycles. Cambridge: MIT Press, 1977, p. 270, Figs. 235, 236, 237). **(B)** *are the average normal and tangential force patterns recorded during five pedalling cycles, using the pedal designed at the Pennsylvania State University (reprinted with permission from Gregor, R.J., P.R. Cavanagh, and M. LaFortune. Knee flexor movements during propulsion in cycling: a creative solution to Lombard's paradox.* J. Biomech. *18:307–316, 1985).* **(C)** *are the force [Fx, Fy, Fz] and moment [Mx, My, Mz] patterns recorded during one pedalling cycle using the pedal illustrated by Hull and Davis (reprinted with permission from Hull, M.L., and R.R. Davis.* Measurement of pedal loading in bicycling—I. Instrumentation. J. Biomech. *14:843–855, 1981).* **(D)** *are the forces Fx, Fy, and Fz, moments [Mz] about a variable and fixed vertical axis in the pedal, and center of pressure [Az, Ay] coordinates in the frontal plane during one pedalling cycle (reprinted with permission from Broker, J.P., and R.J. Gregor. A dual piezoelectric force pedal for kinetic analysis of cycling.* Int. J. Sports Biomech. *6:394–403, 1990).*

plane motion, movement of the limb in the frontal plane is important and has relevance to cycling kinetics and lower extremity injuries. The knee can move medially up to 2 cm during the first half of the pedalling cycle [78]. Movement of the lower extremity in the frontal plane, principally abduction of the thigh early in the power phase, involves tibial and femoral rotation and, ultimately, joint loading. Frontal plane motion and its relevance to frontal plane kinetics are discussed in the following section.

Recent clipless pedal designs (which act like ski bindings and have no straps) focus on permitting the cyclist to rotate the foot on the pedal (about an axis orthogonal to the pedal surface) to minimize stress on the knee and ankle. To date, however, no systematic investigation has been made regarding the effects of these new pedals on lower extremity kinematics and kinetics.

Studies in the early part of this century focused on using estimates of pedalling forces to study load and velocity characteristics of muscle, but few recent reports have expanded on these early interests. Rugg [98] reported muscle-tendon length changes in both knee and ankle flexors and extensors during cycling, and Boutin et al. [6] reported on three-dimensional kinematics and muscle-tendon length changes during cycling. Both studies reported considerable variability between subjects. Additional results have been reported by Hawkins and Hull [51]. One of the most significant observations in muscle-tendon length change

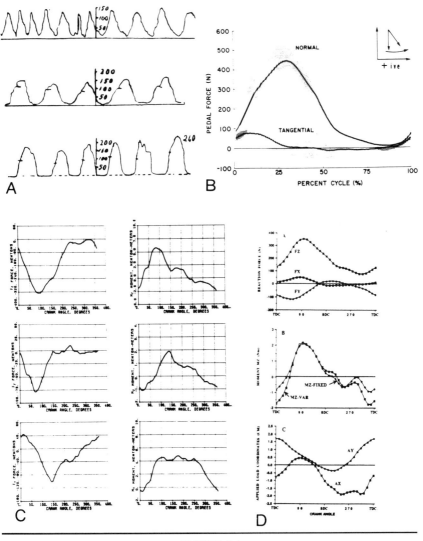

FIGURE 4.4

patterns is the large number of major muscle-tendon units that appear
to experience a stretch-shorten cycle. For example, the gastrocnemius
muscle appears to lengthen actively and then shorten during the power
phase of cycling, taking advantage of the potential storage and reuse
of elastic strain energy in the muscle-tendon unit. The implications of
these data on the involvement of individual muscles and muscle groups
in imparting energy to the bicycle are significant and warrant further
study.

FIGURE 4.5

A modification of the pedal reported by Broker and Gregor [8] to accommodate the more popular "clipless" pedal design. No modifications were made in measurement capabilities.

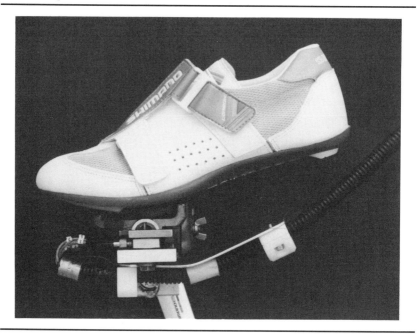

KINETICS

JOINT MOMENT PATTERNS. To understand lower extremity function under varying physiological loads, Gregor [43] employed specially designed bicycle pedals and inverse dynamics to calculate joint moment patterns in a group of five experienced cyclists. Electromyographic data were subsequently added and a final manuscript published by Gregor et al. [45]. Joint moment patterns were examined in relation to the crank moment during propulsion, and it became clear that the hip and knee were performing very different actions during the propulsion phase of cycling. During the first 180° of the pedalling cycle, the hip moment was always extensor, whereas the knee moment was first extensor but became flexor at approximately 100° of the cycle (Fig. 4.7). This observation and its explanation represent the most original aspect of these studies on joint kinetics. The paradoxical muscle action during cycling (knee flexor moment during knee extension—see Lombard [74]) stimulated further research about the function of the lower extremity in the constrained cycling motion [1, 115]. Andrews [1]

FIGURE 4.6

*Schematic of the application of forces to the pedal. (**A**) illustrates angle conventions; (**B**) illustrates normal (Fn), tangential (Ft), and the resultant (Fr) force components applied to the pedal; and (**C**) illustrates the dissection of Fr into effective (Fe) and ineffective or unused (Fp) components with respect to the crank. (Reprinted with permission from Cavanagh, P.R., and D.J. Sanderson. The biomechanics of cycling: studies of the pedalling mechanics of elite pursuit riders. E.R. Burke (ed.).* Science of Cycling. *Champaign, IL: Human Kinetics Pub., 1986, p. 103, Fig. 7).*

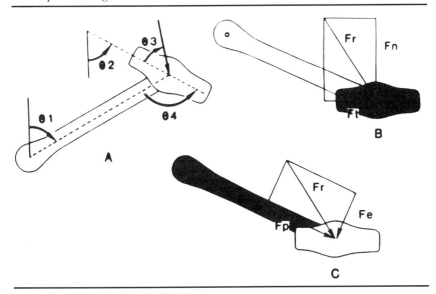

redefined paradoxical muscle action during cycling, basing it on the kinematic role of the lower extremity muscles (the effect that muscle-tendon shortening has on pedal motion). Van Ingen Schenau [115] attempted to describe muscle roles during cycling in light of power production and power distribution by mono- and biarticular lower extremity muscles, respectively.

Studies by Jorge and Hull [62], Redfield and Hull [96], Browning et al. [11], Ericson et al. [34], and Rugg [98], support the data originally presented by Gregor [43] regarding joint moment patterns. Using a planar, five-bar linkage model, Jorge and Hull [62] recorded pedal forces, EMG, and pedal and crank kinematics to evaluate how both pedal forces and different pedalling rates affect lower extremity joint moments during cycling. Redfield and Hull [95] showed that peak knee flexor moments increased as cadence decreased (from 100 to 63 rpm), whereas the transition from an extensor to a flexor knee moment occurred earlier in the power phase. The total hip moment was more

FIGURE 4.7

Average joint moment patterns for five pedalling cycles at the ankle, knee, and hip (thigh). Shaded area represents the range of values calculated for five subjects. Positive moments represent dorsiflexion, knee extension, and hip flexion. (Reprinted with permission from Gregor, R.J., P.R. Cavanagh, and M. LaFortune. Knee flexor movements during propulsion in cycling: a creative solution to Lombard's paradox. J. Biomech. *18:307–316, 1985.)*

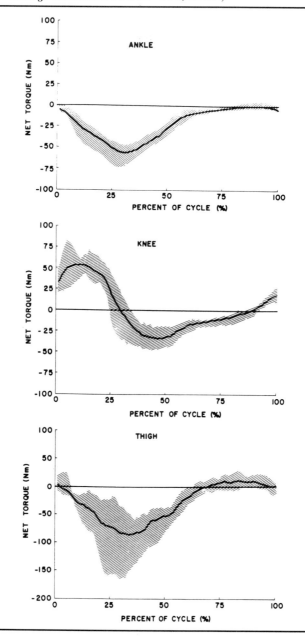

variable (cf. Gregor [43]) with a peak extensor moment increasing from approximately 10 N·m to 60 N·m as cadence decreased from 100 to 63 rpm. Hull and coworkers [96] indicated that average joint moments varied considerably and with changes in cadence, both hip and knee moments showed an average minima near 105 rpm. They suggested that an optimal rotation speed could be determined from a mechanical approach for any given power level and bicycle-rider geometry.

Studying load moments at the hip and knee during ergometer cycling, Ericson et al. [34] presented information that supports previous reports [43, 62, 95]. Hip moments remain extensor throughout the power phase with small flexor moments observed during recovery. Knee moments begin as an extensor moment and change to a flexor moment prior to the limb reaching full extension (180° into the cycle). In addition, Rugg [98] and Browning et al. [11] showed that the net moment at the ankle, although being almost entirely plantar flexor throughout the pedalling cycle, increased in peak magnitude as seat height decreased from 108% of pubic symphysis height to 96% of pubic symphysis height. Additionally, seat height affected the magnitude of peak knee extensor moment as higher peak magnitudes were observed at the 96% pubic symphysis height than at 108% pubic symphysis height. Both Rugg and Browning et al. showed that knee flexor moments occurred earlier in the pedalling cycle (approximately 100°) at 108% pubic symphysis height and later in the pedalling cycle (approximately 145°) at 96% pubic symphysis height. Furthermore, peak knee flexor magnitudes were higher at 108% pubic symphysis height than those reported at either 96% or 102% pubic symphysis height. Changing seat height also affected the peak hip moment. A hip extensor moment of approximately 55 N·m occurred at 108% pubic symphysis height versus approximately 45 N·m at both the 96 and 102% pubic symphysis height conditions. Hip moment patterns displayed high intersubject variability; in fact, some cyclists exhibited hip flexor moments during isolated regions of the power phase [11]. Hip flexor moments during the power phase seem counter-intuitive but intersegmental dynamics indicate that large knee extensor moments occurring early in the power phase may necessitate coincident large hip flexor moments. The data on these issues, however, remain sparse with a need for further experimental evidence on variations in joint moments as a function of changing bike geometry and pedalling cadence.

VARUS AND VALGUS LOADS. There is increasing interest in evaluating joint kinetics during cycling in a clinical setting [80]. The bicycle offers an instrument in which demands imposed on the lower extremity (e.g., the knee) can be carefully controlled. Modification of seat height, pedal load, and cadence results in a variety of exercise paradigms useful in rehabilitation of the knee musculature. Ericson et al. [30] reported a varus knee load, caused mainly by a medially directed pedal reaction forces, to be the most dominant load on the knee joint during the pedalling cycle. Because these forces and moments were low when compared to walking, Ericson and colleagues concluded that cycling should be the exercise of choice for patients with injuries to the medial collateral ligaments of the knee. McCoy [78] with Gregor [77] investigated the effects of three seat heights and three anterior-posterior seat positions on knee joint forces and moments. In support of Ericson's data, varus knee loads were observed throughout the power phase, peaking at 90° in the cycle coincident with peak knee joint compressive forces (200N). It appears that bicycling offers a relatively benign environment for some structures in the knee while placing significant demands on others. With proper feedback and control, the bicycle may represent a valuable exercise paradigm designated to meet specific demands imposed in the clinical setting.

ELECTROMYOGRAPHY

Muscle activation patterns provide information about how the central nervous system controls movement. These data are important in understanding movement sequences. Because cycling is a continuous task, EMG patterns are generally assumed to be repeatable over a number of pedalling cycles at a constant power output. This may be the case in the laboratory where conditions are more easily controlled, but they are not as common during overground riding when the riders must adjust their output to meet varying environmental demands. To maintain a certain level of performance, the response of the musculature will vary in timing and magnitude as riding conditions change.

Research using EMG has focused primarily on describing the effects of different riding conditions on the recruitment patterns of lower extremity muscles. Muscles typically sampled are the gluteus maximus (GMax), gluteus medius (GMed), rectus femoris (RF), vastus lateralis (VL), vastus medialis (VM), semitendinosus (ST), semimembranosus (SM), biceps femoris (BF), tibialis anterior (TA), gastrocnemius (GA) and soleus (SOL). These superficial muscles represent the prime movers involved in imparting energy to the bicycle. Fine wire electrodes are necessary to establish precisely the activation patterns in deep muscles. Data typically are organized to describe the onset and cessation of activity relative to top dead center (TDC) and by the magnitude of the EMG signal during the pedalling cycle.

Differences between EMG patterns reported in the literature may be the result of variations in electrode preparation and placement, individual differences within and between rider populations, differences in rider-bicycle configuration, and the various methods of data reduction and presentation. Despite the problems inherent in experimental conditions and subject population differences, the similarity in timing reported for some muscles, even across conditions where peak magnitudes may vary, is remarkable.

Most researchers agree that muscle activation patterns are similar, but a close examination of specific data supports the contention that selection of a criterion for onset and cessation of activity can dramatically affect our interpretation of results. Data displayed using "polar plots," for example, can be misleading if the criteria for selection of "on" and "off" are insufficiently described. Expression of magnitudes with respect to a maximal isometric contraction helps our understanding of threshold selection, but this representation [44] also has limitations. When comparisons are made between studies in which both magnitude and timing are shown, variations in activation patterns are observed. An example of such a variation is found in the BF muscle, from which two different patterns emerge (Fig. 4.8). As presented in Figure 4.8, peak activity in pattern A is seen after TDC [44, 99, 100], with activity decreasing to a minimum early during recovery. Activity then rapidly increases again prior to TDC. In contrast, pattern B displays peak activity late in the power phase (between 90° and 180°), with low levels of activity seen prior to and just after TDC. To address the issue of potential crosstalk influence on BF EMG data interpretation, we have used fine wire electrodes to substantiate the BF pattern differences [unpublished observations]. We believe the differences may be related to individual rider pedalling technique or, perhaps, to sensitivity of a person's pedalling technique and associated muscle activation patterning to workload level.

EMG patterns typically reported for cycling are presented in Figure 4.9. There are, however, variations between riders in both timing and magnitude of activity. These patterns should, therefore, only be used as a guide. Recent studies in our laboratory [99, 100] indicate that the one-joint knee extensors VM and VL, and GMax are temporally consistent across a number of experienced riders (N = 18) for a constant workload and cadence (250 W, 90 rpm). The two-joint RF muscle exhibits activation patterns similar to the VL and VM during the early power phase (0 to 120°) but displays an earlier onset of activity during recovery. Across riders, the BF, ST, and SM, as a group, display more variability—with the BF being the most variable. The GA and SOL each display a consistent temporal pattern across riders, with SOL activity consistently beginning just prior to GA activity. The phase shift between these muscles may be due to differences in their articulations and consequently muscle function. The single joint TA is usually active just prior to TDC [24, 32, 44, 55, 63]; however, our data indicate that secondary bursts can occur in the first three quadrants (0 to 270°) [99, 100].

A common assumption made in the development of cycling muscu-

FIGURE 4.8

Examples of two apparently different patterns for the biceps femoris muscle activity during cycling. All amplitudes are in % maximum activity, and all figures begin and end at top dead center (TDC). The top two figures represent one pattern, the bottom three another pattern. (The top left pattern is reprinted with permission from Gregor, R.J., D. Green, and J.J. Garhammer. An electromyographic analysis of selected muscle activity in elite competitive cyclists. A. Morecki, K. Fidelus, K. Kedzior, and A. Wit (eds.). Biomechanics VII. *Baltimore: University Park Press, 1982, pp. 537–541. The bottom left pattern is reprinted with permission from Ericson, M.O., R. Nisell, U.P. Arborelius, and J. Ekholm. Muscular activity during ergometer cycling.* Scand. J. Rehab. Med. *17:53–61, 1985. The bottom center pattern is reprinted with permission from Jorge, M., and M.L. Hull. Analysis of EMG measurements during bicycle pedalling.* J. Biomech. *19:683–694, 1986.)*

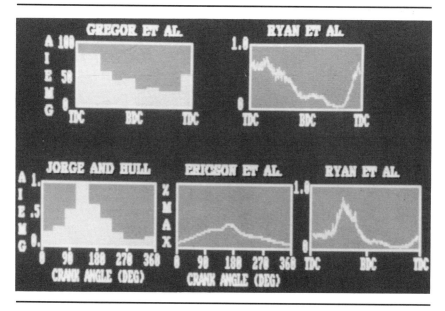

loskeletal models concerns the absence of flexor-extensor coactivation at the knee. This assumption is critical to these cycling models to reduce the number of unknowns and yield a determinant system. This assumption, however, does not apply to all riders. Gregor et al. [44] and others [24, 44, 99, 100, 111] show coactivation between knee flexors and extensors. Specifically, knee flexors and extensors are coactive during the first 90° of the pedalling cycle. Subsequent to this coactivation period, the knee extensors virtually cease activity from 90° to 180° in the cycle, whereas the knee flexors maintain a substantial electrical output. The seemingly counterproductive and paradoxical action of

FIGURE 4.9

Average EMG patterns for the semitendinosus **(ST)**, *semimembranosus* **(SM)**, *biceps femoris* **(BF)**, *gastrocnemius* **(GA)**, *soleus* **(SOL)**, *vastus lateralis* **(VL)**, *vastus medialis* **(VM)**, *rectus femoris* **(RF)**, *gluteus maximus* **(GM)**, *and tibialis anterior* **(TA)** *muscles during the pedalling cycle. Values represent data averaged from 15 cycles across 18 subjects.*

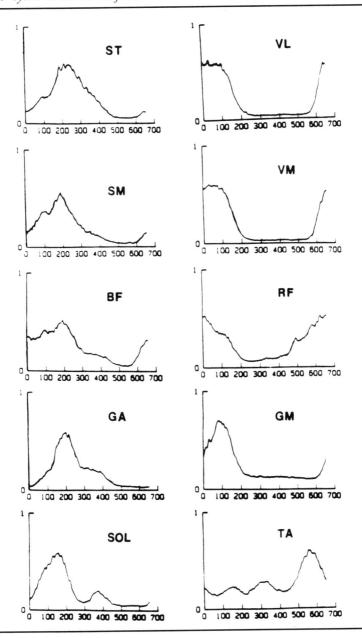

these two muscle groups has been explained by several authors in the description of the role of two-joint muscles [1, 45, 115].

Muscle activity patterns have been used to characterize subject populations from recreational riders [32] to elite cyclists [44, 63]. Although cycling experience would seem to affect EMG, the patterns between the various populations appear similar. Variations in the configuration of loading systems (ergometers, rollers, treadmills, and racing bicycles) and the associated effects on EMG have not been adequately assessed, and a systematic comparison investigating this issue appears warranted. The effects of seat height, cadence, workload, and shoe-pedal interface on muscle activity patterns have been studied and are discussed below.

EMG & SEAT HEIGHT. The effect of seat height on EMG patterns in lower extremity muscles has received considerable attention [24, 32, 55, 63, 98]. Although different measurement methods and ranges of seat heights employed make it difficult to compare directly the effects of seat height manipulation, researchers generally agree that leg muscle activity increases as seat height decreases. This increase appears to be more prevalent in the quadriceps and hamstring muscle groups. Houtz and Fischer [55] reported that a higher seat height allowed the subjects to pedal with greater ease, particularly at higher workloads.

Ericson et al. [32], in contrast to the general finding that high seat heights reduce muscle activity magnitudes, reported that GMed, medial hamstring, and medial GA show increased activity at high seat heights, with insignificant changes in the remaining muscles studied (GMax, VM, RF, SOL, TA, BF and lateral GA). An accurate comparison of seat height measurement technique, referenced to specific anatomical features, may be required to resolve the reported differences. Phase shifts in muscle activation resulting from changes in seat height were reported by Desipres [24] and Rugg [98], but other researchers [32, 55, 63] described no temporal effects.

EMG & CADENCE. Changes in cycling cadence alter the demands imposed on the rider, particularly with respect to the energy required to move the limbs. Consequently, EMG patterns of the muscles used during cycling are expected to change with modifications in cadence. The effects of cadence on lower extremity EMG have been studied by several investigators [32, 42, 82, 111]. Collectively, Ericson et al. [32] and Goto et al. [42] reported increased muscle activity in GMax, GMed, VL, ST, SM, GA, SOL, and TA as cadence was increased (40 to 100 rpm). Although the RF and BF muscles exhibited similar increased activity at higher cadence, the changes were not significant.

Suzuki et al. [111], studying the EMG response to cadence changes between 12 and 60 rpm, reported that RF and BF activity began progressively earlier in the pedalling cycle as cadence increased, each exhibiting double bursts of activity at the higher cadences. The secondary bursts were attributed to biarticular joint function. Coincident activity of BF and RF was evident at the higher cadences. The medial GA shifted in phase as cadence increased, but little change in timing of VM and TA occurred. Interestingly, Suzuki [112] suggests that a preferential and selective activation of faster twitch fibers occurs as cadence increases. Activation of fast-twitch fibers in response to increased workload also may shift the preferred operating conditions for the muscles involved to those associated with higher cadences. Observations regarding "optimal" cadence as a function of workload, outlined in greater detail in the cycling optimization section, support this view [48, 73].

EMG & WORKLOAD. Workload (power output) can be changed by increasing cadence at constant load, increasing load at constant cadence, or increasing both. Most studies have used constant gear ratios and cadence and have varied workload by changing the resistance imposed at the bicycle cranks. At higher loads, EMG magnitudes are expected to be greater and that activation timing would remain the same. Houtz and Fischer [55] reported that as ergometer workload increased, the magnitude of activity in all lower extremity muscles studied (BF, ST, VM, VL, RF, GMax, GMed, TA and GA) increased while activation timing remained constant. Ericson et al. [32] varied ergometer workload from 0 to 240 W at constant cadence (60 rpm) and also found that eight muscles (GMax, GMed, RF, VL, VM, BF, ST or SM, GA, and SOL) showed increased EMG magnitudes as workload increased. Goto et al. [42] reported similar results for GM, VL, GA, and TA, monitored as working resistance increased. There was no reference in either of these studies however, to the effect of workload on activation timing.

Jorge and Hull [63] assessed EMG differences as workload changed by varying gear ratios at a constant pedalling rate on a laboratory bicycle on rollers. At lower power levels (83 and 100 W), timing and magnitude of activity appeared insensitive to changes in workload (17 W). Interestingly, BF, SM, and TA displayed greater activity at 83 W than at 100 W. Their data are averages for six subjects and, consequently, these trends may not represent individual pattern sensitivity to workload. Incidentally, Jorge and Hull [63] state that the greatest variability between subjects, most noticeable in the hamstring group and TA, could be attributed to differences in pedalling technique. As workload increased to 125 W, the magnitude of activity in all muscles except the GA increased substantially. These data support those of Houtz and Fisher [55], Ericson et al. [32], and Goto et al. [42].

EMG & SHOE-PEDAL INTERFACE. How a rider imparts force to the bicycle is dependent on a number of factors, one of which is the interface between the shoe and the pedal. Most recreational riders use soft-soled shoes when cycling; however, more serious cyclists make use of hard-soled cleated or clipless shoes which are uniquely adjusted for function and comfort. Cleated shoes and toe clips (or clipless pedals and associated shoes) permit the application of productive pedal forces through BDC (pulling back) and into recovery (pulling up). Shoe-pedal interfaces, it appears, may affect muscle activation patterns. Ericson et al. [32] compared cycling with and without toe clips and found that muscle activity increased significantly in the RF, BF, and TA muscles when toe clips were used. In contrast, toe clips produced significantly lower activity levels in the VM, VL, and SOL muscles, although the GMax, GMed, GA, and medial hamstring muscles were not significantly different between conditions. Ericson et al. [32], however, did not evaluate the effect of cleated shoes on muscle activation, as only soft-soled shoes were used in their study. The effect of cleated shoes with toe clips versus soft-soled shoes without toe clips were evaluated by Jorge and Hull [63]. These researchers reported that with soft-soled shoes, both the single joint knee extensors (VL and VM) and the hamstring muscles (BF and SM), displayed increased muscle activity during normal regions of peak activity. Associated decreases in magnitude of activity were reported in the GA and the RF muscles. Although the isolated effect of the cleated cycling shoe in the toe-clip interface configuration is not known, current data suggest that the addition of toe clips and cleated cycling shoes modifies the load sharing distribution of lower extremity muscles. The effect of the new clipless shoe-pedal interface on muscle activity patterns, including those with rotational freedom about their vertical axes, has not been studied and warrants investigation.

ACHILLES TENDON FORCES

Early papers by Fenn [37] and Dickinson [26] illustrated the potential use of cycling to understand the function of individual muscles in the lower extremity. Gregor et al. [46] presented exemplar data on Achilles tendon force, gastrocnemius and soleus EMG, and muscle length changes, as well as EMG activity in the vastus medialis and tibialis anterior muscles (Figure 4.10). In an additional manuscript, Gregor et al. [47] described the contribution made by the triceps surae to the residual moment (that produced by muscles and periarticular structures crossing the joint) at the ankle during cycling at three separate power outputs. Results indicated that the Achilles tendon force increased as external resistance increased. As power was increased by increasing cadence alone (at constant workload), peak Achilles tendon force did not change. Results indicated that the impulse generated by the triceps surae was consistently about 65% of the impulse calculated using the *residual muscle moment* at all power levels studied. Electromyograms and muscle length changes recorded by Gregor et al. [47] also support a division of effort between the gastrocnemius and soleus in their con-

FIGURE 4.10

Achilles tendon forces, gastrocnemius **(GAST)** *and soleus* **(SOL)** *EMG and muscle-tendon length-change patterns, and EMG from the vastus medialis* **(VM)** *and tibialis anterior* **(TA)** *for one pedalling cycle in one subject riding at approximately 270 W. (Reprinted with permission from Gregor, R.J., P.V. Komi, and M. Jarvinen. Achilles tendon forces during cycling.* Int. J. Sports Med. *1:S9–S14, 1987.)*

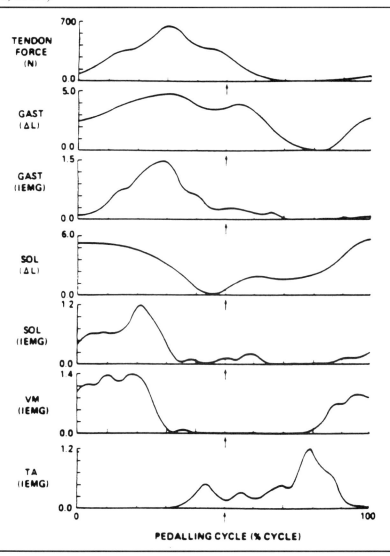

tribution to the Achilles tendon force. Because tendon buckle transducer experiments are invasive, continued experiments in this area will predominantly rely on current techniques in inverse dynamics and optimization modelling.

CYCLING OPTIMIZATION

As previously stated, cycling represents a complex human-machine system, with interactions between the rider and bicycle having a profound effect on the function of the system as a whole. Although an "optimal' cycling system, characterized and defined by specific geometric and operational relationships, theoretically exists, to date this optimal system has not been fully defined. This is true despite the considerable time and energy dedicated by several researchers to define the optimal cycling system.

Cycling optimization usually takes the form of an experimental or an analytical exercise in which critical characteristics (e.g., dimensions and operating parameters of the rider-bicycle system) are defined such that some objective (e.g., maximizing performance or minimizing injury) is achieved. The initial critical step in the process involves defining optimal performance. Optimal performance has been described as that associated with maximizing metabolic or mechanical efficiency, maximizing power output, and minimizing musculoskeletal loads (e.g., joint moments and muscle stresses). Interestingly, physiologically and mechanically based goals differ in their resulting optimal system representations.

A second step in the optimization process involves the selection of parameters to be optimized. Some cycling parameters, e.g., component weights, component efficiencies, and frame design, although critical to system performance, have little influence on rider-bicycle interactions and, therefore, are of more concern to the bicycle engineer and manufacturer than to the biomechanist. System parameters that specifically affect the rider-bicycle interface include: 1) geometric variables such as seat height, crank length, foot position on the pedal (longitudinal and vertical), chainring shape, seat tube angle, and handlebar height (trunk position); and 2) operational variables, such as cadence, ankling patterns, pedal reaction forces, hip motion, and handlebar loading. These geometric and operational variables influence cycling performance through their effects on system kinematics and kinetics.

A third step in characterizing the optimal rider-bicycle system involves validation of the optimal system representation. Here, researchers are faced with the problems of subject performance variability, the high cost of cycling performance instrumentation, and the complexity associated with the analysis of cycling data, particularly in multiparametric optimization studies.

Two approaches have been used in the formulation of optimal cycling characterizations, experimental performance testing, and analytical optimization modelling. Much of the experimental data have already been discussed, so that emphasis here will be placed on the analytical approach with experimental questions focused on optimization.

Experimental Performance Testing

The experimental approach to cycling optimization involves the manipulation of specific variables of interest (e.g., seat height and cadence) while system responses associated with the established goal (e.g., oxygen consumption and muscle activity patterns) are observed. This approach has several advantages. First, experimental observations use data collected on "live" subjects. Consequently, the need for simplifying assumptions inherent in analytical mathematical analyses is dramatically reduced. Also, live-subject data permit the description of multiple responses to single system perturbations (e.g., pedal angle and pedal force application both change in response to an increase in workload) and the evaluation of system perturbations across different subject populations (e.g., elite versus beginner). Second, the experimental approach permits the use of directly measurable physiological responses (i.e., heart rate, oxygen consumption, blood lactate, ventilation) and subjective measures such as perceived exertion in the development of an optimal system representation.

Several disadvantages also are associated with the experimental approach. First, the cost and complexity of analyzing several subjects across multiple system operating conditions can be prohibitive. Variability in physiological, mechanical, and musculoskeletal parameters during cycling between and within subjects (even at the elite level) makes it difficult to assess the consequences of system perturbations, particularly when the perturbations are small. Second, a single mechanical adjustment may influence several performance variables, confounding attempts to isolate specific causal relationships between perturbation and response. Third, experimentally derived optimal system representations may be sensitive to the test equipment used during data collection. For example, most investigators do not recognize the importance of system inertia on pedalling mechanics. Other test equipment characteristics that should be considered include fixed- versus free-front fork (particularly during hill-climbing studies), seat tube angle, pedal configuration (the presence or lack of toe clips and cleated cycling shoes), handlebar position, crank length, and chainring shape.

Despite the problems associated with its approach, experimental observation represents the most viable method of validating the optimal systems defined by analytical mathematical analyses. Several meaningful relationships between the rider-bicycle operating conditions and cycling performance have in fact emerged from these experimental observations.

OPTIMAL SEAT HEIGHT. Optimal seat height has been estimated based on caloric expenditure [49, 88, 108] and power output [49]. These researchers generally agree that oxygen consumption is minimized at approximately 100% of trochanteric height, or 106–109% of pubic symphysis height (measured from the ground while standing barefoot). Elite cyclists generally chose seat heights close to the established optimum [44].

Muscle activity patterns [24, 32, 44, 63], joint force and moment patterns [11, 31, 33, 34], and pedalling force effectiveness [7] also have been reported to vary across seat heights. These relationships, however, have not been used to suggest optimal seat heights. Rugg [98] analyzed muscle activity, joint moment patterns, muscle length changes, and moment arms at the ankle across seat heights in five experienced cyclists. A complex relationship emerged in which seat height changes influenced muscle activity patterns, joint moment profiles and the force-velocity and length-tension operating conditions for the triceps surae muscle group.

OPTIMAL CRANK LENGTH. Although Harrison [50] reported that crank length was relatively unimportant in maximizing power output, optimal crank lengths have been estimated using mean and peak power maximization [61] and oxygen consumption minimization [2]. Inbar et al., [61] reported that maximum power output during a 30-s Wingate Anaerobic test occurred at a crank length of 16.4 to 16.6 cm and varied as a function of subject leg length. Nevertheless, sensitivity within the range of crank lengths commonly used (16.5 to 18.0 cm) was low.

OPTIMAL FOOT-PEDAL INTERFACE. Although it is intuitively obvious that use of cleated cycling shoes and toe clips (or the new "clipless" pedals) permits propulsive torque generation over a greater portion of the pedalling cycle than regular shoes without toe clips, few studies have specifically analyzed the effect of the shoe-pedal interface on pedalling mechanics. Davis and Hull [23] studied torque generation during pedalling using soft-soled shoes alone, soft-soled shoes with toe clips, and cleated cycling shoes with toe clips. Their primary observations indicated that toe clips (independent of shoe type) enhanced efficiency early in the pedalling cycle because of improved normal pedal load utilization, and that the addition of cleated cycling shoes enhanced efficiency still further by permitting effective shear force utilization near bottom dead center (BDC) and throughout recovery. Maximal efficiency occurred when the resultant pedal force was perpendicular to the bicycle crank (generating crank torque). Davis and Hull [23] postulated that toe clips with cleated shoes permitted distribution of the cycling work to the ankle dorsiflexors (around TDC) and the hamstring muscle group (through BDC and into recovery).

Muscle activity patterns have been described across variations in longitudinal foot position and shoe type (soft sole versus cleated shoes with toe clips) [32, 63]. Although muscle activity was not used to suggest optimal foot-pedal interface parameters, changes in muscle activity across interface configurations supported Davis and Hull [23], suggesting that a redistribution of load sharing among lower extremity musculature occurs with the addition of a rigidly coupled foot-pedal connection.

OPTIMAL CHAINRING SHAPE. Recent developments in the design of bicycle transmission systems have included the introduction and use of elliptical chainrings. Elliptical chainrings were originally developed in response to the recognition that crank torque varies systematically during the pedal cycle. Remarkably, the concept of an elliptical chainring and its potential effect on energy transmission from the rider to the bicycle was reported over 90 years ago by Sharp [107]. Intuitively, chainrings that increase the effective gearing during the peak crank torque region of the pedal cycle (45° to 135° beyond TDC) should improve performance [117]. Elliptical chainrings configured in this way (with the minor axis of the ellipse aligned with the cranks) were evaluated across workloads by Henderson et al. [52] using caloric expenditure as the measure of efficiency. No improvements in maximal work capacity could be associated with the elliptical chainring, but the caloric cost decreased slightly, although not significantly.

A more comprehensive approach [90] to the design of elliptical chainrings involved matching the inherent force-velocity characteristics of muscle [53] to pedalling mechanics. Okajima [90] generated an ellipse that varied crank velocity to match more accurately impedance in the rider-bicycle system. Furthermore, Okajima's ellipse decreased the angular velocity of the lower extremity near top and bottom dead center, attempting to minimize losses associated with kinetic energy variations. Interestingly, this design places the minor axis of the ellipse perpendicular to the cranks—exactly opposite to that derived from the intuitive approach.

To date, no experimentally derived scientific evidence exists to suggest that an elliptical chainring improves rider-bicycle system efficiency. Incidentally, professional cyclists and triathletes comment that elliptical chainrings adversely disrupt pedalling mechanics at high cadences (90 to 110 rpm), and that these chainrings may be more suited to mountain bike riding during which pedalling cadences tend to be lower. Not surprisingly, the use of elliptical chainrings as standard equipment on road racing bicycles has decreased dramatically in recent years.

OPTIMAL SEAT TUBE ANGLE AND HANDLEBAR CONFIGURATION. The angle of the seat tube and handlebar configuration interact to define the upper body and pelvic orientation relative to the bicycle. Recently, time trial bicycles and bicycles designed specifically for triathlons have gone to more vertical seat tubes and lower, more forward-positioned handlebars. These changes in bicycle geometry rotate the rider forward relative to the bicycle, dramatically reducing aerodynamic drag. Aerodynamics play a major role in time trial and triathlon racing because drafting is not allowed. Studies are needed to examine the effects of the aerodynamically advantageous riding position on pedal force profiles, musculoskeletal loads and moments, and muscle activity patterns in elite road cyclists and triathletes.

OPTIMAL CADENCE. Cadence, the most widely studied variable in the cycling literature, has attracted such universal attention because it is the one variable that cyclists can freely alter while riding (by changing gears). By definition, there is a direct and linear cadence versus torque trade-off at constant power output, and even beginning riders notice that changing cadence by shifting gears markedly affects pedalling efficiency. Early studies [26] reported the use of 30 rpm on a bicycle ergometer to study muscle mechanics in the lower extremity. Astrand and Rodahl [3] report the most suitable cadence to be 60 rpm, and it is widely reported in the exercise physiology literature that rates between 50 and 60 rpm are most suitable. General observations of competitive cyclists reveal that cadences during flat riding generally range from 80 to 110 rpm, and that more experienced cyclists usually select higher cadences [15, 48, 67, 94, 105, 110, 117]. Hagberg et al. [48] recently reported that at 80% of each subject's maximal aerobic potential (N = 7), cadence varied from 72 to 102 rpm (mean of 92 rpm). Hagberg's group was one of the first to test competitive cyclists on their own racing bicycles, whereas previous reports focused on offering standard working conditions on laboratory ergometers. Experimental evidence on the physiological and mechanical consequences of changing cadence produces conflicting information regarding *optimal cadence*.

Perceived exertion has been used to characterize a person's subjective response to physical work [13, 29, 87, 91]. Several methods of rating perceived exertion exist, but most studies reviewed employed the Borg Scale (a scale from 1 to 20, rating somatic stress from very very light to very very hard). The general belief is that perceived exertion is related to both central (cardiopulmonary) and peripheral (muscle and joint stress) sensations. Lollgen et al. [73] tested both trained and untrained cyclists for perceived exertion across changes in workload and cadence. Both groups preferred high cadences at each workload (maximum cadence allowed was 100 rpm). As workload was increased, perceived exertion minima shifted to higher cadences, suggesting that optimal cadence is workload-specific.

It is generally agreed that by using minimum caloric expenditure to estimate optimal pedalling efficiency, optimal cadence increases with increasing workload. Reported optimal cadences, however, vary considerably (33 to 110 rpm). Several explanations may account for these differences. Most of the investigators used flywheel ergometers, known to have inertial characteristics different from the lightweight racing bicycle ridden overground. Toe clips were used on some of the more recent studies, and it appears that cleated cycling shoes and the subjects' own bicycles were only employed by Hagberg et al. [48]. Second, the different optimal cadences reported may also be attributed to different methods of calculating efficiency. Gaesser and Brooks [39] reported that optimal cadence varied when efficiency was expressed as gross, net, work, or delta efficiency—each accounting for rest level, no load cycling, and loaded cycling oxygen consumption in a different way. Finally, it is generally recognized that competitive cyclists train, race, and are expected to perform more efficiently at higher rpm.

Pedalling mechanics as affected by changes in cadence also have been investigated. Cavanagh and Sanderson [15] reported that pedalling force effectiveness decreases as cadence is increased, specifically during the recovery phase of the pedal cycle (BDC to TDC). The decrease was attributed to increased difficulty in unloading the pedal during recovery at higher pedalling rates. No attempt was made to relate force effectiveness to optimal cadence, and the limitations of force effectiveness measures have been discussed previously.

Kaneko and Yamazaki [64] and Morrisey et al. [83] evaluated internal work (work associated with moving the limbs) during ergometer pedalling at different cadences. Not unexpectedly, internal work increased at higher cadences at constant power. Kaneko and Yamazaki partially attributed changes in internal work across cadence to nonconstant rpm during each pedal cycle (5.5 rad/s variation in crank angular velocity). Interestingly, the effect of nonconstant angular velocity on limb dynamics was first presented by Fenn in 1932 [37].

Hull and Jorge [57], evaluating static (derived from pedal forces) and kinematic (derived from segment accelerations) components of the hip, knee, and ankle joint moments across changes in cadence, showed that kinematic moments increase nonlinearly at the hip and ankle, and linearly at the knee as cadence is increased at constant power. More importantly, however, the total moment response at the hip indicated that the static and kinematic components of the total moment at this joint offset each other and that there existed a cadence at which a minimum mean and/or peak hip moment occurred. Although no optimal cadence was derived from these data, the results strongly suggested that cadence interacts with musculoskeletal dynamics and the associated muscular requirements. These concepts form the basis for an analytical mathematical optimization using joint moments as an objective function.

Muscle activity response to changes in cadence has been reported by several investigators [16, 42, 82, 111]. The general observation is that muscle activation patterns do change in response to changes in cadence at constant power. Citterio and Agostoni [16], and Suzuki [112] suggested that there is a preferential, selective activation of faster twitch fibers as cadence increases. Furthermore, activation of faster twitch fibers in response to increased workload may shift the preferred operating conditions for the muscles involved to those associated with higher cadences. These findings have not been specifically related to the identification of optimal cadence and no data are presented to support this potential change in motorneuronal pools.

OPTIMAL ANKLING AND PEDAL FORCES PATTERNS. The ankling pattern, more technically referred to as the pedal angle, interacts with the normal and tangential components of pedal loading to describe torque generation at the bicycle crank. Ankling pattern recommendations have appeared in the popular literature that contradict biomechanical observations. Sloane [109] suggested that the ankle be in relative dorsiflexion as the pedal moves through the top of the pedal cycle, and plantarflexed through the bottom of the cycle. Ankling patterns of elite cyclists, which vary considerably, illustrate that pedal angle variations during the pedal cycle produce relative dorsiflexion at the ankle during the power phase (45° to 135° beyond TDC) and plantarflexion through BDC and most of the recovery phase (BDC to TDC) [15, 23, 36]. Specific pedal angle profiles have not been associated with optimal cycling.

Pedal force profiles during cycling have been reported by a number of investigators [8, 15, 20, 23, 30, 36, 43, 45, 54, 56, 86]. Maximal pedalling force effectiveness [15, 36, 72] dictates a pedalling style in which the resultant pedal load is oriented perpendicular to the bicycle crank and in the direction of crank rotation at all points within the pedal cycle. Although it is universally recognized that maximal pedalling effectiveness is incompatible with the capabilities of the human-bicycle system, improving force effectiveness during specific regions of the pedal cycle has emerged as a popular performance improvement technique [9, 15, 23, 81, 102]. The relationships, however, between improved force effectiveness at the pedal and overall rider-bicycle system efficiency and performance remain unclear.

OPTIMAL HIP MOTION. Data relating variations in hip motion and handlebar loading to rider-bicycle performance are scarce. Nordeen and Cavanagh [88] claim that hip motion, particularly in the vertical direction, is substantial. Conversely, Hull and Gonzalez [58], in support of a fixed hip assumption used in an analytical model, report that the pelvis is "virtually stationary" (movement of approximately 1 cm) and that measured hip motion is probably a result of incorrect seat height adjustment and improper joint marker placement. Our measurements [11] on elite and experienced cyclists with high-speed film indicate that the hip moves 1 to 2 cm in the anterior-posterior direction and up to 3 cm vertically. Hip motion of this magnitude can affect the calculation of peak hip and knee joint moments by 5–10%. Although coaches recommend that hip motion (particularly that associated with pelvis rocking) should be minimized, the effect that hip motion has on rider-bicycle performance through its effect on musculoskeletal loads, moments, and the potential for energy transfer from the trunk and upper extremity warrants further study.

Analytical Optimization Modeling
The analytical approach to cycling optimization has expanded in recent years. The approach applies optimization concepts developed in the study of human gait [19, 28, 92] to cycling. In general, a mathematical model describing the rider-bicycle system is generated that has any number of modifiable geometric and operational characteristics (e.g., seat height and cadence). Constraints are placed on selected kinematic and physiological features (e.g., no knee hyperextension, limited joint moment or muscle force capacity), and pedal force application patterns as well as pedal angles usually are derived respectively from previously measured pedal force data and mathematical approximations. The approach uses objective (cost) functions, in place of performance measurements, to evaluate parametric manipulations. Optimal system characteristics are associated with minimization or maximization of the chosen objective function (e.g., minimization of joint moments).

The advantages of the analytical optimization approach parallel the disadvantages associated with the experimental approach. First, multi-parametric optimizations are easily and inexpensively performed, permitting simultaneous evaluation of several critical variables. Each variable can be evaluated separately or interactively with other variables, and the effects of small perturbations are determinable. Second, subject variability is eliminated as fixed mathematical representations and fixed input data are used in the model. Third, the sensitivity of the optimal solution to related parameters and simplifying assumptions (e.g., rider segment lengths and body segment parameter approximations) can be assessed.

The disadvantages associated with the analytical optimization approach are not trivial. Numerous assumptions are required to permit simulation of the cycling motion. Some of the assumptions currently employed have only marginal support from experimental observations. Next, the optimal system representations derived from the analytical approach are invalid if the chosen objective function is incorrect. To date, an objective function that accurately characterizes elite cyclist technique (if that is considered optimal) has not been identified. A related problem with the analytical approach is the difficulty in validation. Here, the mathematical representation must rely on experimental observations (with the associated problems of subject variability and experimental complexity) to evaluate differences between optimal system predictions and actual rider-bicycle responses to perturbations.

With a few exceptions [65, 66], most of the studies employing the analytical modelling technique have been conducted by Hull and his associates. Optimal system parameters defined using the analytical approach include cadence, crank length, seat height, seat tube angle, longitudinal foot position, pedal platform height, and pedal forces. The various rider-bicycle optimization analyses share several features with regard to the construct of the cycling model, rider-bicycle parameters studied, simplifying assumptions, and objective functions used. The models, assumptions and objective functions used to simulate and optimize the rider-cycling system will be presented, followed by a discussion of the results.

OPTIMIZATION MODELS, ASSUMPTIONS, AND OBJECTIVE FUNCTIONS. The standard biomechanical model used in the development of analytical optimizations consists of a closed five-bar linkage fixed at both the hip joint and the crank spindle, the links being the bicycle crank, the foot, the shank, the thigh, and the segment joining the hip to the crank spindle (described as a four-bar linkage if the hip-to-spindle segment is not counted) [41, 58, 59, 60, 65, 66, 96, 97]. The system is planar and exhibits two degrees of freedom (crank angle and pedal angle). Input data required to run the model consists of pedal force and pedal angle histories, segment lengths, and lower extremity body segment parameters. In addition, the model developed by Komor et al. [65] includes aerodynamic loading estimates and, therefore, accounts for total body mass and trunk position. Either experimentally measured pedal forces are used to drive the model [41, 58, 59, 60, 65, 66, 96] or pedal forces are mathematically represented by three harmonic Fourier series [97]. Changes in cadence at constant power are handled by scaling pedal forces (both normal and tangential) proportionally with cadence. Pedal angles are represented by sinusoidal approximations based on experimental observations.

Several assumptions are used in the development of mathematical cycling representations. Planar motion of the lower extremity, rigid segments, frictionless hinge joints with fixed axes of rotation, and uniform segment mass parameters represent generally accepted assumptions used in the dynamic analysis of movement. These assumptions are also used in the cycling optimization models. Other assumptions common to all the cycling models reviewed include: (1) constant crank angular velocity, (2) fixed hip joint, (3) sinusoidal pedal angle profile, and (4) scaled pedal force profiles (proportional to cadence). These assumptions are applied over variations in power output, cadence, seat height, seat tube angle, crank length, and pedal platform height. Assumptions specific to isolated cycling optimization studies include Fourier series approximation of pedal forces [97], absence of coactivation, and muscle equivalency (combining muscles into functional groups) [59, 97].

Objective functions used in the cycling studies reviewed include minimization of (1) the sum of the average absolute knee and hip joint moments [96], (2) the sum of the squared knee and hip joint moments [41, 58, 60], (3) the sum of the squared ankle, knee, and hip joint moments [65, 66, 97], and (4) the sum of the squared muscle group stresses [59, 97]. Joint moment- and muscle stress-based objective functions assume that intersegmental moments and muscle stresses correlate well with physiological endurance capabilities. Treating the objective function parameters nonlinearly eliminates the influence of negative moments on the objective function and, more importantly, produces moment and muscle force predictions more physiologically consistent with experimental observations [19, 28].

Before presenting the results of the analytical optimization analyses, a few comments regarding some of the assumptions previously outlined are warranted. First, crank angular velocity varies throughout the pedal cycle and is directly related to variable crank torque observed during the pedalling cycle. Crank angular velocity variations are most likely influenced by changes in cadence, load, crank length, and seat height. Although the effect of crank angular velocity variation on optimal parameter definitions is unknown, at high loads and low cadences the effect may be significant. Inclusion of system rotational inertia in the rider-bicycle model and coupling torque generation at the crank-to-crank angular and system accelerations would eliminate associated nonconstant angular velocity effects.

The assumption that pedal angle can be approximated with a sinusoidal function, *invariant* across manipulations of cadence, power, seat height, crank length, longitudinal foot position, and pedal platform height must be evaluated more closely. Observations of elite cyclists reveal that considerable variability in ankling patterns exist. In support of the fixed pedal angle profile assumption, Newmiller et al. [86] reported that pedal angle undergoes a phase shift of 5% and an offset amplitude of less than 10% in response to changes in cadence. Redfield and Hull [95] conducted a sensitivity analysis of joint moments as affected by changes in offset pedal angle and phase shifts of $\pm 10\%$ and also found minimal effects. Pedal angle offsets and phase shifts, and perhaps even the sinusoidal characteristic, are altered ($>10\%$), however, by modest changes in seat height, seat tube angle, crank length, longitudinal foot position, and pedal platform height. Experimental measurements describing pedal angle variations in response to these optimized parameters are necessary to clarify this issue.

Finally, scaling pedal forces to match constant power output with cadence has been shown by Hull and his associates to be reasonably accurate during the first half of the pedal cycle, and inaccurate during the second half [41, 60]. The lack of productive torque generation during the recovery phase of cycling (BDC to TDC) has never been completely explained. Redfield and Hull [97] reported that muscle stress-based cost functions more accurately predict recovery phase pedalling mechanics than do joint moment-based cost functions. If recovery phase pedalling technique is to be fully understood and realistically optimized, models (such as Redfield and Hull's) that account for specific musculoskeletal capabilities should be used more extensively.

ANALYTICAL OPTIMIZATION PREDICTIONS. Optimal cadence has been estimated analytically in several studies [41, 58, 59, 96]. Kinematic (segment acceleration-based) and quasistatic (pedal force-based) contributions to joint moments at the hip, knee, and ankle characterize the sensitivity of joint moment and muscle stress-based cost functions to pedalling rate [57]. Derived optimal cadences were found to vary from 95 to 115 rpm, and interacted with crank length [41, 58], seat height, seat tube angle, and longitudinal foot position [41]. These estimates agree well with observations of experienced cyclists [15, 48, 67, 94, 105, 110, 118] and with experimentally derived optimal cadence measured on elite cyclists [48].

Analytically defined optimal crank lengths range from 140 mm [41] to roughly 170 mm [58, 66]. Crank lengths used in standard practice range from 165 mm to 185 mm. Gonzalez and Hull [41] reported that crank length is second only to cadence in its effect on joint moment cost. Crank length optimums also were reported to interact with cadence, seat height, seat tube angle, longitudinal foot position, and rider anthropometry (heavier riders requiring longer cranks).

Optimal seat height and seat tube angle have been estimated analytically [41, 65, 66]. Only Komor [66] and Komor et al. [65] included the interaction between seat tube angle, trunk position, and aerodynamic loading. Gonzalez and Hull [41] found that seat height optimums interacted with cadence, crank length, seat tube angle, and longitudinal foot position. Optimal seat height was determined for a rider of average anthropometry pedalling at 115 rpm at 200 W to be 97% of greater trochanteric height (GTH) [41], very close to the 100% GTH optimal determined during experimental observations [49, 89, 108]. Pedal-angle sensitivity and any associated effects on optimal predictions were ignored.

Optimal longitudinal foot position and pedal platform height were studied by Gonzalez and Hull [41] and by Hull and Gonzalez [60]. Longitudinal foot position and pedal platform height optimums were placed at 54% of foot length from the heel and 2 cm above the pedal spindle. Both of these variables, however, were considered relatively insignificant in their effect on joint moment cost.

Finally, pedal force profiles have been analytically optimized using both joint moment-based [65, 66, 97] and muscle stress-based cost functions [97]. Redfield and Hull [97] reported that optimized pedal force histories (normal and tangential) were similar to those observed experimentally. Komor [65] and Komor et al. [66] also reported reasonable agreement between optimal and measured pedal force patterns (power-phase only), and they displayed power-phase, pedal force optimal patterns, and measured pedal force patterns to cyclists in a feedback environment to "enhance" cycling performance. Recovery-phase optimal pedal force profiles (only estimated by Redfield and Hull [97]) do not correlate well with measured profiles, because optimal patterns overestimated effective crank loading, particularly when the joint moment-based cost function was employed.

BIOMECHANICAL FEEDBACK

The majority of cycling studies conducted over the past 30 years have focused on either physiological response or mechanical response, or a combination of these responses. As discussed, these studies have helped to characterize the optimal rider-bicycling system, stimulating and motivating the development of methods to modify selected cycling characteristics to match those associated with optimal performance. Recent developments in rapid on-line data acquisition systems and data processing software now permit the use of the real-time biomechanical feedback in the modification of cycling mechanics. The presentation of kinetic parameters describing pedalling mechanics to the cyclist has been used in the laboratory [65, 81, 102] and "on the road." Komor [66] trained cyclists to modify the pedalling technique in accordance with a subject's specific optimal pedal force pattern determined from mathematical simulation. Only Sanderson [102], however, has questioned whether the modified pedalling pattern represent learned capabilities. In essence, we are faced with a situation in which information can be given to a subject, but what information to present and how that information should be packaged are unclear.

Broker et al. [9] studied the effect of two different feedback schedules on the retention of cycling kinetic patterns. Of particular interest was the potential for feedback dependency. Inexperienced cyclists (n = 18) practiced a pedalling kinetic pattern, emphasizing "effective" shear-force application centered about BDC. Half of the subjects assigned to a concurrent-feedback group received feedback during the final 30 seconds of each of 50 one-minute practice trials. The remaining subjects, assigned to a summary feedback group, received averaged feedback during the final 30 seconds of 1-minute rest periods interposed between each practice trial. Retention was evaluated during a no-feedback test conducted 1 week following the practice trials. Results indicated that both groups improved significantly during the practice phase of the experiment and that performance decay in retention (without feedback) was negligible. Feedback dependency was not apparent in either group, indicating that information-processing strategies used by subjects in each group, although probably quite different, were highly effective. There is a definite need to continue the exploration of how existing theories in motor learning affect our capability to modify cycling performance, whether it be in a performance or clinical setting.

FINAL COMMENTS

The long-standing interest in cycling mechanics is linked to efforts to understand alternate forms of transportation as well as musculoskeletal mechanics. Early insight into bicycle design, methods of measuring rider-induced loads, and the effect of these loads on the human musculoskeletal system have stimulated a great deal of research in the past 100 years. Although recent advances in technology have permitted additional insight, much remains to be accomplished in understanding the correct rider-bicycle interface that optimizes available human resources to power the bike effectively.

REFERENCES

1. Andrews, J.G. The functional roles of the hamstrings and quadriceps during cycling: Lombard's paradox revisited. *J. Biomech.* 20:565–575, 1987.
2. Astrand, P.O. Study of bicycle modifications using a motor driven treadmill. *Arbeitsphysiol.* 15:23–32, 1953.
3. Astrand, P.O. and K. Rodahl. *Textbook of work physiology.* New York: McGraw-Hill, Inc., 1970.
4. Bolourchi, F., and M.L. Hull. Measurement of rider induced loads during simulated bicycling. *Int. J. Sports Biomech.* 1:308–329, 1985.
5. Borg, G. Perceived exertion as an indicator of somatic stress. *Scand. J. Rehab. Med.* 2:92–98, 1970.
6. Boutin, R.D., G.T. Rab, and I.A.G. Hassan. Three dimensional kinematics and muscle length changes in bicyclists. *Proceedings 13th Annual Meeting ASB.*, Burlington, VT: UVM Conferences, 460 S. Prospect St., 1989, pp. 94–95.
7. Broker, J.P., R.C. Browning, R.J. Gregor, and W.C. Whiting. Effects of seat height on force effectiveness in cycling. *Med. Sci. Sports Exerc.* 20:583, 1988.
8. Broker, J.P., and R.J. Gregor. A dual piezoelectric force pedal for kinetic analysis of cycling. *Int. J. Sports Biomech.* 6:394–403, 1990.
9. Broker, J.P., R.J. Gregor, and R.A. Schmidt. Extrinsic feedback and the learning of kinetic patterns in cycling. *Human Movement Sci.* (In review).
10. Brooks, A.N., and B. Hibbs. Some observations on the energy consumption of human powered vehicles. A.V. Abbot (ed.). *Proceedings of the 1st Human Powered Vehicle Scientific Symposium.* Anaheim, CA: International Human Powered Vehicle Association, 1981, p. 42.
11. Browning, R.C., R.J. Gregor, J.P. Broker, and W.C. Whiting. Effects of seat height changes on joint force and movement patterns in experienced cyclists. *J. Biomech.* 21:871, 1988.
12. Burke, E.R., F. Cerny, D.L. Costill, and W. Fink. Characteristics of skeletal muscle in competitive cyclists. *Med. Sci. Sports Exerc.* 9:109–112, 1977.

13. Cafarelli, E. Peripheral and central inputs to the effort sense during cycling exercise. *Eur. J. Appl. Physiol.* 37:181–189, 1977.

14. Cavanagh, P.R., and K.S. Nordeen. Biomechanical studies of cycling: instrumentation and application. *Med. Sci. Sports Exerc.* 8:61–62, 1976.

15. Cavanagh, P.R., and D.J. Sanderson. The biomechanics of cycling: studies of the pedalling mechanics of elite pursuit riders. E.R. Burke (ed.). *Science of Cycling.* Champaign, IL: Human Kinetics Pub., 1986, pp. 27–30.

16. Citterio, G., and E. Agostoni. Selective activation of quadriceps muscle fibers according to bicycle rate. *J. Appl. Physiol.* 57:371–379, 1984.

17. Coast, J.R., and H.G. Welch. Linear increase in optimal pedal rate with increased power output in cycle ergometry. *Europ. J. Appl. Physiol.* 53:339–342, 1985.

18. Croisant, P.T., and R.A. Boileau. Effect of pedal rate, brake load and power on metabolic responses to bicycle ergometer work. *Ergonomics* 27:691, 1984.

19. Crowninshield, R.D., and R.A. Brand. A physiological based criterion of muscle force production in locomotion. *J. Biomech.* 14:793–301, 1981.

20. Dal Monte, A., A. Manoni, and S. Fucci. Biomechanical study of competitive cycling. S. Cerquiglini, A. Venerando, J. Wartenweiler (eds.). *Biomechanics III.* Basel: Karger, 1973, pp. 434–439.

21. Daly, D.J., and P.R. Cavanagh. Asymmetry in bicycle ergometer pedalling. *Med. Sci. Sports Exerc.* 8:204–208, 1976.

22. Davies, C.T.M. Effect of air resistance on the metabolic cost and performance of cycling. *Europ. J. Appl. Physiol. Occupat. Physiol.* A5:245–254, 1980.

23. Davis, R.R., and M.L. Hull. Measurement of pedal loading in bicycling: II. Analysis and results. *J. Biomech.* 14:857–872, 1981.

24. Desipres, M. An electromyographic study of competitive road cycling conditions simulated on a treadmill. R.C. Nelson and C. Morehouse (eds.). *Biomechanics IV.* Baltimore, MD: University Park Press, 1974, pp. 349–355.

25. Di Prampero, P.E., G. Cortili, P. Mognoni, and F. Saibene. Equation of motion of a cyclist. *Eur. J. Appl. Physiol.* 47:201–206, 1979.

26. Dickinson, S. The efficiency of bicycle-pedalling as affected by speed and load. *J. Physiol.* 67:242–255, 1929.

27. Dill, D., J. Seed, and F. Marzulli. Energy expenditure in bicycle riding. *J. Appl. Physiol.* 7:320, 1954.

28. Dul, J., M.A. Townsend, R. Shiavi, and G.E. Johnson. Muscular synergism—I. On criteria for load sharing between muscles. *J. Biomech.* 17:663–673, 1984.

29. Ekblum, B., and A.N. Goldbarg. The influence of physical training and other factors on the subjective rating of perceived exertion. *Acta Physiol. Scand.* 83:399–406, 1971.

30. Ericson, M.O., R. Nisell, and J. Ekholm. Varus and valgus loads on the knee joint during ergometer cycling. *Scand. J. Sports Sci.* 6:39–45, 1984.

31. Ericson, M.O., J. Ekholm, O. Svensson, and R. Nisell. The forces on ankle joint structures during ergometer cycling. *Foot and Ankle* 6:135–142, 1985.

32. Ericson, M.O., R. Nisell, U.P. Arborelius, and J. Ekholm. Muscular activity during ergometer cycling. *Scand. J. Rehab. Med.* 17:53–61, 1985.

33. Ericson, M.O. On the biomechanics of cycling. A study of joint and muscle load during exercise on the bicycle ergometer. *Scand. J. Rehab. Med.* 16:1–43, 1986.

34. Ericson, M.O., A. Bratt, R. Nisou, G. Nemeth, and J. Eicholm. Load moments about the hip and knee joints during ergometer cycling. *Scand. J. Rehab. Med.* 18:165–172, 1986.

35. Faria, I., G. Sjojaard, and F. Bonde-Petersen. Oxygen cost during different pedalling speeds for constant power output. *J. Sports Med.* 22:295–299, 1982.

36. Faria, I.E., and P.R. Cavanagh. *The Physiology and Biomechanics of Cycling.* New York: John Wiley and Sons, 1978.

37. Fenn, W.O. Zur mechanik des radjahrens in vergleich zu der des laufens. *Pflügers Arch. Ges. Physiol.* 229:354, 1932.

38. Firth, M.S. Equipment note: A sport-specific training and testing device for racing cyclists. *Ergonomics* 7:565–571, 1901.

39. Gaesser, G., and G. Brooks. Muscular efficiency during steady state exercise: effects of speed and work rate. *J. Appl. Physiol.* 38:1132, 1975.

40. Garry, R.C., and G.M. Wishart. On the existence of most efficient speed in bicycle pedalling, and the problem of determining human muscular efficiency. *J. Appl. Physiol.* 72:426–437, 1931.

41. Gonzalez, H., and M.L. Hull. Multivariable optimization of cycling biomechanics. *J. Biomech.* 22:1151–1161, 1989.

42. Goto, S., S. Toyoshima, and T. Hoshikawa. Study of the integrated EMG of leg muscles during pedalling of various loads, frequency, and equivalent power. E. Asmussen, K. Jorgensen (eds.). *Biomechanics VI-A*. Baltimore: University Park Press, 1976, pp. 246–252.

43. Gregor, R.J. A biomechanical analysis of lower limb action during cycling at four different loads. Unpublished doctoral dissertation, Pennsylvania State University, 1976.

44. Gregor, R.J., D. Green, and J.J. Garhammer. An electromyographic analysis of selected muscle activity in elite competitive cyclists. A. Morecki, K. Fidelus, K. Kedzior, and A. Wit (eds.). *Biomechanics VII*. Baltimore: University Park Press, 1982, pp. 537–541.

45. Gregor, R.J., P.R. Cavanagh, and M. LaFortune. Knee flexor moments during propulsion in cycling: a creative solution to Lombard's paradox. *J. Biomech.* 18:307–316, 1985.

46. Gregor, R.J., P.V. Komi, and M. Jarvinen. Achilles tendon forces during cycling. *Int. J. Sports Med.* S1, 8:S9–S14, 1987.

47. Gregor, R.J., P.V. Komi, R. Browning, and M. Jarvinen. Comparison of the triceps surae moment and the residual muscle moment during cycling. *J. Biomech.* (In press).

48. Hagberg, J.M., J.P. Mullin, M.D. Giese, and E. Spitznagel. Effect of pedalling rate on submaximal exercise responses of competitive cyclists. *J. Appl. Physiol.: Respirat. Environ. Exercise Physiol.* 51:447–451, 1981.

49. Hamley, E.J., and V. Thomas. Physiological and postural factors in the calibration of the bicycle ergometer. *J. Physiol.* 191:55p–57p, 1967.

50. Harrison, J.Y. Maximizing human power output by suitable selection of motion cycle and load. *Human Factors* 12:315–329, 1970.

51. Hawkins, D., and M.L. Hull. Muscle-tendon kinematics of the lower extremity during cycling. Applied Mechanics Division, ASME. P.A. Torzilli and M.H. Friedman (eds.). *Proceedings Biomechanics Symposium*, Vol. 98, July 9–12, 1989.

52. Henderson, S.C., R.W. Ellis, G. Klimovitch, and G.A. Brooks. The effects of circular and elliptical chainwheels on steady-state cycle ergometer work efficiency. *Med. Sci. Sports Exerc.* 9:202–207, 1977.

53. Hill, A.V. The heat of shortening and the dynamic constants of muscle. *Proc. Roy. Soc.* 126:136–195, 1938.

54. Hoes, J.J., R.A. Binkhorst, A.E. Smeekes-Kuyl, and A.C. Vissers. Measurement of forces exerted on pedal and crank during work on a bicycle ergometer at different loads. *Int. Zeitschrift fur Ang. Physiol.* 26:33–42, 1968.

55. Houtz, S.J., and F.J. Fischer. An analysis of muscle action and joint excursion during exercise on a stationary bicycle. *J. Bone Jt. Surg.* 41-A:123–131, 1959.

56. Hull, M.A., and R.R. Davis. Measurement of pedal loading in bicycling—I. Instrumentation. *J. Biomech.* 14:843–855, 1981.

57. Hull, M.L., and M. Jorge. A method for biomechanical analysis of bicycle pedalling. *J. Biomech.* 18:631–644, 1985.

58. Hull, M.L., and H.K. Gonzalez. Bivariate optimization of pedalling rate and crank arm length in cycling. *J. Biomech.* 21:839–849, 1988.

59. Hull, M.L., H.K. Gonzalez, and R. Redfield. Optimization of pedalling rate in cycling using a muscle stress-based objective function. *Int. J. Sports Biomech.* 4:1–20, 1988.

60. Hull, M.L., and H.K. Gonzalez. The effect of pedal platform height on cycling biomechanics. *International J. Sports Biomech.* 6:1–17, 1990.

61. Inbar, O., R. Dotan, T. Trousic, and Z. Dvir. The effect of bicycle crank-length variation upon power performance. *Ergonomics* 26:1139–1146, 1983.

62. Jorge, M., and M.L. Hull. Biomechanics of bicycle pedalling. J. Terauds, K. Barthels, E. Kreighbaum, R. Mann, and J. Crakes (eds.). *Sports Biomechanics*. Del Mar, CA: Research Center for Sports, 1984, pp. 233–246.

63. Jorge, M., and M.L. Hull. Analysis of EMG measurement during bicycle pedalling. *J. Biomech.* 19:683–694, 1986.

64. Kaneko, M., and T. Yamazaki. Internal mechanical work due to velocity changes of the limb in working on a bicycle ergometer. E. Asmussen and K. Jorgensen (eds.). *Biomechanics VI-A*. Baltimore: University Park Press, 1978, pp. 86–92.

65. Komor, A.J., A. Dal Monte, M. Faina, and L. Leoneredi. An attempt of modelling and computer simulation in optimization of an athlete's performance during cycling (Part I): *Report to the Institute of Sports Science*. Rome, 1985.

66. Komor, A.J. Methodological aspects of modelling and computer simulation applied to analysis and optimization of cycling performance. *Report to the Congress on Medical and Scientific Aspects of Cycling*. Rome: Abano Terme, 1989.

67. Kroon, H. The optimum pedalling rate. *Bike Tech.* 2:1–5, 1983.

68. Kyle, C.R. Mechanical factors affecting the speed of a cycle. E. Burke (ed.). *Science of Cycling*. Champaign, IL: Human Kinetics Pub., 1986, pp. 123–136.

69. Kyle, C.R. The aerodynamics of handlebars and helmets. *Cycling Science* 1:22–25, 1989.

70. Kyle, C.R. Wind tunnel tests of bicycle wheels and helmets. *Cycling Science* 2:27–30, 1990.

71. LaFortune, M.A., and P.R. Cavanagh. Effectiveness and efficiency during bicycle riding. H. Matsui and K. Kobayashi (eds.). *Biomechanics VIII-B*. Champaign, IL: Human Kinetics Pub., 1983, pp. 928–936.

72. LaFortune, M.A. Cycling from a biomechanical perspective. *Sport Sci. Med. Q.* 2:8–10, 1986.

73. Lollgen, H., H.V. Ulmer, R. Gross, G. Wilbert, and G.V. Meding. Methodical aspects of perceived exertion rating and its relation to pedalling rate and rotating mass. *Europ. J. Appl. Physiol.* 34:205–215, 1975.

74. Lombard, W.P. The action of two-joint muscles. *Am. Phys. Ed. Rev.* 8:141–145, 1903.

75. McCartney, N., G.J.F. Heigenhauser, A.J. Sargeant, and N.L. Jones. A constant-velocity cycle ergometer for the study of dynamic muscle function. *J. Appl. Physiol.: Respirat. Environ. Exerc. Physiol.* 55:212–217, 1983.

76. McCole, S.D., K. Claney, J.-S. Coute, R. Anderson, and J.M. Hagberg. Energy expenditure during bicycling. *J. Appl. Physiol.* 68:748–753, 1990.

77. McCoy, R.W., and R.J. Gregor. The effect of varying seat position on knee loads during cycling. *Med. Sci. Sports Exerc.* 21:579, 1989.

78. McCoy, R.W. The effect of varying seat position on knee loads during cycling. Unpublished doctoral dissertation, University of Southern California, Los Angeles, 1989.

79. McKay, G.A., and E.W. Banister. A comparison of maximum oxygen uptake determination of bicycle ergometry at various pedalling frequencies and by treadmill running at various speeds. *Eur. J. Appl. Physiol.* 35:191–200, 1976.

80. McLeod, W.D., and T.A. Blackburn. Biomechanics of knee rehabilitation with cycling. *Am. J. Sports Med.* 8:175–180, 1980.

81. McLean, B., and M.A. LaFortune. Improving pedalling technique with "real time" biomechanical feedback. *Excel* (Australian Institute of Sport Publication), 5:15–18, 1988.

82. Miller, N., and A. Seireg. Effect of load, speed and activity history on the EMG signal from intact human muscle. *J. Bioeng.* 1:147, 1977.

83. Morrissey, M., R. Wells, R. Norman, and R. Hughson. Internal mechanical and total mechanical work during concentric and eccentric cycle ergometry. D.A. Winter, R.W. Norman, R.P. Wells, K.C. Hayes, and A.E. Patla (eds.). *Biomechanics IX-B.* Baltimore: University Park Press, 1985, pp. 549–554.

84. Moulton, A. The moulton bicycle. *Proc. R. Instn. Gr. Br.* 46:217–233, 1973.

85. Muller, E.A., T. Hettinger, and G.F. Kuhn. Arbeitphysiologische versuche über das radfahren mit einem kuntstbein. *Z. Orthop.* 84:462, 1953.

86. Newmiller, J., M.L. Hull, and F.E. Zajac. A mechanically decoupled two force component bicycle pedal dynamometer. *J. Biomech.* 21:375–386, 1988.

87. Noble, B.J., K.F. Metz, K.B. Pandol, C.W. Bou, E. Cafavelli, and W.E. Sime. Perceived exertion during walking and running—II. *Med. Sci. Sports Exerc.* 5:116–120, 1973.

88. Nordeen, K.S., and P.R. Cavanagh. Simulation of lower limb kinematics during cycling. P.A. Komi (ed.). *Biomechanics V-B.* Baltimore: University Park Press, 1975, pp. 26–33.

89. Nordeen-Snyder, K.S. The effect of bicycle seat height variation upon oxygen consumption and lower limb kinematics. *Med. Sci. Sports Exerc.* 9:113–117, 1977.

90. Okajima, S. Designing chainwheels to optimize the human engine. *Bike Tech.* 2:1–7, 1983.

91. Pandolf, K.B., and B.J. Noble. The effect of pedalling speed and resistance changes on perceived exertion for equivalent power outputs on the bicycle ergometer. *Med. Sci. Sports Exerc.* 5:132–136, 1973.

92. Patriarcs, A.G., R.W. Mann, S.R. Simon, and J.M. Mansours. An evaluation of the approach of optimization models in the prediction of muscle forces during human gait. *J. Biomech.* 14:513–525, 1981.

93. Pons, D.L., and C.L. Vaughan. Mechanics of cycling. C.L. Vaughan (ed.). *Biomechanics of Sport.* Boca Raton, FL: CRC Press, 1989, pp. 289–315.

94. Pugh, L.G.C.E. The relation of oxygen intake and speed in competition cycling and comparative observations on the bicycle ergometer. *J. Physiol.* 241:795–808, 1974.

95. Redfield, R., and M.L. Hull. Joint moments and pedalling rates in bicycling. *Biomechanics.* J. Terauds, K. Barthels, E. Kreighbaum, R. Mann, and J. Crakes (eds.). *Sports Mechanics.* New York: Academic Publishers, 1984, pp. 247–258.

96. Redfield, R., and M.L. Hull. On the relation between joint moments and pedalling rates at constant power in bicycling. *J. Biomech.* 19:317–329, 1986.

97. Redfield, R., and M.L. Hull. Prediction of pedal forces in bicycling using optimization methods. *J. Biomech.* 19:523–540, 1986.

98. Rugg, S.R. Muscle mechanics of the triceps surae and tibialis anterior muscles during ankle dorsi- and plantarflexion. Unpublished doctoral dissertation. University of California, Los Angeles, 1989.

99. Ryan, M.M., R.J. Gregor, and J.A. Hodgson. Neural patterning of lower extremity muscles during cycling at a constant load. *J. Biomech.* 21:854, 1988.

100. Ryan, M.M., R.J. Gregor, and B. Healy. Use of surface and fine wire electromyography in the study of lower extremity flexors during cycling. *J. Biomech.* 22:991, 1989.

101. Sanderson, D.J., and P.R. Cavanagh. An investigation of the effectiveness of force application in cycling. *Med. Sci. Sports Exerc.* 17:222, 1985.

102. Sanderson, D. An application of a computer based real-time data acquisition and feedback system. *Int. J. Sports Biomech.* 2:210–214, 1986.

103. Sargeant, A.J., and C.T.M. Davies. Forces applied to cranks of a bicycle ergometer during one- and two-leg cycling. *J. Appl. Physiol.: Respirat. Environ. Exerc. Physiol.* 42:514–518, 1977.

104. Sargeant, A.J., A. Charters, C.T.M. Davies, and E.S. Reeves. Measurement of forces

applied and work performed in pedalling a stationary bicycle ergometer. *Ergonomics* 21:49–53, 1978.

105. Seabury, J.J., W.C. Adams, and M.R. Ramey. Influence of pedalling rate and power output on the energy expenditure during bicycle ergometry. *Ergonomics* 20:491–498, 1977.

106. Schwandt, D.F., M.R. Zomlefer, C.C. Boylls, J.H. Ongski, L.A. Cohen, and F.E. Zajac. An apparatus for studying the neural control and biomechanics of bilateral coordination in conventional versus novel pedalling. *S.A.E. Int. Congress, Technical Paper No. 840029.* 1984.

107. Sharp. A. *Bicycles and Tricycles.* London: Longmans Green and Co., 1986; reprinted Cambridge: M.I.T. Press, 1977, pp. 268–270.

108. Shennum, P.L., and H.A. DeVries. The effect of saddle height on oxygen consumption during bicycle ergometer work. *Med. Sci. Sports Exerc.* 8:119–121, 1976.

109. Sloane, E.A. *The New Complete Book of Cycling.* New York: Simon and Schuster, 1974.

110. Soden, P.D., and B.A. Adeyefa. Forces applied to a bicycle during normal cycling. *J. Biomech.* 12:527–541, 1979.

111. Suzuki, S., S. Watanabi, and S. Homma. EMG activity and kinematics of human cycling movements at different constant velocities. *Brain Research* 240:245–258, 1982.

112. Suzuki, Y. Mechanical efficiency of fast- and slow-twitch muscle fibers in man during cycling. *J. Appl. Physiol. Respirat. Environ. Exerc. Physiol.* 47:263–267, 1979.

113. Tate, J., and G. Sherman. Toe-clips: how can they increase pedalling efficiency. *Bicycling* 18:57, 1977.

114. Thomas, V. Scientific setting of saddle position. *Am. Cycling* June:12, 1976.

115. Van Ingen Schneau, G.J. From rotation to translation: constraints on multi-joint movements and the unique action of bi-articular muscles. *Human Mov. Sci.* 8:301–337, 1989.

116. Warner, B., L.C. Hager, and J.S. Alylen. The evolution of a hand-powered tricycle. *Bike Technol.* 2:10, 1983.

117. Whitt, F.R., and D.G. Wilson. *Bicycling Science.* Cambridge: MIT Press, 1974.

5
Demand vs. Capacity in the Aging Pulmonary System

BRUCE D. JOHNSON, Ph.D.
JEROME A. DEMPSEY, Ph.D.

The primary focus of this review is on the remarkable capacity of the healthy pulmonary system, even the significantly compromised system, for gas transport during exercise in the older adult (60–80 yrs of age). Numerous structural and functional changes in the lung, chest wall, respiratory muscles, and vasculature occur with age [9, 27, 38, 82, 74, 139]. These changes encroach significantly on the reserve of the healthy pulmonary system to produce expiratory airflow and inspiratory muscle pleural pressure, to ensure diffusion equilibrium of alveolar and end-capillary partial pressure of oxygen (PO_2), to uniformly distribute inspired gas, and to maintain a low pulmonary vascular resistance in the face of high pulmonary blood flow. Nonetheless, the healthy pulmonary system, even in the later years of life (>70 years of age) continues to meet the extraordinary demands placed on it by heavy exercise to maintain arterial blood gas and pH homeostasis. Even in the highly trained and fit older athlete capable of achieving very high maximal metabolic requirements, these reserves are further reduced, but only in extremely rare instances are they surpassed [61, 62]. The only major, consistent consequence of the aging process may be the degree of efficiency and, therefore, metabolic cost with which exercise hyperpnea is achieved [61].

In the first decade of life the respiratory system undergoes extensive growth and development [106, 129, 117]. By the second decade cellular proliferation ceases and only hypertrophy of existing structures occurs, reaching maturity between the 20th and 25th years of life [70, 71, 106]. Following these developmental years the aging process begins, apparently affecting the majority if not all the tissues of the respiratory system. Although the process is extremely gradual during most of adulthood, the process may accelerate in the later years, beyond the age of 60 to 65 [71, 95, 117].

Because the aging process mimics so closely changes in lung tissue that are associated with a disease process (i.e., emphysema) [108, 142] it often is difficult to factor out changes associated with aging alone versus accelerated changes caused by a history of exposure to environ-

171

FIGURE 5.1

Representative FEV_1 for healthy 30- and 70-year-old adults and for 70-year-old adults with moderate and severe chronic obstructive pulmonary disease expressed as a percent of predicted for 30-year-old adults. The loss of lung recoil with aging causes FEV_1 to move towards the disease state; however, the aging affect alone is substantially less than that resulting from the disease process.

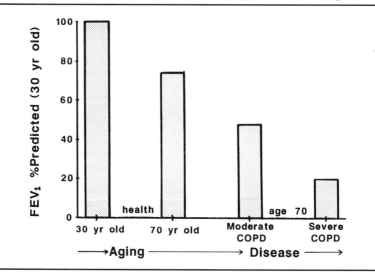

mental pollutants, pulmonary infections, and differences in lifestyle, such as smoking habits [134]. Although the aged lung appears to fit on a continuum leading to the disease state as shown in Figure 5.1, the nonsmoking, aging lung (in this case showing the forced expiratory volume in one second, FEV_1) falls much closer to the healthy state than the diseased state. The majority of studies dealing with aging also are cross-sectional, which, when compared to longitudinal studies, may tend to overestimate declines in respiratory function with age [71, 134, 44, 28]. The aim of this review is to examine the changes in pulmonary function and airway mechanics that are associated with aging, discuss morphological correlates for these changes and how they might alter the normal ventilatory response to exercise, and review what actually is known about the response of the respiratory system to exercise in an aging population. We frequently will refer to data from our own studies [61, 62] of 30 healthy, physically active older persons.

MAJOR RESPONSES OF THE PULMONARY SYSTEM TO EXERCISE IN THE HEALTHY, UNTRAINED YOUNG ADULT

The pulmonary system in the young adult (20 to 30 yrs of age) responds to exercise by a precise neuromechanical regulation of alveolar venti-

FIGURE 5.2
Typical ventilatory response to progressive exercise in an untrained young adult. The solid lines represent the flow:volume (on the left) and pressure:volume (on the right) response at rest and during mild-, moderate-, heavy-, and maximum-intensity work loads. Loops were placed on the volume axis according to a measured end expiratory lung volume (EELV). The flow:volume loops are placed within the maximum volitional postexercise (dashed line) flow:volume loop, and the tidal pressure:volume loops are placed within the shaded area, representing the maximal effective pressures on expiration (Pmax$_e$) and the capacity for inspiratory muscle pressure generation (Pcap$_i$) at the volume and flow rate at which peak pressure occurred during tidal inspiration.

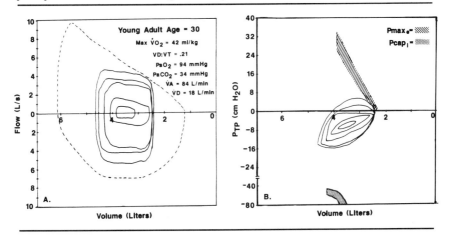

lation matched to metabolic demand [24], as well as through myriad changes that occur to optimize the transfer of oxygen from alveolar gas to arterial blood [21]. Figure 5.2 summarizes the normal flow:volume (f:v) and pleural pressure:volume (p:v) response to exercise in the young adult and lists the normal gas exchange parameters obtained at maximal exercise in this group of subjects.

Four key mechanical responses occur as exercise progresses from mild to maximal. First, the lung volume at the end of expiration (EELV) decreases with progressive exercise because of recruitment of expiratory muscles [56, 64]. The energy stored in the abdominal wall because of the active expiration provides some passive recoil at the initiation of the ensuing inspiration [49]. A more optimal (longer) length also is achieved for tension development by the diaphragm [29, 113]. Second, tidal volume (V$_T$) is increased by encroaching equally on inspiratory and expiratory reserve volume, avoiding the less compliant areas of the lung and chest wall [56, 145]. Third, maximum flow rates achieved during tidal breathing are well within the maximum available flow rates

[100]. Pleural pressure development during expiration only approaches flow-limiting pressures ($Pmax_e$) near EELV [100, 57]. That is, for a given lung volume, pleural pressure development does not reach a pressure that causes airways to narrow and therefore limit expiratory airflow. Fourth, on inspiration, peak pleural pressure reaches only 50% of the estimated capacity for pressure generation ($Pcap_i$) as determined at the lung volume and flow rate at which peak pressure was obtained [2, 79]. The result of these major mechanical responses to exercise is a highly efficient increase in alveolar ventilation with substantial reserve available to increase ventilation ($\dot{V}E$) even at maximal levels of exercise.

Several major adjustments in the pulmonary system occur to optimize gas transfer. The distribution of ventilation (VA) to perfusion (Qc) remains uniform during exercise [43] and overall VA/Qc rises substantially, both of which minimize the chances of arterial hypoxemia. Pulmonary capillary blood volume increases threefold with exercise, assuring an adequately long red blood cell transit time and diffusion surface area for alveolar to end-capillary O_2 equilibrium as cardiac output increases [21, 112]. Any rise in pulmonary arterial pressures that cause an increased turnover of lung water during exercise is matched by an increase in lung lymph flow, which assures that the lung stays dry [14]. Despite these significant adjustments to optimize gas transfer during exercise in the young adult, the alveolar-to-arterial-oxygen difference widens two- to threefold during exercise. This has been attributed to slight intraregional VA/Qc inhomogeneities, a 1% anatomical shunt with mixed venous blood composition [42], and a potential diffusion disequilibrium for oxygen in end-capillary blood even at work loads requiring only 3 L/min $\dot{V}O_2$ [135, 136].

AGE-DEPENDENT STRUCTURAL CHANGES IN THE RESPIRATORY SYSTEM

Pulmonary Mechanics

Four major changes appear to affect lung function, pulmonary mechanics, and expiratory flow rates as aging occurs. The primary change is a decrease in elastic recoil of the lung tissue [40, 39, 60, 104, 105, 133] and to a lesser extent a stiffening of the chest wall [115, 94, 96], a decrease in intervertebral spaces [32, 90], and an apparent loss of respiratory muscle strength [7].

These changes result in the age-related declines in lung volumes and flow rates as shown in Figure 5.3, which describes the mean volitional maximal flow:volume loop (MFVL) for 30 older subjects (age = 70, range 61 to 79) tested in our laboratory [62] compared to that predicted for height- and weight-matched 30-year-old adults. The smaller loop within the MFVL represents the resting tidal breaths for each age

FIGURE 5.3

Expiratory Reserve. *Changes in lung mechanics with age. The figure on the left shows the MFVL for 30 older subjects (average age = 70 ± 2 yrs, solid line) versus the MFVL for height- and weight-matched 30-year-olds (predicted, Knudson et al. [71] dashed line). The smaller loops represent the resting tidal loops for the older and younger subjects placed at their respective functional residual capacity (FRC). The dotted vertical lines represent the closing capacity in each age group, with the line at the highest lung volume representing the older subjects. The figure on the right shows the flow and pleural pressure relationship at a single lung volume of 60% total lung capacity (TLC) in the older (solid) and younger (dashed) subjects (Iso-volume, pressure flow curves). Maximal effective pressure (Pmax$_e$) occurred at 12 cm H_2O vs 21 cm H_2O in the older and younger subjects, respectively. Values were obtained from the following regression equations: Young:Pmax$_e$ = 0.93 * (Lung Volume, %TLC) − 34.4, r = .84), Old: Pmax$_e$ = 1.02 * (Lung Volume, %TLC) − 48.6, r = .83). Note the evidence for reduced lung elastic recoil in the older fit subject: elevated FRC and closing capacity, reduced maximal expiratory flow (MEF) 50%, and lower expiratory pressure (and higher lung volume) at which airways are dynamically compressed and flow rate becomes effort-independent.*

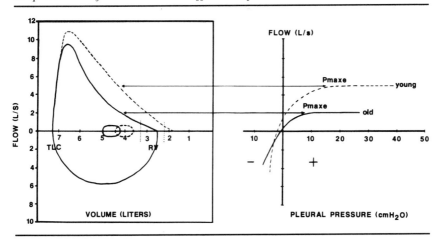

group. As shown, vital capacity (VC) and maximal expiratory flow rates (MEF) decreased, and functional residual capacity (FRC), residual volume (RV), and closing capacity (CC, dotted lines) increased. Total lung capacity (TLC) showed little change with aging.

Although a dominant mechanical change in the intact lung, which leads to the changes in pulmonary function, appears to be the loss of elastic recoil (increased compliance), biochemical correlates with elastin and collagen content (the predominant structural proteins in the lung) and structural changes within the matrix of these components are still not conclusive [74, 4, 36, 76, 77]. Because of the lack of evidence showing specific changes in the content of these proteins, there may be simply a disorganization of the normal crosslink patterns with age [102, 107, 111, 118]. More recent work using immune histochemical techniques shows a decrease in elastic fibers along the alveolar walls, together with an increase in type III collagen with age [25]. No variations of these components were noted in the alveolar ducts or in the respiratory bronchioles. Of the elderly subjects studied [25] (mean age = 76 yrs) who died of nonrespiratory causes, some also showed an increase in the thickness of the alveolar basement membrane. Modifications of the surfactant in the aging lung appear to be minimal [121, 143].

The loss of elastic recoil of the lungs has classically been shown by a shift to the left of the static p:v relationship of the lung [15, 40, 133]. At a given percentage of the TLC, therefore, the recoil pressure is less in the aged lung. Conversely, the compliance characteristics of the chest wall reveal that with aging the chest wall is compliant at any given lung volume, which yields a higher recoil pressure. The increased recoil of the chest wall has been attributed primarily to calcification of the costal cartilages [32, 94]. During ventilatory maneuvers over the range of the VC, it appears that older persons expand the rib cage less than do younger persons, resulting in a greater reliance on the diaphragm for ventilation [115]. This skeletal alteration of the costal cartilages apparently reduces the mobility of the rib cage more during expiration below FRC than during inspiration above FRC [115]. The balance of these two forces (i.e., the recoil of the lung tending towards collapse and the outward pull of the cest wall) yields the resting FRC, which (when measured by means of body plethysmography) usually increases with aging [82].

Changes in the intervertebral spaces, along with decalcification of the vertebrae, lead to decreased height in the elderly and an increase in anterior-posterior diameter. This could account for some decreases in TLC reported in the literature in older subjects [32]. Changes in TLC with age are variable (usually decrease or no change) and are the balance of the ability of the respiratory muscles to inspire versus the recoil of the lung and chest wall.

Some controversy persists over the major reason why RV rises with age and VC declines. A loss of lung recoil and air trapping, as well as a decreased chest wall compliance or decreased expiratory muscle strength [80], would account for this rise [5]. Chest wall strapping studies performed on aging and young adults tend to favor the loss of elastic recoil as the major mechanism [60].

The fall in VC and FEV_1 averages from 27 to 41 mL/yr and 21 to 51 mL/yr, respectively, in cross-sectional studies and significantly lower, 6 to 12 mL/yr, for both variables in longitudinal studies [134, 44, 71].

The apparent discrepancies between cross-sectional and longitudinal studies, however, have not been resolved but may be related to younger adults today being generally taller than their counterparts 50 years ago, or to statistical methodology or equipment changes [134].

Maximal expiratory airflow rates between RV and approximately 75% of TLC (effort independent region of the MFVL) also are reduced with age primarily because of the loss of elastic recoil. As one exhales forcefully, the pressure created outside the lung in the thoracic cavity causes large increases in airflow. The recoil pressure within the airways maintains airway pressure above the thoracic pressures and keeps the airway open; the recoil pressure is reduced as long volume falls during expiration. The radius of the airways and turbulent flow cause a resistance to airflow, which also causes airway pressure to fall below thoracic pressure as air is exhaled. At the "equal pressure point", expiratory air flow becomes effort-independent and any additional pressure generated by expiratory muscles is ineffective. The older adult reaches this "equal pressure point" at a higher lung volume than a younger adult because the recoil pressure within the airway is reduced from the start of an exhalation, therefore reducing the maximal flow rate at a given lung volume.

We demonstrated [61] this principle in a group of 12 older subjects representative of the 30 tested in our laboratory. We determined the largest pleural pressure generated ($Pmax_e$) to obtain maximal expiratory airflow at various lung volumes (50–75% of TLC) according to the methods of Olafsson and Hyatt [100]. We compared their response to young adults (age = 26) also tested in our laboratory. As shown in Figure 5.3, at a given lung volume, in this case 60% of TLC, the maximum pleural pressure generation achieved at the point expiratory air flow levels off is lower in the older adults than in the younger adults. The amount, therefore, of maximal expiratory air flow achieved at any lung volume within the effort-independent region is reduced. These measurements of maximal effective pressure generation in each of the older subjects were later used to determine how close tidal breaths during exercise came to flow limiting pressures.

The loss of elastic recoil also is manifested in the lung volume at which airways "close", or at least markedly narrow (closing volume, CV). In the young adult the closing capacity (RV + CV) occurs at 30% of TLC; at age 70 it occurs at 45% of TLC, a rise of approximately 250 ml/decade [17, 13, 5, 78].

In summary, the major changes in resting lung function associated with aging appear to be due to the loss of elastic recoil of the lung. This leads to the dynamic narrowing or closure of airways during expiration at elevated lung volumes relative to younger adults. In turn, this limits the maximum available expiratory flow rates, causes a mild hyperinflation, and increases the volume of trapped alveolar gas in dependent regions of the aging lung, especially at the lower lung volumes.

Respiratory Muscles

Age-related changes noted in some rodent locomotor skeletal muscles (i.e., decreased isometric and dynamic strength) [11, 30, 33, 132] appear to be attenuated in the diaphragm muscle [123]. Type II muscle fiber size or distribution does not appear to change with age [30, 46]. Capillary density also appears to remain constant in the diaphragm muscle from rats 4 to 27 months old [46]. There appears to be no apparent age-related differences in myosin heavy chain and light chain between old and young rats [123, 124]. Diaphragmatic neuromuscular coupling also is not significantly altered by the normal aging process [123, 124].

Indicators of respiratory muscle strength in humans, such as the maximal amount of mouth pressure that can be developed on inspiration against an occlusion, either do not show any significant changes [91], or show a moderate decline with increasing age [7]. Maneuvers such as this are volitional and highly variable and recruit muscles that probably do not normally play a major role in ventilation. It is difficult, therefore, to assess what is happening in the major respiratory muscles with age.

We attempted to better define inspiratory muscle strength in the twelve older subjects referred to previously that were tested in our laboratory [61]. Maximal pleural pressure development (measured with an esophageal balloon) was determined in duplicate over six different lung volumes from RV up to TLC to determine the effect of lung volume (length-tension relationship) on maximal pleural pressure [79]. In addition, the effect of flow rate (velocity of shortening) on pleural pressure development was determined at rest by having subjects perform maximal inspiratory efforts with different resistances so that the flow rate varied [79]. These measurements were later compared with the inspiratory pleural pressure development during tidal breathing in exercise to determine its proximity to the available capacity for pressure development ($Pcap_i$). Maximal inspiratory pressure development against an occlusion was greatest (-97 cmH_2O) from approximately 40–60% of TLC in the older subjects, which compared to 35–59% of TLC (-110 cmH_2O) in the younger adults tested in our laboratory using an identical protocol. The effects of lung volume and flow rate on inspiratory pressure development are shown in Figure 5.4 together with regression equations showing the combined effect of flow rate and lung volume on the inspiratory pleural pressure development. As shown, neither the effect of increasing lung volume nor the effect of increasing flow rate on pressure generation by inspiratory muscles was significantly different between the younger and older subjects.

Considering the animal studies and the limited amount of human work, it appears that age-related changes in the respiratory muscles are

FIGURE 5.4

Inspiratory Reserve. *The effect of lung volume and flow rate on pleural pressure development by inspiratory muscles in older (n = 12, age = 70 ± 2) and younger (n = 8, age = 26 ± 2) subjects. The effect of lung volume is shown from values obtained during occlusion (zero flow) and the effect of flow rate is shown from values obtained at 70% of TLC. The combined effect of lung volume and flow rate are summarized in the following regression equations: Young: $Pcap_i$ (% of max occlusion pressure) = 113 − 0.65 * (Lung Volume, %TLC) − 5.21 * (Flow rate L/s), r = .83. Old: $Pcap_i$ = 140 − .97 * (Lung Volume, %TLC) − 6.0 * (Flow rate L/s), r = .80.*

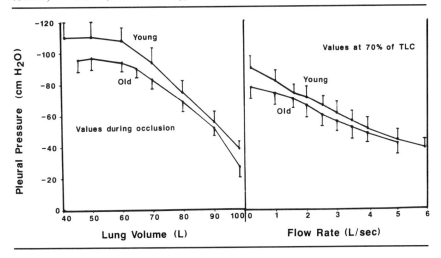

minimal. In older sedentary subjects, the potential for atrophy of accessory muscles and motivation level may play a factor in age-related changes associated with common volitional tests.

Alveolar to Arterial Gas Exchange

Five major changes potentially could affect gas exchange as aging occurs: (1) a loss of elastic recoil of the lung [58, 5, 133], (2) decreased surface area of the lung [130], (3) decreased pulmonary capillary blood volume [18, 34], (4) increased dead space ventilation [10, 109, 114, 89], and (5) decreased distensibility of the pulmonary arterial vasculature [110].

The loss of recoil in the lung not only effects the static lung volumes and MEF rates but also effects how ventilation is distributed. As the lung ages, the decline in recoil throughout the lung is most likely not a uniform process. This results in regions of the lung that may be more or less compliant than other regions, which causes areas of unequal mechanical time constants so that distribution of a breath is most likely not as uniform as in youth [53, 31, 58, 98, 72, 137]. Topographically, at rest, in the normal tidal breathing range ventilation in an older person may not be preferential to the lower regions of the lung as in the young adult [31]. This is presumably due to airway narrowing or closure in these dependent areas of the lung. These topographical differences with age were made worse with a forced expiration preceding the measurement of VA distribution and abolished with augmented inspiratory flow rates [31]. Blood flow to the apex of the lung is higher in the older adult relative to the younger one; however, like the younger adult, the majority of blood flow in the older adult is still directed to the lung base [58, 73].

The inert gas technique quantifies intraregional distribution of VA/Qc. To date, a small number of measurements in a few older, healthy adults showed a greater nonuniformity of VA/Qc relative to the young [137]. In no cases, however, was the VA/Qc distribution abnormal (i.e., markedly skewed to extremely low or high VA/Qc) such as occurs with a diseased state [137].

Structural changes in the aging lung lead to a decrease in alveolar capillary surface area (75 m^2 age 20 to 60 m^2 age 70) [130, 128]. The alveolar septa decrease and the alveolar duct diameter increases [99, 131], resulting in a decreased surface area for diffusion of gases into the pulmonary capillaries. In fact, the lung weight at autopsy is approximately 20% lighter in the aged adult [74]. The decreased surface area results in a decrease in the diffusion capacity for carbon monoxide of the lung, DLCO (approximately 4–8% per decade) [59, 18, 37], a measure of alveolar-capillary interface.

The reduction of pulmonary capillary interface as well as a stiffening of the pulmonary arteries and capillaries result in an age-related decrease in pulmonary capillary blood volume. The decline, however, appears to be small, resulting in a fall in this volume of approximately 2 to 5 ml per decade [18, 45]. In the normal young adult (20–30 yrs) this volume averages 75 ml and in the 70-year-old adult 50–65 ml.

The increased stiffness of the pulmonary vasculature with age has little or only a mild effect (increased slightly) on pulmonary arterial pressure (Ppa) with age at rest [47, 48, 34] which, although small, could account for the increased perfusion to the apex of the lung in the elderly as previously noted.

There appears to be a slight but significant age-dependent rise in dead space ventilation at rest in the aged adult, which has been attributed to the increased diameter of the large airways (anatomical) as well as to increases in areas of the lung that are over ventilated, i.e., high VA/Qc regions (physiological dead space) [109, 127].

Numerous regression equations have been published which describe an age-related decrease in arterial oxygen tension and the resulting widening of the alveolar to arterial oxygen difference (A-a Do_2) [125,

109, 93, 6, 67, 98, 86, 87, 140]. The change in partial pressure of oxygen in the arterial blood (PaO_2) with age appears to be variable, however, ranging from very little change (<1 mmHg per decade) to substantial decline (>5 mmHg per decade). Reasons for the discrepancies are undetermined but may be because many studies were not controlled for body position, smokers and nonsmokers, and general health status of the subjects.

SUMMARY

Figure 5.5 summarizes the potential effects that the structural and functional changes in the respiratory system with age may have on the response to exercise. Clearly, the available reserve for increasing V_T and expiratory air flow and inspiratory muscle pressure during exercise in the elderly person is reduced. In addition, the established rise in closing volume and decreased surface area of the lung (i.e., DLCO) may limit the available strategies of the aging respiratory system for meeting the demands imposed by heavy exercise. Of course, the effect of these changes with age on the exercise response will depend greatly on the demand imposed by the severity of the exercise. These responses are now discussed in detail throughout the remainder of the review.

RESPONSE OF THE RESPIRATORY SYSTEM TO EXERCISE IN THE ELDERLY

Although a good deal of literature describes ventilatory responses in the elderly during exercise [20, 55, 54, 26, 3, 41, 50, 84], few data address pulmonary mechanics and gas exchange. We now discuss these topics based on our recently completed comprehensive study [61, 62] in an older population of 30 relatively fit, healthy older subjects (see Table 5.1). Data have already been presented from this group of subjects on resting lung and chest wall function (see Table 5.2 and Fig. 5.3).

Mechanics, Breathing Pattern, Ventilatory Work, and Cost
The flow, pleural pressure, and volume response to progressive exercise in 12 of the older subjects (representative of the group tested in our laboratory, age = 70, $\dot{V}O_2$max = 44 ml/kg/mn, max HR = 165 bpm, max $\dot{V}E$ = 110 L/mn) is shown in Figure 5.6 and Table 5.3. These are contrasted with those in the 30-year-old untrained subject who reaches about the same mean $\dot{V}O_2$max and $\dot{V}E$max (see Fig. 5.1). The habitually active and relatively fit older subjects showed the usual age-related changes in pulmonary function and mechanics. Like the young adult, the older subjects tended to increase $\dot{V}E$ primarily through increases in

FIGURE 5.5

Summary of potential aging effects on the response of the respiratory system to exercise. The numerous structural changes that occur in the pulmonary system with aging potentially reduce the capacity of the pulmonary system for responding to the increased need for gas transport.

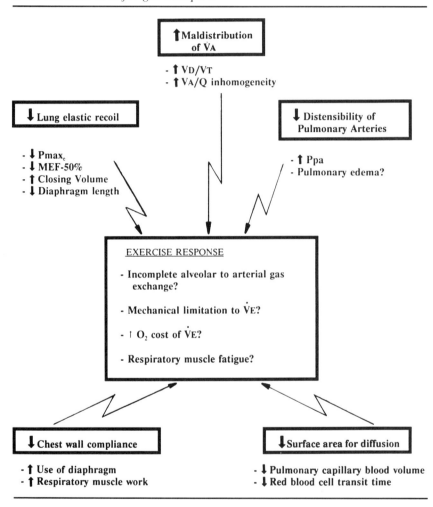

V_T during the lighter exercise loads, with a leveling off of V_T at 58% of VC (75% of $\dot{V}_{O_2}$max), which is slightly greater than that normally reported in younger adults (although the range is substantial, see Table 5.3). After 75% of $\dot{V}_{O_2}$max, primarily a frequency of breathing (fb) response to exercise is noted. These findings are similar to those reported by DeVries and Adams [26]. Ventilatory timing variables (i.e.,

TABLE 5.1
Subject Characteristics and Maximal Exercise Performance In Older, Physically Active Adults (N = 30)

	Age (yrs)	Ht (cm)	Wt (kg)	Max $\dot{V}_{O_2}$ (ml/kg/mm)	Pred* (%)	Max HR (bpm)	Pred† (%)	Wlk/Rn (mi/wk)
Mean	70	173.0	66.8	43.7	199	165	100	28
SEM	1	1.3	1.8	1.7	9	2	2	3
Range	61–79	162–194	54–86	25–62	116–306	148–184	89–112	12–60

* Normal predicted values for $\dot{V}_{O_2}$max based on age, from Jones et al. [66].
† Normal predicted values for maximal heart rate (HR) based on age, from Lange-Anderson et al. [75].

expiratory and inspiratory time) were similar to those in younger subjects at rest and throughout exercise.

The older person appears to have a higher ventilatory response at a given submaximal metabolic demand, so that in our subjects and in other studies [41, 55] the $\dot{V}_E/\dot{V}_{O_2}$ and $\dot{V}_E/\dot{V}_{CO_2}$ relationship is elevated, although in some studies the reported differences are small [144, 52]. This higher $\dot{V}_E/\dot{V}_{CO_2}$ relationship, combined with a higher dead space ventilation, gives the older subjects a near identical $\dot{V}_A/\dot{V}_{CO_2}$ and Pa_{CO_2} to the younger subjects at any given $\dot{V}_{CO_2}$. The fitness level of the older subject, like the younger subject, also will determine the magnitude of the ventilatory response to heavier exercise, because the onset of metabolic acidosis (and the coincidental compensatory hyperventilation) occurs at a higher work load in the trained person [65]. Accordingly, physical training causes a decrease in the $\dot{V}_E/\dot{V}_{O_2}$ relationship in older persons [144, 119, 120].

End expiratory lung volume decreased significantly from rest with mild (50% $\dot{V}_{O_2}$max) and moderate exercise (75% $\dot{V}_{O_2}$max) in a similar manner to that described in the young adult. Unlike the young adult,

TABLE 5.2
Preexercise Lung Volumes and Flow Rates in Older Subjects (Age = 70 yrs)

Preexercise (N = 29)	Actual ($\bar{x} \pm SEM$)	% PRED (70 yr olds)	% PRED (30 yr olds)
TLC (L)	6.98 ± .17	105*	99*
VC (L)	4.28 ± .13	109*	84*
FRC (L)‡	4.07 ± .11	100*	118*
RV (L)	2.68 ± .08	90*	123*
CC (L)	3.33 ± .10	99†	150†
$FEV_{1.0}$ (L)	3.07 ± .09	101**	74**
MEF-50% (L/s)	3.26 ± .20	90**	65**

‡ Values obtained in a body plethysmograph.
** Normal predicted values for maximal expiratory air flow rates and $FEV_{1.0}$ based on age and height, from Knudson et al. [71].
* Normal predicted values for lung volumes based on age, height, and weight, from Needham et al. [97].
† Normal predicted values for CC based on age and height, from Cherniack [13].

FIGURE 5.6

Group mean ventilatory response to exercise in older adults (n = 12, age = 70 ± 2 yrs). The solid lines represent tidal breathing, flow: and pleural pressure: volume loops plotted according to a measured EELV at rest through maximal exercise. The flow: volume loops are plotted within the pre- (solid) and post- (dotted) maximal volitional flow: volume loops. The dashed vertical line represents the closing capacity for the group as measured at rest. On the right, the tidal pressure: volume loops are plotted with respect to the dotted areas representing the maximal effective pressures on expiration and the capacity for pressure development on inspiration. Also shown are relevant arterial blood gas and ventilatory parameters obtained at max exercise (see Figs. 5.3 and 5.4 for explanation of mechanical parameters).

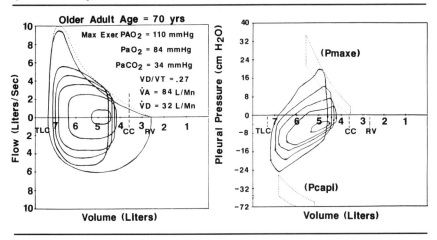

however, flow limitation and maximal effective pressure generation are approached at these lower submaximal exercise levels. To achieve greater expiratory flow with increased metabolic demand, EELV is increased, thus moving a portion of the tidal pressure and flow: volume breath away from flow limitation. During maximal exercise, this results in an EELV that is significantly elevated (60% of TLC) relative to the young adult (40% TLC). This results in a less optimal operating length of the diaphragm in the older person when the demand for inspiratory air flow is near maximal. These changes in lung volumes and capacities for rest, moderate, and maximal exercise are shown in Figure 5.7 for the 30 older subjects tested and compared to the volume changes in $\dot{V}O_2$ matched younger subjects. The rising EELV and constant V_T over the highest work intensities cause mean end inspiratory lung volume (EILV) to rise to 93% of TLC and the capacity for pressure generation by inspiratory muscles to fall. As shown in Figure 5.6, peak inspiratory pressure comes within 80% of the capacity of the inspiratory muscles

TABLE 5.3
Metabolic, Ventilatory, and Timing Variables During Exercise in Older Subjects (Age = 70 yrs)

$n = 30$	Rest ($\bar{x} \pm SEM$)	Moderate (75%)*	Max (100%)*	Range (at max)
$\dot{V}O_2$ (ml/kg/m)	4.2 ± .2	31.3 ± 1.1	42.8 ± 1.6	25.6–62.0
$\dot{V}E$ (L/mm)	11.3 ± .84	71.5 ± 3.4	113.6 ± 4.8	64.5–158
$\dot{V}E/\dot{V}O_2$	40.3 ± .9	34.2 ± 1.1	38.1 ± 1.6	24.7–50.5
$\dot{V}E/\dot{V}CO_2$	47.5 ± .9	32.4 ± .6	35.5 ± 1.4	22.5–53.1
f (bpm)	14 ± 1	29 ± 1	46 ± 1.2	32–58
VT (L)	.82 ± .05	2.43 ± .11	2.45 ± .08	1.41–3.4
Ti/Ttot	.47 ± .02	.48 ± .01	.48 ± .01	.43–.61
VT/Ti (l/sec)	.42 ± .04	2.47 ± .12	3.75 ± .15	2.16–5.88
VT/VC	.20 ± .02	.57 ± .02	.58 ± .03	.43–.86
EELV (L)	4.07 ± .11	3.69 ± .13	4.04 ± .15	2.84–5.44
$\dfrac{n = 12}{\text{Cdyn}}$ (l/cm H_2O)	.24 ± .02	.25 ± .03	.17 ± .01	.08–.24
RLe (cmH_2O/l/sec)	3.17 ± .18	3.61 ± .40	5.20 ± .38	3.6–7.6
RLi (cmH_2O/l/sec)	2.86 ± .20	2.46 ± .20	3.17 ± .21	2.4–5.1

* Represents approximate percent of $\dot{V}O_2$max.
Cdyn = dynamic compliance, RLe = expiratory pulmonary resistance, RLi = inspiratory pulmonary resistance. Resistance calculated at peak flow [92].

for pressure generation and is actually reached in 4 of the 12 subjects tested. This is in contrast to younger, untrained subjects who reach <50% of this pressure generation capacity (as shown in Figure 5.1) at this level of ventilation [79]. Without the rise in EELV in the older subjects, peak inspiratory pressure would have reached only 65% of the capacity for pressure generation. In summary, owing to decreased reserve for expiratory flow rate, EELV is elevated, reducing the length:tension relationship of the inspiratory muscles, and causing the capacity for inspiratory pressure generation to fall.

Despite the rising EELV, flow limitation still occurred over >40% of the VT at maximal exercise, and expiratory pressure generation reached maximal effective pressures over 25% of the VT. The large, positive expiratory pressures indicate a significant recruitment of expiratory muscles, greatly adding to the ventilatory work. Like the younger adult, however, the older adult generally does not develop excessive expiratory pleural pressure (i.e., pressure without increased flow); as a result, highly inefficient breathing is avoided. Expiratory resistance rises as a result of the disproportionate rise in pleural pressure for the given flow rate because of dynamic airway narrowing. This is unlike the younger adult who shows no significant rise in resistance at this level of ventilation (see Fig. 5.2) [145, 56]. Dynamic compliance of the lung (Cdyn) falls in the elderly subjects, especially over the top two work loads, most likely because the EILV reached such a high percentage of the TLC and an alinear portion of the pressure:volume relationship of the lung and chest wall. The younger adult also shows a progressive

FIGURE 5.7

Changes in lung volumes during exercise in older (n = 30, age 70 ± 2 yrs) and $\dot{V}_{O_2}$ max matched younger (age = 30) subjects. $\dot{V}_{Emax}$ is also similar for young (100 L/min) and older (115L/min) subjects. Shaded areas represent the tidal volume. Starting from the bottom of each bar graph the first line represents RV, the second line, CC, third line EELV, fourth line EILV, and the top line TLC. Note in the older subjects the increased EELV and end-inspiratory lung volumes at rest and exercise.

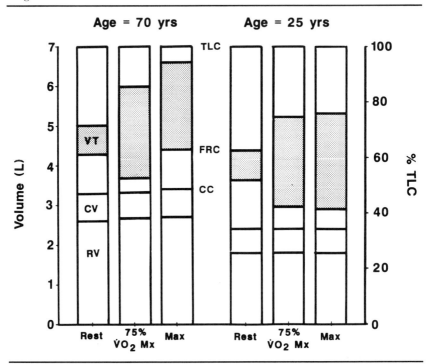

decrease in the Cdyn during exercise, although EILV achieves only 75 to 85% of the TLC [56]. This decrease in Cdyn is attributable to the tidal breath reaching the less compliant portion of the elderly person's lung and chest wall owing to a high inspiratory volume as well as a reduced EELV [56].

The expiratory flow limitation and concomitant increase in expiratory resistance (flow resistive work) and decreased Cdyn (elastic work) in the older subject cause the ventilatory work ($\dot{W}_v$) to increase curvilinearly with exercise. This curvilinear increase is out of proportion to the increase in work determined in younger adults at similar levels of ventilation [1, 101]. Because the measurement of work (i.e., integrated p:v loops) does not take into account several components of ventilatory

FIGURE 5.8

Ventilatory work ($\dot{W}_v$) and the estimated respiratory muscle $\dot{V}O_2$ (ml/min) in fit older subjects (n = 12, age = 70 ± 2) and $\dot{V}O_2$ matched younger subjects [1] and in younger athletes at a much higher $\dot{V}O_2$max. The work and cost of ventilation increases disproportionately at a lower ventilation in the older subjects versus the younger adults who require a greater percent of the total body $\dot{V}O_2$ at any given $\dot{V}E$ to support the muscles of respiration. At maximal exercise the $\dot{V}O_2$max devoted to ventilation was 13% (range 7 to 23%) in the older subjects, 6% (range 5–8%) in the younger untrained subjects, and 13% (range 10–16%) in the younger athletes. Ventilatory work was measured in all cases from the pressure:volume loops. $\dot{V}O_2$ of maximal exercise ventilation was estimated from ventilatory work according to the relationship defined by Aaron et al. [1]: $\dot{V}O_2$ of the respiratory muscles during exercise − the resting $\dot{V}O_2$ = .081 + .001 * (exercise $\dot{W}_v$ − rest $\dot{W}_v$).

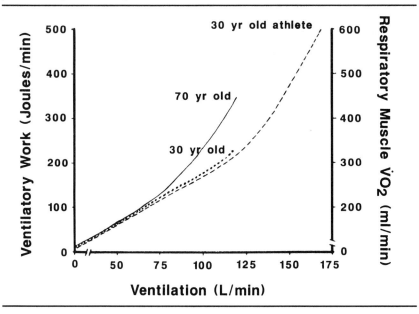

work (such as chest wall distortion, etc.), which are exaggerated in the elderly, our calculated $\dot{W}_v$ values are low. Figure 5.8 shows the differences in $\dot{W}_v$ between young and older adults tested in our laboratory.

We estimated the O_2 cost of breathing based on a regression equation derived on young adults from the increase in $\dot{V}O_2$ required when the mechanical characteristics and respiratory muscle recruitment patterns achieved during exercise were mimicked at rest [1]. The oxygen cost of breathing in our older subjects averaged 13% of the total body $\dot{V}O_2$ at maximal exercise, with values as high as 15–23% in the fittest subjects with the greatest ventilatory responses. This compares with approximately 5–7% for the same $\dot{V}_E$ in the younger adult [1]. The relationship of the change in respiratory muscle oxygen consumption to the change in ventilation appears to increase dramatically as mechanical limits for flow and pressure development are approached [16]. This represents a significant increase in the need for blood flow to the respiratory muscles and would theoretically compromise blood flow to the working locomotor muscles.

The postexercise MFVL of the elderly subjects shown in Figure 5.6 shows a significant rise in the MEF rates relative to preexercise. The apparent bronchodilation which occurs during exercise allows an additional 10 to 15 L/min of ventilation during maximal exercise. This significant effect on airway diameter helps to counteract some of the rise in the flow resistive work of breathing in these subjects [141]. The exercise-induced bronchodilation occurs in both young and old, but was greater in the older subjects tested in our laboratory.

Pulmonary Vasculature
Minimal literature exists on the hemodynamic changes in the pulmonary vasculature in the healthy aged subject [47, 48, 51, 110]. The data available describe changes in pulmonary arterial pressure (Ppa), pulmonary wedge pressure (Ppw), and the resultant pulmonary vascular resistance (PVR) (Ppa-Ppw/Q) with exercise. There is some debate over the accuracy of Ppw as an indicator of left atrial pressure, mainly because of intrathoracic pressure changes associated with hyperpneic states such as exercise, which yield erroneously high results. Figure 5.9 shows the changes in Ppa in response to supine exercise in a group of older subjects (61–83 years) relative to that determined on younger adults [47, 110]. At rest in the supine position, Ppas are only slightly elevated in the older adults as are Ppws and the estimated PVR. To increase blood flow through the lung, one must increase vascular driving pressure from the pulmonary artery to the left atrium. During heavy exercise in the older subjects, the Ppa increases (i.e., 100% from rest) out of proportion to those determined at a similar $\dot{V}_{O_2}$ and Q in younger adults (50%). Similarly, Ppw increases 120% in the older subjects versus only 25% in the younger adults. The pressure difference Ppa-Ppw was similar in both age groups and, therefore, PVR was similar in both groups. Although the older adults were more hypertensive than the younger ones at a given $\dot{V}_{O_2}$ and Q, the younger adults were able to achieve much higher metabolic work rates and therefore reach Ppas and Ppws similar to those achieved in the older adults at lower workloads. Measurements obtained in the sitting position at rest and during exercise reveal similar trends between the old and young, although differences are not as striking as while supine [47]. We emphasize that despite the relative pulmonary hypertension, we have no evidence for accumulation

FIGURE 5.9

Pulmonary hemodynamics with age. Shown are the pulmonary arterial pressures with increased cardiac output from rest to exercise in the supine position in 14 healthy older men aged 61 to 83 years (solid regression line) and in young men and women (dashed regression line). From Reeves et al. [110] and Granath et al. [47].

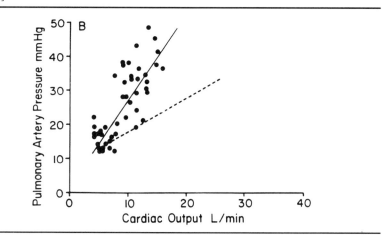

of extra vascular lung water in the older subjects, even during very heavy exercise, at least as judged indirectly by means of the A-a D_{O_2} during exercise (see below). Furthermore, we were unable to detect any change in lung volume subdivisions, closing volume, or diffusion capacity immediately following maximal exercise in our older subjects.

Pulmonary Gas Exchange

We investigated the adequacy of pulmonary gas exchange in 19 of our sample of 30 elderly subjects, as described earlier. Tonometered blood was used to ensure accurate calibration of blood gas electrodes. Three to six arterial blood samples were obtained in the steady-state at rest and at each workload in each subject and averaged to best represent each condition; all exercise samples were corrected for changes in core temperature. Individual subject values for PaO_2 at rest and at maximal exercise are shown in Figure 5.10, together with a comparison with average values for untrained 30 year olds at rest and at their max $\dot{V}O_2$ and with highly trained younger athletes.

In general, at rest and during all exercise loads through maximum, alveolar to arterial gas exchange and arterial blood gas homeostasis showed very little effect of aging in our group of healthy, fit subjects. Note the following evidence. At rest in the sitting posture, PaO_2 averaged in the high 80s, with a mean $PaCO_2$ of 38–40 mmHg. Only 3 of the 19

FIGURE 5.10

Arterial Po_2 and A-a Do_2 values in 19 older subjects (age = 70 ± 2) at rest and during maximal exercise. These values are shown relative to the resting and maximal exercise values in $\dot{V}o_2$ matched young adults and in young endurance athletes at higher max $\dot{V}o_2$max (n = 24) [21, 23]. The mean values for the older subjects are shown by the horizontal dashes.

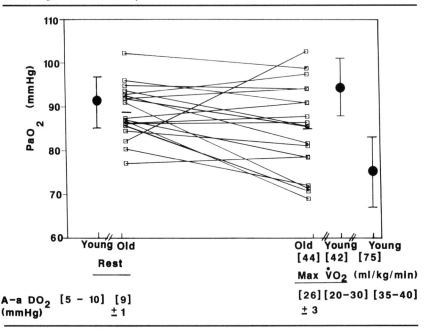

subjects showed a PaO_2 of less than 85 mmHg, and this was due to mild hypoventilation ($PaCO_2$ 43–44 mmHg). Thus, in almost all cases, our older subjects fit well within the 95% confidence limits of resting arterial blood gases for younger adults. The alveolar to arterial O_2 difference (A-a DO_2) was more variable but remained only slightly wider (2–5 mmHg) than the usual mean values for younger subjects; only 3 of the 19 older subjects exceeded 15 mmHg. The dead space to tidal volume ratio (VD/VT) was consistently higher by 15–20% in the older subjects, but extreme values, i.e., greater than 0.5 VD/VT, did not occur. During exercise the group mean A-a DO_2 gradually widened to about three times rest at $\dot{V}o_2$max; PaO_2 remained within 5 mmHg of resting values. The mean A-a DO_2 was within the upper range of the average values achieved by younger untrained adults at a similar max $\dot{V}o_2$. The A-a DO_2 exceeded 30 Torr in 8 of the 19 subjects tested, but the accompanying hyperventilatory response was usually sufficient to raise alveolar PO_2 high enough so that arterial hypoxemia was prevented. As described earlier, V_D/V_T was elevated (relative to younger subjects) at any given $\dot{V}_{O_2}$, but fell progressively with exercise; when combined with a vigorous ventilatory response, this ensured that alveolar hyperventilation was usually sufficient at all work loads for adequate CO_2 elimination (see Fig. 5.6). In only 4 of 19 subjects was there evidence of exercise-induced hypoxemia as PaO_2 fell to less than 75 mmHg and SaO_2 to less than 92% at max exercise. These subjects were characterized by wider A-a DO_2 in the 35 to 45 mmHg range, and only one of the four had an alveolar PO_2 less than the average value (see subject RA, Fig. 5.14). During submaximal exercise, PaO_2 was reduced to less than 75 mmHg in four subjects; this usually coincided with a hypoventilatory response, with $PaCO_2$ in the 42–46 mmHg range.

These data support the conclusion that alveolar to arterial gas exchange and blood gas homeostasis during even markedly intense exercise is, for the most part, almost independent of the aging process. Theoretically, one might predict otherwise, given the propensity for maldistribution of ventilation secondary to the older subjects' high closing capacity and the age dependent decline in pulmonary diffusion surface area. Under conditions of controlled, inspiratory flow rate and tidal volume, initiating inspiration from within the closing volume does cause a clear maldistribution of ventilation [35, 19]. Accordingly, some studies do report markedly widened A-a DO_2 (greater than 20 mmHg) and PaO_2 only 70–75 mmHg range at rest in some groups of otherwise healthy adults greater than 60 years of age; however, others support the findings in our group of a barely measurable aging effect or no change from the young [69, 93, 98, 109]. Perhaps more surprising is our finding that alveolar to arterial PO_2 differences only rarely widened markedly in the older subject, even at extremely high workloads. During moderate to heavy exercise, 11 of our subjects did reduce their EELV so that inspiration was initiated below their closing capacity, an average of 0.26L (0.07–0.6L); thus, about 15–20% of their V_T occurred within their closing capacity. The A-a DO_2 or V_D/V_T in 9 of these 11 subjects was not abnormally increased. To study this further, we examined the effects of posture in 10 subjects and found that closing capacity fell an average of 169 ml and end expiratory lung volume fell 435 ml from upright to supine position at rest, so that all subjects, even at rest, were breathing very close to or slightly within their closing capacity. Again, the A-a DO_2 at rest or during heavy exercise in the supine position remain very similar to that shown in these same subjects while upright; V_D/V_T was actually reduced slightly in the supine position both at rest and during exercise.

Given these findings on A-a DO_2, we speculate that distribution of ventilation during exercise must have been relatively unaffected by the aging effect of elastic recoil on airway closure—at least to the extent that would be manifested in overall pulmonary gas exchange. On the one hand, breathing at these low lung volumes must certainly bring into play a maldistribution of mechanical time constants among peripheral airways [35, 19]. Perhaps, during exercise, these effects are over-ridden by the homogeneity in ventilation distribution promoted by inspiratory flow rates that are 8 to 10 times the resting level, and the fact that the greater majority of the augmented tidal inspiration still occurs above closing volume, and probably on the linear portion of the pressure:volume relationships of most of these open airways. Furthermore, as exercise intensity increased, expiratory flow limitation caused most of these subjects to raise their EELV, thereby moving their tidal breath not only away from flow limitation (see Fig. 5.6) but also well above their closing capacity. Furthermore, although the aging effect on alveolar-capillary diffusion surface area is significant (shown by the 30% decrease in single breath DLCO from age 30 to 70 years at rest), the available reserve for diffusion and pulmonary-capillary blood volume in the healthy elderly subject is apparently sufficient to meet the demands for pulmonary oxygen transport imposed by their max $\dot{V}o_2$, as well as to ensure sufficiently long red cell transit time in the pulmonary-capillary bed to provide alveolar to end pulmonary-capillary O_2 equilibrium at their maximum pulmonary blood flow. In most elderly, healthy, fit adults, therefore, the widened A-a DO_2 with heavy exercise is, as in the young, probably explained by a small but significant exercise-induced increase in the nonuniformity of VA:Qc distribution and by the contributions from a normal anatomical shunt of about 1% of total cardiac output containing reduced O_2 content similar to that in mixed venous blood [42, 43].

Finally, we note a significant portion of the group did show some significant problems with gas exchange at maximal exercise; 8 of the 19 subjects had an A-a DO_2 > 30 mmHg, and four of the eight had significant hypoxemia with PaO_2 < 75 mmHg and A-a DO_2 in the 35 to 45 mmHg range. These subjects were not necessarily those with the highest $\dot{V}o_2$max values; 6 of the 8 subjects had a $\dot{V}o_2$max > than the group mean, but an *equal number* of subjects with a $\dot{V}o_2$max in this 45–55 ml/kg/min range had A-a DO_2 < 25 mmHg. A significant but weak correlation existed between lung closing capacity and max A-a DO_2 (r = 0.48, p < .05) and seven of eight subjects with A-a DO_2 > 30 mmHg were among those with the highest closing capacities. These relationships may be an indirect indication of propensity toward nonuniformity in ventilation distribution. Resting DLCO was not abnormally low in any of these subjects. We believe these cases in the young or old are examples of the demand for oxygen transport and more rarely, CO_2 transport, exceeding capacity [21]. More specifically, in the case of the older athlete, these subjects have reached an appropriate position on the demand versus capacity continuum, in which either the negative aging effects on diffusion surface or the mechanical characteristics of the small airways, or both, have surpassed the negative aging effects on the more primary determinants of $\dot{V}O_2$max, such as the dimensions of the cardiovascular system and the aerobic capacity of locomotor skeletal muscle. This disparity in the relative capacities of the organ systems may, of course, occur with continued physical training in the elderly, if the training stimulus had a greater effect on the cardiovascular-skeletal muscular dimensions than it did on the lung. These concepts are developed further in the remaining sections of this review.

EXERCISE DEMAND VERSUS RESPIRATORY SYSTEM CAPACITY

We have viewed the aging process as a reduction in the capacity or available reserve of the respiratory system to adjust to the increased demands imposed on it through exercise. As the degree of fitness increases because of either a training effect on the cardiovascular and skeleto-muscular systems or a genetic endowment, the reduced capacity of the aging respiratory system may present a greater relative influence on $\dot{V}O_2$max or exercise performance. We now address this balance between the demands placed on the respiratory system and the ability or capacity of the system to respond. This concept applies either to the ability and cost to the lung and chest wall to generate airflow or to the capability of the system to exchange alveolar gas.

Four representative examples showing variations in the aging effect on the lung and chest wall versus the level of fitness as defined by the $\dot{V}O_2$max are shown in Figure 5-11 and exemplifies the responses observed in the 30 older subjects tested.

LESS FIT ($\dot{V}O_2$max 23–43 ml/kg/min): Compare subject SK to subject JH. JH experienced a much larger effect of aging on elastic recoil. Subject SK had a relatively low ventilatory demand during maximal exercise compared to the normal amount of airflow reserve available (MEF–50% = 125% predicted); subject JH also had a very low absolute ventilatory demand but a significant demand relative to his more limited reserve (i.e., MEF–50% = 35% of predicted). The major difference between these two subjects is related to the apparent aging effect on the lung, specifically affecting the available maximal expiratory flow rates.

HIGHLY FIT ($\dot{V}O_2$max = 44–62 ml/kg/min): Subject WA represents someone with normal lung function for his age (78 yrs), but with an extraordinarily high $\dot{V}O_2$max and thus substantial demand for ventilation and flow rate. Subject WA had to increase his EELV over the last three workloads to continue increasing flow rates; as a result his EILV reached 95% of his TLC at end inspiration. Subject EE also is highly fit and has a tremendous ventilatory demand; however, he has

FIGURE 5.11

Ventilatory demand versus capacity in the aged lung. Tidal flow:volume loops (solid loops) from progressive exercise tests (demand) *in four older subjects plotted according to measured EELV within the maximal volitional flow:volume loops* (capacity). *Note the variability in V̇o₂max (and therefore airflow and volume demand) relative to the available reserve for flow and volume in these four subjects.*

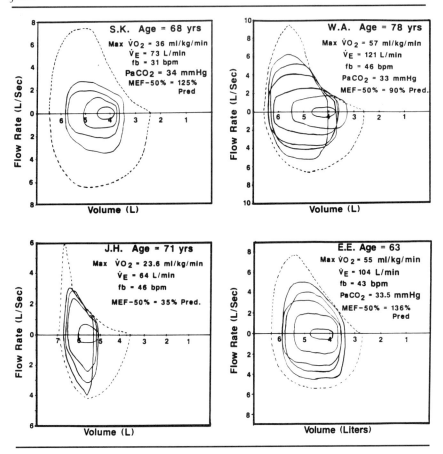

much better than normal lung function for his age, so that his ventilatory response to exercise and his flow and volume reserve at maximal exercise look similar to that noted in a younger adult (i.e., decreased EELV, little flow limitation) (see Fig. 5.2).

Contrast the large differences in V̇o₂max between subjects EE and JH. Despite his low ventilatory demand, subject JH is very close to reaching the limits for generating airflow because of a substantial aging effect on the MEF–50%. Subject EE, however, still has significant room to increase $\dot{V}_E$ at maximal work because, even though his ventilation and flow requirements are much higher than JH, his aging effect on elastic recoil is virtually nonexistent. This substantial reserve at maximal work is even greater in a few additional subjects with lower levels of fitness who also showed (like subject EE) little effect of aging on lung mechanics.

Subject EE also represents an older subject with extreme metabolic demands, yet who demonstrates an adequate hyperventilatory response at maximal exercise sufficient to decrease $PaCO_2$ to 33.5 mmHg. He also demonstrates very effective gas exchange because he has a small A-a DO_2 (14 mmHg) during maximal exercise. This is in contrast to subject RA (Fig. 5.14), who not only shows an inadequate hyperventilatory response to exercise ($PaCO_2$ = 38.5 mmHg) but an extremely widened A-a DO_2 at a similar $\dot{V}O_2$max and $\dot{V}E$max. Although subject RA had a MEF–50% that was normal for his age, it is significantly reduced relative to subject EE; in view of his widened A-a DO_2, his lung must have greater inhomogeneity in VA/Qc or approach a diffusion limitation for O_2 transfer owing to his extreme level of metabolic demand.

The balance struck, therefore, between ventilatory demand versus the capacity of the respiratory system to respond in the healthy elderly subject shows a great deal of variability among subjects. It depends critically on the contrast of aging effects on the morphological dimension of the pulmonary system *versus* exercise capacity.

What Role does Training or Fitness Have in Modulating the Aging Effects on the Pulmonary System?

There is limited evidence from cross-sectional studies that training or fitness may somehow influence lung volumes and airway mechanics both in older and in younger subjects [52]. Although our data represent cross-sectional information, we can make some inferences from our data to this question. Our subjects as a group represent a high level of fitness relative to their age predicted maximum (i.e., $\dot{V}O_2$max = 199 ± 10% of predicted). Despite this relatively fit population, the lung volumes (i.e., VC, FRC, CC, RV), MEF rates at 50% and 75% of VC, and gas exchange surface area as indicated by the DLCO still show the usual age-related changes. As a result, our group mean values average 100% of predicted values for their age. The data clearly show, therefore, that our highly fit group as a whole has undergone a significant aging effect on lung function. However, it is more difficult to determine any significant effect of "fitness" on this process because the normative predicted equations are based on broad ranges in the normative population.

A more definitive approach to this question takes advantage of the substantial variation in fitness in our group. Even though most of our

FIGURE 5.12

Relationship between lung function (i.e., MEF–50% and DLCO) expressed as a percent of age-predicted normal values and fitness level (i.e., V̇o₂max) in 30 older adults (age = 70 ± 2 yrs).

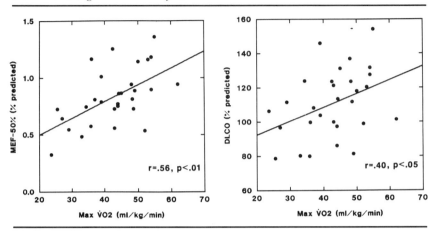

subjects exceed 150% of their predicted V̇o₂max, the range extended from 110–306% or 23 mL/kg per minute to 62 mL/kg per minute (Fig. 5.12). Within our group there were significant correlations (Fig. 5.12) between either % predicted MEF–50% or $FEV_{1.0}$ and V̇o₂max (mL/kg per min) (r = .56, p < .01) as well as with % predicted DLCO and V̇o₂max (mL/kg/per min) (r = .40, p < .05). Although these correlations are rather low, they tend to support the concept that either training or the level of fitness somehow does modulate or coincide with exceptional lung function. This impression is further demonstrated by taking the highest fit subjects (n = 15) and the lowest fit subjects (n = 15) in our group of older subjects and comparing mean values as shown in Table 5.4.

MEF–50% is 10% higher in the most fit group, as was the DLCO. The A-a DO_2 was similar at rest and had a tendency to be higher during submaximal exercise at 50–60% of V̇o₂max in the less fit group. At V̇o₂max the A-a DO_2 was similar in the two groups, but the fitter group achieved this at a substantially higher V̇o₂max.

The mechanical differences in lung function between the two groups (i.e., reduced MEF – 50%) were further manifested at a given V̇E during submaximal exercise by a greater degree of expiratory flow limitation and hyperinflation in the least fit subjects. However, owing to the reduced maximal V̇o₂ and therefore ventilatory demand in the least fit group, the degree of expiratory flow limitation during maximal exercise was similar regardless of the fitness level. If the less fit subjects had the

TABLE 5.4
The Effect of Fitness Level on Lung Function in Older Adults
(Mean ± SEM) (N = 30)

	$\dot{V}O_2max >43$ ml/kg/min (n = 15)		$\dot{V}O_2max <44$ ml/kg/min (n = 15)	
	Absolute Value	*% Pred*	*Absolute Value*	*% Pred*
Max $\dot{V}O_2$ (ml/kg/min)	50 ± 1	229 ± 10	35 ± 2	160 ± 9*
(L/min)	3.28 ± .12		2.44 ± .14	
MEF-50% (L/s)	3.41 ± .18	98 ± 5	2.75 ± .25	78 ± 6*
CC (L)	3.32 ± .10	100 ± 4	3.33 ± .17	98 ± 4
FRC (L)	3.92 ± .13	95 ± 3	4.24 ± .17	105 ± 3*
VC (L)	4.20 ± .15	111 ± 3	4.25 ± .21	110 ± 4
DLCO (ml/min/mmHg)	28.9 ± .6	116 ± 5	26.5 ± 1.2	106 ± 4
A-a DO$_2$ (mmHg):				
rest	8.4 ± 1.3		9.1 ± 1.2	
50% $\dot{V}O_2$	9.8 ± 1.6		14.9 ± 2.6	
Max	25.0 ± 2.9		25.8 ± 2.6	

* Significant difference between the two groups (p < .05).

maximum ventilatory demands of the higher fit group, this would had to have been achieved through greater hyperinflation, a reduced V_T and greater tachypnea, and much more severe expiratory flow limitation. Undoubtedly, within our group, there are those less fit subjects with the extremes of reduced MEF–50% who could not have achieved the level of maximum $\dot{V}E$ that some of the more fit subjects achieved no matter what the strategy they attempted.

There was a consistent tendency among our group for those subjects with the highest level of fitness to have better lung function and more efficient pulmonary gas transport. At the same time, the effect of aging on lung elastic recoil was still very evident in the lungs of the highly trained person. The aging process occurred across all fitness ranges. There is no consistent evidence of training-induced changes in lung function as studied in younger subjects or animals [22, 112, 8], nor do many groups of young adult athletes show superior pulmonary function relative to their untrained contemporaries. We propose, then, that the most likely explanation for this tendency in our older healthy sample is that $\dot{V}O_2$max and lung elastic recoil are both good indicators of the physiological aging process. The fitter subjects may therefore be thought of as having a certain genetically based resistance to aging.

Is Maximal Exercise Ventilation Mechanically Limited in the Active Older Adult (Demand > Capacity)?
All but four subjects reached a significant degree of flow limitation during maximal exercise (40–90% of V_T occurred along the expiratory boundary of the MFVL). Of the 30 subjects, 22 also reached a significant degree of flow limitation during submaximal exercise (>25% of V_T at

75% of $\dot{V}O_2$max), causing EELV to increase with further increases in ventilatory demand. Despite this degree of mechanical limitation, the submaximal and maximal ventilation and CO_2 elimination for the metabolic demand was adequate, because on the average the group showed a significant hyperventilation and compensatory arterial hypocapnia.

In a subgroup of six subjects representative of the group of subjects tested in fitness levels and degree of mechanical limitation during maximal exercise, we increased the fractional percent of the inspired CO_2 concentration ($FICO_2$) in an attempt to stimulate ventilation further during maximal exercise to determine if V_E was truly at a "physiological" limit. In subjects who had achieved flow limitation over >40% of their maximal air breathing V_T and had reached the capacity for pressure generation at peak inspiratory pressure, we found that $\dot{V}_E$ did not increase further. Generally only the fittest older subjects ($\dot{V}O_2$max > 45 mL/kg/per min) tended to show this level of mechanical limitation to ventilation, which was compatible with an inability to increase ventilation with further chemical stimulation at maximal levels of exercise. As previously noted in Figure 5.11, however, some subjects showed much greater age-dependent declines in resting lung function and achieved significant mechanical limitation at very low maximal oxygen uptakes (25 to 35 mL/kg/per min). It appears, therefore, that in the majority of older, especially highly fit subjects, maximal oxygen uptake is achieved *just prior to* or more usually, *commensurate with* attainment of the mechanical limits to ventilation. This is reflected by the significant alveolar hyperventilation in most subjects, so that as a group the capacity of the respiratory system for airflow and pulmonary gas transport is adequate to meet the maximal metabolic demand.

We investigated whether mechanical flow limitation or respiratory muscle pressure development in our older subjects was manifested in perceptions of dyspnea or shortness of breath. Our older subjects rated their perceived level of breathlessness as well as total body effort according to a 10-point scale [68] which asked how "heavy" the work was. During maximal exercise, dyspnea ratings averaged 7.1 ("very heavy" work to breathe), which was similar to that reported for total body effort (7.0). In all 30 subjects for $\dot{V}O_2$max maximal ventilatory output, peak inspiratory or expiratory pleural pressure development, degree of expiratory flow limitation, and tidal volume limitation (EILV as a % TLC), we found no significant correlations with the perceived level of dyspnea or the ratio of dyspnea to total body effort. The subjects who used the greatest percentage of their reserve, however, for inspiratory muscle pressure development during tidal breathing at maximal exercise (peak inspiratory pressure/Pcap$_i$, see Fig. 5.6) did show a significant tendency to have the highest rates of dyspnea to total effort ($r = 0.66$, $p < .05$). (This was determined in a smaller subset of

12 subjects in which Pcap$_i$ was measured.) Our limited data in the older, fit subjects do show, therefore, that a relatively high level of dyspnea is manifested at maximal exercise and that the degree of dyspnea is positively correlated with the percent of maximal inspiratory muscle pressure used, but not with the magnitude of expiratory flow limitation or ventilatory output. We cannot determine if these dyspneic sensations contributed significantly to exercise limitation in our subjects.

Respiratory Muscle Fatigue
Any decline in respiratory muscle power output would decrease the capacity of the inspiratory muscles for pressure development. In younger subjects, the issue of respiratory muscle fatigue during exercise is unclear. Some studies claim reductions in maximal inspiratory pressure following exhaustive exercise or fatigue-like changes in diaphragmatic electromyographic (EMG) frequency spectra during exercise [81, 12, 83, 85], but the validity of these indices of fatigue is questionable either because of the volitional nature of the tests, the interpretation of the EMG changes [122], or the problem of EMG analysis of an electrocardiogram-contaminated EMG signal. Because of the stiffened rib cage which causes an increased reliance on the diaphragm, as well as shortened inspiratory muscles due to flow limitation and a rising EELV, and the use of >80% of the capacity of the inspiratory muscles for pressure generation (increased work), one would consider the aged diaphragm as a prime candidate for fatigue. At least in short-term heavy work (3 minutes), however, it is apparent that pressure generation by inspiratory muscles is maintained and even rises over this time in the older subjects we tested. Furthermore, the peak inspiratory pleural pressure generated during tidal breathing at maximal exercise during air breathing or with increased levels of FICO$_2$ often equalled the capacity for pressure generation by the "fresh" inspiratory muscles (as determined at rest) (for example, see Fig. 5.14). Moreover, there was no indication from the arterial blood gases that there was a failure in achieving the appropriate alveolar hyperventilation for the metabolic demand. In the subjects we tested whose respiratory muscles required an estimated 13% and perhaps as high as 23% of the total body $\dot{V}O_2$, it is evident that these muscles were very capable of responding to the demands for pressure development placed on them. The situation might be quite different during endurance, high-intensity exercise in the older athlete, who must sustain these high-ventilatory responses and pressure generation in the face of shortened inspiratory muscle length and a high metabolic cost of breathing.

What Portion of the Pulmonary System Appears to be the Most Vulnerable to the Aging Process in the Exercise Response?
From the results of our mechanics and gas exchange data, there may be a disparity within the pulmonary system concerning the effect of

aging on the exercise response. The decline in the mechanics of lung function (i.e., reduced flow and vital capacity) has significant effects on the available strategies an older subject can choose from to increase minute ventilation, and it forces an increased metabolic cost for a given level of ventilation. Potential factors that could affect gas exchange, the high closing volume, maldistribution of mechanical time constants, the decline in DLCO, loss of diffusion surface area with age, and the rise in V_D/V_T, do not exert profound effects, however, even at maximal levels of exercise. The healthy pulmonary system is vigilant in its protection against hypoxemia and CO_2 retention. Accordingly as the lung ages either through the failure of sufficient age-related change or because of the large reserve present in youth, gas exchange is maintained and hypoxemia is prevented, even at extraordinary demands for gas transport (with few exceptions, see below). Although V_D/V_T increases, therefore, a relatively high overall V_A/Q relationship throughout the aged lung must be maintained and the number of regions with low V_A/Q ratios could not have been any greater than in a healthy young adult. That DLCO falls with age and yet A-a DO_2 at rest or maximal exercise does not widen abnormally exemplifies the substantial reserve of the pulmonary capillary blood volume and the limited minimum time required for complete end-capillary equilibration of alveolar and end-capillary blood [126]. Although there were a significant number of cases in which A-a DO_2 at maximal exercise widened greater than the upper range of normal in the young (at the same $\dot{V}_{O_2}$max), most of these persons even compensated with sufficient alveolar hyperventilation to avoid hypoxemia.

A disparity is therefore apparent between the influence that aging has on pulmonary gas exchange versus the mechanical cost and efficiency of breathing. That is, the loss of lung recoil, increased work of breathing, and increased V_D/V_T greatly influence the metabolic cost of V_E; however, overall alveolar ventilation and alveolar to arterial O_2 exchange remain sufficient to maintain an adequate arterial HbO_2 saturation and CO_2 elimination.

How Does the Fit Older Athlete Compare to the Young Athlete?
Our comparisons to this point have contrasted the older, physically active person and the untrained younger adult with a comparable $\dot{V}_{O_2}$max and $\dot{V}_E$; major differences in flow limitation, FRC regulation, and the work of breathing were noted. When comparing the degree of mechanical limitation, however, in the older fit subjects we tested to that in younger athletes, the latter, operating at a $\dot{V}_{O_2}$max and $\dot{V}_E$ which were 70% and 45% higher, respectively, had a remarkably similar degree of mechanical limitation (see Figure 5.13). Because the young athletes approach flow limitation at a much greater metabolic demand than in the older adults, they also increase EELV, and ventilatory work

FIGURE 5.13

Mean ventilatory response to progressive exercise in young endurance athletes (n = 8). Tidal flow (on the left) and pressure (on the right) volume loops (solid lines) are plotted from rest through maximal exercise. The flow:volume loops are plotted within the pre- (solid) and postexercise (dashed) maximal volitional flow:volume loops relative to a measured EELV. The tidal pressure:volume loops are plotted relative to the maximal effective pressures on expiration and the capacity for pressure generation on inspiration $\dot{V}o_2 max = 74 \pm 1$ ml/kg/min (range 66 to 80). Also shown are relevant maximal exercise blood gas and ventilatory parameters. Because of the much greater $\dot{V}E$ demand in the young athletes, they approach a level of mechanical limitation similar to that noted in the older, relatively fit adult during maximal exercise at a much lower $\dot{V}o_2 max$ (Fig. 5.6).

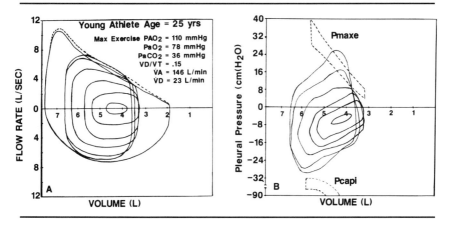

rises disproportionately. The work of breathing and the oxygen cost of ventilation approach those of the elderly at maximal exercise; but, of course, a much greater ventilatory response is required. Both groups therefore use virtually all their mechanical capacity for the generation of flow rate and inspiratory muscle pressure. In both groups it also is a rare occurrence that alveolar hyperventilation or CO_2 elimination at max work is inadequate. The widening A-a Do_2 at maximal exercise becomes even more extreme in the young athletes than in the older subjects. The additional drop in PaO_2 in the young and their higher incidence of exercise-induced hypoxemia is attributed to a diffusion disequilibrium due to shortened red cell transit times secondary to a combination of normal maximal pulmonary capillary blood volume with an extraordinarily high cardiac output [21, 136]. It appears that although the capacity of the lung for diffusion and flow rate are much greater in the young athlete, in a significant number of these athletes the demand for gas transport is increased disproportionately.

In summary, there are some key similarities but also important

FIGURE 5.14

Demand exceeds capacity. Subject RA showed the usual age-related declines in lung function (i.e., MEF–50% = 100% predicted, DLCO = 109% of predicted). With progressive exercise, the mechanical limits to $\dot{V}_E$ are reached at a submaximal exercise load. During both heavy (but submaximal) and maximal exercise, the maximal effective expiratory pressures were significantly exceeded, the capacity for inspiratory pressure development was reached at peak pressure, the cost of breathing approached an estimated 23% of the total body $\dot{V}O_2$, and PaO_2 fell to 59 mmHg, and $PaCO_2$ rose throughout the final work load.

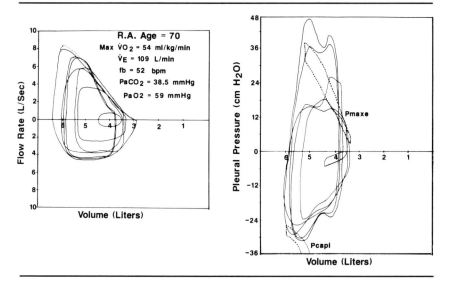

differences in where the young versus the older athlete reside on their respective continuums of maximal demand versus capacity. In the younger and older subjects alike the mechanical constraints and metabolic cost of ventilation during heavy and maximal exercise are excessive relative to the less fit subject. The incidence of inadequate pulmonary O_2 transport, however, is probably significantly greater in the younger athlete, suggesting that demand for pulmonary gas transport more often exceeds capacity in the young. With aging, lung function (i.e., MEF–50%, CV, VC, DLCO) declines at a rate similar to the rate of decline in $\dot{V}O_2$max (20–40% from age 25 to age 70) [116].

Failure: Does Demand Ever Exceed Capacity in the Healthy Aging Respiratory System?

Figure 5.14 shows one of the fittest older athletes we studied. This older athlete failed to increase $\dot{V}_E$ over the highest two work intensities he performed. With the addition of CO_2 to the inspired air, the $\dot{V}_E$ did not increase further during maximal exercise. He reached the capacity of his inspiratory muscles for developing pressure during tidal breathing and reached expiratory flow limitation over 80% of the V_T. This subject used virtually all of his maximal flow:volume loop available to him at a very heavy but submaximal work load. Nonetheless, he was capable of completing yet another workload with little further increase in total body $\dot{V}o_2$. In addition, during maximal exercise the partial pressure of alveolar O_2 (P_{AO_2}) failed to increase above 100 mmHg and arterial P_{CO_2} even started to rise throughout the highest work load. The extremely widened A-a DO_2 also showed a failure for complete gas exchange, and probably contained a significant component of diffusion disequilibrium. This subject represents a rare point of intersection on the continuum of demand versus capacity, in which the cardiovascular and musculoskeletal systems response capabilities are able to push the aging, healthy respiratory system to the point of failure. Our studies with added inspired CO_2 at maximal exercise do show the coincidence of mechanical limitation to flow and pressure generation and ventilation at maximal exercise, which occurs in many highly fit older and especially younger athletes. It is the rarity with which this point of intersection between capacity and demand is exceeded that is so remarkable. Perhaps the incidence of this "failure" in the slightly younger 55 to 65-year-old "master athlete" competing at an international level with $\dot{V}o_2$max values commonly in excess of 60–65 mL/kg/per minute might be significantly different [3].

SUMMARY—AGING, FITNESS AND LIMITATIONS TO $\dot{V}o_2$ MAX

Do the significant aging effects on lung mechanics and on gas exchange mean that the pulmonary system may "become" a significant limitation to max O_2 transport, as it does in some younger athletes. Theoretically, in a very limited sense this does occur; the 30-year old, highly trained athlete clearly could not achieve his max $\dot{V}o_2$ with the lungs of most fit, healthy 70-year olds. In reality, however, because aging also affects all links in the chain of O_2 transport and utilization, the pertinent question becomes, To what extent is the capacity of the pulmonary system curtailed by the aging process *relative to* that of the capacity of the cardiac pump, the total blood volume and its distribution, capillary-to-muscle mitochondria diffusion capacity, and metabolic capacity of locomotor muscle? As we have seen, the margin between demand and capacity in the pulmonary system does indeed narrow with age, especially in the highly fit adult in whom the selective effect of the training "stimulus" on the pulmonary system seems relatively small or negligible. This narrowing of the demand *versus* capacity margin does require some degree of compensatory response, as well as a mechanically inefficient and higher cost of exercise hyperpnea in the older athlete. Nonetheless, in all but the rarest cases, the pulmonary system capacity continues to exceed (or at least precisely meet) demand throughout the aging process.

ACKNOWLEDGEMENTS

Research supported by NHLBI, USARDC and the WI Heart Association. We are indebted to our subjects who gave extraordinary amounts of their time and effort and who never lost their spirit of cooperation nor their sense of humor. The aging process clearly builds character.

REFERENCES

1. Aaron, E., B. Johnson, D. Pegelow, and J. Dempsey. The oxygen cost of exercise hyperpnea: a limiting factor? *Am. Rev. Resp. Dis.* 141:4, A122, 1990.
2. Agostoni, E., and W.O. Fenn. Velocity of muscle shortening as a limiting factor in respiratory air flow. *J. Appl. Physiol.* 15:349–353, 1960.
3. Allen, W.K., D.R. Seals, B.F. Hurley, A.A. Ehsani, and J.M. Hagberg. Lactate threshold and distance-running performance in young and older endurance athletes. *J. Appl. Physiol.* 58:1281–1284, 1985.
4. Andreotti, L., A. Bussotti, D. Cammelli, et al. Connective tissue in aging lung. *Gerontology* 29:377–387, 1983.
5. Anthonisen, N.R., J. Danson, P.C. Roberton, et al. Airway closure as a function of age. *Respir. Physiol.* 8:58–65, 1970.
6. Bachofen, H., H.J. Hobi, and M. Scherrer. Alveolar-arterial N_2 gradients at rest and during exercise in healthy men of different ages. *J. Appl. Physiol.* 34:137–142, 1973.
7. Black, L.E., and R.E. Hyatt. Maximal respiratory pressures: normal values and relationship to age and sex. *Am. Rev. Resp. Dis.* 99:696–702, 1969.
8. Blomquist, G., R.L. Johnson, and B. Saltin. Pulmonary diffusion capacity limiting human performance at altitude. *Acta Physiol. Scand.* 76:284–287, 1969.
9. Brandsetter, R.D., and H. Kazemi. Aging and the respiratory system. *Med. Clin. North Am.* 67:419–431, 1983.
10. Brischetto, M.S., R.P. Millmen, D.D. Peterson, D.A. Silage, and A.I. Pack. Effect of aging on ventilatory response to exercise and CO_2. *J. Appl. Physiol.* 56:1143–1150, 1984.
11. Brooks, S.V., and J.A. Faulkner. Contractile properties of skeletal muscles from young, adult, and aged mice. *J. Physiol.* (London) 404:71–82, 1988.
12. Bye, P.T., G.A. Farkas, and C. Roussos. Respiratory factors limiting exercise. *Ann. Rev. Physiol.* 45:439–51, 1983.
13. Cherniak, R.M. *Pulmonary Function Testing*. Philadelphia:WB Saunders 1977, p. 249.
14. Coates, G.H., H. O'Bradovich, A.L. Jerreries, and G.W. Gray. Effects of exercise on lung lymph flow in sheep and goats during normoxia and hypoxia. *J. Clin. Invest.* 74:133–141, 1984.
15. Colebatch, H.J.H., I.A. Greaves, and C.K.Y. Ng. Exponential analysis of elastic recoil and aging in healthy males and females. *J. Appl. Physiol.* 47:683–691, 1979.
16. Collett, P.W., and C.A. Engel. Influence of lung volume on oxygen cost of resistive breathing. *J. Appl. Physiol.* 61:16–24, 1986.

17. Craig, D.B., W.M. Wahba, H.F. Don, J.G. Couture, and M.R. Becklake. "Closing volume" and its relationship to gas exchange in seated and supine positions. *J. Appl. Physiol.* 31:717–721, 1971.

18. Crapo, R.O., A.H. Morris, and R.M. Gardner. Reference values for pulmonary tissue volume, membrane diffusing capacity, and pulmonary capillary blood volume. *Bull. Europ. Physiopath. Resp.* 18:893–899, 1982.

19. Crawford, A.B.H., D.J. Cotton, M. Paiva, and L.A. Engel. Effect of lung volume on ventilation distribution. *J. Appl. Physiol.* 66:2502–2510, 1989.

20. Cunningham, D.A., E.A. Nancekievill, D.H. Paterson, A.P. Donner, and P.A. Rechnitzer. Ventilation threshold and aging. *J. Gerontol.* 40:703–707, 1985.

21. Dempsey, J.A. Is the lung built for exercise? *Med. Sci. Sports Exerc.* 18:143–155, 1986.

22. Dempsey, J.A., and R. Fregosi. Adaptability of the pulmonary system to changing metabolic requirements. *Am. J. Cardiol.* 55:59D–67D, 1985.

23. Dempsey, J.A., B.D. Johnson, and W.M. Bayly. Constraints on the ventilatory response to maximum exercise in health. *Hypoxia: The Adaptations.* J.R. Sutton, G. Coates, and J.E. Remmers (eds.). Canada: B.C. Decker, Inc., 1990, pp. 178–181.

24. Dempsey, J.A., E.H. Vidruk, and G.H. Mitchell. Pulmonary control systems in exercise: update. *Fed. Proc.* 44:2260–70, 1985.

25. D'Errico, A., P. Scarani, E. Colosimo, M. Spina, W.F. Grigioni, and A.M. Mancini. Changes in the alveolar connective tissue of the ageing lung. *Virchows Archiv. A Pathol. Anat.* 415:137–144, 1989.

26. DeVries, H.A., and G.M. Adams. Comparison of exercise responses in old and young men. II. Ventilatory Mechanics. *J. Geronotol.* 27:349–352, 1972.

27. Dhar, S., S. Shastri, and R. Lenora. Aging and the respiratory system. *Med. Clin. North Am.* 60:1121–1136, 1976.

28. Dockery, D.W., F.E. Speizer, B.G. Ferris, J.H. Ware, T.A. Louis, A. Spiro III. Cumulative and reversible effects of lifetime smoking on simple tests of lung function in adults. *Am. Rev. Resp. Dis.* 137:286–292, 1988.

29. Druz, W.S., J.T. Sharp. Activity of respiratory muscles in upright and recumbent humans. *J. Appl. Physiol.* 51:1522–1561, 1981.

30. Eddinger, T.J., R.G. Cassens, and R.L. Moss. Mechanical and histochemical characterization of skeletal muscles from senescent rats. *Am. J. Physiol.* (Cell Physiol.) 152:C421–C430, 1986.

31. Edelman, N.H., C. Mittman, A.H. Norris, and N.W. Shock. Effects of respiratory pattern on age differences in ventilation uniformity. *J. Appl. Physiol.* 24:49–53, 1968.

32. Edge, J.R., F.J. Millard, L. Reid, et al. The radiographic appearance of the chest in persons of advanced age. *Br. J. Radiol.*, 37:769, 1964.

33. Edstrom, L., and L. Larsson. Effects of age on contractile and enzyme-histochemical properties of fast- and slow-twitch single motor units in the rat. *J. Physiol.* 392:129–145, 1986.

34. Emirgil, C., B.J. Sobol, S. Campodonico, W.M. Herbert, and R. Mechkati. Pulmonary circulation in the aged. *J. Appl. Physiol.* 23:631–640, 1967.

35. Engel, L. Gas mixing within the acinus of the lung. *J. Appl. Physiol.* 54:609–618, 1983.

36. Eyre, D.R., M.A. Paz, and P.M. Gallop. Crosslinks in elastin and collagen. *Annu. Rev. Biochem.* 53:717–748, 1984.

37. Farney, R.J., A.H. Morris, R.M. Gardner, and J.D. Armstrong Jr. Rebreathing pulmonary capillary and tissue volume in normals after saline infusion. *J. Appl. Physiol.: Resp. Environ. Exercise Physiol.* 43:246–253, 1977.

38. Fowler, W.S., E.R. Cornish, Jr., and S.S. Kety. Lung function studies. VIII. Analysis of alveolar ventilation by pulmonary N_2 clearance curves. *J. Clin. Invest.* 31:40–50, 1952.

39. Frank, N.R., J. Mead, and B.G. Ferris Jr. The mechanical behaviour of the lungs in healthy elderly persons. *J. Clin. Invest.* 36:1680–1687, 1957.

40. Gibson, G.J., N.B. Pride, C. O'Cain, et al. Sex and age differences in pulmonary mechanics in normal nonsmoking subjects. *J. Appl. Physiol.* 41:20–25, 1976.

41. Gladden, L.B., J.W. Yates, W. Stremel, and B.A. Stanford. Gas exchange and lactate anaerobic thresholds: inter and intra evaluater agreement. *J. Appl. Physiol.* 58:2082–2089, 1985.

42. Gledhill, N., A.B. Forese, F.J. Buick, and A.C. Bryan. Va:Qc inhomogeneity and AaDO$_2$ in man during exercise: effect of SF$_6$ breathing. *J. Appl. Physiol.* 45:512–515, 1978.

43. Gledhill, N., A. Froese, and J. Dempsey. Ventilation to perfusion distribution during exercise in health. *Muscular Exercise and the Lung.* J. Dempsey and C. Reed (eds.). Madison: University of Wisconsin Press, 1977, pp. 325–344.

44. Glindmeyer, H.W., J.E. Diem, R.N. Jones, et al. Noncomparability of longitudinally and cross-sectionally determined annual change in spirometry. *Am. Rev. Resp. Dis.* 125:544–548, 1982.

45. Georges, R., G. Saumon, and A. Loiseau. The relationship of age to pulmonary membrane conductance and capillary blood volume. *Am. Rev. Resp. Dis.* 117:1069–1078, 1978.

46. Gosselin, L.E., T. Bohlmann, and D.P. Thomas. Effects of age and endurance training on capillary density and fiber type distribution in rat diaphragm muscle. *Med. Sci. Sports Exerc.* 20:59, 1988.

47. Granath, A., B. Jonsson, and T. Strandell. Circulation in healthy old men, studied by right heart catheterization at rest and during exercise in supine and sitting position. *Acta Med. Scand.* 176:425–446, 1964.

48. Granath, A., and T. Strandell. Relationships between cardiac output, stroke volume, and intracardiac pressures at rest and during exercise in supine position and some antropometric data in healthy old men. *Acta Med. Scand.* 176:447–466, 1964.

49. Grassino, A.E., J.P. Derenne, J. Almirall, J. Milic-Emili, and W. Whitelaw. Configuration of the chest wall and occlusion pressures in awake humans. *J. Appl. Physiol.* 50:134–142, 1981.

50. Grimby, G., and B. Saltin. Physiological analysis of physically well-trained middle-aged and old athletes. *Acta Med. Scand.* 179:513–526, 1966.

51. Gurtner, H.P., P. Walser, and B. Fassler. Normal values for pulmonary hemodynamics at rest and during exercise in man. *Prog. Resp. Res.* 9:295–315, 1975.

52. Hagberg, J.M., J.E. Yerg II, and D.R. Seals. Pulmonary function in young and older athletes and untrained men. *J. Appl. Physiol.* 65:101–105, 1988.

53. Harf, A., and J.M.B. Hughes. Topographical distribution of VA/Q in elderly subjects using krypton-81 m. *Respir. Physiol.* 34:319–327, 1978.

54. Hartley, R.H., Grimby, G., Kilbom, A., et al. Physical training in sedentary middle aged and older men. *Scand. J. Clin. Lab. Invest.* 24:335–344, 1969.

55. Heath, G.W., J.M. Hagberg, A.A. Ehsani, and J.O. Holloszy. A physiological comparison of young and older endurance athletes. *J. Appl. Physiol.* 51:634–640, 1981.

56. Henke, K.G., M. Sharratt, D. Pegelow, and J.A. Dempsey. Regulation of end-expiratory lung volume during exercise. *J. Appl. Physiol.* 64:135–146, 1988.

57. Hesser, C.M., D. Linnarsson, and L. Fagraeus. Pulmonary mechanics and work of breathing at maximal ventilation and raised air pressure. *J. Appl. Physiol.* 50:747–53, 1981.

58. Holland, J., J. Milic-Emili, P.T. Macklem, et al. Regional distribution of pulmonary ventilation and perfusion in elderly subjects. *J. Clin. Invest.* 47:81–92, 1968.

59. Horvath, S.M., and J.F. Borgia. Cardiopulmonary gas transport and aging. *Am. Rev. Resp. Dis.* 129:568–571, 1984.

60. Islam, M.S. Mechanism of controlling residual volume and emptying rate of the lung in young and elderly healthy subjects. *Respiration* 40:1–8, 1980.
61. Johnson, B.D., W.G. Reddan, K.C. Seow, and J.A. Dempsey. Mechanical constraints on exercise hyperpnea in a fit aging population. *Am. Rev. Resp. Dis.* 1990 (accepted for publication).
62. Johnson, B.D., W.G. Reddan, D.F. Pegelow, K.C. Seow, and J.A. Dempsey. Flow limitation and regulation of FRC during exercise in a physically active aging population. *Am. Rev. Resp. Dis.* (accepted for publication).
63. Johnson, B.D., W.G. Reddan, D.F. Pegelow, and J.A. Dempsey. Aging effects on expiratory flow limitation during exercise. *FASEB J.* 3:4, 6248, 1989.
64. Johnson, B.D., K.C. Seow, D.F. Pegelow, and J.A. Dempsey. Adaptation of the inert gas FRC technique for use in heavy exercise. *J. Appl. Physiol.* 68:802–809, 1990.
65. Jones, N.L. Normal values for pulmonary gas exchange during exercise. *Am. Rev. Resp. Dis.* 129:Suppl. 544–546, 1984.
66. Jones, N.L., and E.J.M. Cambell. *Clinical Exercise Testing, 2nd Edition.* Philadelphia: WB Saunders, 1982, p. 249.
67. Kanber, G.J., F.W. King, Y.R. Eshchar, and J.T. Sharp. The alveolar-arterial oxygen gradient in young and elderly men during air and oxygen breathing. *Am. Rev. Resp. Dis.* 97:376–381, 1968.
68. Killian, K.J. Breathlessness: the sense of respiratory muscle effort. *The Perception of Exertion in Physical Work.* G. Borg, D. Ottasan (eds.). London: Macmillan Press Ltd., 1985, pp. 71–82.
69. Kitamura, H., Sawa, T., and E. Ikezono. Postoperative hypoxemia: The contribution of age to the maldistribution of ventilation. *Anesthesiology* 36:244–252, 1972.
70. Knudson, R.J., D.F. Clark, T.C. Kennedy, et al. Effect of aging alone on mechanical properties of the normal adult human lung. *J. Appl. Physiol.* 43:1054–1062, 1977.
71. Knudson, R.J., M.D. Lebowitz, C.J. Holberg, and B. Burrows. Changes in the normal maximal expiratory flow-volume curve with growth and aging. *Am. Rev. Resp. Dis.* 127:725–734, 1983.
72. Kronenberg, R.S., C.W. Drage, R.A. Ponto, and L.E. Williams. The effect of age on the distribution of ventilation and perfusion in the lung. *Am. Rev. Resp. Dis.* 108:576–586, 1973.
73. Kronenberg, R.S., P.O. L'Heurex, and R.A. Ponto. The effect of aging on lung-perfusion. *Ann. Intern. Med.* 76:413–421, 1972.
74. Krumpe, P.E., R.J. Knudson, G. Parsons, and K. Reiser. The aging respiratory system. *Clin. Ger. Med.* 1:143–175, 1985.
75. Lange-Anderson, K., R.J. Shepherd, and H. Denolin. *Fundamentals of Exercise Testing.* Geneva: World Health Organization, 1971.
76. Last, J.A., T.E. King, Jr., A.G. Nerlich, and K.M. Reiser. Collagen cross-linking in adult patients with acute and chronic fibrotic lung disease. *Am. Rev. Resp. Dis.* 141:307–313, 1990.
77. Last, J.A., P. Summers, K.M. Reiser. Biosynthesis of collagen crosslinks. II. In vivo labelling, stability and turnover of collagen in the developing rat lung. *Biochim. Biophys. Acta* 990:182–189, 1989.
78. Leblanc, P., F. Ruff, and J. Milic-Emili. Effects of age and body position of "airway closure" in man. *J. Appl. Physiol.* 28:448–481, 1970.
79. Leblanc, P., E. Summers, M.D. Inman, N.L. Jones, E.J.M. Campbell, and K.J. Killian. Inspiratory muscles during exercise: a problem of supply and demand. *J. Appl. Physiol.* 64:2482–2489, 1988.
80. Leith, D.E., and J. Mead. Mechanisms determining residual volume of the lungs in normal subjects. *J. Appl. Physiol.* 23:221–227, 1967.
81. Levine, S., and D. Henson. Low frequency diaphragmatic fatigue in spontaneously breathing humans. *J. Appl. Physiol.* 64:672–680, 1988.

82. Levitzky, M.G. Effects of aging on the respiratory system. *The Physiologist* 27:102–106, 1984.

83. Loke, J., D. Mahler, and A. Virgulto. Respiratory muscle fatigue after marathon running. *J. Appl. Physiol.* 52:821–824, 1982.

84. Makrides, L., G.F. Heigenhuser, N. McCartney, and N.L. Jones. Physical training in young and older healthy subjects. *Sports Medicine for the Master Athlete.* J.R. Sutton and R.M. Brock (eds.). Indianapolis: Benchmark Press, 1986, pp. 363–373.

85. Maron, M.B., L.H. Hamilton, and M.B. Maksud. Alterations in pulmonary function consequent to competitive marathon running. *Med. Sci. Sports* 2:244–249, 1979.

86. Marshall, B.E., P.J. Cohen, C.H. Klingenmaier, and S. Aukberg. Pulmonary venous admixture before, during and after halothane-oxygen anesthesia in man. *J. Appl. Physiol.* 27:653–657, 1969.

87. Marshall, B.E., and R.A. Millar. Some factors influencing post-operative hypoxemia. *Anesthesiology* 20:408, 1965.

88. Masoro, E.J. (ed.). *CRC Handbook of Physiology in Aging.* Boca Raton, Florida: CRC Press, 1984.

89. Martin, C.J., S. Das, and A.C. Young. Measurement of the dead space volume. *J. Appl. Physiol.* 47:319–324, 1979.

90. Mauderly, J.L., and F.F. Hahn. The effects of age on lung function and structure of adult animals. *Adv. Vet. Sci. Comp. Med.* 26:35–77, 1982.

91. McElvaney, G., S. Blackie, J. Morrison, P.G. Wilcox, M.S. Fairbarn, and R.L. Pardy. Maximal static respiratory pressures in the normal elderly. *Am. Rev. Resp. Dis.* 39:277–281, 1989.

92. Mead, J., and J.L. Whittenberger. Physical properties of human lungs measured during spontaneous respiration. *J. Appl. Physiol.* 12:779–796, 1953.

93. Mellemgaard, K. The alveolar-arterial oxygen difference: its size and components in normal man. *Acta Physiol. Scan.* 67:10–20, 1966.

94. Mittman, C., N.H. Edelman, A.H. Norris, et al. Relationship between chest wall and pulmonary compliance and age. *J. Appl. Physiol.* 20:1211–1216, 1965.

95. Morris, J.G., A. Koski, and L.C. Johnson. Spirometric standards for healthy nonsmoking adults. *Am. Rev. Resp. Dis.* 103:57–67, 1971.

96. Muiesan, B., C.A. Sorbini, and V. Grassi. Respiratory function in the aged. *Bull. Physio-Pathol. Respir.* 7:973–1003, 1971.

97. Needham, C.D., M.C. Hogan, and F. McDonald. Normal standards for lung volumes, pulmonary gas mixing and maximum breathing capacity. *Thorac* 9:313–325, 1954.

98. Neufeld, O., J.R. Smith, and S.L. Goldman. Arterial oxygen tension in relation to age in hospital subjects. *J. Am. Ger. Soc.* 21:4–9, 1973.

99. Niewoehner, D.E., and J. Kleinerman. Morphologic basis of pulmonary resistance in the human lung and effects of aging. *J. Appl. Physiol.* 36:412–418, 1974.

100. Olafsson, S., R.E. Hyatt. Ventilatory mechanics and expiratory flow limitation during exercise in normal subjects. *J. Clin. Invest.* 48:564–573, 1969.

101. Otis, A.B. The work of breathing. *The Handbook of Physiology* Section 3: *Respiration,* Volume I. W.O. Fenn, and H. Rahn (eds.). Philadelphia: Waverly Press Inc, 1964, pp.463–476.

102. Palecek, F., and E. Jezova. Elastic properties of the rat respiratory system related to age. *Physiologia Bohemoslovaca* 37:39–48, 1988.

103. Peterson, D.D., A.I. Pack, D.A. Silage, and A.P. Fishman. Effects of aging on ventilatory and occlusion pressure responses to hypoxia and hypercapnia. *Am. Rev. Resp. Dis.* 124:387–391, 1981.

104. Pierce, J.A. Tensile strength of the human lung. *J. Clin. Invest.* 66:652–658, 1965.

105. Pierce, J.A., and R.V. Ebert. Fibrous network of the lung and its change with age. *Thorax* 20:469–476, 1965.

106. Polgar, G., and T.R. Weng. The functional development of the respiratory system. From the period of gestation to adulthood. *Am. Rev. Resp. Dis.* 120:625–695, 1979.

107. Prockop, D.J., K.I. Kivirikko, and L. Tuderman. The biosynthesis of collagen and its disorders. *N. Engl. J. Med.* 302:13–23, 77–95, 1979.
108. Pump, K.K. Emphysema and its relation to age. *Am. Rev. Resp. Dis.* 114:5–13, 1976.
109. Raine, J.M., and J.M. Bishop. A-a difference in O_2 tension and physiological dead space in normal man. *J. Appl. Physiol.* 18:284–288, 1963.
110. Reeves, J.T., J.A. Dempsey, and R.F. Grover. Pulmonary circulation during exercise. *Pulmonary Vascular Physiology and Pathophysiology.* E.K. Weir and J.T. Reeves, eds. New York: Marcel Dekker, Inc., 1989, pp. 107–133.
111. Reiser, K.M., S.M. Hennessy, and J.A. Last. Analysis of age-associated changes in collagen crosslinking in the skin and lung in monkeys and rats. *Biochim. Biophys. Acta* 926:339–348, 1987.
112. Reuschlein, P.L., W.G. Reddan, J.F. Burpee, J.B.L. Gee, and J. Rankin. The effect of physical training on the pulmonary diffusing capacity during submaximal work. *J. Appl. Physiol.* 24:152–158, 1968.
113. Road, J.D., S. Newman, J.P. Derenne, and A. Grassino. The in vivo length-force relationship of the canine diaphragm. *J. Appl. Physiol.* 60:63–70, 1986.
114. Rubin, S., M. Tack, and N.S. Cherniack. Effect of aging on respiratory responses to CO_2 and inspiratory resistive loads. *J. of Gerontol.* 37:306–312, 1982.
115. Rizzato, G., and L. Marazzini. Thoracoabdominal mechanics in elderly men. *J. Appl. Physiol.* 28:457–460, 1970.
116. Saltin, B. The aging endurance athlete. *Sports Medicine for the Mature Athlete.* J.R. Sutton and R.M. Brock (eds.). Indianapolis: Benchmark Press, 1986, pp. 59–80.
117. Schoenberg, J.B., G.T. Beck, and A. Bouhuys. Growth and decay of pulmonary function in healthy blacks and whites. *Respir. Physiol.* 33:367–393, 1978.
118. Schofield, J.D. Connective tissue aging: differences between mouse tissues in age-related changes in collagen extractability. *Exp. Gerontol.* 15:113–119, 1979.
119. Seals, D.R., J.M. Hagberg, B.F. Hurley, A.A. Ehsand, and J.O. Holloszy. Endurance training in older men and women. I. Cardiovascular responses to exercise. *J. Appl. Physiol.: Respirat. Environ. Exercise Physiol.* 57:1024–1029, 1984.
120. Seals, D.R., B.F. Hurley, J. Schultz, and J.M. Hagberg. Endurance training in older men and women II. Blood lactate response to submaximal exercise. *J. Appl. Physiol.: Respirat. Environ. Exercise Physiol.* 57:1030–1033, 1984.
121. Shimura, S., E.S. Boatman, and C.J. Martin. Effects of aging on the alveolar pores of Kohn and on the cytoplasmic components of alveolar type II cells in monkey lungs. *J. Pathol.* 148:1–11, 1986.
122. Sieck, G.C., and M. Fournier. Changes in diaphragm motor unit EMG during fatigue. *J. Appl. Physiol.* 68:1917–1926, 1990.
123. Smith, D.O. Physiological and structural changes at the neuromuscular junction during aging. *The Aging Brain: Cellular and Molecular Mechanisms in the Nervous System.* E. Giacobini, G. Filogamo, G. Giacobini, A. Vernadakis (eds.). New York: Raven Press, 1982, pp. 123–137.
124. Smith, D.O., and J.L. Rosenheimer. Aging at the neuromuscular junction. *Aging and Cell Structure* J.E. Johnson, Jr. (ed.). New York: Plenum Press, 1984, pp. 111–137.
125. Sorbini, C.A., V. Grassi, E. Solinas, and G. Muiesan. Arterial oxygen tension in relation to age in healthy subjects. *Respiration* 25:3–13, 1968.
126. Sue, D.Y., Oren, A., Hansen, J.E., and K. Wasserman. Diffusing capacity for carbon monoxide as a predictor of gas exchange during exercise. *New Engl. J. Med.* 316:1301–1306, 1987.
127. Tenney, S.M., and R.M. Miller. Dead space ventilation in old age. *J. Appl. Physiol.* 9:321–327, 1956.
128. Terry, P.B., R.J. Traystman, H.H. Newball, G. Batra, and H.A. Menkes. Collateral ventilation in man. *N. Engl. J. Med.* 298:10–15, 1978.

129. Terry, P.B., H.A. Menkes, and R.J. Traystman. Effects of maturation and aging on collateral ventilation in sheep. *J. Appl. Physiol.* 62:1028–1032, 1987.

130. Thurlbeck, W.M. The internal surface area of non-emphysematous lungs. *Am. Rev. Resp. Dis.* 95:765–773, 1967.

131. Thurlbeck, W.M. The effect of age on the lung. *Aging—Its Chemistry.* A.A. Dietz (ed.). Washington: Association for Clinical Chemistry, 1980, pp. 88–109.

132. Trounce, I., E. Byrne, and S. Marzuki. Decline in skeletal muscle mitochondrial respiratory chain function: possible factor in ageing. *Lancet* 1:637–639, 1989.

133. Turner, J.M., J. Mead, and M.E. Wohl. Elasticity of human lungs in relation to age. *J. Appl. Physiol.* 25:664–671, 1968.

134. Vollmer, W.M., L.R. Johnson, L.E. McCamant, and A.S. Buist. Longitudinal versus cross-sectional estimation of lung function decline-further insights. *Statistics in Medicine,* 7:685–696, 1988.

135. Wagner, P.D. Influence of mixed venous PO_2 on diffusion of O_2 across the pulmonary blood:gas barrier. *Clin. Physiol.* 2:105–115, 1982.

136. Wagner, P.D., G.E. Gale, R.E. Moon, J. Torre-Bueno, B.W. Stolpe, and H.A. Saltzman. Pulmonary gas exchange in humans at sea-level and simulated altitude. *J. Appl. Physiol.* 61:260–270, 1986.

137. Wagner, P., R. Laravuso, R. Uhl, and J.B. West. Continuous contributions of ventilation-perfusion ratios in normal subjects breathing air at 100% O_2. *J. Clin. Invest.* 54:54–68, 1974.

138. Wahba, W.M. Body build and preoperative arterial oxygen tension. *Can. Anaesth. Soc. J.* 22:653–658, 1975.

139. Wahba, W.M. Influence of aging on lung function—clinical significance of changes from age twenty. *Anesth. Analg.* 62:764–76, 1983.

140. Ward, R.J., A.G. Tolas, R.J. Benveniste, J.M. Hansen, and J.J. Bonica. Effect of posture on normal arterial blood gas tensions in the aged. *Geriatrics*:139–143, 1966.

141. Warren, J.B., S.T. Jennings, and T.J.H. Clark. Effect of adrenergic and vagal blockade on the normal human airway response to exercise. *Clin. Sci.* 66:79–85, 1984.

142. Wilson, R.M., R.S. Meadow, B.E. Jay, and E. Higgins. The pulmonary pathologic physiology of persons who smoke cigarettes. *N. Engl. J. Med.* 262:956–961, 1960.

143. Yasuoka, S., H. Manabe, T. Oaki, and E. Tsubura. Effect of age on the saturated lecithin contents of human and rat lung tissues. *J. Gerontol.* 32:387–391, 1977.

144. Yerg, J.E. II, D.R. Seals, J.M. Hagberg, and J.O. Holloszy. Effect of endurance exercise training on ventilatory function in older individuals. *J. Appl. Physiol.* 58:2082–89, 1985.

145. Younes, M., and G. Kivinen. Respiratory mechanics and breathing pattern during and following maximal exercise. *J. Appl. Physiol.* 57:1773–1782, 1984.

6
Community Intervention for Promotion of Physical Activity and Fitness

ABBY C. KING, Ph.D.

INTRODUCTION

An accumulating body of epidemiological, clinical, and basic research underscores the importance of regular physical activity to a broad array of physical and psychological processes which influence health and functioning [23]. Particularly compelling evidence has been collected supporting an independent role of physical activity in the primary prevention of cardiovascular disease, notably coronary heart disease (CHD) [94, 115, 124]. Results from a number of large-scale epidemiological studies in this area point to the importance of even moderate levels of physical activity in the prevention of CHD [94, 103]. Similar findings have been reported when either the level of physical activity or the actual assessment of physical fitness has been the major outcome of interest [19, 45, 94, 115]. The influence of regular physical activity on obesity and long-term weight control, as well as hypertension, also has been consistently demonstrated [16, 25, 61, 74, 116, 144].

Regular physical activity has further been linked, albeit in a less well-demonstrated manner, with prevention of the amelioration of a number of other diseases, including noninsulin-dependent diabetes mellitus [156], osteoporosis [140], and cancer [1, 19]. Exercise also appears to improve some aspects of mental health and emotional well-being [80, 102, 148], as well as more general processes of aging. Indeed, the often observed age-related declines in physical functioning noted in the U.S. population have been increasingly attributed to sedentary lifestyles, rather than to senescence per se [150].

Taken together, the above data support the legitimacy of developing orchestrated efforts to promote regular physical activity across a broad segment of the population as an aid to chronic disease prevention and control [153]. Notable among such efforts is the growing interest in community-level approaches to promotion of physical activity. The purpose of this chapter is to review the concepts underlying community approaches to health behavior change and current efforts in physical activity. Finally, limits and challenges facing community approaches to promotion of physical activity and possible future directions will be discussed.

211

THE CASE FOR APPLYING A COMMUNITY APPROACH TO THE PROMOTION OF PHYSICAL ACTIVITY

The past several decades have witnessed a burgeoning of health promotion programs that cover a variety of health behaviors, physical activity among them. Most programs have used personal or interpersonal approaches to promoting such behaviors; that is, the health professional meets with a person or group at a designated time and place where face-to-face counseling or training subsequently occurs. This approach, which emphasizes reliance on a health professional and individual responsibility for health, reflects the type of medical or clinical model of health care delivery that is most familiar to both this country's health professionals and the American public. Such an approach is consonant with the notions of personal responsibility and individual control over relevant health behaviors which have been emphasized by a number of leaders in the health community during the 1970s and 1980s [83].

Personal and interpersonal interventions have a number of advantages. They include the targeting of persons who have been either self-identified or identified by a health professional as in need of a health behavior change; the potential application of an array of motivational strategies that stem from the direct personal encounter with a health professional; the greater convenience of such intervention programs for the health professional, who typically chooses both the time and the location of the program; and the ability of the health professional to assess change in a relatively direct fashion.

Notwithstanding the advantages of the medical or clinical model, the fact remains that the most significant achievements in advancing the health of the American public have been the result of public health rather than medical approaches to health care programming and delivery [62]. Indeed, the case for applying a public health approach to eliminating our nation's current major health threats has been convincingly argued [85]. The public health approach uses a population-based, prevention-oriented perspective typically lacking in the medical or clinical model. As part of this perspective, methods for reaching broader segments of the population that extend beyond the personal and interpersonal arenas (e.g., mass media, environmental change, community organization) are frequently used. The use of such "higher order" levels of intervention provides a natural complement to more individually based interventions.

Given the somewhat unique aspects of physical activity promotion in this country, the use of larger scale community approaches may be especially important. Relative to many other health behaviors, a much greater percentage of the American public is falling short of what is currently considered to be an optimal level of regular physical activity.

Indeed, although more of the American public reports being involved in physical activity today than a decade ago [143], recent reviews of the literature suggest that as much as 40% of the population may be completely sedentary, with another 30% or more irregularly active [29, 143]. Based on the large number of inactive persons as well as current data indicating that cardiovascular risk can be reduced through relatively modest increases in physical activity, some researchers have further argued that community-wide increases in physical activity could actually result in greater population-based cardiovascular risk reduction than could be achieved through similar endeavors in other risk factor areas such as cigarette smoking or blood pressure control [114].

Although a large number of persons could benefit from increases in their levels of physical activity, the number of health professionals working in the physical fitness field is relatively small. Reliance, therefore, on face-to-face contact with health professionals as the principal means for promoting ongoing participation remains inadequate for achieving widespread change. This is particularly true given the frequently made observation that the majority of the American public prefers to exercise outside of a formal class or group [69, 79]. At the other end of the continuum, health professionals also are constrained by the lack of appropriate regulatory or passive prevention approaches (i.e., strategies that do not require individual action to be successful, such as changing the content of products during the manufacturing process or enforcing laws regulating product use). Although such strategies do exist for some important health behaviors such as smoking cessation and dietary change, relatively little can be undertaken in this regard in the physical activity area that currently would be feasible or acceptable to the majority of the American public. One relevant example of a passive prevention approach that *has* been undertaken by some communities involves blocking off sections of town to motor traffic, thereby resulting in increased pedestrian and bicycle traffic.

The use of a broad approach to physical activity promotion that taps multiple levels of analysis and intervention as well as expertise from a range of health fields is strongly indicated. Community-based approaches are one means of reaching more of the population than is presently occurring. Another mechanism is to use methods of risk reduction that apply to the natural environments in which persons live and that draw on available opportunities for diffusion and social support [49]. Current community-based efforts for promoting physical activity are reviewed and future directions discussed in the remaining portion of this chapter. Because of the contribution of large-scale physical activity approaches as a potentially important means for preventing a number of the major chronic diseases facing this nation, *primary prevention* activities that are occurring at the community level are the focus.

COMPONENTS OF A COMMUNITY APPROACH TO INTERVENTION

Communities can be defined structurally, as geographical entities, or ecologically, as a set of interactive social and institutional relationships bound together by a common sense of identity or "community" [30]. The two definitions often are combined in delineating a locale or entity on which to intervene.

The goal of community-based interventions is to achieve risk reduction across a broad segment of the community. To achieve this goal, a variety of strategies are used to reach a number of different target groups which extend beyond those that are the typical focus of personal or interpersonal programs. Targets of change include the person, organizations (e.g., worksite or school health programs), the environment (e.g., development of walking or bicycle paths in community parks), and public policies (e.g., innovative physical activity curricula in the public schools).

The principle underlying the use of such strategies is that an orchestrated effort to support individual behavioral change that spans all levels of intervention will result in longer term behavioral change across a more diversified portion of the community for potentially less cost [50, 126]. In applying a preventive stance in initiating health behavior change, the community approach uses seeking mode interventions (i.e., the health professional uses methods to seek out portions of the community at risk), in addition to the waiting mode interventions more typical of individual approaches to health behavior change [164]. In the latter case, the person comes to the health professional with a problem. Evidence suggests, however, that most Americans, although able to benefit from preventive measures such as increased physical activity, do not seek help from traditional sources (e.g., physicians and other health professionals) [98].

Health professionals who have undertaken community programming have drawn on a diverse theoretical literature that spans several disciplines [52, 111]. These theoretical perspectives and approaches include the following:

Learning Theory
Learning theory and its more recent derivations (i.e., applied behavioral analysis, cognitive-behavioral theory, social learning and social cognitive theories) [8, 162] have long been applied on the individual and interpersonal levels to the problem of achieving increased, sustained participation with notable success [97]. Strategies derived from such theories have included population-specific reinforcers (e.g., contests, lotteries, competitions) [46], self-monitoring, goal-setting, and feedback [71, 110, 142], training in problem-solving, decision-making, and relapse prevention skills to aid maintenance [75,

159], and the application of varying types of social support [42, 96]. More recently, the principles from such theories have been expanded to achieve institutionally based and environmentally influenced increases in physical activity [3, 26, 82, 99].

In light of the accumulating evidence that suggests that different social, psychological, and behavioral processes may be in operation at different stages of behavioral change (i.e., exercise adoption versus maintenance) [130], some researchers have emphasized that such a stage approach needs to be taken into account when exercise programming in the community is being developed [91, 92, 164]. The issue of a stage approach to achieving increases in physical activity in the community will be addressed later in this chapter.

Communication Theory
Research based on communication theories seeks to identify the factors that have a major impact on how successfully information relevant to health is transmitted to and received by the community. Relevant factors that influence the communication of health messages include the characteristics of both the senders and potential receivers of the message, the construction of the message itself, and the types of channels used to transmit the message [128]. Relevant channels may include electronic and print media as well as face-to-face communication, aimed either at the populace or at members of organizational or political structures within the community.

Diffusion of Innovations
A special type of communication, diffusion has been defined as "the process by which an innovation is communicated through certain channels over time among the members of a social system" [128, p. 5]. An innovation can be an object (e.g., a product or new technology), an idea (e.g., an attitude or belief), or, most relevant to the current discussion, a practice (e.g., health-related behavior). Research on diffusion has resulted in the identification of a number of characteristics of innovations that help to explain how rapidly an innovation may be adopted by a community. These include relative advantage (is the innovation perceived as better than the idea or practice already in operation?); compatibility (is the innovation perceived as being consistent with the past experiences and existing values of potential adopters?); complexity (is the innovation perceived as too difficult to understand or accomplish?); trialability (can the innovation or new practice be "tried out" or experimented with on a limited basis initially?); and observability (to what extent are the results of the innovation or new behavior visible to others?) [128]. In addition, research on diffusion has underscored the importance of identifying and securing the help of group opinion leaders in influencing the adoption of new behaviors among the group [128].

Community Organization Perspectives
Derived from several disciplines, including public health, community psychology, and social work, the community organization perspective emphasizes an understanding of community leadership and power structures in attempting to promote behavior change. Community mobilization and adoption principles include consensus development across a wide array of community organizations and agencies, social action perspectives focusing on activation of the political process and community 'ownership' of the health programs, and social planning perspectives to achieve systemwide change [49, 58].

Social Marketing
Social marketing approaches aim to apply basic marketing principles to achieve health-related change. Central to this approach is the development of programs that are *tailored* to the needs and preferences of the consumer, rather than the use of prepackaged programs that fit the preconceived notions held by the health professional [84]. Tailoring involves segmenting the community into more homogenous subgroups, based on demographic factors and other behavioral and psychological variables related to health. The needs and preferences of these segments are then determined, using surveys or other data-gathering methods, with respect to the health area of interest. Once this needs analysis is accomplished, the information it provides can aid the health professional in developing the right health program or "product" for each segment, delivered in the right "place" (including the most appropriate channels of communication), using the right promotional strategies, and offered at the right "price" (both economically and psychologically). The information-gathering activities described above have typically been referred to, along with message or program pretesting activities, as *formative* evaluation or research.

Contextual or Systems Approach
A systems perspective suggests that a reductionist approach to intervention, which breaks down the system into its component parts rather than attempting to study the system as a whole, results in a picture of the problem that is incomplete and often invalid. Identifying the social context in which health behaviors occur is imperative if community programs are to be successful. Understanding the social context involves an understanding of the other forces present in the community that may have an impact on health behaviors. These other sources of information, influence, and support include the mass media, schools, private sector, health professional organizations, community political structure, and other community organizations.

In researching methods for achieving community-wide changes in health behaviors important to reducing health risk, most researchers have attempted to incorporate at least some aspects of many or all of the theories and approaches described above. This typically requires bringing together a variety of different disciplines to form a multidisciplinary team. By developing programs that incorporate a mix of such approaches, it is hoped that a broader community audience will be reached, more powerful changes will be observed, and longer term institutionalization of the programs as part of the ongoing community structure will be achieved.

ISSUES TO BE ADDRESSED IN DEVELOPING COMMUNITY INTERVENTIONS FOR PHYSICAL ACTIVITY

In developing programs for exercise promotion, several issues specific to this important health behavior have been receiving increasing attention and debate by the health community. These issues require attention by health professionals seeking to intervene on individual as well as community levels. Several of the more salient of these issues are discussed briefly below.

The Goal of Physical Activity versus Fitness

The differential contributions of physical activity participation and actual improvement in physical fitness to health remain unclear. Although much of the epidemiological evidence showing a relationship between exercise and health outcomes such as cardiovascular disease has used physical activity levels as the primary measure [94, 103, 115], recent findings show a significant relationship between physiological measures of fitness and morbidity and mortality [19, 45]. Given that physical fitness, although strongly influenced by exercise patterns, also has a significant genetic component, it is probably reasonable to assume that physical activity is the important stimulus in health promotion and disease prevention, rather than the absolute levels of physical fitness achieved [14]. Because there is still much to learn in this area, however, it is perhaps most prudent to try to measure both the behavioral and the physiological components of a physical activity program in the community. Currently fitness might best be viewed as an objective marker for physical activity in general, and changes in physical activity level in particular.

Measurement of Physical Activity and Fitness

Accurate measurement of both physical activity and fitness outcomes remains a challenging task. Collection of information on physical activity participation typically is easier and less expensive to accomplish across a wider segment of the community. Yet such self-report measures are potentially fraught with a number of problems, including recall, sampling, reactivity (the behavior being assessed over time changes as a consequence of the assessment itself), and difficulties in attempting to secure accurate reports of exercise intensity [14, 86]. Although these limitations may hinder the use of such measures in clinical or related health settings where accurate individual data are needed, measures that allow for sensitive, reliable assessment of change in group physical activity patterns may suffice for community intervention studies [14]. For a more complete review of exercise and physical fitness assessment issues, the reader is directed to other sources [14, 86, 163].

Despite the potential limitations of self-report methods, several have been developed that appear to meet criteria adequately on a group basis in the areas of sensitivity, reliability, and validity, and thus could be useful for evaluating community interventions. These include the Minnesota Leisure Time Physical Activities Questionnaire [149], Montoye's quantitative history survey [101], Bouchard and colleagues' daily recall survey [23], and the seven-day physical activity recall [17]. These surveys provide a means of calculating total energy expenditure, an important variable in the determination of health outcomes [14].

In theory the assessment of physical fitness probably provides a more objective measure than the assessment of physical activity participation through self-report. But the measurement of physical fitness can be a difficult task, particularly on the large scale that would be appropriate for community interventions. Laboratory assessments involving measurement of maximum oxygen uptake ($\dot{V}O_2max$), the most widely accepted standard measure of physical fitness, are infeasible to administer on a community basis. Alternatively, submaximal testing procedures supplying estimates of O_2 uptake are reliable and valid, relatively simple to obtain, and require limited equipment and personnel [14]. Examples of such submaximal tests that can be used successfully in the field include Cooper's 12-minute walk-run [33], step tests [137], and bicycle ergometer tests [136]. The use of appropriate safety procedures, such as careful screening for eligibility to take the test (accomplished through administration of questionnaires such as the PAR-Q [6]), and the application of conservative criteria for stopping the test, minimize the development of problems as a consequence of testing [133]. Indeed, field tests such as the BIKE TEST (a low-level bicycle physical fitness test) and the Canadian home fitness test [6] have been administered without direct medical supervision to thousands of adults without serious complications [14]. As an alternate means for estimating physical fitness, Blair and colleagues [18] have demonstrated that, in lieu of more direct measures of fitness, the addition of sedentary traits measurements (i.e., obesity, resting tachycardia, low vital capacity) to a simple physical activity measure can provide a valid estimate of fitness in community-based studies.

The above discussion underscores that effective assessment of both physical activity patterns and physical fitness is achievable in the community, although it does require effort. The reader is referred to the National Center for Health Statistics' (Public Health Service) manual on physical activity measurement [107] and the report of the recent National Heart, Lung, and Blood Institute (Public Health Service) workshop physical activity and fitness assessment [163] for further discussion of types of measurement in this area.

How Much is Enough?

Another important issue concerns the type of exercise stimulus that is necessary or optimal for achieving health benefits. It often has been assumed that exercise undertaken at a sufficient intensity, frequency, and duration to achieve substantial improvement in physical fitness was the necessary stimulus required to promote resistance to disease. Recent discussions in this area, however, have led to increased questioning of this tenet [64]. Although it is possible that the effects of physical activity on health status may be mediated primarily through the biological changes achieved through increased fitness [141], it also is possible that the physical activity-induced biological changes that lead to positive health outcomes may be largely independent of changes responsible for increase in fitness [64]. This would help to explain the accumulating epidemiological data that demonstrate a significant relationship between light- and moderate-intensity activities and all-cause mortality as well as cause-specific mortality for cardiovascular disease, stroke, cancer, and respiratory disease [94, 103, 114].

It also is quite possible that the optimal type of exercise regimen (with respect to type of activity, intensity, frequency, and duration) for achieving one sort of health outcome (e.g., weight loss, decreased cardiovascular disease, decreased manifestations of osteoporosis, psychological benefits) may differ from that required to achieve another health outcome [64]. Unfortunately, much remains to be learned concerning relevant exercise parameters (e.g., intensity, duration) and such health outcomes. Given that in addition to the conditioning effects achieved through sufficiently vigorous exercise, health benefits also may accrue through frequent participation in low-intensity exercise that is inadequate for increasing fitness, both should be encouraged in the community. Participation in low-intensity activities (e.g., gardening, routine activities such as walking or climbing stairs) may be particularly important for the very sedentary portion of the population, for whom more intensive exercise remains distasteful or infeasible.

Issues of Adherence

Initial participation in and long-term adherence to physical activity programs is a major challenge that, like the issues of measurement and prescription definition discussed above, continues to be an important subject of study. As noted previously, much of the focus of adherence investigations in the physical activity area has been on personal and interpersonal strategies, based largely on social learning theory and similar approaches. Although a number of these strategies have resulted in promising outcomes with respect to program adherence once the individual has enrolled [40, 42, 109], few studies have attempted to apply such strategies on a larger scale or across a broader segment of the population [111]. In addition, less attention has been focused on methods for increasing initial participation rates as well as on strategies for extending adequate adherence beyond the 3- to 6-month period, the typical length of most investigations.

Interventions aimed at achieving adequate participation and adherence must account for factors related to the person, the exercise regimen itself, and the environment. In the personal arena, a host of demographic and health-related variables have been found to be associated with both initial participation levels as well as subsequent adherence. These include gender (women tend to participate less in physical activity, particularly of a vigorous nature, than men), age (older persons tend to participate less than younger persons), occupational status (blue-collar workers less active than white collar workers), and being either a current smoker or overweight [42, 109]. Also included is the presence of skills that allow one to cope with the challenge of routinely engaging in an activity that at times can be physically uncomfortable, psychologically unrewarding, and difficult to fit into an already busy schedule [41, 75].

With respect to the exercise regimen, it is clear that, for a large segment of the U.S. population, regimens that involve exercise that is perceived to be too intense or inconvenient can have a negative effect on initial participation and longer term adherence [41, 79, 132]. Moreover, regimens that allow the person to exercise outside if he or she chooses can be undertaken in one's own rather than in a formal class, but for many persons would entail some structure while allowing for flexibility [42, 77].

The environmental variable that probably has received the most attention to date concerns the level and type of social support received for engaging in physical activity. Studies indicate that support administered across a variety of sources (family members, exercise instructor, exercise partners, co-workers, employer) as well as channels (face-to-face, telephone, mail) can have a positive impact on both participation and adherence rates [38, 81, 96]. Use of strategically placed environmental prompts [26, 99] as well as inducements or incentives to exercise (e.g., contests, lotteries) [3, 46, 82, 99] have also resulted in positive outcomes. These latter sorts of environmental approaches offer particular promise for community interventions and should be targeted for additional formal investigation. In addition, the use of community submaximal fitness testing may provide an incentive for encouraging increased exercise participation across individuals of varied ages and fitness levels [108].

Some of the factors being discussed appear to operate both during the initial participation or "joining" phase and during the subsequent adherence or maintenance phase (e.g., smoking status, regimen intensity, level of overweight, at least some types of contests or competitions). Others appear to be most influential during one or the other such phase. For instance, attitudes and beliefs concerning exercise appear to influence greatly a person's decision to begin to exercise, rather than subsequent adherence [91–92]. In contrast, the impact of problem-solving and related skills will be felt largely during the adherence or maintenance phase. Continuing efforts, therefore, to develop interventions that are tailored to each phase as well as to supply a bridge between the two phases are strongly needed. This is particularly true for community approaches, to which little formal attention has been paid to date.

REVIEW OF COMMUNITY PROGRAMS AND APPROACHES

Current community-based efforts to promote physical activity and fitness can be divided into three groups: those advocating a comprehensive package of programs with the ultimate goal of influencing the community at large; those targeting special populations within the community; and those focusing on setting-specific approaches to physical activity promotion. Because many of the large number of such programs that have been developed over the past several decades have never been evaluated, the review will focus on representative programs from each category that have undergone or are currently undergoing formal evaluation.

Comprehensive, Integrated Community-Based Interventions

Comprehensive, integrated approaches to promoting community-wide increases in physical activity have generally involved an orchestrated series of physical activity interventions which cover multiple targets (e.g., health care providers, the elderly, adults in general) channels (e.g., print and broadcast media, face-to-face instruction) and settings (neighborhoods, worksites, schools). Such efforts are represented in the work undertaken as part of the four major multicommunity cardiovascular risk reduction studies in the United States: The Stanford Five-City Project, the Minnesota Heart Health Project, the Pawtucket Heart Health Project, and the Pennsylvania-based Community Health Improvement Project. Although all four studies are currently ongoing, descriptions of their efforts to date provide useful information on how such multiintervention community efforts can be undertaken.

THE STANFORD FIVE-CITY PROJECT. The first of the four U.S. multi-community cardiovascular risk reduction studies to receive funding, the Stanford Five-City Multifactor Risk Reduction Project is an outgrowth of the previous encouraging results achieved through the Stanford Three-Community Study [51]. The Three-Community Study provided the first formal demonstration that a community-wide approach to cardiovascular risk reduction and behavior change could result in significant community-wide improvements in risk factors [51]. The principal method used for obtaining behavior change in the two intervention communities was mass media, supplemented in one of the communities by intensive face-to-face instruction of high-risk individuals. The third community served as a reference.

The goals of the Stanford Five-City Project are to evaluate more comprehensive community-based efforts to modify cardiovascular risk factors and behaviors across larger, more socially complex communities, with measurement of actual cardiovascular disease event rates included [48]. Outcomes from two intervention communities are being compared with those from three assessment-only reference communities located in the central California region.

Begun in 1978, the Stanford Five-City Project has developed extensive community-wide campaigns to foster change across a number of health behaviors influencing cardiovascular disease (CVD). Targeted health behaviors have been organized into educational "waves," which serve to focus the community's (and intervention team's) attention on a particular risk factor or health behavior.

The major goals of the physical activity component of the intervention have been to enhance the general level of activity in the target communities irrespective of the type of intensity of the activity, and to increase the percentage of individuals performing more vigorous endurance activities on a regular basis. During the first two years of the intervention, program goals focused on increasing awareness and knowledge related to the need to exercise regularly, benefits of regular physical activity, and ways of carrying out a physical activity program that would be safe and effective. Programs delivered during this time included the creation of print and broadcast media on exercise (developed in English and Spanish); the delivery of talks, seminars, and workshops by health professionals who supplied relevant information on physical activity; and the organization of community events in this area to enhance awareness. The latter included community walking events and races and the development of the neighborhood-based Heart and Sole Exercise Program, which provided supervised exercise opportunities near the home. Community-based fitness assessments also were made available to community members at minimal cost.

During Years 3 and 4, the programs described above were expanded and tailored further to reach special populations, including women, older adults, and ethnic minorities (e.g., Hispanics). Efforts included the development of electronic mass media (e.g., public service announcements, a series accompanying the evening news) for these population segments.

During Years 5 and 6, worksites were targeted through a multiworksite contest (Coming Alive) which promoted regular participation in physical activity. Interested persons also were enrolled in a Healthy Living Program which provided low-level fitness assessments, walking and jogging kits, and announcements throughout the year of exercise programs in the community. During this time, relevant information was distributed to elementary school children and their parents through a school-based "Race to Health" series, and exercise booklets were distributed to libraries, worksites, and other organizations throughout the community.

During Year 6, increasing efforts were directed toward the institutionalization of the above programs to enhance their maintenance beyond the life of the grant funding period. To date, programs such as the Heart and Sole Race, Heart and Sole classes, and Coming Alive, as well as stable mechanisms for distribution of written materials such as the Walking and Jogging Kits, have been fully or largely adopted by the communities. Efforts to promote institutionalization of the exercise interventions, as well as community action for exercise (additional walking and bicycle paths, Par courses where strength and endurance exercises are laid out in an exercise "route" which the person traverses) will continue over the next two years.

Community-based assessments completed to date show significantly greater participation in routine and moderate activities in the intervention compared to the control communities [47]. Congruent with the self-report measures, resting pulse rates (one indicator of fitness level) were found to be significantly decreased in treatment versus control communities following initiation of the intervention program. Further, evaluations of the effectiveness of specific programs that have been completed have been promising. For instance, findings from the worksite Coming Alive exercise contest show significant increases in physical activity participation and indices of increased fitness derived from field testing (e.g., endurance as measured by three-minute step test; percent body fat as measured from skinfolds) in the intervention worksites relative to matched control worksites [3].

THE MINNESOTA HEART HEALTH PROGRAM (MHPP). Begun in 1980, MHHP, like its sister study at Stanford, is a community-based research project aimed at reducing coronary risk across the communities being targeted for intervention [13]. The MHHP is currently taking place in three pairs of communities in Minnesota as well as North and South Dakota. Physical activity has been targeted as one of several risk-related behaviors receiving systematic attention and effort. The general goal of such efforts has been to increase physical activity-related motivation and skills and to decrease barriers to regular activity. This has been sought through a focus on information aimed at increasing motivation to exercise (e.g., physical activity can facilitate weight loss), increased availability of exercise facilities in the community, as well as a more general influence on community values and behavioral norms in the physical activity area [36].

Steps that have occurred in influencing community exercise patterns include increasing community organization efforts in this area through establishment of a community physical activity task force which comprises community leaders and relevant organizations; the mounting of community-wide mass media campaigns to increase awareness and knowledge; the use of screening methods to provide individual feedback and incentive to change; the development of programs targeted for specific audience segments, including youth and their parents, health professionals, and worksites; and the use of more general campaigns (e.g., city walks and "fitfests") aimed at the community at large. All such efforts, generally organized as a series of intervention "waves," are being evaluated for their impact on awareness, knowledge, attitudes and beliefs, and participation levels [36].

Specific interventions implemented by the MHHP have included general campaign events, such as City Walk for the community at large, and a "Fitfest" which involved a series of participative physical activity events occurring during the community's annual summer festival; a "Shape Up" television series on how to begin an exercise program; a "Job-N-Log" program for all elementary school children; a self-training brochure, distributed through physicians' offices and other community settings, which focused on helping individuals begin an exercise program; the development of "little" media products such as slide or tape programs on fitness and exercise; and a "Shape Up Challenge" or exercise competition organized in local worksites [22].

Evaluation of the above programs in one of the intervention communities during 1983 resulted in a number of interesting findings with respect to the utility of different interventions for promoting distinct, targeted outcomes [22]. For instance, overall community awareness was most influenced by the more generic campaign events such as the City Walk and Fitfest, particularly in women and older adults. In contrast, actual physical activity participation was greatest for setting-specific events, such as the school or worksite programs, which encouraged groups of individuals to work toward common physical activity goals. The greatest cost-effectiveness per participant was achieved through interventions administered in existing community settings (schools, worksites). Such interventions reached typically underexposed community segments, and provided an effective means for inducing relatively large groups of individuals to participate in physical activities for a sustained period of time. The authors argue, however, that probably all aspects of such a multiple-intervention approach are useful in promoting an enhanced community milieu for regular physical activity.

In addition to these program-specific findings, the experiences to date from the MHHP indicate that it is feasible and productive to actively involve communities in health programming focused on physical activity. Significant awareness of appropriate physical activity information and messages was achieved in approximately 1 to 2 years, and participation rates in many of the programs described above are encouraging [36]. As with the Stanford project, changes in fitness and other relevant health indices (e.g., weight) are being evaluated through a series of community assessments, although the results are not yet available. In addition, this comprehensive, integrated community approach to physical activity and other targeted health behaviors has been successfully implemented in three different communities, supporting the generalizability of such approaches to other communities.

THE PAWTUCKET HEART HEALTH PROGRAM (PHHP). Similar to the Stanford and Minnesota programs, the Pawtucket Heart Health Program is a community-wide, multiple-risk-factor intervention study that is based on principles derived from a range of disciplines and theories, including social learning theory, community organization and community psychology approaches, and diffusion theory [93]. An important feature of the PHHP is its extensive use of volunteers for program delivery and its innovative use of community organizations such as churches to enhance the reach of its interventions into the community. Its church-based physical activity program is described in a subsequent section. Programming in areas such as physical activity, blood pressure control, and weight control have taken advantage of these features in promoting change.

Institutionalization of program delivery within the community to ensure continuation of activities following the end of the federal grant period is a major goal of the PHHP [87]. One way in which this has occurred in the area of physical activity has been through the establishment of formal links with the Pawtucket Parks and Recreation Department. As part of its ongoing relationship with this organization, the PHHP has played a major role in training a number of aerobic dance instructors and establishing other health behavior classes through the Parks and Recreation Department's ongoing ExerCity program. Since the start of the PHHP's collaborative relationship with the ExerCity program, the number of participants enrolled in this program has approximately tripled [87].

The PHHP also has established important links to other community organizations including health-related agencies such as the American Heart Association and the American Cancer Society; health professional organizations; social organizations such as the Rotary Club and the

Lions Club; local libraries, where health-related classes are delivered and accurate health education materials are housed; and local colleges and universities, which provide both resources and a range of interested students and personnel. Similar to the other community-wide heart health projects, media-based messages that promote physical activity and other health behaviors are being delivered in an ongoing fashion through a variety of channels, including promotional and public service announcements on local radio and television, a regular newspaper column, and a PHHP-produced exercise show on cable television.

THE PENNSYLVANIA COUNTY HEALTH IMPROVEMENT PROGRAM (CHIP). Like the other three programs described, CHIP is a community-based multiple risk factor intervention study aimed at decreasing CVD-related morbidity and mortality in a county with a population of 118,000 in north central Pennsylvania [147]. CHIP shares with the other U.S. community intervention trials a standardized set of epidemiological surveillance procedures to ensure comparability of outcomes. In contrast to the other three programs, which have been reasonably well funded through the National Institutes of Health, CHIP's budget has been considerably smaller. The types of interventions the CHIP investigators have developed reflect their goal of keeping costs sufficiently low so as to make the program widely replicable [147]. These have included early, formal involvement of community representatives, and the identification and use of existing resources and facilities. The long-term goal of this program, similar to the others, is to create a permanent community-owned program.

Although physical activity programming was initially accorded a relatively low priority, experience in the field, which indicated the strong popularity of physical activity programs among both residents and organizations, led to its receiving a higher priority [147]. The channels being used for promotion of physical activity and other health behaviors include the mass media, an extensive worksite health promotion campaign, programs for health professionals and voluntary organizations, and, most recently, school-based interventions.

Early evaluations of the amount of health promotion activities being undertaken in the experimental and control counties have been encouraging. During a three-year period the number of organizations in the reference county that offered health promotion programs fell by 42% (possibly owing to economic factors), the number of programs in the experimental county during the same period doubled [147].

Community-based Exercise Programming Efforts in Other Countries
In addition to the U.S. community studies, a number of community-based, multifactor health education programs recently have been completed or currently are underway in other countries throughout the world. These include the North Karelia Project in Finland [127], the

North Coast Project in Australia [44], and the South African Study [129]. The programs vary considerably in the amount of systematic intervention and evaluation that has been undertaken in the physical activity area. Community intervention efforts in two countries will be highlighted.

THE NORTH KARELIA PROJECT. The most fully reported project occurring outside of the U.S. is the Finnish North Karelia Project, launched in 1972 [126]. The 10-year findings from this project have indicated a significant decrease in the incidence of cardiovascular disease mortality in the intervention county (24%) compared to a decrease of only 12% in the control county and a national decrease of only 11% [126]. This appears to be due largely to the significant changes that were achieved in the areas of smoking, serum cholesterol, and blood pressure control.

The strengths of this effort included a well-conducted mass media program as well as significant involvement and mobilization of community organizations such as local heart associations, physicians, and the Finnish housewives' organizations in areas such as nutrition education [127]. Relatively little systematic attention was given to physical activity programming, however, in comparison with the three major risk factor areas noted above, so that few conclusions can be made with respect to that particular area.

AUSTRALIAN INTERVENTION PROJECTS. Although the multifactor Australian North Coast Project's success was achieved largely in the area of smoking cessation [52], a number of promising approaches to community-based physical activity programming have been initiated by researchers from other parts of the Australian continent. Several of these investigations, undertaken by Lee and Owen [90, 111–113], underscore the potential utility of systematic applications of behavioral science theory and techniques to widespread promotion of physical activity. The strategies they investigated include the systematic training of self-management techniques designed to promote generalization of exercise across time and to settings in addition to regular fitness classes [113]. They also demonstrated the feasibility of using mediated self-instructional training methods (e.g., single mailings, correspondence courses) for aerobic exercise [112]. As noted by these investigators, researchers in the field need to continue to explore methods of ongoing instruction and support that allow for a broader reach into the population (e.g., mediated approaches) and which place increased emphasis on integrating physical activity into the normal routine of daily living [111].

Strengths and Limitations of Comprehensive, Integrated Community-based Approaches

There are a number of potential strengths and integrated community-based approaches to exercise and other health behaviors. These strengths include the ability to (1) reach a larger, more diverse number of persons in a community; (2) deliver a health message in a repeated fashion through a variety of communication channels and settings, leading potentially to the augmentation and reinforcement of the message which in turn may result in a greater impact; (3) reach persons in the natural, daily settings in which they live; (4) combine programs for one health behavior with those for others which they may naturally influence or complement (e.g., exercise and dietary intake); and (5) utilize all four levels of potential impact (personal through legislative).

In addition to their strengths, however, comprehensive community approaches also have a variety of limitations, with respect to both their execution and their evaluation. These include (1) dependence typically on quasiexperimental research designs, which limit the extent to which causal inferences can be applied; (2) inability to keep the investigators blinded to the experimental conditions; (3) difficulty in developing and evaluating strategies that can be administered across a large number of people and that can be successfully tailored to meet the heterogeneous needs of the many subgroups comprised in most communities; (4) difficulty in being able to isolate the effects of one intervention from another, both within and between health behaviors (for instance, if exercise participation increases along with dietary change as a consequence of a multifactor intervention program, it becomes difficult to separate the importance of the dietary change interventions from the change observed in exercise); and (5) financial, political, and logistical constraints involved in attempting such comprehensive approaches in many portions of the United States. In addition, many of the current community-wide projects have placed more effort on evaluating the overall impact of the combination of interventions implemented in a specific risk factor area rather than on the outcomes specific to any one intervention program. This increases the difficulty of determining which of the many programs undertaken in the physical activity area are most likely to lead to successful outcomes in other communities. It is also worth noting that for the majority of such community efforts, the overall effort spent in conducting physical activity programming was generally less than that put into behavioral change in other risk factor areas (i.e., smoking cessation, blood pressure control, dietary change, weight control).

A related issue is that although both broadcast and print media that focused on physical activity have been incorporated into the ongoing informational campaigns launched by these community projects, disentangling the effects of this potentially powerful community strategy from other intervention approaches remains difficult. Just how effective different types of media may be for promoting either initial adoption or subsequent maintenance of physical activity is unclear. Findings from the few systematically evaluated national media campaigns launched in this health area are equivocal. For instance, an evaluation was completed recently of the U.S. Department of Health and Human Services' Healthstyle, a national health promotion media campaign which included physical activity as one of its six target health behaviors [37]. The campaign was implemented in 1981 in nine test communities across the U.S. Although there was some indication of increases in both awareness and knowledge related to physical activity, a more rigorous comparison of one of the test communities with a control community yielded no statistically significant differences in awareness, beliefs, attitude, or intentions with respect to exercise. The best predictor of exercise levels following the campaign was precampaign exercise levels. An Australian national campaign for physical activity entitled "Life–Be In It," launched in 1977, appears to have produced similarly ambiguous results [69]. Clearly, more effort needs to be placed in determining the most effective uses of media in the physical activity area.

Notwithstanding the limitations of comprehensive community approaches noted above, the current findings suggest that community-wide interventions in the physical activity area are feasible, acceptable to community residents, and potentially effective in bringing about change in at least some indices of physical activity and fitness.

Community Programming for Special Populations
In addition to comprehensive programming for the general community, several large-scale projects have been undertaken which have been targeted for minority segments of the population normally underserved in the health promotion area. Two of the better documented efforts in this area are presented below.

THE COMMUNITY HEALTH ASSESSMENT AND PROMOTION PROJECT (CHAPP). Supported by the Centers for Disease Control, CHAPP has sought to modify health behaviors relevant to hypertension and obesity in approximately 400 women from a predominantly black community in Atlanta [89]. The project consisted of two 2-hour sessions per week across a 10-week period that included a choice of several types of moderate-intensity physical activity (e.g., walking, water exercises, low-impact aerobic dance) as well as instruction in a number of other health topics (e.g., nutrition, weight control). Participants underwent a health screening and were required to commit to spending at least 4 hours per week across the 10-week period in program activities. Individual goals were established in several health areas, including exercise, weight reduction, and blood pressure control, and social support and incentives were used to promote continued participation.

The exercise program was specifically tailored to be culturally relevant to this population. For instance, consideration was given to the special needs of this population with respect to safety and privacy (e.g., security escorts were provided for groups walking in dangerous neighborhoods;

curtains were installed on windows in the exercise room to ensure privacy). In addition, free transportation and child care were offered and home visits undertaken to encourage continued participation.

Follow-up information at 4 months is encouraging [89]. Participation rates continue to be approximately 60–70%, and significant pre- and posttest reductions have been noted in weight and blood pressure. Successful participation has been attributed to the personal attention received from project staff and ongoing community support for the project. The formation of a community coalition has been identified as a critical component for the success of CHAPP. The coalition brought together a number of community organizations (e.g., the YMCA, churches, local teen centers) which are working to maintain the program. In addition, health professionals from Emory University, Grady Hospital, and the Centers for Disease Control (CDC) have recently developed a handbook to help educate others in the methods for mobilizing minority communities to reduce cardiovascular disease risk factors, including inactivity [32].

This effort provides an excellent example of how interventions tailored to the needs of a particular population segment and involving the support of community organizations can have a worthwhile impact on physical activity and other health behaviors. It also underscores the point that, counter to what some health professionals may think, physical activity programs and related preventive efforts are of substantial interest to less fortunate, lower socioeconomic groups and need not be limited to the domain of the middle- and upper-class for whom they are typically targeted.

THE ZUNI DIABETES PROJECT. Although the major goal of the Zuni Diabetes Project (exercise as a means for aiding control of noninsulin-dependent diabetes mellitus or NIDDM) places it more correctly within the realm of treatment rather than prevention, the methods used to intervene could be readily transferred to preclinical populations. Begun in 1983 by the Indian Health Service, the purpose of the project was to implement a community-based physical activity program that would provide instruction and motivation to Zunis with NIDDM as a means for helping them to become more fit and achieve normal body weight [95].

Begun as two one-hour aerobic exercise sessions per week, the program has since expanded to 48 sessions per week, which occur at several sites throughout the Zuni community in New Mexico. Promotion for the program, which includes a general community advertisement and informational campaign and recruitment through health professionals, has been geared specifically to Zuni Indians with NIDDM as well as to the general public. To reduce barriers to participation, open enrollment is maintained for the sessions, which are offered continuously. In addition, community ownership of the exercise program has been enhanced through having 48 Zuni Indians, trained in exercise and group leadership methods, help in the coordination of the program. A two-year evaluation using retrospective comparisons with a group of nonparticipants during the same period who were matched for age, gender, residence, health care provider, and duration of NIDDM, has recently been completed [67]. The findings are encouraging with respect to mean weight loss, fasting blood glucose values, and compliance with diabetes medication regimens [67]. A further interesting outcome of the project was that the physical activity message being promulgated appeared to have diffused into the Zuni community: 18% of nonparticipants who had been inactive prior to the program subsequently initiated home exercise during the course of the study.

The findings from these two community intervention projects, although preliminary, support the feasibility and acceptability of community-based physical activity interventions for minority populations, provided that they are *tailored* to the needs of those populations. Program tailoring can be enhanced through using the principles drawn from social marketing described earlier. Future research using stronger prospective, controlled designs and more extensive physiological, behavioral, and psychological assessment will continue to shed light on the most effective programming strategies for what has typically been an underserved, though risk-laden, portion of the population.

Setting-specific Approaches to Physical Activity Promotion
In addition to the multisetting, multiorganizational approaches to community-based physical activity promotion already described, a number of systematic efforts to increase physical activity and fitness levels have occurred within specific settings. As indicated by the findings from the Minnesota Heart Health Program, programs anchored to a particular setting appear to promote greater participation than those conducted outside of a specific setting [22]. This may be due in part to the greater availability of an array of communication channels and types of support (both formal and informal) found in such settings.

Although all communities offer a range of settings through which physical activity programming can, and does, occur, three major community settings will be discussed in detail here: worksites, schools, and places of worship. Given the burgeoning amount of programming that is occurring in or through the auspices of each of these organizational settings, an exhaustive review of each of them is beyond the scope of this article. Instead, specific examples of programming efforts that serve to highlight the opportunities available through such settings will be discussed. The reader is directed to sources such as the CDC's *Promoting Physical Activity Among Adults: A Community Intervention Handbook* [154] for further references concerning programming efforts in these and other settings.

WORKSITES.The workplace remains an important setting for reaching a large percentage of the population. This is true now more than ever as the number of women and elderly seeking work continues to increase [11]. Among the many potential advantages that may accompany worksite-based health promotion programs are increased accessibility to a large percentage of Americans, convenience for both employees and health promotion staff, availability of an array of existing communication and health care channels, the opportunity to utilize both coworkers and employer social support and influence, and the ability to replicate and generalize program findings across other worksites and employee populations [164]. In addition, worksite health promotion programs have a wide degree of appeal among employees [65].

For the employer, the potential for reaping benefits in areas such as employee productivity, job satisfaction, morale, and health status, as well as reductions in health insurance costs, absenteeism, and turnover have made such programs particularly attractive [21, 134–135]. Notably, however, empirical support for many of the positive claims associated with such health promotion programs, including physical activity, remains relatively scarce [160]. It is hoped that this situation will continue to improve as a greater number of findings from systematic investigations in these areas become available [10, 134].

The potential advantages of physical activity and other health promotion programming have not been lost on either employers or the health community, as is evidenced by the presence of physical activity programs throughout a growing number of American workplaces [55, 135]. Yet the majority of such programs continue to employ a clinical model in conducting such programs. That is, their programs consist primarily of supervised exercise classes that typically are attended by relatively small numbers of highly motivated employees [34]. An alternative approach consists of treating the worksite as a community, with the goal of trying to increase both formal and informal types of physical activity across the entire worksite population. Three examples of programs in which this type of public health model was applied in a worksite context to achieve increased physical activity participation will be discussed briefly.

THE JOHNSON & JOHNSON LIVE FOR LIFE PROGRAM. The best example to date of a comprehensive public health approach to enhancing employee physical activity participation is the Johnson & Johnson companies' Live for Life program. Four Johnson & Johnson companies received the complete Live for Life program, which consisted of an annual health assessment, a highly visible health education campaign using newsletters, contests, health fairs, and informational displays in hallways, cafeterias, and restrooms, and a series of health promotion seminars and exercise classes [161]. Exercise participation and health outcomes in employees from these companies were compared to those from employees in three comparison companies who received the annual health assessment only.

The findings reported at the end of the first 24-month period were impressive. During that time, the amount of vigorous activity engaged in more than doubled in the intervention companies, compared with only a 33% increase among employees at the comparison companies [20]. The changes in physical activity patterns were corroborated using estimates of Vo_2max obtained from a submaximal bicycle ergometer test. In addition, significant associations were found between positive changes in body weight, levels of body fat, systolic blood pressure, and psychological outcomes (e.g., feelings of general well-being) and increases in estimated maximal oxygen uptake. An added strength of this study was the high participation rates obtained for the baseline and posttest evaluations in both intervention and comparison companies (i.e., approximately 75% for both groups at baseline, and approximately 96% of the original sample of employees from both groups who were still employed at Johnson & Johnson at 24 months).

The findings from this study underscore the feasibility of obtaining significant increases in physical activity and fitness across all levels of a large workforce. As noted by Blair and colleagues [20], the promise for achieving the U.S. Surgeon General's objectives for the nation in exercise and physical fitness lies with the continued development of such public health approaches for reaching large numbers of individuals.

THE TEAM HEALTH PROGRAM. The Team Health Program at Hunt Consolidated, Inc., in Dallas, Texas, represents another type of effort, using a public health approach, to promote health behavior changes across an entire workforce [82]. The program, managed by a worksite coordinator from the Institute for Aerobics Research and an on-site committee of employee volunteers, has focused on the implementation of a range of health promotion activities that are relevant for that worksite (employee population = 500+).

An initial needs assessment survey of the largely white-collar workforce indicated their desire for help in increasing their levels of current physical activity. In light of the lack of space available for on-site exercise classes and related programs, it was decided to focus on a physical activity in which all employees at this 50-story, high-rise workplace could participate—stair-climbing. To increase interest in and motivation for engaging in such an activity, a stair-climbing contest was instituted, referred to as "Mountain Climb Month." Employees were helped in their efforts through use of weekly tracking cards (to log stair climbing activities), stair climbing safety tips which were posted on all stairwell doors throughout the building, a series of prompts to use the stairs posted next to all elevators, and regular incentives (e.g., formal acknowledgement of their efforts) contingent on making progress towards their stair-climbing goals.

The findings have been quite encouraging. A significant number of employees (approaching 50%) signed up for the contest, and approximately 33% of the total company workforce accumulated 200 or more flights of stairs during the 1-month period. In addition, of the two-thirds of participants who responded to a post-program survey, 94% indicated that they would participate in the event again if it were offered the following year [82]. Efforts to maintain participation in the program following the initial contest have resulted in the development of regular "stair-climbing" clubs and the continued distribution of low-cost incentives (e.g., certificates, T-shirts, desk clocks) based on participation levels.

Although lacking the experimental rigor and more extensive evaluation found in the Johnson & Johnson study, the Team Health exercise intervention program represents an innovative, low-cost approach for encouraging a significant percentage of a workforce to increase their energy expenditure levels on a regular basis.

INCREASING PHYSICAL ACTIVITY PARTICIPATION IN THE BLUE-COLLAR WORKERS. Despite the large number of worksite physical activity programs currently available, few have specifically targeted blue-collar employees, a segment of the workforce that could potentially benefit significantly from such programs [59]. In the majority of programs that have been designed to include all employees, blue-collar employees often are found to be less likely to participate than white-collar and better educated employees [42, 120].

A systematic effort to increase physical activity participation in blue-collar employees was recently undertaken at Stanford University [73]. Although comprising approximately 16 percent of the university workforce, less than 1% of blue-collar employees were participating in on-campus aerobic exercise programs prior to the start of the intervention.

The program began with a formative assessment of the physical activity habits, needs, and preferences of this segment of the workforce. Based on the results of the assessment, employees were offered a fitness evaluation which occurred on the premises where they worked, and then were invited to participate in a 15-week exercise course which focused on the use of a nearby worksite parcourse. To encourage ongoing participation, monthly contests were conducted, in which working groups competed against one another for the best exercise participation levels. Most of the prizes used in the contests were donated by local area merchants. All participants also were encouraged to log their exercise sessions on publicly displayed charts located in their work areas, so that group members could observe their progress. An enthusiastic member from each work area was enlisted to aid in the accurate completion of the charts.

Approximately 25% of the university's blue-collar workforce participated in the exercise course during the 4-month intervention [73]. Self-reported exercise was significantly related to improvement in fitness as assessed by a 3-minute step-test. Course attendees showed significant increases in fitness and decreases in weight relative to nonattendees. In addition, an increase in awareness of regular exercise as an important component of health was noted across the target population.

Similar to the Team Health program, this program suggests the utility of tailoring interventions to the needs and interests of the particular workforce of interest, as well as using environmental strategies in addition to program-based methods for enhancing physical activity levels.

Worksite Approaches—Conclusions
Although the types of physical activity programming being undertaken throughout our nation's worksites continue to expand, a number of challenges remain in program development, implementation, and evaluation in this important community setting. They include practical constraints on the use of true experimental designs and extensive measurement that reduce experimental control and limit the strength of study findings; an overreliance, as mentioned earlier, on clinical approaches that often involve expensive exercise facilities, an item that can be ill afforded by the nation's smaller worksites that continue to employ the majority of Americans; and a focus on offering a number of health promotion programs at one time which, without appropriate guidance, can be overwhelming to employees uncertain about which programs may be best for them. Johnson & Johnson's Live for Life program and others such as Staywell, which is offered to CDC employees and their spouses [106], have addressed this concern through implementation of substantial screening procedures and subsequent matching of employees to programs based on their needs. As part of Staywell's computer-managed program, their employees are matched to appropriate interventions on an ongoing basis (i.e., the program adapts information and suggestions based on each person's participation and success to date). Additional questions remain concerning the cost benefit and cost effectiveness of worksite health promotion programs, including those for physical activity, and the most effective methods for setting up and maintaining such programs for smaller as well as larger workforces [53].

As underscored by the success of the Johnson & Johnson program, continued efforts to intervene across all four levels of analysis (personal, interpersonal, environmental, institutional) as part of a more comprehensive public health approach to programming is strongly indicated. As is true for the more comprehensive community programming efforts, worksite programs that use environmental strategies in addition to personal and interpersonal approaches can have a potentially larger impact across the entire workforce. In addition, although institutional-level worksite policies may be more difficult to develop on physical fitness activity than on other health behaviors such as smoking, continued exploration of such high-level strategies is worthwhile.

Schools

Research suggests that, given the insidious, progressive nature of most chronic diseases, their prevention optimally should begin early in life [57]. This is particularly true with behavioral risk factors, given that the early experiences one has with health-related behaviors such as physical activity can play a major role in how that behavior is perceived and engaged in later in life. Consequently, schools, a major caretaker of our nation's children throughout their formative years, become a critical setting for developing (or discouraging) these important health behaviors [145, 146].

Unfortunately, school curricula in physical fitness remain focused largely on drills and competitive sports. Such activities often do not adequately instill in students an appreciation of physical activity as a life-long program to be engaged in by everyone, not just the athletically gifted. This may partly explain why at present most physical activity programs engaged in by youth occur outside of school [155].

Neither are children equipped with the skills for carrying on a physical activity program once leaving school. Indeed, although naturally active as children, they start to decrease their energy expenditure in early to mid-adolescence, with the drop particularly striking in girls [2, 56]. These and other recent findings underscore concerns that this country's children are poorly prepared for lifetime physical activity [155].

One research project currently underway to modify the type and amount of physical activity youngsters engage in both during and outside of school physical education classes is Project SPARK in San Diego. A goal of this 5-year study is to increase the amount of vigorous physical activity elementary-school children experience during their regular physical education classes, as well as to encourage family involvement and skill training to foster exercise outside of school [Sallis, personal communication, May 1990]. A program similarly aimed at modifying the physical education curriculum, the Go For Health program in Texas [139], is described subsequently.

In most cases, however, rather than modifying or replacing the traditional physical education curricula available in the schools, public health efforts to increase physical activity in youth have been viewed as complementing the physical education curriculum by focusing on skills that may be better transferred to adulthood. Several of these programs have been carried out as part of the major community-based, multiple risk-factor projects described earlier [121–122, 125]. These approaches have frequently used contests and other hands-on activities (e.g., logging of exercise behavior; involvement of parents in home assignments) to encourage both interest and increased participation. Because they have been conducted as part of a larger multi-intervention project, specific outcome evaluations for individual interventions have often been less rigorous than those for the interventions considered as a group.

Efforts to increase exercise in children or adolescents independent of such comprehensive community-based programs also have been undertaken, with mixed success [31, 72, 123]. Several examples of such programs are described below.

THE SCHOOL-BASED KNOW YOUR BODY INTERVENTION TRIALS. The Know Your Body (KYB) project, initiated in 1975 with funding from the National Heart, Lung, and Blood Institute and the National Cancer Institute, was developed to bring about favorable risk-factor change in demographically diverse populations of elementary school children [157]. Field tested in two populations of children in the New York City area, the program is primarily classroom-based and focuses on dietary and physical activity changes and cigarette smoking prevention. Some parent education and periodic health examinations have occurred as well.

The KYB program was organized around the PRECEDE health education planning model [60]. One of the two populations used to evaluate the program comprised fourth-grade students in all 22 elementary schools of a school district in the Bronx, a low-income borough of New York City. The other population consisted of fourth grade students in four school districts in Westchester County, a middle- and upper-income suburb of New York City [157]. The Bronx elementary schools were randomly assigned by school and the Westchester schools by district to either an intervention or a nonintervention condition. Outcome measures included postexercise pulse recovery rate, dietary intake using a 24-hour dietary recall interview, blood pressure, skinfold thickness as a measure of body composition, saliva continine, and measurement of plasma lipoprotein levels.

After 5 years of intervention, positive changes in knowledge were noted in both population groups receiving the intervention, and favorable changes in dietary intake and plasma total cholesterol levels were noted in the Westchester intervention group relative to the control group [157]. By the end of the sixth year of intervention a net reduction in the rate of initiation of cigarette smoking also was found, which reached statistical significance in the Westchester population [157]. Notably, however, the program appeared to have little effect on physical fitness levels, body mass index, or blood pressure in either population.

In light of indications that economically disadvantaged children may be at particular risk for the development of chronic disease [158], increased efforts to reach that segment of the population are particularly warranted. A successful effort to do so was reported recently by Bush and colleagues [28]. In 1983 they undertook a longitudinal study of the effectiveness of the KYB program for cardiovascular risk-factor reduction among over 1000 elementary school-aged black students in the District of Columbia. During the first 4 years of intervention, measurable improvements were observed in the intervention groups relative to the control group for systolic and diastolic blood pressure, HDL cholesterol, total cholesterol/HDL cholesterol ratio, fitness based on recovery pulse after a controlled bout of exercise, and smoking based on serum thiocyanate levels. In addition, this study revealed a significant relationship between decreases in systolic blood pressure and increases in fitness from baseline to 2-year follow-up similar to that reported in the New York KYB study after the first year of intervention [68].

Even though the authors [28] note the difficulty of obtaining uniform delivery of the curriculum across teachers and schools, their findings and those of others [157, 158] nevertheless provide favorable evidence for the utility of the KYB curriculum across diverse school populations. They also provide some indication that physical activity levels may be positively enhanced through such programs, although more systematic efforts are required, with respect to both intervention and assessment.

THE HEART HEALTH PROGRAM. A pioneering multicomponent program for systematically modifying health behaviors that influence cardiovascular risk among children, the Heart Health Program focused on changing eating and physical activity patterns in elementary school students [31]. The program included individualized goal-setting and feedback, classroom instruction, participatory classroom activities, use of a reward system, and family involvement by way of parent handouts and information. The experimental design consisted of a time-series analysis across three classes in each of two schools. Assessment included self-report measures as well as direct observations of eating and activity behaviors at school. The investigators reported impressive changes in knowledge about heart health as well as eating patterns as measured by food preferences, observed eating behavior at school, and parents' reports of family eating patterns. These changes were found to persist over the summer vacation period. In contrast, observed changes in physical activity as a consequence of the intervention were minimal. The changes in physical activity that were observed were related largely to seasonal sports activities.

These findings indicate that, in at least some school-age populations, interventions adequate for obtaining dietary change may be less effective in promoting physical activity change. The authors suggest that a focus on increases in vigorous playground activities that are already *naturally* occurring among children rather than on the more traditional cardiovascular fitness activities (e.g., use of a Parcourse) emphasized in the current curricula could prove worthwhile.

THE GO FOR HEALTH PROGRAM. The Go For Health Program is a school-based health promotion program focused on increasing healthful diet and exercise behaviors in elementary school children (third and fourth grades) [118]. Two schools were assigned to intervention and two others served as control sites. The intervention consisted of social learning theory-based strategies and organizational strategies for increasing physical activity both as part of ongoing physical education classes and outside of such classes. At baseline, observations of students attending physical education classes revealed that children moved continuously for an average of only about 2 minutes per class period, underscoring the need for such a program [117]. The program objectives included increasing the amount of physical education class time spent in moderate to vigorous physical activity to at least 50% of available class time, and increasing students' knowledge, confidence, and skills (behavioral capacity) related to undertaking physical activity both in and outside of school. Health education classes were used to accomplish the latter objectives.

Results from evaluations of the program have been generally encouraging, although less consistent for physical activity relative to dietary outcomes. At the first evaluation 1 year after the start of the intervention, children attending the schools who had been assigned to receive the intervention program were found to engage in fitness activities during their physical education classes approximately 41% of the available class time, compared with about 21% of the time in the control schools [139]. Baseline class-based activity percentages had been approximately 17% for all four schools. The program also was found to have an impact on exercise-related behavioral capacity and self-efficacy in the older children being evaluated [118]. In the dietary area, significant changes were found for diet behavioral capacity, self-efficacy and behavioral expectations, and use of salt. On the organizational level, at the 1-year evaluation point both the amounts of sodium and fat in selected foods served in the school cafeteria were reduced substantially.

The findings underscore the feasibility and potential utility of incorporating both personal- and organizational-level methods for achieving health-related changes in this age group. They further highlight the challenges of undertaking organizational changes within an often complex school structure. Because of the variation of results found within treatment groups between schools, the authors have recommended the use of school as the major unit of analysis in future studies [118].

THE SAN DIEGO FAMILY HEALTH PROJECT. In recognition of the important role the family plays in shaping the early health behaviors of children, the San Diego Family Health Project targets the family as a major focus of intervention for bringing about improvements in dietary and physical activity behaviors in elementary school-aged children [105]. The importance of the family's influence on physical activity has been underscored through data collected by the investigators on a multiethnic sample of families with elementary school-aged children; they found that parental role-modeling related to physical activity can have an impact on child physical activity habits that extends beyond the actual home environment itself [131].

Over 200 healthy, low-to-middle-income families have been recruited to participate in the major portion of the project, which, similar to other studies in this area, uses techniques derived from social learning theory [7]. An additional important aspect of this study is its focus on developing strategies tailored specifically to the needs of the Anglo and Mexican-American segments of its target population.

Twelve San Diego elementary schools were randomly assigned to either intervention or control conditions, with those Hispanic and Anglo families that contained a fifth- or sixth-grade child subsequently recruited to participate in the 2-year study [105]. The intervention consisted of 12 weekly sessions in which groups of families participated, followed by six maintenance sessions occurring during the subsequent 9-month period. The goal of the intervention was to instruct the families in methods for achieving long-term lifestyle changes in the areas of dietary intake and physical activity, and to facilitate both intra- and interfamilial interactions around these topics.

At 24-month follow-up, both Mexican- and Anglo-American families randomized to the experimental condition showed significant improvement in knowledge concerning making changes in both the dietary and physical activity areas relative to controls [104]. In addition, although there were no significant group differences found in tested cardiovascular fitness levels or reported physical activity, direct observation of physical activity levels in a structured environment (e.g., a family outing at the local zoo) suggested that some enhancement of this health behavior had occurred [119]. Positive changes in eating habits were reflected by significant improvement on a food frequency index for both ethnic groups, and significant reductions in LDL cholesterol for Anglo-American adults in the intervention, compared to the control, condition. In addition, significant group differences in blood pressure measures that favored the intervention condition were found for all subgroups.

The results suggest that using school-based resources to involve families in making health behavior changes is both feasible and effective. However, similar to the other studies that have been described, the findings were more impressive for dietary change than for physical activity change. The investigators recommend that future studies focus on developing approaches for combining family strategies with other types of school health education programs [104].

THE TENTH GRADE, MULTIPLE RISK FACTOR, SCHOOL-BASED PROGRAM. The Tenth Grade Youth Study represents one of the first controlled efforts to improve cardiovascular risk factors, including the amount of physical activity, in high school students [72]. Subjects were tenth grade students from two high schools. Within each of two school districts, one high school was randomly assigned to receive a 20-session risk-reduction intervention and another was assigned to be an assessment-only control. In the schools receiving the special intervention, students underwent instruction, based on social-cognitive theory [8], which focused on cognitive and behavioral skills development and problem-solving to aid behavior change. In addition to other health behaviors, students completed pre- and postintervention evaluations, reporting the types and amount of physical activity in which they were currently engaged. Students who reported engaging in one or more endurance activities for at least 20 minutes continuously three or more times per week were classified as aerobic exercisers.

Postintervention findings indicated that the intervention had a positive impact on both physical activity knowledge and reported exercise behavior [72]. In addition, both boys and girls in the intervention group had a measurable reduction in resting heart rate relative to their control group counterparts. Positive treatment effects were also observed for body mass index and body composition measured using skinfolds.

Of note, the general similarity of the study sample to other regional and national samples on a number of relevant variables bodes well for the generalizability of the results to other school districts. Questions with respect to the longer-time stability of the changes achieved (students were evaluated at a 2-month follow-up) remain, however.

FITNESSGRAM YOUTH FITNESS ASSESSMENT PROGRAM. In contrast to programs involving classroom instruction, FITNESSGRAM, sponsored by the Campbell Soup Company and designed and implemented by the Institute for Aerobics Research in Dallas, is a physical fitness assessment and feedback program designed to increase awareness and encourage increased involvement in physical activity [15]. The first test of its kind in widespread use in the U.S. that uses a standard approach to fitness testing, the current form of the test uses age- and sex-specific acceptable health fitness standards to aid test interpretation [15]. The program includes a microcomputer software package that aids data compilation and provides individual and group reports of student physical fitness status. As part of these reports, exercise-related feedback and recommendations are provided based on the student's fitness status. An exercise log is also provided, which can be sent to FITNESSGRAM to qualify the student for participation awards. Good fitness-related performance is acknowledged, but the FITNESSGRAM awards program also stresses the importance of health-related behaviors that are obtainable by all students.

FITNESSGRAM is currently being implemented in numerous school districts, YMCAs, hospitals, and recreation centers throughout the United States. Preliminary evaluations of the program have been published [15], which suggest that the program offers an effective, practical means for evaluating children's fitness levels in a standardized way, and for providing incentive for future gains. The findings further suggest that most children and youth do currently meet current physical fitness standards as established by the FITNESSGRAM project. How such programs may influence the decline in fitness and physical activity currently observed in this country as children grow up remains to be investigated.

Schools—Conclusions
Although school settings provide a potentially powerful opportunity to positively influence the long-term physical activity pattern of our nation's youth, their promise in this area has yet to be realized. Health education programs typically have demonstrated increases in knowledge and changes in attitudes relevant to the practice of regular exercise, but evidence for their efficacy in achieving actual behavior change has been inconsistent. Possible reasons for this include the following: (1) school-based programs typically have involved a focus on several health behaviors at one time, with physical activity being only one of them and often not the behavior that is most strongly targeted; it is possible that making physical activity change the primary target of a health promotion effort could result in more powerful intervention effects; (2) adherence to a program of physical activity may require the child or adolescent to adopt behaviors that are counter to the prevailing habits of his or her peer group, which increases the difficulty of implementing the program; (3) the health-related incentives for engaging in regular exercise are typically less potent for younger age groups, who do not perceive themselves to be at immediate risk; and (4) attempts to permanently modify the child's health habits may require that other family members be included as well to achieve success.

To place greater emphasis on physical activity within the school-based program may be particularly useful. For instance, the Australian Health and Fitness Study has been one of the few randomized controlled intervention studies involving physical activity promotion in school children that has been able to demonstrate significant increases in fitness and reductions in body fat [43]. The study intervention consisted of an intensive daily physical activity program carried out in 10-year-old children.

Important challenges remain in area of research design, in which, like worksites, true randomized, controlled studies are difficult to execute, as well as in the areas of assessment, including the continued development of accurate tools for measuring children's habitual activity

[9], and follow-up, including the use of evaluations spanning longer periods (i.e., a year or more). Moreover, finding ways to use family and peer influences to help promote habitual physical activity across all phases of a child's schooling is an important goal that has received relatively little systematic attention to date.

In addition to aiding behavioral change in the student, it is possible that school-based health education programs that involve parents could potentially lead to positive changes in parents' health beliefs, behaviors, and verbalizations about health [31, 35]. It also is possible that children could benefit indirectly, through modeling and other channels, from comprehensive worksite approaches to physical activity promotion that targets teachers and other school personnel [21]. At present relatively few successful efforts to reach either group have been reported [122, 138].

It is clear that a different strategy or series of strategies for promoting physical activity in children, most likely ones that combine programs based within and outside of schools, will need to occur if the current national objectives for youth [153] are to be reached.

Places of Worship

Even though recent findings indicate that our nation's schools do not place a strong emphasis on physical education programs (i.e., only 36% have daily physical education classes), over 80% of school-aged children report engaging in physical activities through other community organizations [152]. Some of these community organizations include churches and other places of worship.

Although places of worship have not traditionally played a leading role in health promotion programming, such community settings offer a number of advantages. These include large memberships, with community residents often living within relatively close proximity to the church or synagogue; the ability to reach an entire family through program efforts—often a difficult task to accomplish [138]; a history of "helping" in a wide range of activities including family counseling, community improvement projects, and health; and a presence in virtually every community throughout the U.S., which can aid program dissemination efforts [100]. Two such church-based projects are briefly described.

THE FITNESS THROUGH CHURCHES PROJECT. The Fitness Through Churches Project, funded by the American Heart Association and sponsored by the University of North Carolina at Chapel Hill, is a demonstration project that promotes aerobic exercise together with education on other health behaviors to African-American residents of North Carolina [66]. The goals of the project include (1) training 30 persons chosen by pastors of ten inner-city churches to serve as organizers and instructors of aerobic exercise classes as well as advisors in other areas of heart health (e.g., nutrition, smoking cessation); (2) assisting the congregations of their churches in developing regular exercise classes and other health education activities in their churches; and (3) developing and evaluating a model for health promotion that will be culturally acceptable and generalizable to other black communities throughout the country [66]. A pilot study has been completed which demonstrates that such a program is both feasible and attractive to the community in general and to church pastors and their congregations in particular. Based on the findings from this pilot study, more formal implementation and evaluation of the project is underway. In addition, methods have been investigated for encouraging more permanent institutionalization of the program in the churches, through, for example, its being made a part of the designated activities being fostered by already active church committees.

The investigators note that the multiple community roles traditionally played by black churches make them a particularly fitting venue for culturally appropriate lifestyle programming, including physical activity, for this population [66].

THE HEALTH AND RELIGION PROJECT (HARP) OF RHODE ISLAND. Begun in 1983, HARP is affiliated with the Pawtucket Heart Health Program [88]. Similar to the Fitness Through Churches Project, a primary goal of HARP has been to evaluate the effectiveness of volunteers as providers of health programs within their own churches. To test the effectiveness of varying levels of professional involvement as well as the need for training special task forces to coordinate the health promotion activities within each church, 20 churches representing a variety of denominations have been randomly assigned to five experimental conditions.

The information collected thus far supports the feasibility and utility of encouraging churches to play an active role in behavioral change programming, including physical activity, to improve health. The project was successful in recruiting almost two-thirds of the churches in the state of Rhode Island that were eligible for the study, and all of these churches have remained involved in the project for at least a two and a half year period [88]. Future findings from this project will provide valuable information on methods for effectively using places of worship to bolster community-wide programming in the health promotion area.

Places of Worship—Conclusions

As understood by these two projects, places of worship provide promising avenues for innovative programming in physical activity and other health areas. Such settings can offer programming opportunities at all levels of intervention, including personal and interpersonal (e.g., church-based physical activity classes, family walking programs), environmental (e.g., provision of health education information using church bulletins), and institutional levels (e.g., establishment of a network of churches or synagogues to promote interfaith physical activity programs, involvement and training of religious leaders in the promotion of physical activity to their congregations) [100].

ISSUES ACCOMPANYING HEALTH PROMOTION PROGRAMMING

Health promotion programming, whether it be in a specific setting or in the community at large, invariably brings with it a number of important ethical issues. Becoming or remaining aware of these issues can prevent the health professional from creating situations that may have a detrimental effect on program outcomes. Included among such issues are the potential victim-blaming that may accompany interventions that emphasize personal responsibility for health and illness; the tendency to "oversell" health behaviors in the face of available evidence that, although promising, typically is far from conclusive; the need to be aware of the costs of health promotion programs, both monetarily and psychologically, as well as their benefits; and the continuing need for sensitivity to the fact that what may be a high priority for health professionals may not be so for other individuals or groups (i.e., may not be valued or desired by them).

In addition to such issues, the potential advantages versus disadvantages of multiple- versus single-risk-factor interventions require further investigation [147]. Notwithstanding the difficulties created in attempting to assess program effectiveness when several health behaviors are being intervened on at the same time, there are compelling reasons for undertaking physical activity intervention as part of a broader multiple-risk-factor intervention. These include the potential for gaining a "bigger bang for the buck," given that many of the major risk factors for CHD, cancer, and other chronic diseases are influenced by a relatively small group of health behaviors (e.g., smoking, dietary patterns, physical activity habits). The potentially complementary and synergistic nature of many of the health behaviors, both physiologically and behaviorally, also supports the development of multi-risk-factor programs [138]. For instance, in the weight control area, it has become increasingly clear that to combine systematic dietary change and increases in physical activity is generally the most optimal method for promoting both initial weight loss and longer term maintenance [27]. A further argument in favor of multiple-risk-factor intervention programs is that risk factors for chronic diseases such as CHD tend to cluster within the population [12].

The potential problem of such programs being overwhelming to both participants and staff can be reduced by staging interventions in consecutive "waves," as has typically been done in the multiple-risk-factor community intervention trials described earlier.

PROMOTION OF PHYSICAL ACTIVITY AND FITNESS IN THE COMMUNITY—FUTURE DIRECTIONS

A promising start has been made in the development of physical activity interventions in the community, but numerous areas for future investigation remain. Several of the more important areas that could benefit from continued or expanded efforts are discussed briefly below.

Coordination of Programs Across All Levels of Analysis and Intervention
There is, as noted earlier in this chapter, a continuing need to develop a coordinated set of interventions that extend beyond the personal and interpersonal approaches that constitute most of the nation's physical activity intervention efforts to date. Strategies developed at institutional, environmental, and regulatory levels can be used to complement face-to-face approaches, enhancing awareness and motivation for change and reaching currently underserved population segments. For instance, a potentially promising environmental and institutional approach that has been underused in the physical activity area is "life path points" in which goods and services are distributed to the population-at-large. Examples of such life path points include supermarkets, banks, drug-stores, clinics, shopping centers, and libraries.

The use of alternate channels for program delivery (e.g., the telephone or mail) may provide an additional means for applying potentially powerful personal-level strategies (e.g., individualized instruction, feedback, support) to a broader audience [70, 81, 112]. In a recently completed clinical trial, home-based physical activity programs, in which ongoing staff supervision was delivered via telephone and mail, resulted in significantly better 18-month adherence to aerobic exercise in a large group of middle-aged adults than a standard, class-based exercise program [78]. Telephone- and mail-based systems of support allow for more convenient, flexible modes of exercise participation and instruction which health care providers and the American public alike desire [69]. This preference for convenient physical activity programming has been found in men and women across a range of ages and cultural backgrounds [79, 89].

Examples of the types of programs that can be delivered across different levels of interventions are shown in Table 6.1. As illustrated, decisions about levels of intervention influence a number of other variables, including the targets of the intervention(s), delivery channels, and specific program strategies. In choosing different intervention

TABLE 6.1

Examples of Physical Activity Programs, by Level of Intervention, Channel, Target, and Strategy

Level of Intervention	Channel	Target	Strategy
Personal	Face-to-face: physician's office; health clinic; health spas and clubs.	Patients, clients	Information on risk, health benefits; counselor support; personal monitoring and feedback; problem-solving (relapse prevention).
	Mediated/Not face-to-face: telephone, mail (feedback systems, correspondence courses; self-help kits and booklets).		Same as above.
Interpersonal	Classes; telephone/mail systems; health spas and clubs; peer-led groups.	Patients, healthy individuals, families, peers.	Information; peer, family & counselor support; group affiliation; personal or public monitoring and feedback; group problem-solving.
Organizational/ Environmental	Schools; worksites; neighborhoods; community facilities (e.g., par courses, walk/bike paths); churches, community organizations; sites for activities of daily living (public stairs; shopping malls, parking lots).	Student body; all employees; local residents; social norms or milieu.	Curricula; point-of-choice education and prompts; organizational support; public feedback; incentives.
Institutional/ Legislative	Policies; laws; regulations.	Broad spectrum of the community or population.	Standardization of exercise-related curricula; insurance incentives for regular exercisers; flexible work time to permit exercise; monetary incentives for the development of adequate public facilities for exercise; Surgeon General's report on physical activity and health.

levels, trade-offs occur with respect to program intensiveness and tailoring on the one hand, and its subsequent reach into the population on the other. Clearly, the use of a *mix* of strategies from all four levels of intervention, targeted to meet the needs of the different subgroups in a community, is most likely to have a measurable impact on the community as a whole.

In theory the use of such multilevel, comprehensive approaches across an entire community should result in more effective outcomes. Yet the striking paucity of data on community-wide approaches to physical activity sharply curtail the conclusions that presently can be made in this area. It remains unclear whether such comprehensive approaches, and the increased complexity they entail, would lead to more cost-effective results than smaller scale, setting-specific approaches which make up the majority of efforts undertaken in this area to date.

Training of Health Professionals in Community Intervention Methods
As should be evident from the earlier portions of this chapter, the use of a multidisciplinary approach is essential if the successful promotion

of physical activity in the community is to be achieved. This means at least two things; first, that curricula and training methods specific to each health discipline are required if that discipline is to bring its unique perspectives and position in the community to bear in this health area; and second, strategies for promoting cooperative efforts *across* disciplines need to occur so that the delivery of contradictory messages can be minimized and development of the most potent strategies accomplished.

With respect to the first of these two points, systematic efforts to provide specific guidance relevant to different health professions are beginning to emerge. An example of this is the U.S. Preventive Services Task Force's recent article outlining the physician's role in promoting physical activity in the clinical setting [63]. The American College of Sports Medicine continues its important role in supplying exercise professionals with up-to-date developments in exercise testing and prescription guidelines as well as in important health areas related to physical activity [4]. Health professionals at the Centers for Disease Control also have taken the lead in developing a series of guidebooks for public health professionals in a number of health promotion areas, including physical activity and fitness. Their handbook *Promoting Physical Activity Among Adults* [154] is designed to assist program planners in gathering relevant information from their own communities, and subsequently applying this information in developing intervention priorities for their constituency. The handbook also outlines the types of interventions that can be implemented at different sites throughout the community as well as methods for aiding program evaluation. It can be supplemented with an available evaluation guide [151], which describes assessment tools that can be used in physical activity program evaluation. A manual for the promotion of physical activity in the community also has been developed by the Stanford Center for Research in Disease Prevention in cooperation with the Henry J. Kaiser Family Foundation [76]. Its purpose is to provide community health professionals with a brief overview of the scientific basis and rationale for community-based physical activity promotion, and practical steps to take in developing community-based exercise programming.

Increased communication across health disciplines is evident from promising activities that have begun to surface in the form of interdisciplinary training programs, such as those offered at the pre- and postdoctoral levels in affiliation with some of the federally funded community intervention projects. In addition, some professional health organizations have continued to promote a multidisciplinary membership. Yet substantially more needs to be done to bring the combined expertise of exercise physiologists, trainers, physicians, behavioral scientists, nurses, and public health professionals to bear on the problem of physical activity participation in this country.

The Utility of a Life-span (Developmental) Approach to Community Intervention

As noted previously, researchers in the health area increasingly have conceptualized health behavior change as processes or stages [39]. The exercise area is no exception, as recent evidence continues to shed light on factors that influence initial adoption as well as ongoing maintenance of physical activity [92]. Although useful, such an approach could be enhanced through consideration of aspects of change relevant to stages of human development in addition to stages of exercise participation. A developmental perspective allows for an increased understanding of life periods and transitions when behaviors such as physical activity may be markedly affected [54, 164]. For example, adolescence represents a period of biological, psychological, and social turbulence when gender differences in physical activity participation become noticeable. The transition from school to the workforce, as well as other issues such as parenthood, retirement, widowhood, and relocation are other examples of milestones which may have a significant effect on both the ability and desire of a person to participate in regular exercise. Understanding the consequences of such milestones, in addition to the more general developmental course of physical activity participation throughout the lifespan, may enhance the relevance and effectiveness of efforts to keep Americans active as a way of life.

Table 6.2 outlines some of the specific features associated with several such milestones and their potential consequences with respect to physical activity programming.

Increased Tailoring of Programs to Specific Population

Underlying efforts to use different levels of intervention and understand the effects of developmental milestones on exercise involvement is the goal of tailoring programs to meet the needs and preferences of different portions of the community. To date, a "kitchen sink" approach has been generally implemented by which an array of strategies are delivered throughout the community or community setting, such as a worksite, with the hope that something will "catch." With the knowledge, from programs such as Life for Life, that systematic efforts to intervene can have a positive impact on physical activity patterns, attention now needs to be focused on identifying the critical elements for different segments of the community or community setting. In addition to the systematic dismantling of multi-intervention programs to determine what works, the use of formative evaluation and other social marketing strategies in concert with behavioral science principles can help health professionals hone interventions to meet the needs of both people and budgets. Further, in collecting information on persons' time allocations, travel patterns, and the groups or entities with whom they identify, new ways of defining "mini-communities" within a larger jurisdiction

TABLE 6.2
Features and Examples of Physical Activity Programs for Several Major Developmental Milestones

Milestone (critical period)	Specific Features	Goals/Strategies
Adolescence	Rapid physical and emotional changes	Exercise as part of a program of healthy weight regulation (both sexes)
	Increased concern with appearance and weight	Noncompetitive activities that are fun, varied
	Need for independence	Emphasis on independence, choice
	Short-term perspective	Focus on proximal outcomes (e.g., body image, stress management)
	Increased peer influence	Peer involvement, support
Initial Work Entry	Increased time and scheduling constraints	Choice of activities that are convenient, enjoyable
	Short-term perspective	Focus on proximal outcomes
	Employer demands	Involvement of worksite (environmental prompts, incentives)
		Realistic goal-setting/injury prevention
		Coeducational noncompetitive activities
Parenting	Increased family demands and time constraints	Emphasis on benefits to self and family (e.g., stress management, weight control, well-being)
	Family-directed focus	Activities appropriate with children (e.g., walking)
	Postpartum effects on weight, mood	Flexible, convenient, personalized regimen
		Inclusion of activities of daily living
		Neighborhood involvement, focus
		Family-based public monitoring, goal-setting
		Availability of child-related services (child care)
Retirement Age	Increased time availability and flexibility	Identification of current and previous enjoyable activities
	Longer term perspective on health; increased health concerns, "readiness"	Matching of activities to current health status
	Caregiving duties, responsibilities (parents, spouse, children or grandchildren)	Emphasis on mild- and moderate-intensity activities, including activities of daily living
		Use of "life path point" information and prompts
		Emphasis on activities engendering independence
		Garnering support of family members, peers
		Availability of necessary services (e.g., caretaking services for significant other)

may emerge. This, in turn, may aid subsequent efforts to match programs to people.

Tailoring of strategies becomes particularly important when underserved or hard to reach groups (e.g., smokers, ethnic minorities, the disadvantaged), as well as other special populations (e.g., teenagers, elders) are the targets of intervention efforts. As noted in the discussion of CHAPP earlier, it often is hardest to reach subgroups that have the most to gain, both physically and emotionally, from successful engagement in positive health-related behaviors. In this regard, we may benefit from the experience of health professionals in other cultures. Some of these individuals have taken advantage of the natural interest in health concerns shown by segments such as the elderly in establishing partnerships, initiated at the grass-roots level, to promote increases in physical activity [5]. By being sensitive to the cultural milieu of each subgroup, as has been done in projects like CHAPP and the San Diego Family Health Project [104], the probability of attaining successful outcomes can be enhanced.

CONCLUSIONS

In light of the relationship of regular physical activity to health and the significant prevalence of underactivity in the U.S. population, community approaches provide a potentially important, though as yet relatively untested, means for enhancing physical activity levels across diverse populations. Although the long-term cost effectiveness of such approaches remains to be determined, the short-term benefits that can be gained from increases in physical activity in areas related to daily functioning and well-being, weight control, and overall functional capacity provide a solid rationale for further community-based efforts in this area. The challenge remains to develop methods for helping persons maintain adequate levels of activity throughout all stages of their lives, as well as to find ways to reach the significant numbers of Americans who have yet to begin participating at all.

ACKNOWLEDGEMENTS

The author would like to thank Steven N. Blair, P.E.D., and William L. Haskell, Ph.D., for their helpful comments on earlier drafts of this manuscript. The preparation of this review was supported in part by Public Health Service grant #AG-00440 from the National Institute on Aging.

REFERENCES

1. Albanes, D., A. Blair, and P.R. Taylor. Physical activity and risk of cancer in the NHANES I population. *Am. J. Public Health* 79:744–750, 1989.
2. Alpert, B.S., N.L. Flood, W.B. Strong, et al. Response to ergometer exercise in a healthy biracial population of children. *J. Pediatrics* 101:538, 1982.
3. Altman, D.G., A.J. Evans, J.A. Flora, et al. A worksite exercise contest. *Proceedings of the Society of Behavioral Medicine Seventh Annual Scientific Sessions;* March, 1986, San Francisco. Washington, DC: Society of Behavioral Medicine, 1986.
4. American College of Sports Medicine. *Resource Manual for Guidelines for Exercise Testing and Prescription.* Philadelphia: Lea & Febiger, 1988.
5. Attig, G.A., and K. Chanawongse. Elderly people as health promoters. *World Health Forum* 10:186–189, 1989.
6. Bailey, D.A., R.J. Shephard, and R.L. Mirwald. Validation of a self-administered home test of cardio-respiratory fitness. *Can. J. Applied Sport Sci.* 1:67–78, 1976
7. Bandura, A. Social learning theory. Englewood Cliffs, NJ: Prentice-Hall, 1977.
8. Bandura, A. *Social Foundations of Thought and Action: A Social Cognitive Theory.* Englewood Cliffs, NJ: Prentice-Hall, 1986.

9. Bar-Or, O. Discussion: growth, exercise, fitness, and later outcomes. In C. Bouchard, R.J. Shephard, and T. Stephens, et al. (eds.). *Exercise, Fitness, and Health: A Consensus of Current Knowledge.* Champaign, IL: Human Kinetics Books; 1990, pp. 655–660.

10. Baun, W.B., E.J. Bernacki, and S.P. Tsai. A preliminary investigation: effect of a corporate fitness program on absenteeism and health care cost. *J. Occup. Med.* 28:18–22, 1986.

11. Bezold, C., R.J. Carlson, and J.C. Peck. *The Future of Work and Health.* Diver, MA: Auburn House, 1986.

12. Blackburn, H. Multifactor preventive trials (MPT) in coronary heart disease. In G.T. Stewart (ed.). *Trends in Epidemiology: Application to Health Services Research and Training.* Springfield, IL: Charles C. Thomas, 1972, pp. 212–230.

13. Blackburn, H., R.V. Luepker, F.G. Kline, et al. The Minnesota Health Program: a research and demonstration project in cardiovascular disease prevention. In J.D. Matarazzo, S.M. Weiss, J.A. Herd, et al. (eds.). *Behavioral Health: A Handbook for Health Enhancement and Disease Prevention.* New York: John Wiley and Sons, 1984, pp. 1171–1178.

14. Blair, S.N. How to assess exercise habits and physical fitness. In J.D. Matarazzo, S.M. Weiss, J.A. Herd, et al. (eds.). *Behavioral Health: A Handbook of Health Enhancement and Disease Prevention.* New York: John Wiley & Sons, 1984, pp. 424–447.

15. Blair, S.N., D.G. Clark, K.J. Cureton, and K.E. Powell. Exercise and fitness in childhood: implications for a lifetime of health. In C.V. Gisolfi and D.R. Lamb (eds.). *Perspectives in Exercise Science and Sports Medicine, Volume 2: Youth, Exercise, and Sport.* Indianapolis: Benchmark Press, 1989, pp. 401–430.

16. Blair, S.N., N.N. Goodyear, L.W. Gibbons, et al. Physical fitness and incidence of hypertension in healthy normotensive men and women. *J.A.M.A.* 252:487–490, 1984.

17. Blair, S.N., W.L. Haskell, P. Ho, et al. Assessment of habitual physical activity by a seven-day recall in a community survey and controlled experiments. *Am J. Epidemiol.* 122:794–804, 1985.

18. Blair, S.N., W.B. Kannel, H.W. Kohl, et al. Surrogate measures of physical activity and physical fitness: evidence of sedentary traits of resting tachycardia, obesity, and low vital capacity. *Am. J. Epidemiol.* 129:1145–1156, 1989.

19. Blair, S.N., H.W. Kohl III, R.S. Paffenbarger Jr, et al. Physical fitness and all-cause mortality: a prospective study of healthy men and women. *J.A.M.A.* 262:2395–2401, 1989.

20. Blair, S.N., P.V. Piserchia, C.S. Wilbur, et al. A public health intervention model for worksite health promotion: impact on exercise and physical fitness in a health promotion plan after 24 months. *J.A.M.A.* 255:921–926, 1986.

21. Blair, S.N., M. Smith, T.R. Collingwood, et al. Health promotion for educators: impact on absenteeism. *Prev. Med.* 15:166–175, 1986.

22. Blake, S.M., R.W. Jeffery, J.R. Finnegan, et al. Process evaluation of a community-based physical activity campaign: the Minnesota Heart Health Program experience. *Health Educ. Res.* 2:115–121, 1987.

23. Bouchard, C., et al. A method to assess energy expenditure in children and adults. *Am. J. Clin. Nutr.* 37:461–467, 1983.

24. Bouchard, C., R.J. Shephard, T. Stephens, et al. (eds.). *Exercise, fitness, and health: A consensus of current knowledge.* Champaign, IL: Human Kinetics Books, 1990.

25. Bray, G.A. Exercise and obesity. In C. Bouchard, R.J. Shephard, T. Stephens, et al. (eds.). *Exercise, fitness, and health: A consensus of current knowledge.* Champaign, IL: Human Kinetics Books, 1990, pp. 497–510.

26. Brownell, K.D., A.J. Stunkard, and J.M. Albaum. Evaluation and modification of exercise patterns in the natural environment. *Am. J. Psychiatry* 137:1540–1545, 1980.

27. Brownell, K.D., and T.A. Wadden. Behavior therapy for obesity: modern approaches and better results. In K.D. Brownell, J.P. Foreyt (eds.). *Handbook of eating disorders:*

Physiology, psychology, and treatment of obesity, anorexia, and bulimia. New York: Basic Books Inc., 1986, pp. 180–197.

28. Bush, P.J., A.E. Zuckerman, V.S. Taggart, et al. Cardiovascular risk factor prevention in black school children: the 'Know Your Body' evaluation project. *Health Educ. Q.* 16:215–227, 1989.

29. Caspersen, C.J., G.M. Christenson, and R.A. Pollard. Status of the 1990 physical fitness and exercise objectives—evidence from NHIS 1985. *Public Health Rep.* 101:587–592, 1986.

30. Chavis, D.M., and J.R. Newbrough. The meaning of 'community' in community psychology. *J. Community Psychology* 14:335–340, 1986.

31. Coates, T.J., R.W. Jeffery, and L.A. Slinkard. Heart healthy eating and exercise: introducing and maintaining changes in health behaviors. *Am. J. Public Health* 71:15–23, 1981.

32. The Community Health Assessment and Promotion Project. Mobilizing a minority community to reduce risk factors for cardiovascular disease: an exercise nutrition handbook. Atlanta: Centers for Disease Control, 1989.

33. Cooper, K.H. A means of assessing maximal oxygen intake. *J.A.M.A.* 203:201–204, 1968.

34. Cox, M., R.J. Shephard, and P. Corey. Influence of an employee fitness program upon fitness, productivity, and absenteeism. *Ergonomics* 24:795–806, 1981.

35. Crockett, S. The family team approach to fitness: a proposal. *Public Health Rep.* 102:546–551, 1987.

36. Crow, R., H. Blackburn, D. Jacobs, et al. Population strategies to enhance physical activity: the Minnesota Heart Health Program. *Acta. Med. Scand., Suppl.* 711:93–112, 1986.

37. David, M.F., and D.C. Iverson. An overview and analysis of the Health Style campaign. *Health Educ. Q.* 11:253–272, 1984.

38. DeBusk, R.F., N. Houston, W.L. Haskell, et al. Exercise training soon after myocardial infarction. *Am. J. Cardiol.* 44:1223–1227, 1979.

39. DiClemente, C.C., and J.O. Prochaska. Processes and stages of change: Coping and competence in smoking behavior change. In S. Shiffman and T. Wills (eds.). *Coping and substance use.* New York: Academic Press, 1985, pp. 319–344.

40. Dishman, R.K. Compliance/adherence in health-related exercise. *Health Psychology* 1:237–267, 1982.

41. Dishman, R.K. (ed.). *Exercise adherence: Its impact on public health.* Champaign, IL: Human Kinetics, 1988.

42. Dishman, R.K., J.F. Sallis, and D.R. Orenstein. The determinants of physical activity and exercise. *Public Health Rep.* 100:158–171, 1985.

43. Dwyer, T., W.E. Coonan, D.R. Leetch, et al. An investigation of the effects of daily physical activity on the health of primary school students in South Australia. *Int. J. Epidemiol.* 12:308–313, 1983.

44. Egger, G., W. Fitzgerald, G. Frape, et al. Results of large scale media antismoking campaign in Australia: North Coast 'Quit for Life' programme. *Br. M. J.* 287:1125–1128, 1983.

45. Ekelund, L.G., W.L. Haskell, J.L. Johnson, et al. Physical fitness as a predictor of cardiovascular mortality in asymptomatic North American men. *New Engl. J. Med.* 319:1379–1384, 1988.

46. Epstein, L.H., et al. Attendance and fitness in aerobics exercise: the effects of contract and lottery procedures. *Behav. Modif.* 4:465–479, 1980.

47. Farquhar, J.W., S.P. Fortmann, J.A. Flora, et al. The Stanford Five-City Project: effects of community-wide education on cardiovascular disease risk factors. *J.A.M.A.* 264:359–365, 1990.

48. Farquhar, J.W., S.P. Fortmann, N. Maccoby, et al. The Stanford Five-City Project: design and methods. *Am. J. Epidemiol.* 122:323–334, 1985.

49. Farquhar, J.W. Community-based health promotion: lessons from field research. *Evaluation Practice.* (In press).

50. Farquhar, J.W., S.P. Fortmann, P.D. Wood, et al. Community studies of cardiovascular disease prevention. In N. Kaplan and J. Stamler, (eds.). *Prevention of coronary heart disease.* Philadelphia: W.B. Saunders Co., 1983, pp. 170–181.

51. Farquhar, J.W., N. Maccoby, P.D. Wood, et al. Community education for cardiovascular health. *Lancet* 1:1192–1195, 1977.

52. Farquhar, J.W., N. Maccoby, and P.D. Wood. Education and community studies. In W.W. Holland, R. Detels, and G. Knox (eds.). *Oxford Textbook of Public Health.* vol. 3. Oxford, London: Oxford University Press, 1985, pp. 207–221.

53. Felix, M.R.J., A.J. Stunkard, R.Y. Cohen, et al. Health promotion at the worksite: A process for establishing programs. *Prev. Med.* 14:99–108, 1985.

54. Felner, R.D., S.S. Farber, and J. Primavera. Transitions and stressful life events: A model of primary prevention. In R.D. Fenler, et al. (eds.). *Preventive psychology: Theory, research, and practice.* Elmsford, NY: Pergamon Press, 1983.

55. Fielding, J.E. Health promotion and disease prevention at the worksite. *Annu. Rev. Public Health* 5:237–265, 1984.

56. *Fitness Profile in American Youth. A report on 1981–83 fitness tests involving more than 4 million boys and girls in over 10,000 schools.* East Hanover, NJ: Nabisco Brands, 1983.

57. Fraser, G.E. *Preventive Cardiology.* New York: Oxford University Press, 1986.

58. Gesten, E.L., and L.A. Jason. Social and community interventions. *Annu. Rev. Psychology* 38:427–460, 1987.

59. Godin, G., and R.J. Shephard. Physical fitness promotion programmes: effectiveness in modifying exercise behavior. *Can. J. Applied Sports Science* 8:104–113, 1983.

60. Green, L.W., M.W. Kreuter, S.G. Deeds, and K.B. Partridge. *Health education planning: A diagnostic approach.* Palo Alto, CA: Mayfield Press, 1980.

61. Hagberg, J.M. Exercise, fitness, and hypertension. C. Bouchard, R.J. Shephard, and T. Stephen, et al. (eds.). *Exercise fitness, and health: A consensus of current knowledge.* Champaign, IL: Human Kinetics Books, 1990, pp. 455–466.

62. Hanlon, J.J., and G.E. Pickett. *Public health: Administration and practice (8th ed.).* St. Louis, MO: Mosby, 1984.

63. Harris, S.S., C.J. Caspersen, G.H. DeFriese, et al. Physical activity counseling for healthy adults as a primary preventive intervention in the clinical setting: report for the U.S. Preventive Services Task Force. *J.A.M.A.* 261:3590–3598, 1989.

64. Haskell, W.L. Physical activity and health: Need to define the required stimulus. *American J. Cardiol.* 55:4D–9D, 1985.

65. Haskell, W.L., and S.N. Blair. The physical activity component of health promotion in occupational settings. *Public Health Rep.* 95:109–118, 1980.

66. Hatch, J.W., A.C. Cunningham, W.W. Woods, et al. The Fitness Through Churches Project: Description of a community-based cardiovascular health promotion intervention. *Hygie* 5:9–12, 1986.

67. Heath, G.W., B.E. Leonard, R.H. Wilson, et al. Community-based exercise intervention: Zuni diabetes project. *Diabetes Care* 10:579–583, 1987.

68. Hofman, A., J.H. Walter, P.A. Connelly, et al. Blood pressure and physical fitness in children. *Hypertension* 9:188–191, 1987.

69. Iverson, D.C., M.E. Fielding, R.S. Crow, et al. The promotion of physical activity in the United States population: The status of programs in medical, worksite, community, and school settings. *Public Health Rep.* 100:212–224, 1985.

70. Juneau, M., F. Rogers, V. De Santos, et al. Effectiveness of self-monitored, home-based moderate-intensity exercise training in middle-aged men and women. *Am. J. Cardiol.* 60:66–70, 1987.

71. Keefe, F.J., and J.A. Blumenthal. The life fitness program: A behavioral approach to making exercise a habit. *J. Behav. Ther. Exp. Psychiatry* 11:31–34, 1980.

72. Killen, J.D., M. Telch, T. Robinson, et al. Cardiovascular risk reduction for tenth graders: a multiple factor school-based approach. *J.A.M.A.* 260:1728–1733, 1988.

73. King, A.C., F. Carl, L. Burkel, et al. Increasing exercise among blue-collar employees: the tailoring of worksite programs to meet specific needs. *Prev. Med.* 17:357–365, 1988.

74. King, A.C., B. Frey-Hewitt, D. Dreon, et al. Diet versus exercise in weight maintenance: the effects of minimal intervention strategies on long-term outcomes in men. *Arch. Intern. Med.* 149:2741–2746, 1989.

75. King, A.C., and L.W. Frederiksen. Low-cost strategies for increasing exercise behavior: relapse preparation training and social support. *Behav. Modif.* 8:3–21, 1984.

76. King, A.C., W.L. Haskell, N. Miller, et al. (eds.). *Promotion of physical activity in the community: A manual for community health professionals.* Stanford University School of Medicine: Stanford Center for Research in Disease Prevention and the Henry J. Kaiser Family Foundation, 1988.

77. King, A.C., and J.E. Martin. Adherence to exercise. American College of Sports Medicine. *Guidelines for exercise testing and prescription: Reference manual.* Philadelphia: Lea and Febiger, 1988, pp. 335–344.

78. King, A.C., C.B. Taylor, and W.L. Haskell. Expanding methods for achieving sustained participation in community-based physical activity. *The First International Congress of Behavioral Medicine;* June, 1990, Uppsala, Sweden. International Society of Behavioral Medicine.

79. King, A.C., C.B. Taylor, W.L. Haskell, et al. Identifying strategies for increasing employee physical activity levels: findings from the Stanford/Lockheed exercise survey. *Health Educ. Q.* 17:269–285, 1990.

80. King, A.C., C.B. Taylor, W.L. Haskell, et al. Influence of regular aerobic exercise on psychological health: a randomized, controlled trial of health middle-aged adults. *Health Psychology* 8:305–324, 1989.

81. King, A.C., C.B. Taylor, W.L. Haskell, et al. Strategies for increasing early adherence to and long-term maintenance of home-based exercise training in healthy middle-aged men and women. *Am. J. Cardiol.* 61:628–632, 1988.

82. Knadler, G.F., and T. Rogers. Mountain climb month program: a low-cost exercise intervention program at a high-rise worksite. *Fitness in Business.* Oct.: 64–67, 1987.

83. Knowles, J.H. The responsibility of the individual. J.H. Knowles (ed.). *Doing better and feeling worse: Health in the United States.* New York: Norton, 1977, pp. 53–71.

84. Kotler, P. *Marketing for nonprofit organizations* (2nd ed.). Englewood Cliffs, NJ: Prentice-Hall, 1982.

85. Kottke, T.E., P. Puska, J.T. Salonen, et al. Projected effects of high risk versus population-based prevention strategies in coronary heart disease. *Amer. J. Epidemiol.* 121:697–704, 1985.

86. LaPorte, R.E., H.J. Montoye, and C.J. Caspersen. Assessment of physical activity in epidemiologic research: problems and prospects. *Public Health Rep.* 100(2):131–146, 1985.

87. Lasater, T.M., R.A. Carleton, and R.C. Lefebvre. The Pawtucket Heart Health Program: V. Utilizing community resources for primary prevention. *Rhode Island Med. J.* 71:63–67, 1988.

88. Lasater, T.M., B.L. Wells, R.A. Carleton, et al. The role of churches in disease prevention research studies. *Public Health Rep.* 101:125–131, 1986.

89. Lasco, R.A., R.H. Curry, V.J. Dickson, J. Powers, S. Menes, and R.K. Merritt. Participation rates, weight loss, and blood pressure changes among obese women in a nutrition-exercise program. *Public Health Rep.* 104:640–646, 1989.

90. Lee, C., and N. Owen. Community exercise programs: Follow-up difficulty and outcome. *J. Behav. Med.* 9:111–117, 1986.

91. Lee, C., and N. Owen. Exercise persistence: Contributions of psychology to the promotion of regular physical activity. *Aust. Psychologist* 21:427–466, 1986.

92. Lee, C., and N. Owen. Uses of psychological theories in understanding the adoption and maintenance of exercising. *Aust. J. Sci. Med. in Sport* 18:22–25, 1986.

93. Lefebvre, R.C., T.M. Lasater, R.A. Carleton, et al. Theory and delivery of health programming in the community: the Pawtucket Heart Health Program. *Prev. Med.* 16:80–95, 1987.

94. Leon, A.S., J. Connett, D.R. Jacobs Jr, et al. Leisure-time physical activity levels and risk of coronary heart disease and death: the Multiple Risk Factor Intervention Trial. *J.A.M.A.* 258:2388–2394, 1987.

95. Leonard, B., C. Leonard, and R. Wilson. Zuni diabetes project. *Public Health Rep.* 101:282–288, 1986.

96. Martin, J.E., P.M. Dubbert, A.D. Katell, et al. The behavioral control of exercise in sedentary adults: studies 1 through 6. *J. Consult. Clin. Psychology* 52:795–811, 1984.

97. Martin, J.E., and P.M. Dubbert. Exercise applications and promotion in behavioral medicine: Current status and future directions. *J. Consult. Clin. Psychology* 50:1004–1017, 1982.

98. Matarazzo, J.D. Behavioral health's challenge to academic, scientific, and professional psychology. *Am. Psychologist* 37:1–14, 1982.

99. Mayer, J., and E.S. Geller. Motivating energy efficient travel: A community-based intervention for encouraging biking. *J. Environ. Systems* 12:99–112, 1982–83.

100. Miller, N. Using places of worship for health promotion programs. In A.C. King, W.L. Haskell, N. Miller, et al. (eds.). *Promotion of physical activity in the community: A manual for community health professionals.* Stanford University School of Medicine: Stanford Center for Research in Disease Prevention and The Henry J. Kaiser Family Foundation, 1988, p. 67.

101. Montoye, H.J. Estimation of habitual physical activity by questionnaire and interview. *Am. J. Clin. Nutr.* 24:1113–1118, 1971.

102. Morgan, P.P., and S.E. Goldston. *Exercise and mental health.* Washington, D.C.: Hemisphere Publishing Corporation, 1987.

103. Morris, J.N., M.G. Everitt, R. Pollard, et al. Vigorous exercise in leisure-time: protection against coronary heart disease. *Lancet* 8206:1207–1210, 1980.

104. Nader, P.R., J.F. Sallis, T.L. Patterson, et al. A family approach to cardiovascular risk reduction: results from the San Diego Family Health Project. *Health Educ. Q.* 16:229–244, 1989.

105. Nader, P.R., J.R. Sallis, J. Rupp, et al. San Diego family health project: Reaching families through the schools. *J. School Health* 56:227–231, 1986.

106. Naditch, P. The Staywell Program. J.D. Matarazzo, S.M. Weiss, J.A. Herd, et al. (eds.). *Behavioral health: A handbook of health enhancement and disease prevention.* New York: Wiley, 1984, pp. 1071–1078.

107. National Center for Health Statistics. *Assessing physical fitness and physical activity in population-based surveys.* Thomas F. Drury, ed. Washington, DC: U.S. Government Printing Office, 1989, DHHS Pub. No. (PHS) 89-1253.

108. Nutbeam, D., and J. Catford. The Dorset Get-fit Campaign—community fitness testing programme. *Br. J. Sports Med.* 19:5–7, 1985.

109. Oldridge, N.B. Compliance and exercise in primary and secondary prevention of coronary heart disease: a review. *Prev. Med.* 11:56–70, 1982.

110. Oldridge, N.B., and N.L. Jones. Improving patient compliance in cardiac rehabilitation: effects of written agreement and self-monitoring. *J. Cardiac Rehab.* 3:257–262, 1983.

111. Owen, N., and T. Dwyer. Approaches to promoting more widespread participation in physical activity. *Community Health Stud.* 12:339–347, 1988.

112. Owen, N., C. Lee, L. Naccarella, et al. Exercise by mail: a mediated behavior-change program for aerobic exercise. *J. Sport Psychology* 9:346–357, 1987.

113. Owen, N., C. Lee, and A.W. Sedgwick. Exercise maintenance: integrating self-management guidelines into community fitness programs. *Aust. J. Sci. Med. in Sports* 19:8–12, 1987.

114. Paffenbarger, Jr, R.S., R.T. Hyde, A.L. Wing, et al. A natural history of athleticism and cardiovascular health. *J.A.M.A.* 252:491–495, 1984.

115. Paffenbarger, Jr, R.S., R.T. Hyde, A.L. Wing, et al. Physical activity, all-cause mortality, and longevity of college alumni. *New Engl. J. Med.* 314:605–613, 1986.

116. Paffenbarger Jr, R.S., A.L. Wing, R.T. Hyde, et al. Physical activity and incidence of hypertension in college alumni. *Am. J. Epidemiol.* 117:245–257, 1983.

117. Parcel, G.S., B.G. Simons-Morton, N.M. O'Hara, et al. School promotion of healthful diet and exercise behavior: an integration of organizational change and social learning theory interventions. *J. School Health* 57:150–156, 1987.

118. Parcel, G.S., B. Simons-Morton, N.M. O'Hara, et al. School promotion of healthful diet and physical activity: impact on learning outcomes and self-reported behavior. *Health Educ. Q.* 16:181–199, 1989.

119. Patterson, T., J. Sallis, P. Nader, et al. Direct observation of physical activity and dietary behaviors in a structured environment: effects of a family-based health promotion program. *J. Behav. Med.* 11:447–458, 1988.

120. The Perrier Study. *Fitness in America.* New York: Perrier-Great Waters of France, Inc., 1979.

121. Perry, C.L., G. Griffin, and D.M. Murray. Assessing needs for youth health promotion. *Prev. Med.* 14:379–393, 1985.

122. Perry, C.L., R.V. Luepker, D.M. Murray, et al. Parent involvement with children's health promotion: a one-year follow-up of the Minnesota Home Team. *Health Educ. Q.* 16:171–180, 1989.

123. Petchers, M.K., E.Z. Hirsch, and B.A. Bloch. A longitudinal study of the impact of a school heart health curriculum. *J. Community Health* 13:88–93, 1988.

124. Powell, K.E., P.D. Thompson, C.J. Caspersen, et al. Physical activity and the incidence of coronary heart disease. *Annu. Rev. Public Health* 8:253–287, 1987.

125. Puska, P. Possibilities of a preventive approach to coronary heart disease starting in childhood. *Acta Paediatr. Scand. Suppl.* 318:229–233, 1985.

126. Puska, P., A. Nissinen, J.T. Salonen, et al. Ten years of the North Karelia Project: results with community-based prevention of coronary heart disease. *Scand. J. Soc. Med.* 11:65–68, 1983.

127. Puska, P., J. Tuomilehto, J.T. Salonen, et al. *Community control of cardiovascular diseases: The North Karelia Project.* Copenhagen: World Health Organization, 1981.

128. Rogers, E.M. *Diffusion of innovation (3rd edition).* New York: Free Press, 1983.

129. Russouw, J.E., P.L. Jooste, J.P. Kotze, et al. The control of hypertension in two communities: An interim evaluation. *South African Med. J.* 60:208, 1981.

130. Sallis, J.F., W.L. Haskell, S.P. Fortmann, et al. Predictors of adoption and maintenance of physical activity in a community sample. *Prev. Med.* 15:331–341, 1986.

131. Sallis, J.F., T.L. Patterson, T.L. McKenzie, and P.R. Nader. Family variables and physical activity in preschool children. *J. Dev. Behav. Pediatr.* 9:57–61, 1988.

132. Sallis, J.F., M.F. Hovell, C.R. Hofstetter, et al. Does access to exercise facilities facilitate exercise? A geographical analysis. *Public Health Rep.* 105:179–185, 1990.

133. Shephard, R.J. The current status of the Canadian home fitness test. *Br. J. Sports Med.* 14:114–125, 1980.

134. Shephard, R.J. *Economic benefits of enhanced fitness.* Champaign, IL: Human Kinetics Publishers, 1986.

135. Shephard, R.J. *Fitness and health in industry.* Basel: Karger, 1986.

136. Siconolfi, S.F., E.M. Cullinane, R.A. Carleton, et al. Assessing VO2max in epidemiologic studies: modification of the Astrand-Ryhming test. *Med. Sci. in Sports and Exer.* 14:335–338, 1982.

137. Siconolfi, S.F., C.E. Garber, T.M. Lasater, et al. A simple valid step test for estimating

maximal oxygen uptake in epidemiologic studies. *Am. J. Epidemiol.* 121:382–390, 1985.

138. Simons-Morton, B.G., N.M. O'Hara, and D.G. Simons-Morton. Promoting healthful diet and exercise behaviors in communities, schools, and families. *Family and Community Health* 9:1–13, 1986.

139. Simons-Morton, B.G., G.S. Parcel, and N.M. O'Hara. Implementing organizational changes to promote healthful diet and physical activity at school. *Health Educ. Q.* 15:115–130, 1988.

140. Smith, E.L., K.A. Smith, and C. Gilligan. Exercise, fitness, osteoarthritis, and osteoporosis. C. Bouchard, R.J. Shephard, T. Stephens, et al. (eds.). *Exercise, fitness, and health: A consensus of current knowledge.* Champaign, IL: Human Kinetics Books, 1990, pp. 517–528.

141. Sobolski, J., M. Kornitzer, G. DeBacker, et al. Protection against ischemic heart disease in the Belgian Physical Fitness Study: physical fitness rather than physical activity? *Am. J. Epidemiol.* 125:601–610, 1987.

142. Stalonas, P.M., W.G. Johnson, and M. Christ. Behavior modification for obesity: the evaluation of exercise, contingency management, and program adherence. *J. Consult. Clin. Psychol.* 46:463–469, 1978.

143. Stephens, T., D.R. Jacobs Jr, and C.C. White. A descriptive epidemiology of leisure-time physical activity. *Public Health Rep.* 100:147–158, 1985.

144. Stern, J.S., and P. Lowney. Obesity: the role of physical activity. K.D. Brownell and J.P. Foreyt (eds.). *Handbook of Eating Disorders: Physiology, Psychology, and Treatment of Obesity, Anorexia, and Bulimia.* New York: Basic Books, 1986, pp. 145–158.

145. Stone, E.J. (ed.). School health research. *The National Conference on School Health Education Research in the Heart, Lung, and Blood Areas;* Sept. 15–16, 1983; Bethesda, Maryland. Washington, D.C.: USDHHS, 1983.

146. Stone, E.J., C.L. Perry, and R.V. Luepker. Synthesis of cardiovascular behavioral research for youth health promotion. *Health Educ. Q.* 16:155–169, 1989.

147. Stunkard, A.J., M.R.J. Felix, and R.Y. Cohen. Mobilizing a community to promote health: the Pennsylvania County Health Improvement Program (CHIP). J.C. Rosen and L.F. Solomon (eds.). *Prevention in Health Psychology.* Hanover, NH: University Press of New England, 1985, pp. 143–190.

148. Taylor, C.B., J.F. Sallis, and R. Needle. The relation of physical activity and exercise to mental health. *Public Health Rep.* 100:195–202, 1985.

149. Taylor, H.L., D.R. Jacobs Jr, B. Schucker, et al. A questionnaire for the assessment of leisure time physical activities. *J. Chronic Dis.* 31:741–755, 1978.

150. U.S. Department of Health and Human Services. Surgeon General's workshop on health promotion and aging: summary recommendations of the physical fitness and exercise working group. *M.M.W.R. (Centers for Disease Control).* 38(October 20):700–707, 1989.

151. USDHHS, CDC. *Program evaluation handbook: Physical fitness promotion.* Los Angeles: IOX Assessment Associations, 1988.

152. USDHHS, PHS. *Prevention Report.* Washington, D.C.: U.S. Government Printing Office, Dec. 1989.

153. USDHHS, PHS. *Promoting health/preventing disease: Year 2000 objectives for the nation.* Washington, D.C.: U.S. Government Printing Office, Sept. 1989.

154. USDHHS, PHS, Centers for Disease Control. *Promoting physical activity among adults: A CDC community intervention handbook.* Atlanta: Centers for Disease Control; 1988.

155. USDHHS, PHS. Summary of findings from the national children and youth fitness study. *JOPERD.* January: 44–90, 1985.

156. Vranic, M., and D. Wasserman. Exercise, fitness, and diabetes. C. Bouchard, R.J. Shephard, T. Stephens, et al. (eds.). *Exercise, fitness, and health: A consensus of current knowledge.* Champaign, IL: Human Kinetics Books, 1990, pp. 467–490.

157. Walter, H.J. Primary prevention of chronic disease among children: the school-based 'Know Your Body' intervention trials. *Health Educ. Q.* 16:201–214, 1989.

158. Walter, H.J., and A. Hofman. Socioeconomic status, ethnic origin, and risk factors for coronary heart disease in children. *Am. Heart J.* 113:812–818, 1987.

159. Wankel, L.M. Decision-making and social support strategies for increasing exercise involvement. *J. Cardiac Rehab.* 4:124–135, 1984.

160. Warner, K.E. Selling health promotion to corporate America: uses and abuses of the economic argument. *Health Educ. Q.* 14:39–55, 1987.

161. Wilbur, C.S. The Johnson & Johnson program. *Prev. Med.* 12:672–681, 1983.

162. Wilson, G.T., and C.M. Franks (eds.). *Contemporary behavior therapy: Conceptual and empirical foundations.* New York: Guilford Press, 1982.

163. Wilson, P.W.F., R.S. Paffenbarger Jr, J.N. Morris, et al. Assessment methods for physical activity and physical fitness in population studies: Report of a NHLBI workshop. *Am. Heart J.* 111:1177–1192, 1986.

164. Winett, R.A., A.C. King, and D.G. Altman. *Health psychology and public health: An integrative approach.* New York: Pergamon Press, 1989.

7
The Annual Survey of Catastrophic Football Injuries: 1977–1988

FREDERICK O. MUELLER, Ph.D.
ROBERT C. CANTU, M.D.

INTRODUCTION

In 1977 the National Collegiate Athletic Association funded the first Annual Survey of Catastrophic Football Injuries. Frederick O. Mueller, Ph.D., and Carl S. Blyth, Ph.D., both professors in the Department of Physical Education at the University of North Carolina at Chapel Hill, were selected to conduct the research. The Annual Survey is part of a concerted effort by many persons and research organizations to reduce the steady increase in football head and neck injuries that had been occurring since the late 1950s. The primary goal of these annual studies has been to make the game of football safer.

In the first investigation of serious head and neck football injuries, Schneider [3] reported that 30 high school and college football players had suffered permanent cervical spinal cord injuries during the five seasons from 1959 through 1963. Torg [4] later reported that a total of 99 high school and college players were similarly disabled in the 5 years from 1971 through 1975. In continued research, Torg [4] reported an all-time high of 34 high school and college permanent cervical cord injuries in 1976. According to one study [1], the incidence of neck injuries based on roentgenographic evidence was as high as 32% in a sample of 104 high school and 75 college freshman football players in Iowa [1].

In response to the rising incidence of serious head and neck injuries, the National Collegiate Athletic Association and the National Federation of State High School Associations implemented rule changes in 1976 to prohibit players from using the head as the initial contact point when blocking and tackling. The American Football Coaches Association Ethics Committee also went on record as opposing blocking and tackling with the head. Other efforts to minimize head and neck injuries included emphasis on complete physical examinations and improved physical conditioning programs. As a result, by 1984 the total number of permanent cervical spinal cord injuries among high school and college players had fallen to five [2].

DATA COLLECTION

Since 1977 when this research first began, catastrophic football injuries were defined as those that resulted in permanent brain or spinal cord disability. In 1984 the report was enlarged to include all catastrophic injuries that resulted in permanent disability. Although all catastrophic injuries involve some type of disability, some have resulted in full recovery following a period of rehabilitation. Injuries that have resulted in death are not included in this report.

Data are compiled with the assistance of high school and college coaches, athletic directors, school administrators, physicians, athletic trainers, executive officers of state and national athletic organizations, sporting goods dealers and manufacturers' representatives, a national newspaper clipping service, and professional associates of the researchers. Data collection would have been impossible without the help of the National Federation of State High School Associations. The research is funded by a grant from the National Collegiate Athletic Association.

On receiving information concerning a possible catastrophic football injury, researchers contact by telephone, personal letter, and questionnaire the injured player's coach, physician, and athletic director. The questionnaire provides background information on the athlete (age, height, weight, athletic experience, previous injury, etc.), as well as the circumstances surrounding the accident and injuries caused, immediate and postaccident treatment, and equipment data. A telephone follow-up was added to the study protocol in 1978 to provide information on the status and prognosis of the injured player.

In 1987, a joint endeavor was initiated with the Section on Sports Medicine of the American Association of Neurological Surgeons. The purpose of this collaboration was to enhance the collection of medical data. Dr. Robert C. Cantu, Chairman of Surgery and Chief of Neurosurgery Service at Emerson Hospital in Concord, Massachusetts, has been responsible for contacting the neurosurgeon involved in each case. Through telephone communication and questionnaire, medical data are collected for all catastrophic football injuries.

DISCUSSION

During the years 1977 through 1988, a total of 116 football players received permanent cervical cord injuries (Table 7.1). An overwhelming majority of these injuries occurred among high school players (96), with 15 of the remaining 20 injuries occurring among college players. According to these data, the number of permanent cervical cord injuries declined when compared to Torg's report [4] of injuries from 1971 through 1975.

Approximately 1.3 million players participate in junior and senior

TABLE 7.1
Permanent Cervical Cord Injuries 1977–1988*

Year	Sandlot	Pro and Semi-pro	High School	College	Total
1977	0	0	10	2	12
1978	0	1	12	0	13
1979	0	0	8	3	11
1980	0	0	11	2	13
1981	1	0	6	2	9
1982	1	1	7	2	11
1983	0	0	11	1	12
1984	1	0	5	0	6
1985	0	0	6	2	8
1986	0	0	3	0	3
1987	0	0	8	0	8
1988	0	0	9	1	10
Total	3	2	96	15	116

* Figures are updated annually due to new cases investigated after publication.

high school football and 75,000 in college football today. Table 7.2 illustrates the incidence of permanent cervical cord injuries among these players from 1977 through 1988. The rates per 100,000 players are low for both groups, averaging over the 12 years 0.62 per 100,000 high school players and 1.66 per 100,000 college players. Most injuries continue to occur during regular games rather than practice. Seven of the 10 catastrophic injuries in 1988 took place during regular games.

Table 7.3 shows that when comparing permanent cervical cord injuries to offensive and defensive players, offensive football is safer than defensive football. From 1977 through 1988 nearly 71% (82) of

TABLE 7.2
Incidence per 100,000 Participants
1977–1988*

Year	High School	College
1977	0.77	2.67
1978	0.92	0.00
1979	0.62	4.00
1980	0.84	2.67
1981	0.46	2.67
1982	0.54	2.67
1983	0.84	1.33
1984	0.38	0.00
1985	0.46	2.67
1986	0.23	0.00
1987	0.62	0.00
1988	0.69	1.33

* Based on 1,300,000 high school (including junior high) players and 75,000 college players.

TABLE 7.3
Offensive vs. Defenseive Football 1977–1988*

Year	Offense	Defense	Unknown	Total
1977	0	7	5	12
1978	2	10	1	13
1979	1	5	5	11
1980	3	8	2	13
1981	3	5	1	9
1982	3	8	0	11
1983	2	10	0	12
1984	1	4	1	6
1985	1	7	0	8
1986	0	3	0	3
1987	2	6	0	8
1988	1	9	0	10
Total	19	82	15	116

* Figures updated with availability of new information.

the 116 players with permanent cervical cord injuries were playing defense. In 1988, this was the case among 90% of the players.

Most catastrophic injuries also occur during defensive tackles. Since 1977, two-thirds of all such injuries have resulted from tackles (Table 7.4); 80% of the injured players in 1988 were tackling. Although coaches are teaching players to tackle with their heads up, many players persist in lowering their heads before making contact.

Statistics further reveal that defensive backs are injured at a higher rate than players in other positions (Table 7.5). In 1988, of the 10 injured players, three were defensive backs, two were tackling on a kick-off, three were linebackers, one was diving for a fumble on a punt return, and one was unknown.

TABLE 7.4
Catastrophic Injuries 1977–1988: Type of Activity

Activity	Number	Percent
Tackling	46	39.6
Tackling Head Down	27	23.2
Tackling on Punt	2	1.7
Tackling on Kick-Off	6	5.1
Tackled	8	6.9
Tackled on Kick-Off	1	0.9
Collision	3	2.6
Blocking on Kick	3	2.6
Blocking	1	0.9
Contact After Interception	2	1.7
Blocked	1	0.9
Hitting Tacklematic Machine	1	0.9
Unknown	15	13.0
Total	116	100.0

TABLE 7.5
Catastrophic Injuries 1977–1988: Position Played

Position	Number	Percent
Defensive Back	38	32.8
Kick-Off Team	14	12.1
Defensive Line	7	6.0
Linebacker	10	8.6
Kick-Off Return	5	4.3
Defensive End	5	4.3
Offensive Back	5	4.3
Quarterback	3	2.6
Flanker	2	1.7
Wide Receiver	2	1.7
Punt Coverage	1	0.9
Punt Return	1	0.9
Drill	1	0.9
Unknown	22	18.9
Total	116	100.0

In tracking the number of cerebral injuries or subdural hematomas to players from 1984 through 1988 (Table 7.6), three of the 18 injuries resulted in permanent disability, all to high school players. A number of catastrophic injuries do not, in fact, result in permanent disability because the players either fully recover or are in the process of full recovery. Each year approximately 20 to 25 additional injuries to the head or cervical spine occur from which the players fully recover. In 1988, eight high school and college players with fractures to the cervical spine recovered, as did five players with spinal stenosis injuries with transient cord symptoms, and another five players with subdural hematomas (Table 7.7). One other player had to have his leg amputated below the patella from a serious knee injury during practice.

RECOMMENDATIONS

As stated earlier, the number of permanent cervical cord injuries has declined when compared to earlier data [4]. The 1988 data continue to

TABLE 7.6
Cerebral Injuries 1984–1988: Permanent Disability

Year	Sandlot	Pro and Semi-pro	High School	College	Total
1984	0	0	5	2	7
1985	0	0	3	1	4
1986	0	0	2	0	2
1987	0	0	2	0	2
1988	0	0	3	0	3
Total	0	0	15	3	18

TABLE 7.7
Catastrophic Injuries 1988 (No Disability)

Injury	High School	College	Total
Subdural Hematoma	3	2	5
Spinal Stenosis Transient Cord Symptoms	3	2	5
Cervical Spine Fracture	5	3	8
Total	11	7	18

show a major reduction in cervical cord injuries when compared to data collected from the early seventies. An average of 9.6 permanent cervical cord injuries occurred yearly from 1977 through 1988. This reduction is the result of efforts from the entire athletic community working to ensure the safety of its players. Greatest credit is owed to the 1976 rule changes which eliminated the head as the initial point of contact during blocking and tackling, improved medical care both at the game site and in medical facilities, and improved coaching techniques in teaching the fundamentals of tackling and blocking.

In an effort to further reduce the number of head and cervical cord injuries, we offer several suggestions.

1. Vigilant enforcement of the rule changes initiated for the 1976 football season which eliminated the head as a primary and initial contact area for blocking and tackling is of utmost importance. Coaches should drill the players in the proper execution of the fundamentals of football, particularly blocking and tackling. *Players should block and tackle with their shoulder. Keep the head out of football.*

2. Coaches and officials should discourage players from using their heads as battering rams when blocking and tackling. The rules that prohibit spearing should be enforced in practice and in games. Players should be taught to respect the helmet as a protective device; it should not be used as a weapon.

3. Athletes must be given proper conditioning exercises that will strengthen their necks to enable them to hold their heads firmly erect while making contact during a tackle or block.

4. All coaches, physicians, and trainers should take special care to ensure that the players' equipment is properly fitted, particularly the helmet.

5. It is important, whenever possible, for a physician to be on the field of play during a game and practice. When this is not possible, arrangements must be made in advance to obtain a physician's immediate services when emergencies arise. Each institution should have a team trainer who is a regular member of the institution's staff and who is qualified in the emergency care of both treating and preventing injuries.

6. Coaches must be prepared for a possible catastrophic head or neck injury. Everyone involved must know what to do. Their being prepared and knowing what to do may be the difference that prevents permanent disability.

7. When a player has experienced or shows signs of a head injury (loss of consciousness, visual disturbances, headache, inability to walk correctly, obvious disorientation, memory loss), he should receive immediate medical attention and should not be allowed to return to practice or a game without permission from the proper medical authorities.

8. Both past and present data show that the football helmet does not cause cervical cord injuries but that poorly executed tackling and blocking technique is the major problem.

Football catastrophic injuries may never completely be eliminated, but studies, by revealing problems and the adequacy of preventive measures, have resulted in rule changes, equipment standards, improved medical care both on and off the playing field, and changes in teaching the fundamental techniques of the game. These changes have been a united effort by coaches, administrators, researchers, equipment manufacturers, physicians, trainers, and players. Continued research based on reliable data and a redoubling of efforts by the entire football community are essential if progress is to proceed.

CERVICAL CORD CATASTROPHIC INJURY CASE REPORTS

High School
A 16-year-old football player fractured cervical vertebrae while diving for a fumble and striking his head with another player as he hit the ground. The accident happened on a punt return. The player is now a quadriplegic.

A player fractured a cervical vertebra while making a tackle after an interception. He is quadriparetic.

A 17-year-old player fractured two cervical vertebrae while making a tackle on a kick-off; he is quadriplegic.

An 18-year-old middle linebacker who tackled with his head down fractured two cervical vertebrae while making a tackle in a game at an All Star summer camp. The player is quadriplegic.

A 17-year-old football player fractured a cervical vertebra while tackling the ball carrier on a kick-off and is now quadriplegic.

A 16-year-old player was injured in a game after making a tackle; he is quadriplegic.

A 15-year-old player suffered a subluxation injury to cervical vertebrae 5 and 6 while making a tackle in a scrimmage. He was fighting off a blocker when the ball carrier ran over him. The player is quadriplegic.

A 17-year-old player fractured his fourth cervical vertebra while making a tackle and at the same time being hit by another defensive player. He is quadriplegic.

A 17-year-old middle linebacker dislocated a cervical vertebra and thoracic vertebrae in a pile-up during an off-tackle play; he is quadriplegic.

College

A community college football player was injured in a game while making a tackle with his head down. Contact was with the top of the head. The player is quadriparetic.

CEREBRAL CATASTROPHIC INJURY CASE REPORTS

High School

A 16-year-old player received a severe head injury during a game and was in a coma for 7 weeks. Now home after 6 months in the hospital, he suffers memory loss, has no left peripheral vision, and has left lower extremity weakness.

A 17-year-old player collapsed on the practice field while participating in tackling drills. He remains in a coma.

An 18-year-old foreign exchange student collapsed during a scrimmage after being tackled. He is presently in a comatose critical condition.

REFERENCES

1. Albright, J.P., J.M. Moses, H.G. Feldick, et al. Nonfatal cervical spine injuries in interscholastic football. *J.A.M.A.* 236:1243–1245, 1976.
2. Mueller, F.O., and R.D. Schindler. Annual Survey of Football Injury Research 1931–1987. Overland Park, Kansas. National Collegiate Athletic Association and American Football Coaches Association, 1987.
3. Schneider, R.C. Head and Neck Injuries in Football. Baltimore: Williams and Wilkins, 1973.
4. Torg, J.S., R. Trues, T.C. Quedenfeld, et al. The national football head and neck injury registry. *J.A.M.A.* 241:1477–1479, 1979.

8
The Plasticity of Skeletal Muscle: Effects of Neuromuscular Activity

ROLAND R. ROY, Ph.D.
KENNETH M. BALDWIN, Ph.D.
V. REGGIE EDGERTON, Ph.D.

INTRODUCTION

A prevailing hypothesis in the neuromuscular literature is that the patterns of impulses that reach a muscle dictate the quantity and quality of contractile (myosin and troponin isoforms) and metabolic (oxidative and glycolytic enzymes) proteins that it expresses [55, 104, 114, 138, 163]. These biochemical properties, in turn, determine the force, velocity, and fatigue characteristics of the muscle. This contention is based primarily on those studies that report that a typical "fast" muscle stimulated chronically (up to 24 hours per day) at a relatively low frequency of activation (e.g., 5–10 Hz) acquires physiological, biochemical, and morphological properties that resemble those found in a typical "slow" muscle [114, 138]. Other factors may be equally important, however. For example, Buller et al. [19, p. 438] in their original cross-reinnervation experiments concluded "that the neural influence on muscle speed is not exerted by nerve impulses as such." Rather, these authors postulated that the crossing effect could have been due to some neurotrophic phenomenon. The presence of other influences have been substantiated [47, 108]. For example, humoral factors (thyroid hormone, testosterone) have been shown to have a dramatic effect on the mechanical and biochemical properties of skeletal muscles [65, 66, 99, 182, 183].

For the past decade or so, our working hypothesis has been that many of the properties of a skeletal muscle are strongly modulated by alterations in the generation of muscle force, both active and passive, that result from the activation level and stimulation pattern and not directly from the associated electrical events. In this chapter, we present the results of a series of experiments performed primarily in rats and cats on a variety of models of decreased or increased "mechanical use" (designated as "use" in this review). In particular, the models we discuss deal with the impact of the weight-bearing forces that are manifest during the course of the animal's normal activity. The chapter is not intended to be a comprehensive review of the literature, but a summary of our own data with the additional incorporation of the most relevant data from the literature. Our approach is first to provide a substantial description of each experimental model as an intervention on the neuromuscular activity patterns of the muscles of interest. Second, we describe the effects of each experimental model on the (1) muscle mass and myosin type, as well as (2) the metabolic and (3) physiological properties of the muscles. Third, we present the effects of interventions designed to ameliorate or prevent those adaptations that accompany chronic decreased use or interventions that modify the effects of increased use. Finally, we offer a general summary of our view of the functional implications of the findings from these studies.

OVERALL DESIGN OF THE EXPERIMENTS

Results from five experimental models that involve an alteration in the amount and/or pattern of neuromuscular activity are discussed in this review. In all five models, the basic element of neuromuscular control, i.e., the motor unit defined as a motoneuron and all the muscle fibers it innervates, is maintained intact. We selected the five models to investigate the separate and combined effects of a reduction or elevation in the electrical and mechanical (weight-bearing) activity on the morphological, biochemical, and physiological properties of the affected muscles. The range in the alteration of the chronic neuromuscular activity level includes virtually no electrical or mechanical activity (spinal isolation); a reduction in both electrical and mechanical activity (spinal transection); a reduction in the mechanical and no change in the electrical activity (hindlimb suspension and, most likely, spaceflight); and an elevation in both mechanical and electrical activity (functional overload). The results from these studies are used to highlight the critical role of mechanical (weight-bearing) activity in maintaining skeletal muscle properties.

In some experiments, neuromuscular activity, defined herein as the amount and pattern of muscle activation and/or force in vivo, was quantified using (a) electromyography (EMG) to measure activation and (b) tendon strain transducers to measure force. Bipolar EMG electrodes were implanted intramuscularly in specific regions of the muscle and used for chronic recordings of in vivo activation [1, 2, 35, 96, 97, 139, 152, 161]. Tendon force transducers ("buckles") were implanted on the distal tendons of individual muscles to measure in vivo forces [79, 167, 190]. In large part because of constraints on the transducer elements used, the force measurements have been performed only in cats at this time. The combination of recordings of individual muscle forces and activation during a variety of motor tasks (e.g., posture, normal daily cage activity, treadmill locomotion at various speeds and inclines, swimming in the rat, paw shaking in the cat) have provided the basis for assessing the level of "use" in each experimental model used.

The duration of the experiments to be discussed range from several days to several months, thus providing an assessment and comparison of the time course of adaptations in the morphological, physiological, and biochemical properties across the various models. Terminal experiments included the assessment of whole muscle, motor unit and/or single-fiber properties of selected hindlimb muscles, i.e., usually a combination of the soleus (Sol), medial gastrocnemius (MG), lateral gastrocnemius (LG), tibialis anterior (TA) and plantaris (Plt), although other muscles were included in some analyses, e.g., extensor digitorum longus (EDL), flexor hallicus longus (FHL), vastus intermedius (VI), vastus lateralis (VL), quadratus femoris (QF), and adductor longus (AL). The rationale for selecting these muscles was to allow the comparison of the relative adaptability among predominantly slow (Sol) and fast (MG, LG, and Plt) extensor and fast flexor (TA) muscles.

The evaluation of the mechanical properties of a muscle included some combination of the following parameters: muscle mass (wet weight); physiological cross-sectional area (PCSA) calculated as follows: (muscle mass) (cosine of the angle of fiber pinnation)/(mean fiber length) (muscle density) [30, 144, 154, 156, 159, 162]; isometric properties to include contraction time (CT), half-relaxation time (HRT), maximum twitch tension (Pt), frequency-tension response to stimulation rates ranging from 1 to 200 Hz, and maximum tetanic tension (Po); specific tension (Po/PCSA); isotonic determination of the maximum rate of shortening (Vmax) using a series of afterloaded contractions and Hill's equation [89] to extrapolate Vmax [88, 139, 154, 159, 191]; and fatigue characteristics based on a fatigue index initially described by Burke et al. [21] for motor units. In some cases, the same properties, except for the Vmax, were determined in single-motor units isolated by means of ventral root teasing techniques [17]. In addition, repetitive stimulation was used to glycogen deplete and subsequently identify the fibers of individual motor units on tissue cross-sections using PAS (glycogen) staining (see below). This procedure makes it possible to study fiber adaptations within a motor unit, and thus determine if the effect of the perturbation of the motor unit activity level affects all fibers similarly. In these studies, motor units were classified according to the tetrapartite classification system of Burke [20], i.e., fast fatigable (FF), fast fatigue intermediate (FI), fast fatigue resistant (FR), and slow (S) based on their fatigue properties and presence or absence of "sag", i.e., a decrease in force production after an initial rise during the determination of the frequency-tension response. Finally, in some cases, the area and succinate dehydrogenase (SDH) activities of lumbar spinal motoneurons were determined as described by Chalmers and Edgerton [22].

Biochemical determinations included a thorough analysis of the myosin molecule to include some combination of the following: myosin adenosine triphosphatase (ATPase) activity, native myosin expression using pyrophosphate gel electrophoresis and light chain composition on denaturing gels [176, 177, 179–181]. In some models, homogenates of portions of whole muscles or muscle regions were used to determine activities of a series of oxidative (e.g., citrate synthase [CS]) and glycolytic (e.g., alpha glycerophosphate dehydrogenase [GPD]) marker enzymes [6–8, 11, 12, 14]. Quantitative histochemical techniques were used to determine the cross-sectional area (CSA) and the metabolic (SDH and GPD) and contractile (myosin ATPase) protein profiles of individual fibers from specific muscle regions or from single motor units [84, 85, 88, 74–76, 92, 100–102, 118–121, 141, 151]. The verification of the quantitative analyses for SDH and GPD activities in frozen tissue cross-sections are detailed in Martin et al. [121]. Fiber types were assessed as follows: (1) typed as fast glycolytic (FG), fast oxidative glycolytic (FOG) or slow oxidative (SO) using the qualitative histochemical procedures described by Peter et al. [137]; (2) typed as dark or light ATPase based on their staining reaction for myosin ATPase, alkaline preincubation [132]; and/or (3) classified as fast or slow based on the qualitative or quantitative staining reaction for myosine ATPase at an alkaline preincubation and/or immunohistochemical reaction to fast or slow myosin heavy chain (MHC) monoclonal antibodies [100, 102].

MODELS OF DECREASED "USE"

Spinal Transection

NEUROMUSCULAR ACTIVITY. The chronic effects of complete spinal cord transection at the junction of T12–T13 has been studied in cats transected either at two weeks of age or as adults. This is a model of decreased use of the hindlimb muscles due to the loss of supraspinal input to the lumbar region of the spinal cord. EMG recordings monitored over 24-hour periods showed a 75% decrease in the total integrated EMG and a 66% decrease in the total duration of muscle activity ("on time") in the Sol muscle 5 to 6 months after transection at two weeks of age compared to control [1]. In contrast, in the LG (and presumably the MG) the total amount of activity was unchanged, whereas the duration of activity was decreased by 66% (the same amount as in the Sol). These observations suggest that this predominantly fast muscle had shorter, high amplitude bursts of activity following transection. Although similar data were not collected from adult transected cats, it is reasonable to assume that the effects would be similar in both age groups.

Some of the spinalized cats from each age group were trained to locomote on a motorized treadmill for ≈30 minutes per day, 5 days per week. Briefly, the exercise was performed with the trunk of the cat supported in a harness and the forelimbs placed on a platform above the treadmill belt for support and balance. The hindlimbs then were positioned on the rotating belt and assisted (by positioning the tail) in stepping at speeds ranging from ≈0.1 to 1.0 meters per second. These procedures are described in detail elsewhere [1, 51–53, 115, 116]. In general, the exercise bout accounted for ≈10–40% of the total daily EMG activity of either the Sol or LG (and presumably the MG) [1]. Another group of adult spinal cats were trained to stand continuously, i.e., support the weight of the hindquarters in a standing position, for ≈30 minutes per day using a similar harness arrangement for the trunk [78, 136].

During the final two weeks of these 6-month experiments, force transducers were implanted on the distal tendons of the Sol and MG [79, 116, 167, 190]. Kinematic analyses in the first group of treadmill-trained spinal cats that were transected at two weeks of age indicated that the forces being produced in the Sol and MG during stepping were small, which suggests that the assistance given during the treadmill training was not allowing for full weight support of the hindquarters by these cats [de Guzman, Roy, Hodgson and Edgerton, unpublished observations]. Consequently, the muscles in the hindlimb were activated (based on the EMG) sufficiently to produce a rhythmical stepping pattern, but small muscle forces were being produced. Further, it has been assumed that the forces produced in the hindlimb muscles, in particular the ankle extensors, during cage activity were less than normal, because the hindlimbs were usually dragged with the ankle in an extended position, which tends to further unload the extensors.

In a similar experiment in cats transected as adults, production of full weight-bearing stepping was prioritized rather than the rate cycling of the hindlimbs during the daily treadmill training [155]. Sensory stimulation around the base of the tail was found to be effective in enhancing performance, especially during the early training sessions. As the trained spinal cats showed significant improvement in their locomotor capability during the 5-month training period, the necessity to use the hypersensitivity of the tail to enhance locomotion was eliminated. In this group of spinal cats, the forces recorded during locomotion in the last 2 weeks of the experiment were dramatically higher than those recorded from the 2-week spinal cats that had been given abundant support by the trainers (see above). In fact, in many of the cats the forces recorded from the Sol were similar in amplitude to those recorded from normal cats during locomotion [78, 79, 91, 116, 190]. Thus, the hindlimb muscles in this group of cats experienced increased active force production during the training sessions. Similar observations that were made in two cats that were transected at 2 weeks of age and trained using full weight-bearing also support the criterion for success [de Guzman, Roy, Hodgson and Edgerton, unpublished data].

NEUROMUSCULAR ADAPTATIONS. *Atrophy and myosin type adaptations.* Spinal transection results in a general atrophic response below the level of the lesion in a variety of muscles in humans [81], dogs [83, 131], cats [122, 128, 150, 158, 159, 188], guinea pigs [106], and rats [94, 125, 112, 113]. The degree of atrophy is muscle-specific, i.e., extensors atrophy more than flexors, and predominantly slow extensors are affected more than predominantly fast extensors [150, 188]. In addition, atrophy occurs whether the transection occurs at an early age of development [188] or as an adult [150]. For example, the Sol and MG atrophy by $\approx 45\%$ and 30%, respectively in cats transected at 2 weeks of age [188] and by $\approx 45\%$ and 15%, respectively in cats transected as adults [150]. In both of these experimental groups, the TA, an ankle flexor, was minimally affected. These flexor–extensor relationships are consistent for muscles functioning at the ankle, knee and/or hip joints [150, 188]. In general, the predominant fiber type in any given muscle is usually affected most by the decreased use regardless of the age of transection [150, 188, 112].

Almost all muscles studied show an increase in the percentage of fast fibers and a decrease in the percentage of slow fibers following spinal cord transection [12, 92, 100, 101, 112, 150, 188]. For example, in the Sol of control cats, almost all fibers react only with a slow MHC antibody, whereas as many as 50% of the fibers react with only a fast MHC, and a small percentage ($\approx 5\%$) of the fibers react with both a fast and a slow MHC antibody following transection in adult cats [100, 101]. The fast fibers tended to be found disproportionately at the boundaries of the fascicles, suggesting that myogenic spatial factors had influenced the ATPase conversion of these fibers [71]. The myosin ATPase activity of the Sol and MG increased by $\approx 52\%$ and 30%, respectively in the adult transected [10, 13] and by $\approx 53\%$ and 18%, respectively in the two-week transected cats [159]. Based on single fiber, quantitative, histochemical analyses, there is about a twofold difference between the ATPase activities of the light and dark ATPase fibers in either the Sol or the MG of control cats [100, 101]. This differenc was maintained following transection in adult cats, which indicates that the increase in the myosin ATPase activity in muscle homogenates reflects the increase in the percentage of fast fibers rather than an increase in the activities of individual fibers of either ATPase type. Native isomyosin electrophoretic profiles of the Sol muscle of the spinal transected compared to control cats show a down-regulation of the slowest migrating myosin isoform and an up-regulation of two "faster" migrating slow myosin isoforms [10, 13]. In the MG, there was a down-regulation of slow and intermediate myosin expression and a concomitant increase in the expression of the fast myosin isoforms. Together, these data demonstrate that in addition to becoming smaller the extensor muscles are becoming "faster" following transection. It does not appear, however, that the severity of the atrophy in a given fiber is related to the relative degree of up-regulation of fast and down-regulation of slow myosin. Other contractile proteins also are affected by spinal transection. For example, 8 months after transection there is a 16% increase in the fibers that react for the fast form of troponin I in the Sol [58].

Metabolic adaptations. Based on muscle homogenates from cats transected at 2 weeks of age, CS activity is significantly higher in the Sol and unchanged in the MG (13% decrease, $P > 0.05$) 6 months after transection [12]. When the spinal cord is transected in adult cats, CS activity is maintained at near-normal levels in the Sol but is decreased by $\approx 50\%$ in the MG [160]. Based on quantitative assays of single fibers that were classified according to myosin type in these same cats, SDH activity was similar to control in both the light and dark ATPase fibers of the Sol and MG [92]. Consistent with the enzyme activities in muscle homogenates in cats transected as adults, SDH activity in single fibers was maintained in the Sol [101], but significantly reduced in both light and dark ATPase fibers in the MG [100]. These data suggest muscle and type specificity in the adaptation of oxidative capacity in response to decreased "use". The data further suggest a significant degree of independence of changes in enzymes of the citric acid cycle in response to chronic changes in the level of EMG activity in a muscle.

The glycolytic capacity as indicated by GPD in muscle homogenates was significantly increased in both the Sol and MG 6 months after transection at 2 weeks of age [12] or as adults [160]. In these same muscles of the cats transected at 2 weeks of age, GPD activity in the light and dark ATPase fibers was three- and twofold higher, respectively in transected than control cats [92], which indicates that both fiber types were responsive to decreased use. In contrast, the GPD activity of the light ATPase fibers was 100% higher in the Sol and 50% higher in the MG of cats transected as adults, whereas the GPD activity of dark ATPase fibers was unchanged [100, 101]. These data suggest that the age of transection, as well as the fiber type as defined by myosin properties, can affect the magnitude of the metabolic adaptations at the single fiber level. Further, it is quite clear from these studies that the interrelationship between the glycolytic potential of a fiber and its myosin type that occurs normally in the muscle fiber is maintained after spinal transection.

Physiological adaptations. The adaptations in the physiological properties of the Sol and MG generally are consistent with the adaptations in the quality and quantity of the contractile and metabolic proteins. In the cat Sol, the CT, HRT, frequency tension, and Vmax change in the direction of a "faster" muscle. These changes occur whether the cord transection occurred at 2 weeks of age [159] or as an adult [10, 13, 158, 160]. The elevated Vmax is consistent with the increased myosin ATPase activity, the increased percentage of fast fibers, and the shift towards faster myosin isoforms [12, 159]. In the control cats, the Sol was essentially nonfatigable, and this fatigue resistance was maintained following transection [12, 158, 160]. These data are consistent with the observations that muscle CS activity and fiber SDH activities are either unchanged or elevated following spinal transection. In addition, the specific tension (Po/PCSA) of the Sol was maintained following transection at either age. Similar results have been reported in the rat Sol both 5 weeks [125] and 1 year [112, 113] after spinal transection.

In the cat MG, the twitch speed properties were unaffected, whereas the Vmax was increased following transection at an early age [159] or as adults [160]. This uncoupling adaptation in isometric twitch speed properties and Vmax has been observed in other models of muscle plasticity [65, 154], which emphasizes that Vmax is a reliable measure of contractile speed whereas CT is not. A much strong correlation exists between Vmax and myosin ATPase activity than between CT and myosin ATPase activity [103, 159]. The fatigue properties of the MG reflect the changes in the oxidative metabolic markers described above. The fatigability of the MG was unchanged in the 2-week transected cats [12], but was reduced in the adult transected cats [160]. Specific tension was lower than control in the MG following transection at 2 weeks of age [159], but not in adult transected cats [Roy, Pierotti, Hodgson, Flores and Edgerton, unpublished data]. These latter data suggest that there may be an age-related response to spinalization in the MG.

Adaptations to chronic spinal transection also has been studied at the motor unit and motoneuron level [31, 32, 45, 51, 53, 18, 118, 122, 128, 168]. The Sol of normal cats usually comprises exclusively type S motor units [21]. Three to four months after cord transection at ages ranging from 2 weeks to adult, many of the motor units isolated and tested had acquired characteristics that made them appear fast relative to normal type S units of the Sol [31, 45, 51, 53, 118]. For example, CT and HRT were shorter, the frequency-tension relationship had shifted such that fusion occurred at higher frequencies and sag was present in these units. Possible mechanisms for this "speeding up" of the isometric properties of these motor units may be related to an increase in the density of terminal cisternae indentations, which occurs in the Sol of rats spinally transected at a mid-thoracic level 6 weeks earlier [40], as well as the increase in percentage of fibers that express fast myosin [10, 12, 13]. Based on the maintenance of nonfatigability of the fast units [31, 45, 51, 53, 118], the division of the units into two distinct populations based on a number of electrophysiological properties and the slight increase in the SDH activity of the fibers in these fast units, it was concluded that the fast units in the Sol of transected cats were of the FR type [118]. This finding is interesting when one considers that the activity level of these muscles had been reduced by approximately two-thirds [1], and it suggests that the mitochondrial content of a fiber (at least in the Sol) was largely determined by factors intrinsic to the fiber and not by the level of neuromuscular activity. This interpretation is consistent with the finding that Sol motor units maintain their resistance to fatigue when reinnervated by fast motoneurons [25, 46].

Based on pooled data from cats transected as adults and maintained from 1 week to 7 months after transection, there is an increase in the percentage of FI (from 4% to 9%) and FF (from 48% to 61%) units and a concomitant decrease in FR (from 23% to 10%) and S (from 25% to 19%) units in the cat MG [128]. In cats transected as adults and maintained for 22 to 23 weeks, Mayer et al. (122) showed an increase in the percentage of FI units (from 6% to 19%), no change in FF units, and decreases in FR (from 23% to 17%) and S (from 25% to 17%) units in the cat MG. Together, these data are consistent with the 14% increase in whole muscle fatigability [12], the overall 13% increase in the percentage of fast fibers [12], and the significant decrease in mean fiber SDH activities [100] in the cat MG.

Sol motoneurons in spinal transected cats are less excitable based on passive electrical properties that normal [31], although there appears to be no alteration in resting membrane potential [32]. Some Sol motoneurons in spinal transected cats tended to have electrical characteristics resembling fast motoneurons, e.g., afterhyperpolarization duration was decreased and rheobase and voltage threshold increased four months after transection in adult cats [31]. MG motoneurons associated with each motor unit type in spinal transected cats were similar to control in rheobase, input resistance, afterhyperpolarization, and action potential amplitude [122, 128]. These data, in conjunction with the observation that a shift occurred in the percentage distribution of each unit type following transection (see above), strongly suggest that some units transformed to "faster" types, and that the affected units maintained a close relationship between some motoneuron and muscle properties. Cope et al. (31) observed that, in general, the changes in motoneuron electrophysiological properties were coordinated with changes in the physiological and biochemical properties of the muscle unit. For example, these researchers reported the matching of the SDH and GPD activities of muscle fibers of their glycogen-depleted units in adult transected cats. These properties also matched the changes in the CT and HRT, as well as the electrophysiological properties of the motoneurons, e.g, afterhyperpolarization duration.

Although the SDH activities of at least some of the fibers innervated by these motoneurons were significantly reduced [100], the size and SDH activities of the soma of motoneurons in the lumbar region of the spinal cord were unaffected following spinal transection in adult cats [23]. A dissociation between motoneuron and muscle fiber adaptations in size and SDH activity also has been observed following chronic electrical stimulation (39); i.e., chronic electrical stimulation results in a reduction in the size and an increase in the SDH activity of the muscle fibers in the peroneal muscles, but no change in either parameter in motoneurons located in the spinal cord region that contain the moto- neurons innervating the peroneal muscles. Based on both sets of data, it appears that, (1) motoneurons may be less activity-dependent than the fibers that they innervate, and (2) activity per se is not the sole determinant of the metabolic and size properties of these excitable cells.

EXERCISE COUNTERMEASURES. Some of the adaptations observed in the muscles following transection were effectively ameliorated by in- ducing full weight-bearing in spinalized cats while they were stepping on a treadmill. Although the data are more complete for the adult transected cats, the results from two cats transected at 2 weeks of age and trained with full weight-bearing stepping were similar. In spinal cats trained to step, the atrophic response of the muscles with a high proportion of slow fibers, i.e., the Sol VI, and QF, was reduced significantly [150]. In contrast, treadmill stepping had little effect on the mass of a large number of muscles with a high proportion of fast fibers, e.g., the MG, LG, Plt, and TA. The largest effect was in the Sol and VI, i.e., the extensors at the ankle and knee that would be expected to be more highly recruited during the treadmill exercise [48, 50, 86, 87, 91, 140, 152, 161]. The mass, Po, and specific tension of the Sol muscle in the trained cats were similar to control. As mentioned previously, the magnitude of the forces produced at the Sol tendon while stepping on the treadmill during the last 2 weeks of the experiment were near normal levels [116]. Unlike the spinal cats who were not exercised, the size and percentage of slow fibers in predominantly slow muscles such as the Sol, VI, and QF were near normal in the spinal trained cats. For example, the Sol of the spinal trained cats had, on the average, less than 10% fast fibers compared to ≈45% in the spinal nontrained cats. Also, the SDH activity in muscle homogenates was significantly higher in the treadmill trained spinal cats (both age groups) than either the nontrained spinal cats or the controls. This finding indicates that the Sol maintained the ability to increase its mitochondrial content in response to a minimal amount of training, even when the muscle was placed under conditions of chronic decreased use. Further evidence of the training effect was evident in the activities of myosin ATPase and GPD in Sol homogenates, in which the spinal trained cats had values closer to control values than in the nontrained spinal cats [160]. Similarly, the shifts towards a faster Vmax and frequency-tension response were ameliorated by the treadmill training, whereas the CT and HRT were relatively unaffected [158, 160], which demonstrates an uncoupling of the adaptations in the twitch and dynamic speed properties as noted earlier. Consistent with the observation that the MG of these cats produced minimal forces during the treadmill exercise [116], the mechanical and metabolic characteristics of the MG from the trained and nontrained spinal groups were similar [160].

A second group of spinal transected adult cats were trained to weight support (standing posture) for 30 minutes per day [78, 136]. Interestingly, this type of training resulted in a decline in the locomotor capability of these cats, i.e., three of the five cats trained with this protocol could not generate any stepping pattern 6 months after transection, and the other two cats could walk at only the slowest speeds achieved by the treadmill trained cats [52, 78, 136]. In fact, the performance of the weight-support cats during the testing of treadmill walking during the last 2 weeks of the experiment was less effective than that of the cats who had not been trained for the 6 months [192].

Daily weight-support activity had some beneficial effects on the Sol, although the effects were not as great as daily treadmill training [101, Roy, Pierotti, Hodgson, Flores and Edgerton, unpublished observations]. The mass and Po of the Sol of the weight-support trained cats were ≈20% and 15% higher, respectively than in the nontrained spinal cats. Unlike in the treadmill trained cats, however, these values were still significantly lower than control. Similarly, mean fiber size was ≈10% larger and there were ≈15% fewer fast fibers in the Sol of weight support trained compared to nontrained cats [101]. CT and HRT were not affected by the standing training, whereas the mean Vmax of the Sol was 10% lower, and the frequency tension curve was closer to the curve seen in normal cats in the weight-support trained spinal cats than in the nontrained spinal cats. Quantitative histochemical techniques revealed that the mean myosin ATPase activities of the dark fibers were about double those measured in the light ATPase fibers [101]. This relationship was maintained after transection, with or without standing training. It appears, therefore, that the alterations in the Vmax of the Sol reflect the changes in the percent fiber type distribution rather than changes in the ATPase activity of individual fibers. The fatigue resistance of the Sol in the trained cats was somewhat higher than the nontrained cats, with this muscle maintaining its relative nonfatigability in both groups. Interestingly, the SDH activity of the light ATPase fibers of the Sol of the trained cats was ≈40% higher than the control and spinal transected cats. In contrast to the elevated glycolytic capacities in the treadmill-trained transected cats compared to control cats, the GPD activities of the light ATPase fibers in standing trained cats were similar to control [101].

In general, the mass and mechanical properties of the MG were similar in the standing trained and nontrained spinal transected cats (Roy, Pierotti, Hodgson, Flores and Edgerton, unpublished observations). The percentage of fast fibers, the mean ATPase activities, and cross-sectional areas of either fiber type also were similar in these two spinal groups [100]. Mean SDH activities were significantly reduced in both ATPase fiber types following 6 months of transection. Standing training resulted in SDH activities that were 200% and 100% higher in the light and dark ATPase fibers, respectively, than in the spinal nontrained cats but similar to control. These results, and the data for the Sol reported above, indicate that the muscle fibers in transected cats maintain the capacity to increase their mitochondrial content to increased functional demands, even with the modest amount of time that the neuromuscular activity was elevated in these muscles.

The combined data of the two training studies indicate that the cyclical pattern of force generation associated with treadmill training was much more effective in maintaining the "normal" mechanical and metabolic properties of the Sol muscle than the relatively static contractions associated with weight-support training. These results indicate that the shortening-lengthening phases of a dynamic muscle contraction are an important component of the mechanical response of a muscle. In addition, the changes induced by either training regime were smaller in the MG compared to the Sol. This differential response is most likely related to the division of labor between these slow and fast synergists based on known recruitment patterns during a variety of motor tasks [91, 96, 140, 152, 161, 186]. For instance, the Sol has been shown to be almost fully recruited during quadrupedal posture and low level activity, whereas the MG motor pools are recruited primarily during movements requiring higher force demands. Thus, when the hindlimbs of the spinal transected cats were trained to step on the treadmill or trained to weight support, the Sol was recruited to a relatively higher degree (maybe even close to maximum based on the tendon force data discussed above) than the MG.

Spinal Isolation

NEUROMUSCULAR ACTIVITY. Spinal isolation of the lumbar region of the spinal cord involved transecting the spinal cord in adult female cats at vertebral levels T12-T13 and L7-S1, and severing all dorsal roots intradurally bilaterally between the two transection sites. This preparation often is referred to as the classic "silent preparation" as originally described by Tower [178]. In some cats, the isolation was restricted between L4-L5 and below S3 as described by Eldridge (56). Because data from the two preparations were similar, the results have been pooled. Spinal isolation has been a relatively pure model of disuse in our recent experiments. All supraspinal, infraspinal, and peripheral input is eliminated to the motoneurons isolated in the lumbar portion of the spinal cord. Based on 48 hours of continuous intramuscular EMG recordings from a representative ankle extensor (LG) and a representative ankle flexor (EDL), the muscles innervated by these motoneuron pools are essentially electrically silent, even during passive manipulation [155]. Acute recordings during tactile stimulation of the legs or feet also showed virtually no EMG activity in a variety of hindlimb muscles [57–59, 169]. Moreover, based on observations during cage activity, it can be assumed that minimal forces were generated in these paralyzed muscles.

This spinal isolated model was used to address whether cyclical passive manipulation of one hindlimb through a range of movements mimicking a step cycle ameliorates adaptations to disuse [10, 155]. Passive oscillation of one limb was performed by supporting the trunk of the cat in a harness that allowed both hindlimbs to hang freely while one foot was secured to a pedal mounted on an oscillating arm. The arm then was oscillated at 1 cycle per second and through an excursion of ≈90° at the ankle. The emphasis in joint excursion was at the ankle, thus ensuring that the Sol was passively stretched through a range of motion normally experienced in vivo. The cats were passively exercised for 30 minutes a day, 5 days a week for the 6-month experimental period, beginning 1 to 3 weeks postsurgery. During the week prior to the in situ physiological testing of the muscles, force transducers [79, 167, 190] implanted acutely on the Sol and MG tendons showed that a significant amount of force was generated during the passive stretching of the two muscles [155]. The contralateral limb served as a spinal isolation control.

NEUROMUSCULAR ADAPTATIONS. *Atrophy and myosin type adaptations.* Adaptations in the skeletal muscles innervated by the isolated motor pools generally were similar in direction but larger in magnitude than that accompanying spinal transection alone. For example, the mass of the Sol was ≈45% and 60% smaller than in control muscles six months after spinal transection and spinal isolation in adult cats, respectively [155]. These data are similar to the reported 75% decrease in Sol mass after either 5 or 8 months of spinal isolation [58]. Six to eight months after spinal isolation, a large percentage (mean of 45%) of the fibers in the normally homogeneously slow Sol showed myosin ATPase and MHC characteristic of fast fibers [58, 76]. Both fiber types atrophied, with the light and dark ATPase fibers being 47% and 66% smaller, respectively than the light ATPase fibers in control cats (76). Differential atrophy was observed between fast and slow extensors in that the MG atrophied by 12 and 25% in the spinal transected [102] and spinal-isolated [Roy, Pierotti, Hodgson, Flores and Edgerton, unpublished observation on a large number of spinal isolated cats] groups, respectively. Another fast extensor, the FHL, was reported to atrophy by 41% and after 5 months and 59% after 8 months of spinal isolation

[58]. Based on the staining pattern for myosin ATPase at an alkaline preincubation, there were 64% dark ATPase fibers in the regions sampled in the MG of control cats and 100% in spinal-isolated cats [102]. In addition, essentially all fibers in the MG of the spinal-isolated cats reacted exclusively with a fast MHC antibody. These fiber type data are consistent with the observation that the myosin ATPase activities (muscle homogenates) in spinal-isolated cats are 85% and 30% higher than control in the Sol and MG, respectively [10] and 37% higher in the Sol 9 months after spinal isolation [57]. Further, the myosin ATPase activities in the Sol were 22% higher in spinal isolated compared to spinal transected cats [10]. Spinal isolation also resulted in a shift in the myosin isozyme pattern in the Sol to that resembling a faster muscle, i.e., myosin expression transformed to a more equal distribution of the three slow isoforms and de novo expression of intermediate and some fast myosins. Further, the adaptations in the myosin molecule were more pronounced than that observed in spinal-transected cats [10]. Apparently not all muscles innervated by the isolated motoneurons were affected, however, because myosin ATPase activity was unchanged in the FHL [57]. Eldridge et al. (58) also have shown that 8 months of spinal isolation results in the appearance of the fast form of troponin I in 60% of the fibers of the normally homogeneously slow cat Sol and an increase from 86% to 100% in the FHL. The adaptations in the contractile proteins appear to be even of a greater magnitude after longer periods of inactivity. For example, Steinbach et al. [169] observed that slow-twitch forms of myosin light chains and tropomyosins were absent in the Sol after 2 to 3 years of spinal isolation.

Metabolic adaptations. Chronic inactivity for 6 months had no effect on the mean SDH activities of either light or dark ATPase fibers of the Sol [76]. Because of the large decrease in fiber area, however, the total amount of enzyme, i.e., the total SDH activity, was reduced by 55% in the light and 40% in the dark ATPase fibers of the Sol of spinal-isolated cats compared to control cats. Based on muscle homogenates, CS activity was unaffected in the Sol 8 months after spinal isolation in adult cats [157]. In contrast, the concentration and total amount of SDH enzyme was significantly decreased (by $\approx70\%$) in the fibers (all fast) of the MG of spinal-isolated cats compared to a weighted mean of the light and dark ATPase fibers of controls [102].

Spinal isolation results in an increase in the glycolytic potential of the affected muscles. GPD activity was 340% and 55% higher, respectively, and total GPD 115% higher and 32% lower, respectively in the light and dark ATPase fibers of 6-month spinal-isolated cats than control cats [76]. In addition, both GPD and lactate dehydrogenase activities were elevated in Sol muscle homogenates of cats that had been spinal isolated for 8 months [157]. In the MG of the 6-month isolated cats,

GPD was 120% higher and total GPD 63% higher than in controls [102]. In contrast, after 9 months of spinal isolation, 36% decrease in LDH activity in the FHL was reported [57].

Physiological adaptations. Preliminary data indicate that compared to control, the Po of the Sol and MG were decreased by ≈80% and 50%, respectively after 6 months of spinal isolation [Roy, Pierotti, Hodgson, Flores and Edgerton, unpublished observations]. The decreases in Po were proportionately greater than the reduction in muscle mass, thus specific tension was decreased as well. Specific tension also has been reported to decrease in the Sol muscle in cats 8 months after isolation [157] and in the Sol, gastrocnemius, EDL, and TA 21 days after spinal isolation [42, 43].

CT and HRT were significantly shorter in the Sol [57, 155, 157], whereas these twitch properties were unaffected in the MG [Roy, Pierotti, Hodgson, Flores and Edgerton, unpublished observations] and FHL [57] 6 to 9 months after spinal isolation. Vmax was ≈75 higher in the Sol and 15% higher in the MG of spinal-isolated cats compared to control, which reflects the increase in myosin ATPase activities and alterations in the myosin molecule described above [10]. Unpublished observations from our lab also indicate that the frequency tension curves for both muscles are shifted towards that seen in a faster muscle, with the shift being much larger in the Sol than the MG.

The fatigue properties of the Sol of cats spinally isolated for 8 months were similar to control, whereas the fatigue resistance of FHL was decreased significantly [49]. In a more recent study involving extensive physiological testing of several muscles during the terminal experiment [Roy, Pierotti, Hodgson, Flores and Edgerton, unpublished observations], the fatigue index of the Sol muscle in some of the spinal-isolated cats maintained for 6 months were near normal. In contrast, the MG muscles in these same animals were extremely fatigable (mean fatigue index of 0.05 compared to a control value of 0.36 [Roy, Pierotti, Hodgson, Flores and Edgerton, unpublished observations]). These data, in conjunction with the data from spinal-transected cats discussed above, indicate that the fatigue resistance of the Sol is relatively independent of the amount of electrical activity reaching the muscle, at least for periods of up to 8 months.

Recently, we also have begun to study the effects of spinal isolation on motoneuron size and metabolic properties and on the physiological, morphological, and metabolic properties of motor units. Apparently, complete electrical silence of the motoneurons in the lumbar cord for 6 months (as determined from EMG recordings of muscles innervated by this motoneuron pool [59, 155]) has no effect on the mean cross-sectional area or SDH activity of the soma [23]. These data suggest that action potential activity may not be an important determinant of motoneuron soma size or oxidative capacity. These data, however, do not preclude the possibility of inactivity producing changes in the dendritic arborizations and/or the terminal axonal branches of the motoneuron. In fact, Eldridge et al. [59] have reported the presence of axonal sprouting, multiple innervation of some fibers, and an increase in the density of extrajunctional acetylcholine receptors in a number of hindlimb muscles of the cat after 2 to 3 years of isolation.

Motor units in the TA muscles of the same group of spinal-isolated cats [142] could be physiologically classified into the same categories that are found in control cats [17, 41]. Po values of the FF and FR units were lower than that found in control cats, whereas the Po of the S units remained within the control range. In the spinal-isolated cats, the mean cross-sectional area for the fibers in fast units were 25–50% smaller than control, whereas the mean fiber size in the slow units was similar to control [54, 142]. The variability in fiber size within a unit was greater than that observed in control cats [17, 120]. All other isometric contractile properties were within the control ranges for each unit type. Similarly the relationship between Po and innervation ratio, i.e., number of fibers per motoneuron, reported for TA units in normal cats [17], was maintained in the spinal-isolated cats. The variability in SDH activity among fibers within a motor unit was similar in MUs from control [120] and spinal-isolated [141] cats. Further, the spatial distribution patterns [16, 18] of fibers within the motor unit territory were similar to control [71]. Together, these data indicate that except for the decreases in mass and tension-related properties, inactivity for 6 months had little effect on the functional, metabolic, and morphological properties of single motor units in the cat TA. These data are further evidence that the amount and/or pattern of activity need not dictate the properties of the muscle fibers (or motoneurons) within muscle units.

EXERCISE COUNTERMEASURES. Because spinal isolation was shown to be a reliable model of disuse [57–59, 155], the effects of passive cyclical stretch on the functional and metabolic properties of inactive muscles could be studied. The most dramatic effect of passive stretch in the spinal-isolated cats was the amelioration of the increase in myosin ATPase and Vmax associated with inactivity [10]. These data clearly indicate that mechanical activity, without coupled neural activation, can exert an influence on both the biochemical and the functional properties of the contractile system. In addition, the passive exercise regime had a small effect on most of the functional or metabolic parameters measured at the whole muscle, motor unit, or muscle fiber levels. For example, in comparison to the nonmanipulated leg, the manipulated leg had (1) slightly less atrophy and slightly higher Po values in the Sol and MG in the majority of cats [155 and Roy, Pierotti, Hodgson, Flores, and Edgerton, unpublished observations], (2) a blunting of the transformation of the isomyosin expression towards faster forms [10], and

(3) muscle fiber size, GPD, and SDH activities closer to those observed in control cats [unpublished observations]. A similar small effect of daily passive stretch (≈4 minutes per day for 22 to 23 days) in maintaining muscle mass following spinal isolation was reported by Eccles [43]. The results from these studies are not definitive, however, and the rehabilitative potential of passive, cyclical stretch should be pursued.

Hindlimb Suspension

NEUROMUSCULAR ACTIVITY. Another approach in modifying how muscles are used involves the model of hindlimb suspension. This model results in the elimination of weight-support activity without any surgical intervention compromising the nervous system. In a large series of experiments [2, 13, 74, 75, 84, 85, 88, 139, 151, 153, 174, 176, 177, 179, 180, 182, 183, 191], the hindlimbs of rats were "unloaded" using a modification of the tail suspension technique originally described by Morey [127]. In this model of altered "use", a tail cast was fastened to a harness and attached to the top of the cage by a swivel allowing 360° rotation. The suspension height was adjusted to allow the rats to support their weight and move freely on their forelimbs, while the hindlimbs were not allowed to make contact with any surface. This model has been used extensively as a ground-based model in studying the effects of weightlessness on skeletal muscle properties [173, 129].

The activity patterns of the Sol, MG and TA have been monitored before and during a 1-month period of suspension [2]. EMG was recorded in each rat for 25 minutes of each hour for 24 consecutive hours, 7 and 3 days prior, on the initial day of, and 3, 7, 14, 21, and 28 days during continuous suspension. The total amount of daily EMG activity in the Sol and MG was significantly reduced on the day of suspension, but was similar to control by 7 days postsuspension. Further, the daily EMG levels were near normal for the remainder of the experimental period. Daily EMG levels of the TA were either similar to or above normal for each postsuspension day. In addition, the interrelationships of the EMG amplitude patterns (i.e., a reflection of the recruitment patterns [see 96, 97 for discussion]) between the Sol and MG were altered on the day of suspension, but recovered to a normal pattern by day 7 postsuspension [153]. Although the tension levels in the muscles of suspended rats were not monitored, it is reasonable to assume that the forces were small, in particular in the plantarflexors which seem to have been further unloaded by the extended position in which the ankle was usually observed to be maintained during suspension [2].

NEUROMUSCULAR ADAPTATIONS. *Atrophy and myosin type adaptations.* An excellent review was recently published which thoroughly discusses the effects of "hindlimb unweighting" on the rat Sol muscle [173]. Hindlimb suspension results in a progressive decrease in the mass of some of the muscles in the hindlimb, with the most rapid decrease occurring within the first 2 weeks of suspension [36, 109, 177]. Similar to other experimental models in which atrophy occurs, the magnitude of the atrophic response is greater in predominantly slow extensors, which is greater than in predominantly fast extensors, which is greater than in predominantly fast flexors. The atrophy appears to be due only to a decrease in fiber size, not fiber number [33, 170]. The mean cross-sectional areas of both the light and dark staining ATPase fibers were reduced following suspension, although in most cases the light ATPase fibers atrophy more than the dark ATPase fibers [36, 74, 75, 84, 85, 151 and see Table 2 in 173 for summary data on the Sol].

Hindlimb suspension is accompanied by a progressive decrease in the percentage of slow (Type I) fibers in the Sol [see summary Table 3 in 173], whereas there appears to be little change in fiber type composition of predominantly fast muscles such as the MG and TA [74, 151]. The increase in the percentage of fast fibers, based on myosin ATPase staining reactions at an alkaline preincubation, appear to occur in concert with the changes in fiber GPD activities described above. These results are consistent with the concept that the myosin ATPase and glycolytic capacities of muscle fibers are tightly coupled as shown previously in other models of increased [14] and decreased use [12, 92, 100–102].

Hindlimb suspension is accompanied by a progressive decrease in the concentration of myofibrillar and myosin protein in the Sol muscle [174–177, 179–181]. In addition, there is a shift in myosin isoform expression towards faster forms [174, 176, 177] and an increase in fast MHC composition [145] in the Sol muscle. Myofibrillar ATPase activity [174, 176, 177] and myosin light-chain isoform composition [63, 64, 69, 145, 174, 176, 177] in Sol muscle homogenates and single fibers appear to be unchanged following suspension, but the response appears to be quite variable.

Metabolic adaptations. The oxidative capacity of the fibers in the Sol muscle appears to be maintained or even elevated during suspension. SDH activities (concentration) were either slightly increased or unchanged in the dark and light ATPase fibers of the Sol following 7 days [84] or 28 days [75, 85] of suspension. Because the fibers atrophied, however, the total enzyme activity per fiber (total SDH) was 15–56% lower than in control. Similarly, CS activities of SO fibers in the Sol were significantly higher than control and β-hydroxyacyl-CoA dehydrogenase activities similar to control at 2 and 4 weeks postsuspension [65]. In the MG, SDH activity was unaffected after 7 days of suspension [74] but decreased (7%, light deep, 24% dark deep, and 37% dark superficial) after 28 days of suspension [151]. The total amount of SDH enzyme decreased by 20% in the deep and 32% in the superficial portions of the MG after 7 days of suspension [74]. In contrast, the activities of CS and β-hydroxyacyl-CoA dehydrogenase in both FG and FOG fibers were similar to control after 14 and 28 days of suspension [65]. The TA showed a decrease in SDH activity (about 40% overall) after 28 days of suspension [151]. Although it appears, therefore, that the Sol fibers maintain their oxidative capacity up to 28 days after suspension, the predominantly fast muscles, e.g., the MG and TA, usually have levels lower than control of oxidative marker enzymes.

GPD activity approximately doubles both in fiber types in the Sol [84] and in the deep portion of the MG [151] after 28 days of suspension, whereas there is no effect in the dark ATPase fibers of the superficial region of the MG [151]. Similarly, lactate dehydrogenase and phosphofructokinase activities in SO fibers in the soleus were elevated relative to control 4 weeks after hindlimb suspension when the values are expressed per fiber dry weight [63]. No change in these two glycolytic enzymes were oberved in the FG or FOG fibers of the MG and LG. In the TA, GPD activity was maintained in the fibers of the deep portions of the muscle and elevated in the superficial portions [151]. The data are therefore consistent in indicating that the glycolytic capacity is maintained or elevated in all fiber types of both extensor and flexor muscles.

Physiological adaptations. In the Sol, Po is reduced disproportionately to the decrease in mass following suspension; thus the specific tension is reduced [88, 139, 191 and see summary Table 5 in 173]. These data probably reflect an increase in the relative proportion of noncontractile tissue in the Sol of suspended rats [88, 166, 172]. This decrease in specific tension also could be accounted for by the decrease in the concentration in the myofibril protein that occurs in the Sol muscle of suspended rats [177]. In contrast, specific tension appears to be maintained in predominantly fast muscles, e.g., the MG and TA [88, 139, 191], which is probably associated with the overall lesser effect of suspension on these muscles.

Generally the Sol shows "faster" contractile properties, whereas the predominantly fast muscles are relatively unaffected [65, 88, 93, 139, 171, 172, 191]. Therefore, the following discussion on speed related changes will be restricted to adaptations in the Sol. CT and HRT are decreased [see summary Table 4 in 173], an alteration that may be related to changes in sarcoplasmic reticulum calcium kinetics [65]. The frequency-tension curve indicates a response usually found in a faster muscle [88, 139, 191]. There appears to be an increase in Vmax following suspension, but the data are controversial at this time. Whole muscle Vmax has been reported to increase either 28% [69] or 125% [65] after 2 weeks or to not change (a 4–10% increase) after up to 4 weeks [88, 139, 191] following suspension. A large increase in Vmax would not be expected based on the minor changes in myosin ATPase activity (174, 176, 177), a measure that is highly correlated with Vmax [15]. Single-fiber data show only a small percentage of fibers with an obviously elevated Vmax; i.e., the shortening velocities were similar to control in most of the fibers tested [69, 145]. The fibers demonstrating the fastest Vmax's also had the largest proportions of fast MHCs, which suggests a close relationship between these two parameters [145]. The apparent discrepancies in the Vmax data among the studies across different laboratories has not been resolved.

The normal fatigue resistance of the Sol was maintained at 7 days [62, 88, 139] and 28 days (191) postsuspension. A maintenance of the fatigue properties of the Sol also has been observed in other models of decreased use, i.e., spinal transection [12] and spinal isolation [49]. In contrast, the fatigability of the MG is similar to control after 7 days [88, 139; cf. 62] but significantly increased after 28 days [191] of suspension.

EXERCISE COUNTERMEASURES. A number of studies have clearly demonstrated that many of the effects of unloading can be reversed by allowing the rats to recover under weight-bearing conditions after a period of suspension [37, 177]. The present review, however, will focus on countermeasures used to prevent or ameliorate the effects of unweighting. Recently, Thomason and Booth [173] have emphasized that there is no cause-and-effect relationship between EMG activities [from 2] and myofibrillar protein metabolism [from 174, 176, 177] in the unweighted Sol muscle. In fact, the time courses of protein synthesis or degradation and mean EMG were uncoupled. The authors concluded from these relationships "that the major mechanical factor for maintaining myofibrillar protein in slow-twitch muscle over long periods of time appears to be 'weighted' contraction" [173, p. 9].

Several forms of exercise countermeasures have been shown to be effective in ameliorating the effects of suspension on the hindlimb muscles. Thomason et al [177] showed that 2 or 4 hours of daily stationary ground support for 4 weeks in suspended rats produced a significant reduction in the atrophic response of the Sol, AL, Plt, and VI. Uphill running at 20 meters per minute and a 30% grade for 1.5 hours per day partially ameliorated the atrophy in these muscles. The absolute amount of maintenance of mass was greater in the predominantly slow muscles than the predominantly fast ones, but this could have been related to the fact that these muscles also were the most atrophied. Edgerton and coworkers [85, 88, 139] have demonstrated that much shorter periods of exercise interspersed throughout the day have a similar effect. For example, 10 minute bouts of standing, very slow walking (5 m/min), or moderate running (20 m/min) on a treadmill repeated four times daily (i.e., 40 minutes total of daily exercise) maintained a near normal Sol mass during 7 days of suspension [see Table 4 in 88]. In contrast, these protocols only had a minimal effect in the MG. In addition, climbing a one-meter grid at an 85% incline with 50 to 75% body weight attached for 8 to 10 repetitions, 2 or 4 times per day (≈6 minutes of daily exercise) resulted in a significant retention of Sol and MG mass, although the effect in the MG was somewhat variable [88]. Together, these data indicate that daily periods of load bearing is an effective means of counteracting the atrophic response to hindlimb suspension. Further, it appears that a very small amount of high load bearing per day (as little as 6 minutes) can significantly attenuate the suspension-associated atrophy in the Sol and, to some degree, the MG. Further studies are needed to specify the appropriate types, durations, and intervals of neuromuscular activity required to maintain muscle properties in chronic unloaded conditions.

Spaceflight
  NEUROMUSCULAR ACTIVITY. Weightlessness is a model of decreased use in that the skeletal muscles are chronically unloaded due to the elimination of gravitational effects. Presumably the muscle forces would be minimal under these unloaded conditions, although no muscle force data are available at this time. In humans during spaceflight, the tonic activity (EMG) of the Sol is reduced, whereas the tonic activity of the TA is enhanced during postural adjustments [28, 29, 110, 111]. This reversal of the roles of extensors and flexors normally observed at 1G also has been reported during parabolic flight [27]. These adaptations, however, may be short lived because the tonic activity in both muscles was reduced after 7 days of weightlessness [29]. To our knowledge, no chronic EMG or force data are available on animals during spaceflight. A recent review [44] has been published which addresses many of the critical issues in studying the effects of spaceflight on the skeletal muscle system.
  A confounding variable in many of the spaceflight studies is the amount of time the animals were at 1G before the tissues could be extracted. Most of the data discussed in the present review will be from the following flights, with the duration of the flight followed by the number of hours prior to harvesting the skeletal muscle tissues in parentheses: Space Lab 3 (SL-3, 7 days, 11–17 hours), Cosmos 1887 (12.5 days, 48–53 hours), and Cosmos 1667 (7 days, 4–8 hours). All responses of the muscle should be interpreted in light of the differences in the time between landing and sacrifice. In addition, in many cases, the sample sizes are limited because of obvious reasons; consequently many of the results are trends rather than significant differences in the data.
  NEUROMUSCULAR ADAPTATIONS. *Atrophy and myosin adaptations.* Weightlessness results in a rapid atrophy of rat skeletal muscles, in particular those muscles that predominantly comprise slow fibers [9, 26, 82, 119, 126, 147, 148, 149]. All fiber types show some degree of atrophy following spaceflight, but the relative amount of atrophy in

each fiber type appears to be variable. For example, Martin et al. [119] and Miu et al. [126] report similar decreases, on a percent change basis, for both light and dark ATPase fibers in the Sol after 7 (SL-3) and 12.5 (Cosmos 1887) days of flight, respectively. Riley et al. [148, 149], on the other hand, observed approximately 45% more atrophy in SO compared to FOG fibers in the Sol after 7 days of flight (SL-3) and ≈150% more atrophy in the SO than the FOG fibers in the AL after 12.5 days of flight (Cosmos 1887). The data reported by Martin et al. [119] and Riley et al. [148] from the same flight were from relatively small (243 grams at sacrifice) and large (384 grams at sacrifice) rats, respectively, suggesting an age effect on the atrophic response. The fiber type-specific atrophic response was variable in the mixed fast muscles, although the predominant type of the muscle or region of the muscle appeared to be affected the most [119, 126, 148].

Spaceflights of relatively short durations have a significant impact on the fiber type distributions of hindlimb muscles and muscles regions that are normally predominantly slow. For example, Martin, et al. [119] reported increases in the percentage of dark ATPase (fast) fibers from 39% to 50% and 20% to 46% in the Sol and AL, respectively, after a 7 day flight (SL-3) in rats. In addition, the percentage of fast fibers increased from 76% to 84% in the deep region of the MG, whereas no change in fiber type distribution was observed in the Plt, EDL, or superficial portion of the MG. In contrast, Riley et al. [148] found no change in the fiber type distribution in either the Sol or the EDL of larger rats flown on the same mission, which suggests that there also is an age effect on this response to spaceflight. Riley et al. [149], however, did report a decrease from 83% to 63% in the percentage of SO fibers in the AL and no change in the fiber type distribution in the EDL and Plt after a 12.5-day flight (Cosmos 1887). A decrease in the percentage of slow fibers in the Sol also has been shown after a 7-day Cosmos (1667) biosatellite flight [38]. Further, Miu et al. [126] found an increase from 22% to 40% in the percentage of fibers expressing either fast or fast and slow MHC in the Sol muscle of rats flown for 12.5 days on Cosmos 1887.

These fiber type changes are reflected in alterations in contractile proteins. Baldwin et al. [9] have shown that 12.5 days (Cosmos 1887) of exposure to 0G results in a reduction of the expression of the slower myosin isoforms, a reduction in the concentration of myofibrils, and an increase in myofibril ATPase activity in the VI, a predominantly slow knee extensor, but not the VL, a predominantly fast knee extensor. Similarly, Martin et al. [119] showed a significant increase in the myofibrillar ATPase activity of the Sol, but not the EDL, after 7 days of flight (SL-3). These results in conjunction with the data of Miu et al. (126) from rats flown on the same flight suggest that there is a down-regulation of slow myosin and an up-regulation of fast myosin during spaceflight, at least in some fibers of the Sol.

Metabolic adaptations. Based on single fiber quantitative histochemical determinations, the mean SDH activity (i.e., the enzyme concentration) of the fibers from a number of rat muscles was unchanged after a 7-day (SL-3, 119) or a 12.5-day flight (Cosmos 1887, 126). Because of the larger relative decrease in mean fiber size in the slow versus the fast muscles, however, the total amount of enzyme was decreased in the slow but not the fast muscles. Using single fiber microchemical techniques, Manchester et al. [117] showed no change in the concentration of a battery of oxidative enzymes in the fibers of the Sol, where an increase in these enzyme concentrations did occur in the TA after 7 days of flight (Cosmos 1887). Desplanches et al. [38] reported no change in whole muscle CS activity or capillarization [cf. 130] in the Sol or EDL after a 7-day flight (Cosmos 1667). Thus, it appears that the oxidative potential of muscle fibers is relatively unaffected by these short flights. The effects of longer flights, as planned in the near future, are unknown.

The mean GPD activity was approximately twice that observed in controls in both the light and dark ATPase fibers of the predominantly slow muscles (i.e., the Sol and AL) and generally unchanged in the predominantly fast muscles (i.e., the EDL, Plt and MG) after 7 days of weightlessness (SL-3, 119). After a 12.5-day flight (Cosmos 1887), the results were more variable [126]. Compared to ground based controls, the mean GPD activity of the dark ATPase fibers was 76% higher and the light ATPase fibers unchanged in the Sol, whereas in the MG, the light and dark ATPase fibers were 79% and 26% higher than control. In microdissected fibers of rats from the same flight, the concentrations of a battery of glycogenolytic-glycolytic enzymes were increased in Sol and decreased in TA fibers [117]. LDH activities in muscle homogenates have been reported to increase after 21.5 days of flight (Cosmos 605, 143), but to be unchanged in either the Sol or the EDL after a 7-day flight (Cosmos 1667, 38). Despite the variability in the limited data available, it appears that weightlessness results in a general increase in the glycolytic potential of the skeletal muscles in the rat hindlimb.

Physiological adaptations. There is a paucity of data on the physiological properties of muscles after spaceflight. Based on the atrophic, myosin isoform, and metabolic adaptations described above, however, it seems reasonable to assume that the functional adaptations will be similar to those observed following hindlimb suspension. Thus, the expected major physiological adaptations would include the following: decreased Po, perhaps an increased Vmax, and a shift in the isometric speed-related parameters towards those found in a faster muscle.

EXERCISE COUNTERMEASURES. The effectiveness of existing exercise protocols and the description and recommendation of new exercise protocols based on the actual requirements of astronauts to perform intravehicular and extravehicular activities in microgravity have been reviewed recently [77] and will not be discussed further in this review. For the present review, the most important factor to consider is the animal work in which the ground-based model of hindlimb suspension is being used to help determine the most efficacious manner of maintaining the skeletal muscles in a chronic unloaded condition. These data have been thoroughly discussed in the section on hindlimb suspension.

MODEL OF INCREASED "USE"

Functional Overload

NEUROMUSCULAR ACTIVITY. Functional overload of a muscle is produced by removing its major synergists. The most common model used in our laboratories involves overloading the Plt by complete removal of the Sol, MG and LG bilaterally in rats or cats. Notably, many of the differences in the response to functional overload in the literature are probably due to the method of overloading; i.e., many studies have involved denervation or tenotomy rather than excision of the synergists, and a unilateral rather than a bilateral approach. In this review, we emphasize the results from studies in which the synergists have been removed bilaterally. Under these conditions, the EMG amplitudes of the rat Plt during stepping is elevated compared to preoverload values, which indicates that the recruitment level of the Plt is increased to compensate for the loss of its major synergists [70 and Roy and Edgerton, unpublished observations]. Interestingly, the temporal patterns of activation are unchanged following functional overload of the Plt. Apparently, the amplitude and duration of the EMG activity during posture or stepping in the functionally overloaded Sol is unchanged [90], which probably reflects the fact that the Sol is near maximally recruited even under low-intensity activity periods [2, 96, 161]. Normal weight-bearing activity is a sufficient stimulus to produce a significant hypertrophic response in the overloaded muscles of rats in a relatively short time.

Functional overload in the cat also has been studied extensively in our laboratories, although most of these data remain as unpublished observations. Kinematic data indicate that the cats walk plantigrade for the first 3 to 4 weeks after the functional overload and then regain a normal digitigrade gait pattern (authors' unpublished observations). Similarly, in cats who had the Sol, LG, and MG denervated, Wetzel et al. [189] observed that the ankle was more plantigrade than normal during quadrupedal and bipedal standing, as well as spontaneous walking and trotting. Plantaris tendon force and EMG recordings have been monitored in 4 cats presurgery and between 2 to 12 weeks postsurgery. These results indicate that the forces are significantly higher following functional overload. EMG patterns show similar responses to that reported in the rat; i.e., the magnitude of the signals are increased but the temporal features are relatively unchanged.

The results from our first functional overload experiments with cats emphasized the importance of the muscle-loading characteristics on the hypertrophic response. Six cats had their Plt muscles functionally overloaded bilaterally and were allowed unrestricted activity in large cages. In addition, three of the six cats were exercised at a variety of speeds on a treadmill for less than 10 minutes per day, 3 to 4 days per week. Observation of the cats from both groups in the cages indicated very low levels of activity, with the cats normally spending most of the time lying quietly in the cages. At the end of 12 weeks, the mean mass of the Plt had increased by ≈10% and 65% in the nonexercised and exercised cats, respectively. Based on these data, all functionally overloaded cats in our studies are now periodically exercised on a treadmill at various speeds and grades or induced to perform vigorous play activity, such as jumping and sprinting. Cats who are exercised with the latter exercise protocol show over a 100% hypertrophy 3 months after functional overload (Chalmers, Roy and Edgerton, unpublished observations). The neuromuscular adaptations described below are from functionally overloaded cats who were exercised in one of these manners.

NEUROMUSCULAR ADAPTATIONS. *Hypertrophy and myosin type adaptations.* Following 12 weeks of overload in the rat, the Plt mass doubles [154] and the Sol and MG masses increase by ≈50% [156]. These differences in the amount of hypertrophy appear to be related to two factors: (1) the relative contribution of each muscle to the extensor mass, and (2) the initial percentage of slow fibers in each muscle. The MG, Plt, and Sol represent approximately 36%, 16%, and 6%, respectively of the total mass of the triceps surae-plantaris complex, the major plantarflexors of the leg. The difference in the amount of hypertrophy between the MG and the Plt was probably related to the difference in the relative load placed on these two predominantly fast muscles by the functional overload. The difference in the degree of response between the Sol and the MG or Plt probably reflects a difference in the responsiveness of a muscle that is predominantly slow compared to muscles that are predominantly fast. The Sol is normally heavily recruited even in low-intensity activity periods, whereas the MG (and presumably the Plt) are recruited heavily only when the demands are high [96, 161]. Both slow and fast fibers hypertrophied after overload, although the enlargement was relatively more in the slow than the fast fibers [156]. Compensatory hypertrophy also occurs in fast flexor muscles that are functionally overloaded. For example, after the excision of the TA in the rat, the EDL hypertrophies to ≈130% of control after 28 days and maintains this level of hypertrophy for the next 400 days [67]. The smaller amount of hypertrophy in this fast flexor in comparison to the Plt is probably related to the differences in the loading characteristics of flexors versus extensors; i.e., the extensor must support the weight of the rat during posture and provide propulsion during movement, whereas the main function of the flexor is to recover the limb during the swing phase of the step cycle [73, 140, 161].

An increase in the percentage of slow fibers was observed in each overloaded muscle [12, 156]. The Sol muscle became homogeneously slow, whereas there were regional differences in the response of the MG and Plt. The deep (close to the bone) region of both muscles showed about 50% slow fibers, a three- and twofold increase relative to control in the Plt and MG, respectively. In contrast, the percentage of slow fibers in the superficial (away from the bone) region increased from 3% to 19% in the Plt and was unchanged in the MG (i.e., no slow fibers were present). These data are consistent with the concept of differential recruitment of muscle subregions [60, 61, 161] and with the observation that fiber size is affected more in the deep than in the superficial regions of these muscles in response to the overload condition [156].

Baldwin et al. [12] showed a 25% decrease in the specific activity of myosin and myofibrillar ATPase and an increase in the proportion of slow versus fast myosin heavy and light chains in the Plt 9 to 12 weeks after overload. In addition, myofibrillar and myosin ATPase-specific activities shifted toward that resembling a slower muscle in the overloaded Sol and in the deep, but not the superficial, region of the overloaded MG [156]. Similar adaptations in myosin isozyme patterns were observed in the Plt and Sol after 11 weeks of overload and voluntary wheel running [80]. When voluntary running and overload were combined, the increase in slow myosin was equal to the sum of the increases in the two treatments alone. All of these histochemical and biochemical data are consistent with a conversion of fibers from FG to FOG to SO in functionally overloaded muscles.

The following are preliminary observations from our lab for the cat. The mass of the Plt muscle is ≈65% heavier than control after 3 months of functional overload if the cats are treadmill exercised for short periods every other day [123; also see above]. Compared to control, the percentage of SO fibers was increased from 32% to 55% in the deep region and unchanged in the superficial region of the Plt of these overloaded cats. The mean cross-sectional areas of each fiber type in either muscle region were significantly larger in the overloaded than the control cats, with the relative changes being higher in the deep than the superficial region. Increases in the percentage and size of the slow fibers also have been observed in the cat Plt after 6 weeks of overload produced by denervation of the synergists [189].

Metabolic adaptations. Based on muscle homogenates, Baldwin and coworkers [7, 8, 11] reported a decrease in the CS activity in the Plt after periods of overload ranging from 1 to 12 weeks. This adaptation appears to be occurring in the deep, but not the superficial, region of the muscle [11]. A concomitant increase in key enzymes involved in the ketone oxidation pathway in both whole muscle and deep region homogenates suggests that there actually may be a qualitative change in the composition of the mitochondrial pool in overloaded Plt. A decrease in both CS and the enzymes involved in ketone metabolic pathway has been observed as well in overloaded Sol homogenates [11]. In contrast, SDH and malate dehydrogenase activities appear to be maintained at normal levels in the chronically overloaded Plt [98, 146]. It also has been shown that the enzymatic capacity to oxidize pyruvate, palmitate and glycerophosphate is similar in control and overloaded Plt muscles [11].

Baldwin et al. [7, 8, 14] have shown that the activities of key glycogenolytic enzymes (i.e., phosphorylase, phosphofructokinase, GPD, and lactate dehydrogenase) are significantly reduced in overloaded rat Plt and Sol homogenates. Similar changes were observed in the deep, but not the superficial, portion of the MG [156]. Others have reported no change in phosphorylase after 120 days of overload [146] or phosphofructokinase from 30 to 100 days postoverload in the rat Plt [98]. The reason for these contrasing observations is unclear at this time.

Physiological adaptations. Generally, chronic functional overload results in a compensatory hypertrophy and a shift in the mechanical properties of the overloaded muscle towards those normally observed in slower muscles. After 12 to 14 weeks of overload, the rat Plt mass has increased a relatively larger amount than the Po and, thus, the specific tension was decreased by ≈15% [154; also see 134].

CT and HRT are prolonged, the frequency tension curve has shifted towards the response of a slower muscle, and Vmax has been reduced by ≈45%. The adaptations in the speed properties of the twitch appeared to be closely related to changes in the sarcoplasmic reticulum calcium kinetics, whereas changes in Vmax and myosin ATPase activities were closely interrelated [154].

The overloaded Plt becomes more fatigue resistant than normal [6, 154]. This adaptation may be related to the increase in the percentage of slow (SO) fibers associated with overload [14, 98], because slow fibers have been shown to be more efficient (ATP utilization) in maintaining isometric tension than fast fibers [72, 107].

The effects of functional overload also have been studied at the motor unit level in rats and cats. In the most extensive study on motor units to date, Olha et al. [134] studied the effects of 16 weeks of overload in the rat Plt. FF, FR and S units showed a 30%, 60%, and 80% increase, respectively in mean tension production capability after overload. The mean fiber areas were increased by 110% in slow (Type

I) and 70% fast (Type II) fibers. Each motor unit clearly could be physiologically categorized, which indicates that the transformation of a unit was complete. The overloaded Plt had a higher percentage of FF and S units and a lower percentage of FR and FI units than normal. A composite of the fiber size and motor unit type (fiber type) adaptations suggest that a higher percentage of the aggregate force of the muscle was contributed by the FF units in overloaded compared to control rats. These data further suggest that the higher percentage contribution of the highly fatigable FF units would result in a decreased fatigue resistance in the overloaded Plt. These data are in direct contradiction with the increased fatigue-resistance observed at the whole muscle level [154].

In cats, functional overload of the MG for 14 to 32 weeks resulted in a ≈50% increase in wet weight [187]. Mean tetanic tensions of FF, FI, FR, and S units increased by 40%, 157%, 140%, and 113%, respectively after overload, with the fibers comprising the FR and S units showing a 17% increase in size. No detectable changes in the distribution of motor unit or fiber types were evident. In addition, twitch and fatigue properties were unchanged after overload.

Sixty days after functional overload, the NADH-tetrazolium reductase activity, an indicator of aerobic capacity, was significantly reduced in HRP-labelled motoneurons that innervate the Sol [13%] and in Sol muscle fibers (21%) [135]. Frequency distributions of the enzyme activity in both the motoneurons and the muscle fibers indicate a general downward shift in the oxidative capacity of all cells. GPD activity also showed a general decrease in all muscle fibers after overload [135], in contrast to the large, consistent increase in GPD in muscle homogenates [12, 154]. Recently, Chalmers et al. [24] reported no change in size or SDH activity of Plt motoneurons, but an increase in size and no change in SDH activity of both light and dark ATPase fibers following 3 months of functional overload in cats. In addition, the mean SDH activities of the muscle fibers and the motoneurons within the Plt of control cats were almost identical, a relationship that was maintained after overload [24]. These latter data indicate that although the oxidative potential of the muscle fibers and the motoneurons within the muscle units of a fast muscle are similar, the size and mean SDH activity of each cell can change independently. The reasons for the differences in these results are unknown, although the response may simply be a function of the intrinsic differences between fast and slow muscles.

EXERCISE AND UNLOADING EFFECTS. Endurance training results in either no change [8] or a slight increase [146] in the mass of the overloaded rat Plt and no change in the overloaded Sol [146]. The slow fibers appear to be the most affected by the exercise program [146]. Baldwin et al. [8] showed that endurance walking results in a 74% increase in CS activity levels in the functionally overloaded rat Plt muscle, and Reidy et al. [146], using a more intense endurance running protocol, showed a 60% and 45% increase in SDH activity of the overloaded Plt and Sol, respectively. In contrast, phosphofructokinase activity, a glycolytic marker enzyme, appears to be unaffected by endurance training of overloaded Plt or Sol muscles [8, 146]. Moreover, the myosin ATPase activity was similar in the overloaded Plt of trained and nontrained rats, with both groups exhibiting an $\approx$20% decrease compared to control [8]. Together, these data indicate that functionally overloaded muscles maintain the normal ability to respond to endurance training by elevating mitochondrial protein systems, but do not affect the glycolytic and contractile protein systems.

When rats were subjected to independent and simultaneous functional overload of the Plt and hindlimb suspension for 6 weeks, the mean Plt absolute and relative weight were maintained approximately midway between the weight of only overloaded or only suspended rats [179]. Total protein, total myofibril protein, myofibril protein concentration, and myosin ATPase were similar to control, whereas some of these parameters changed in the only overloaded and only suspended rats. Further, the increases in the expression of slow and intermediate myosin seen with overload were blunted in the overloaded and sus-pended rats. Similarly, 4 weeks of simultaneous Plt overload and hindlimb suspension resulted in muscle weight to body weight ratios that were somewhat larger than those observed in the suspended only group [124]. In addition, 4 hours of weight-support activity per day in the overloaded and suspended group produced a significant hypertro-phy in the Plt, apparently due to a selective increase in the CSA of the slow fibers. Interestingly, the isometric contractile properties of the Plt, such as CT, HRT, fatigue index, and frequency tension response, were similar in the overloaded and suspended rats as well as the only overloaded group. Together, these data indicate that weight bearing is essential in producing the increase in muscle mass and in slow myosin isoform expression, but not the functional changes, associated with functional overload. Further studies on the interactive effects of in-creased and decreased use are warranted.

SUMMARY AND CONCLUSIONS

Regulation of Cell Size

MUSCLE SPECIFICITY. In response to each of the models in which the neuromuscular system is perturbed, a differential atrophy or hypertro-phy occurs among the affected muscles. When some aspect of neuro-muscular activation is reduced by hindlimb suspension, spaceflight, spinalization, or spinal isolation, the relative atrophy among synergists and antagonists is generally as follows: atrophy in the slow extensor is greater than the fast extensor which is greater than the fast flexor. In contrast, when neuromuscular activation is chronically increased by functional overload, the mass of a fast muscle will increase more than in a slow muscle, and the mass of a fast extensor will increase more than a fast flexor.

MUSCLE REGION SPECIFICITY. In addition to the variation in the fiber size adaptations to increased or decreased activity among muscles, there are regional atrophic responses within a muscle. Typically, the deeper portion of the muscle, i.e., the region of the muscle containing the highest percentage of slow and/or high oxidative fibers, atrophies more than the superficial region of a muscle. The deeper region of a muscle also appears to show the greatest hypertrophy after functional overload.

FIBER TYPE SPECIFICITY. The concept of variation in muscle fiber size as a function of myosin type prevails in the literature, in spite of numerous exceptions. For example, it is generally assumed that fibers classified as fast based on their myosin properties, i.e., often referred to as Type II fibers, have larger cross-sectional areas than fibers classified as slow, i.e., Type I, fibers. Although there is a fiber size dependency on myosin type in many muscles, this relationship is not always in the same direction. For example, in most predominantly fast rat muscles, the fast fibers in the superficial region of the muscle are larger than the slow fibers, but the two fiber types are about the same size in the deep region of the same muscle [3]. In predominantly slow muscles such as the rat Sol and AL [3] as well as the cat Sol [118] and VI [151, 188], the fast fibers are consistently smaller than the slow fibers. In humans, the fast fibers of the VL usually are larger than the slow fibers in males, whereas the opposite tends to be the case in females [164]. The atrophic response of Type I and II fibers depends largely on the muscle. In general, the fibers that are the largest in the muscle normally atrophy the most regardless of their type. Further, when the atrophy is expressed as a percent change, the atrophic response is often similar in slow or fast fibers.

RATES OF ATROPHY OR HYPERTROPHY. Within a few days after unloading the hindlimbs of rats by suspension, there are signs of degradation of contractile proteins, particularly slow myosin in the predominantly slow Sol [173, 177]. The fastest rate of atrophy occurs within the first 1 to 2 weeks of hindlimb suspension [109] and may be similar in spaceflight [9, 119, 126, 147–149]. Thereafter, the atrophic rate seems to progress much more slowly. This initial rapid rate of atrophy followed by a virtual plateau has important implications for the strategy of choice in rehabilitative medicine as well as in counter-measures used to prevent muscle atrophy associated with long-term spaceflights by humans.

The rate of hypertrophy in functional overload is less well defined. Although muscle wet weight will increase dramatically within a few days after functional overload, at least for the first week the increased mass has little functional advantage in relation to the force capabilities of the muscle [4, 105]. After this initial acute response, however, the muscle can regain a normal [67, 34, 156] or a near normal [154] force potential per unit cross-sectional area. Both the force potential and the PCSA of the Plt can double in the rat within 4 weeks. As is the case with the rate of atrophy, the rate of hypertrophy after 12 weeks is similar to the effects at 4 weeks [98].

ETIOLOGY. The amount of daily electrical activity imposed on a muscle, as measured by EMG, is poorly related to muscle mass. In most studies in which muscles have been stimulated chronically for several weeks, for example, the mass and force potential of the stimulated muscle is markedly reduced [55, 163]. After an initial reduction, the daily amount of EMG recorded from the Sol and MG of hindlimb suspended rats is similar to control within 7 days of suspension, yet these muscles continue to atrophy [2, 173]. Further, those fibers that are probably the least active based on accepted recruitment patterns [50, 86, 87], i.e., the FG fibers of FF motor units in predominantly fast muscles, usually are the largest fibers in normal animals [3, 5, 150, 188]. Finally, the amount of atrophy that occurs after virtual absence of motoneuron-driven action potentials for 6 months, i.e., after spinal isolation, is only about 15% in fast extensor muscles and 12% in fast flexor muscles (Roy, Pierotti, Hodgson and Edgerton, unpublished observations).

It appears, therefore, that the variable of utmost importance for a muscle fiber to either maintain its usual size or to enlarge is the production of some minimum level of force for some minimum amount of time. Although cyclical passive stretch can effectively induce fiber hypertrophy in in vitro preparations [184, 185], the level of passive forces that can be imposed in vivo with an intact joint may be limited [42, 43, 155]. Consequently, it appears that the activation and the consequential development of force in a fiber is an essential combination of events in maintaining or increasing fiber size. One of the major limitations in maintaining muscle fiber size in response to chronic stimulation may be an inadequate development of tension due to inadequate loading of the appropriate muscles. In no case, to our knowledge, has muscle force been monitored in a study in which chronic stimulation was used to study muscle plasticity.

Fundamental and relevant issues related to the regulation of fiber size that remain inadequately defined are (1) the influences of action potentials on the size of a fiber of a given type; (2) the influences of force on the cross-sectional area of a fiber of a given type; (3) the cross-sectional area of a fiber uninfluenced by either force or activation; and (4) the role of growth factors in influencing fiber size in conjunction with or in absence of either electrical activation or force production, or both.

Regulation of Mitochrondria
Unlike fiber size, the concentration of mitochrondrial enzymes are elevated by increased levels of neuromuscular activity. The clearest demonstrations of this phenomenon have been the documentation of the increase of virtually all mitochrondrial enzymes related to oxidative metabolism in response to chronic exercise training [95]. Subsequently, numerous studies using chronic electrical stimulation have demonstrated large increases in the activity level of mitochondrial enzymes, particularly those associated with oxidative phosphorylation, i.e., enzymes of the citric acid cycle, the electron transport chain, and fatty acid oxidation [138, 163]. Based largely on these findings, the prevailing concept has been that mitochondrial enzyme activities are controlled by the activity patterns and the consequential metabolic demands of the fiber.

This prevailing concept, however, has some limitations. For example, significant heterogeneity in mitochrondrial enzyme levels across fibers persist in muscles that have been inactive for months [76, 102]. After chronic decreases or even elimination of electrical activity by spinal transection [92, 101] or spinal isolation (76), respectively, the cat Sol maintains SDH activities that are near normal. Further, motor units of each of the physiological types usually associated with mammalian skeletal muscle persist after months of inactivity in the cat TA [142] and after months of decreased activity in the cat MG [122, 128]. It therefore, seems clear that electrical activity is only one of many factors that influences mitochondrial enzyme activities. The appropriate conclusions to be drawn from these results seem to be the following: (1) a significant level of heterogeneity in mitochondrial enzyme concentrations persists among muscle fibers even without electrical activity, and (2) an elevation in the activity level of muscle fibers can induce elevated levels of mitochondrial enzymes.

Regulation of Glycogenesis, Glycogenolysis, and Glycolysis
A most striking and consistent finding discussed is that the glycolytic enzyme GPD is modulated upward in the models that unload the muscle and downward in the models that increase the loading of the muscle. Further, the elevation or decrease in GPD is highly fiber-type specific. For example, in response to hindlimb suspension [74, 75, 84, 85, 151], spaceflight [119, 126], spinalization [31, 92, 100, 101, 118], or spinal isolation [76, 102], those fibers that develop the ability to express fast myosin also exhibit the greatest increase in GPD. An interdependence in the regulation of myosin type and glycolysis and undoubtedly the enzymes associated with glycogenolysis and glycogenesis is strong and

persistent. It is not clear whether the change in enzymes of glycolysis of a fiber precedes the myosin type change or vice versa. In either case, the close association between myosin ATPase type and specific activity and the glycogenolytic enzyme levels suggests that there may be some functional advantage to match the maximal rate of glycogen degradation with the maximal rate of ATP degradation, e.g., during conditions of intense brief muscular activity.

Evidence for the coordination of the proteins that regulate the rate of energy expenditures, e.g., myosin, and the immediate rate of replacement of energy by means of glycolysis is compelling. Interestingly, a significant number of glycolytic enzymes are bound to contractile proteins [133]. Perhaps the interdependence of the types of contractile protein and the enzymes associated with glycogen metabolism should be expected in view of the hypothesis that the release of Ca^{++} which initiates the contractile response also could initiate the metabolic processes that accommodate the energy needs obligatory to activation of cross-bridges. Specifically, glycogenolysis is turned on by the activation of phosphorylase by means of a series of intermediate steps simultaneously with the onset of contraction [34]. Because fast myosin can hydrolyze ATP at about twice the rate as slow myosin and because the flux of substrates through glycolysis can increase by several orders of magnitude to meet the demands for ATP, teleologically it seems appealing for the expression of proteins associated with myosin type and the glycolytic potential of a fiber to be so closely linked.

Fatigability of Muscle and Motor Units
The results from the models of neuromuscular adaptation addressed in the present review demonstrate that muscles and motor units can atrophy without having any effect on their fatigability. For example, the Sol muscle from hindlimb-suspended rats maintain their normal high resistance to fatigue even though the muscle atrophies by more than a third [62, 88, 139, 191]. Similarly, the resistance to fatigue is maintained in the Sol muscle of the cat after 6 months of spinalization [12] and in Sol motor units after 3 to 6 months of spinalization [31, 118]. Even after spinal isolation (inactivity) for 6 months, the Sol maintains a very high resistance to fatigue [49]. These results demonstrate the capacity of slow muscle fibers to sustain their ability to metabolically support the amount of contractile proteins remaining in the cells. In the process of atrophy, if the loss of metabolic and contractile proteins are proportional, then no difference in metabolic support enzyme activities, particularly mitochondrial enzymes, will be observed. At the whole body functional level, however, the atrophied muscles will become more easily fatigued during efforts to complete a given task, because more muscle fibers and motor units will be required to complete the task. Further, the additional motor units necessary to complete the

task are likely to be increasingly susceptible to fatigue. A factor that may be an advantage for an atrophied fiber in resisting fatigue, on the other hand, may be its reduced size, because diffusion and transport distances will be shorter.

Regulation of Myosin Isoforms

The collective findings summarized herein suggest that the relative expression of skeletal isomyosins is heavily influenced by the degree of mechanical or weight-bearing stress imposed on the muscle. Under conditions in which the relative force demand on a mixed-fibered fast-twitch muscle is increased, a selective pool of fibers increase the expression of the slower isoforms of myosin (slow and intermediate). This provides a pool of motor units with greater functional effectiveness in meeting the demands imposed by gravity. In contrast, when the influence of gravity and weight-bearing responsibility are reduced (as in spaceflight), those muscles that normally express predominantly the slower isomyosins undergo atrophy and down-regulation of slow myosin expression. The pattern, therefore, of myosin that is expressed in muscle is somewhat plastic and subject to adaptation in accordance with the mechanical stress imposed on the fibers. The mechanisms by which the mechanical stress regulates the myosin genes remain to be resolved.

ACKNOWLEDGEMENTS

The authors would like to thank the numerous co-authors on the manuscripts cited from our laboratories in this review. Dr. S. C. Bodine and Mr. D. J. Pierotti also are thanked for their critical reading and helpful comments on the manuscript. This work has been supported in large part by NIH Grants NS16333 and AR30346 and NASA Grants NCA-1R 390-502 and NAG2-555.

REFERENCES

1. Alaimo, M.A., J.L. Smith, R.R. Roy, and V.R. Edgerton. EMG activity of slow and fast ankle extensors following spinal cord transection. *J. Appl. Physiol.* 56:1608–1613, 1984.
2. Alford, E.K., R.R. Roy, J.A. Hodgson, and V.R. Edgerton. Electromyography of rat soleus, medial gastrocnemius and tibialis anterior during hindlimb suspension. *Exp. Neurol.* 96:635–649, 1987.
3. Armstrong, R.B., and R.O. Phelps. Muscle fiber type composition of the rat hindlimb. *Am. J. Anat.* 171:259–272, 1984.
4. Armstrong, R.B., P. Marum, P. Tullson, and C.W. Saubert IV. Acute hypertrophic response of skeletal muscle to removal of synergists. *J. Appl. Physiol.* 46:835–842, 1979.
5. Armstrong, R.B., C.W. Saubert, IV, H.J. Seeherman, and C.R. Taylor. Distribution of fiber types in locomotory muscles dogs. *Am. J. Anat.* 163:87–98, 1982.

6. Baldwin, K.M., S.L. Hillman, and V. Valdez. Fatigue and metabolic patterns of overloaded fast-twitch rodent skeletal muscle contracting in situ. *Int. Series Sports Sci.* 13:859–863, 1983.
7. Baldwin, K.M., O.M. Martinez, and W.G. Cheadle. Enzymatic changes in hypertrophied fast-twitch skeletal muscle. *Pflugers Arch.* 364:229–234, 1976.
8. Baldwin, K.M., W.G. Cheadle, O.M. Martinez, and D.A. Cooke. Effect of functional overload on enzyme levels in different types of skeletal muscle. *J. Appl. Physiol.* 42:312–317, 1977.
9. Baldwin, K.M., R.E. Herrick, E. Ilyina-Kakueva, and V.S. Oganov. Effects of zero gravity on myofibril content and isomyosin distribution in rodent skeletal muscle. *FASEB J.* 4:79–83, 1990.
10. Baldwin, K.M., R.R. Roy, V.R. Edgerton, and R.E. Herrick. Interaction of nerve activity and skeletal muscle mechanical activity in regulating isomyosin expression. G. Benzi (ed.). *Advances in Myochemistry*. London: John Libbey Eurotext Ltd., 1989, pp. 83–92.
11. Baldwin, K.M., V. Valdez, L.F. Schrader, and R.E. Herrick. Effect of functional overload on substrate oxidation capacity of skeletal muscle. *J. Appl. Physiol.* 50:1272–1276, 1981.
12. Baldwin, K.M., R.R. Roy, R.D. Sacks, C. Blanco, and V.R. Edgerton. Relative independence of metabolic enzymes and neuromuscular activity. *J. Appl. Physiol.* 56:1602–1607, 1984.
13. Baldwin, K.M., D.G. Thomason, H. Phan, R.R. Roy, and V.R. Edgerton. Myosin isoform distribution in mammalian skeletal muscles: effects of altered usage. G. Benzi, L. Packer, and N. Siliprandi (eds.). *Biochemical Aspects of Physical Exercise, Vol. 2*. London: Elsevier Science Publishers, 1986, pp. 15–26.
14. Baldwin, K.M., V. Valdez, R.E. Herrick, A.M. MacIntosh, and R.R. Roy. Biochemical properties of overloaded fast-twitch skeletal muscle. *J. Appl. Physiol.* 52:467–472, 1982.
15. Barany, M. ATPase activity of myosin correlated with speed of muscle shortening. *J. Gen. Physiol.* 50:197–218, 1967.
16. Bodine, S.C., A. Garfinkel, R.R. Roy, and V.R. Edgerton. Spatial distribution of motor unit fibers in the cat soleus and tibialis anterior muscles: local interactions. *J. Neurosci* 8:2142–2152, 1988.
17. Bodine, S.C., R.R. Roy, E. Eldred, and V.R. Edgerton. Maximal force as a function of anatomical features of motor units in the cat tibialis anterior. *J. Neurophysiol.* 57:1730–1745, 1987.
18. Bodine, S.C., A. Garfinkel, R.R. Roy, and V.R. Edgerton. Spatial distribution of muscle fibers within the territory of a motor unit. *Muscle & Nerve* 13:1133–1145, 1990.
19. Buller, A.J., J.C. Eccles, and R.M. Eccles. Interactions between motoneurones and muscles in respect of the characteristic speeds of their responses. *J. Physiol. (London)* 150:417–439, 1960.
20. Burke, R.E.: Motor units: anatomy, physiology and functional organization. J.M. Brookhart and V.B. Mountcastle (eds.). *Handbook of Physiology. The Nervous System. Motor Control*. Bethesda, MD: American Physiological Society, Vol. 2, Part 1, Section 1, 1981, pp. 345–422.
21. Burke, R.E., D.N. Levine, M. Salcman, and P. Tsairis: Motor units in cat soleus muscle: physiological, histochemical and morphological characteristics. *J. Physiol. (London)* 238:503–514, 1974.
22. Chalmers, G.R., and V.R. Edgerton. Single motoneuron succinate dehydrogenase activity. *J. Histochem. Cytochem.* 37:1107–1114, 1989.
23. Chalmers, G.R., R.R. Roy, and V.R. Edgerton. Effect of quantity of action potentials on motoneuron oxidative capacity. *Soc. Neurosci. Abstr.* 15:919, 1989.
24. Chalmers, G.R., R.R. Roy, and V.R. Edgerton. Coordination of succinate dehydro-

genase activity between motoneurons and muscle fibers in the normal and functionally overloaded cat plantaris. *Soc. Neurosci. Abstr.* 16:119, 1990.

25. Chan, A.K., V.R. Edgerton, G.E. Goslow, Jr., H. Kurata, S.A. Rasmussen, and S.A. Spector. Histochemical and physiological properties of cat motor units after self- and cross-reinnervation. *J. Physiol. (London)* 332:343–361, 1982.

26. Chui, L.A., and K.R. Castleman. Morphometric analysis of rat muscle fibers following space flight and hypogravity. *Physiologist* 23:S76–S78, 1980.

27. Clement, G, and C. Andre-Deshays. Motor activity and visually induced postural reactions during two-g and zero-g phases of parabolic flight. *Neurosci. Lett.* 79:113–116, 1987.

28. Clement, G., and F. Lestienne. Adaptive modifications of postural attitude in conditions of weightlessness. *Exp. Brain Res.* 72:381–389, 1988.

29. Clement, G., V.S. Gurfinkel, and F. Lestienne. Mechanisms of posture maintenance in weightlessness. Igarashi and Black (eds.). *Vestibular and Visual Control of Posture and Locomotor Equilibrium.* Basel: Karger, 1983, pp. 158–163.

30. Close, R.I. Dynamic properties of mammalian skeletal muscles. *Physiol. Rev.* 52:129–197, 1972.

31. Cope, T.C., S.C. Bodine, M. Fournier, and V.R. Edgerton. Soleus motor units in chronic spinal transected cat: physiological and morphological alterations. *J. Neurophysiol.* 55:1201–1220, 1986.

32. Czeh, G., R. Gallego, N. Kudo, and M. Kuno. Evidence for the maintenance of motoneurone properties of muscle activity. *J. Physiol. (London)* 281:239–252, 1978.

33. Darr, K.C., and E. Schultz. Hindlimb suspension suppresses muscle growth and satellite cell proliferation. *J. Appl. Physiol.* 67:1827–1834, 1989.

34. Dawson, M.J. The relation between muscle contraction and metabolism: studies by ^{31}P nuclear magnetic resonance spectroscopy. *Adv. Exp. Med Biol.* 226:433–448, 1988.

35. de Guzman, C.P., R.R. Roy, J.A. Hodgson, and V.R. Edgerton. EMG amplitude relationships in hindlimb muscles of adult spinal cats during locomotion. *Med. Sci. Sports Exer.* 22:S117, 1990.

36. Desplanches, D., M.H. Mayet, B. Sempore, and R. Flandrois. Structural and functional responses to prolonged hindlimb suspension in rat muscle. *J. Appl. Physiol.* 63:558–563, 1987.

37. Desplanches, D., M.H. Mayet, B. Sempore, J. Frutoso, R. Flandrois. Effect of spontaneous recovery or retraining after hindlimb suspension on aerobic capacity. *J. Appl. Physiol.* 63:1739–1743, 1987.

38. Desplances, D., M.H. Mayet, E.I. Ilyina-Kakueva, B. Sempore, and R. Flandrois. Skeletal muscle adaptation in rats flown on Cosmos 1667. *J. Appl. Physiol.* 68:48–52, 1990.

39. Donselaar, Y., D. Kernell, and O. Eerbeek. Soma size and oxidative enzyme activity in normal and chronically stimulated motoneurones of the cat's spinal cord. *Brain Res.* 385:22–29, 1986.

40. Dulhunty, A.F., P.W. Gage, and A. Valois. Indentations in the terminal cisternae of slow-and-fast twitch muscle fibers from normal and paraplegic rats. *J. Ultrastruct. Res.* 84:50–59, 1983.

41. Dum, R.P., and T.T. Kennedy. Physiological and histochemical characteristics of motor units in cat tibialis anterior and extensor digitorum longus muscles. *J. Neurophysiol.* 43:1615–1630, 1980.

42. Eccles, J.C. Disuse atrophy of skeletal muscle. *Med. J. Australia* 2:160–164, 1941.

43. Eccles, J.C. Investigations on muscle atrophies arising from disuse and tenotomy. *J. Physiol. (London)* 103:253–266, 1944.

44. Edgerton, V.R., and R.R. Roy. Adaptations of skeletal muscle to spaceflight. S. Churchill (ed.). *Fundamentals of Space Life Sciences.* Cambridge, MA: MIT Press, 1990 (In Press).

45. Edgerton, V.R., R.R. Roy, and G.R. Chalmers. Does the size principle give insight into the energy requirements of motoneurons? M.D. Binder and L.M. Mendell (eds.). *The Segmental Motor System.* New York: Oxford University Press, 1989, pp. 150–164.

46. Edgerton, V.R., G.E. Goslow, Jr, S.A. Rasmussen, and S.A. Spector. Is resistance to fatigue controlled by its motoneurones? *Nature* 285:589–590, 1980.

47. Edgerton, V.R., T.P. Martin, S.C. Bodine, and R.R. Roy. How flexible is the neural control of muscle properties? *J. Exp. Biol.* 115:393–402, 1985.

48. Edgerton, V.R., R.R. Roy, S.C. Bodine, and R.D. Sacks. The matching of neuronal and muscular physiology. K.T. Borer, D.W. Edington, and T.P. White (eds.). *Frontiers of Exercise Biology.* Chicago: Human Kinetics Publishers, 1983, pp. 51–70.

49. Edgerton, V.R., R.R. Roy, L. Eldridge, and M. Liebhold. Maintenance of differences in fatigability of slow and fast muscle with prolonged inactivity. *Med. Sci. Sports Exerc.* 13:87, 1981.

50. Edgerton, V.R., R.R. Roy, R.J. Gregor, C.L. Hager, and T. Wickiewicz. Muscle fiber activation and recruitment. H. Knuttgen, J. Vogel, and J. Poortmans (eds.). *Biochemistry of Exercise, International Series of Sport Sciences.* Chicago: Human Kinetics Publishers, 1983, pp. 31–49.

51. Edgerton V.R., L.A. Smith, E. Eldred, T.C. Cope, L.M. Mendell. Muscle and motor unit properties of exercised and non-exercised chronic spinal cats. D. Pette (ed.). *Plasticity of Muscle.* Berlin: Walter de Gruyter, 1980, pp. 355–371.

52. Edgerton, V.R., C.P. de Guzman, R.J. Gregor, R.R. Roy, J.A. Hodgson, and R.G. Lovely. Trainability of the spinal cord to generate hindlimb stepping patterns in adult spinalized cats. M. Shimamura, S. Grillner, and V.R. Edgerton (eds.). *Neurophysiological Bases of Human Locomotion.* Berlin: Springer-Verlag, 1990 (In Press).

53. Edgerton V.R., D.J. Johnson, L.A. Smith, K. Murphy, E. Eldred, and J.L. Smith. Effects of treadmill exercises on hindlimb muscles of the spinal cat. C.C. Kao, R.P. Bunge, and P.J. Reier (eds.). *Spinal Cord Reconstruction.* New York: Raven Press, 1983, pp. 435–443.

54. Edgerton, V.R., R.R. Roy, S.C. Bodine-Fowler, et al. Motoneurons—muscle fiber connectivity and interdependence. In D. Pette (ed.). The Dynamic State of Muscle Fibers. Berlin: Walter de Gruyter, 1990, pp. 217–231.

55. Eisenberg, B.R., J.M.C. Brown, and S. Salmons. Restoration of fast muscle characteristics following cessation of chronic stimulation: the ultrastructure of slow-to-fast transformation. *Cell Tissue Res.* 238:221–230, 1984.

56. Eldridge, L. Lumbosacral spinal isolation in cat: surgical preparation and health maintenance. *Exp. Neurol.* 83:318–327, 1984.

57. Eldridge, L., and W.F.H.M. Mommaerts. Ability of electrical silent nerves to specify fast and slow muscle characteristics. D. Pette (ed.). *Plasticity of Muscle.* New York: Walter de Gruyter, 1981, pp. 325–337.

58. Eldridge, L., G.K. Dhoot, and W.F.H.M. Mommaerts. Neural influences on the distribution of troponin I isotypes in the cat. *Exp. Neurol.* 83:328–346, 1984.

59. Eldridge, L., M. Liebhold, and J.H. Steinbach. Alterations in cat skeletal neuromuscular junctions following prolonged inactivity. *J. Physiol. (London)* 313:529–545, 1981.

60. English, A.W. An electromyographic analysis of compartments in cat lateral gastrocnemius muscle during unrestrained locomotion. *J. Neurophysiol.* 52:114–125, 1984.

61. English, A.W., and O.I. Weeks. Compartmentalization of single units in cat lateral gastrocnemius. *Exp. Brain Res.* 56:361–368, 1984.

62. Fell, R.D., L.B. Gladden, J.M. Steffen, and X.J. Musacchia. Fatigue and contraction of slow and fast muscles in hypokinetic/hypodynamic rats. *J. Appl. Physiol.* 58:65–69, 1985.

63. Fitts, R.F., C.J. Brimmer, A. Heywood-Cooksey, and R.J. Timmerman. Single muscle

fiber enzyme shifts with hindlimb suspension and immobilization. *Am. J. Physiol.* 256:C1082–C1091, 1989.

64. Fitts, R.H., J.M. Metzger, D.A. Riley, B.R. Unsworth. Models of disuse: a comparison of hindlimb suspension and immobilization. *J. Appl. Physiol.* 60:1946–1953, 1986.

65. Fitts, R.H., W.W. Winder, M.H. Brooke, K.K. Kaiser, and J.O. Holloszy. Contractile, biochemical, and histochemical properties of thyrotoxic rat soleus muscle. *Am. J. Physiol.* 238:C15–C20, 1980.

66. Fitzsimmons, D.P., R.E. Herrick, and K.M. Baldwin. Isomyosin distributions in rodent muscles: effects of altered thyroid states. *J. Appl. Physiol.* 69:321–327, 1990.

67. Freeman, P.L., and A.R. Luff. Contractile properties of hindlimb muscles in rat during surgical overload. *Am. J. Physiol.* 242:C259–C264, 1982.

68. Gallego, R., P. Huizar, N. Kudo, and M. Kuno. Disparity of motoneurone and muscle differentiation following spinal transection in the kitten. *J. Physiol. (London)* 281:253–265, 1978.

69. Gardetto, P.R., J.M. Schluter, and R.H. Fitts. Contractile function of single muscle fibers after hindlimb suspension. *J. Appl. Physiol.* 66:2739–2749, 1989.

70. Gardiner, P., R. Michel, C. Browman, and E. Noble. Increased EMG of rat plantaris during locomotion following surgical removal of its synergists. *Brain Res.* 380:114–121, 1986.

71. Garfinkel, A., R.R. Roy, D.O. Walter, et al. Spatial distribution of dark ATPase fibers in the adult cat soleus muscle six months after spinal transection. *Soc. Neurosci. Abstr.* 15:66, 1989.

72. Goldspink, G., R.E. Larson, and R.E. Davies. The immediate energy supply and the cost maintenance of isometric tension for different muscles in the hamster. *Z. vergl Physiol.* 66:389–397, 1970.

73. Goslow, G.E., R.M. Reinking, and D.G. Stuart. The cat step cycle: hindlimb joint angles and muscle lengths during unrestrained locomotion. *J. Morphol.* 141:1–42, 1973.

74. Graham, S.C., R.R. Roy, E.O. Hauschka, and V.R. Edgerton. Effects of weight support on medial gastrocnemius fibers of suspended rats. *J. Appl. Physiol.* 67:945–953, 1989.

75. Graham, S.C., R.R. Roy, S.P. West, D. Thomason, and K.M. Baldwin. Exercise effects on the size and metabolic properties of soleus fibers in hindlimb-suspended rats. *Aviat. Space Environ. Med.* 60:226–234, 1989.

76. Graham, S.C., R.R. Roy, C. Navarro, et al. Enzyme and size profiles in chronically inactive cat soleus muscle fibers. *Muscle & Nerve* (In Press).

77. Greenleaf, J.E., R. Bulbulian, E.M. Bernauer, W.L. Haskell, and T. Moore. Exercise-training protocols for astronauts in microgravity. *J. Appl. Physiol.* 67:2191–2204, 1989.

78. Gregor, R.J., E.G. Fowler, and R.R. Roy. Motor output capabilities of adult spinal cats following postural training. *Soc. Neurosci. Abstr.* 14:64, 1988.

79. Gregor, R.J., R.R. Roy, W.C. Whiting, R.G. Lovely, J.A. Hodgson, and V.R. Edgerton. Mechanical output of the cat soleus during treadmill locomotion: in vivo vs in situ characteristics. *J. Biomechanics* 21:721–732, 1988.

80. Gregory, P., R.B. Low, and W.S. Stirewalt. Changes in skeletal-muscle myosin isoenzymes with hypertrophy and exercise. *Biochem. J.* 238:55–63, 1986.

81. Grimby, G., C. Broberg, I. Krotkiewska, and M. Krotkiewski. Muscle fiber composition in patients with traumatic cord lesion. *Scand. J. Rehab. Med.* 8:37–42, 1976.

82. Grindeland, R., T. Fast, M. Ruder, et al. Rodent body, organ, and muscle weight responses to seven days of microgravity. *Physiologist* 28:375, 1985.

83. Handa, Y., A. Naito, S. Watanabe, S. Komatsu, and Y. Shimizu. Functional recovery of locomotive behavior in the adult dog. *Tohoku J. Exp. Med.* 148:373–384, 1986.

84. Hauschka, E.O., R.R. Roy, and V.R. Edgerton. Size and metabolic properties of

single muscle fibers in rat soleus after hindlimb suspension. *J. Appl. Physiol.* 62:2338–2347, 1987.

85. Hauschka, E.O., R.R. Roy, and V.R. Edgerton. Periodic weight support effects on rat soleus fibers after hindlimb suspension. *J. Appl. Physiol.* 65:1231–1237, 1988.

86. Henneman, E., and L.M. Mendell. Functional organization of motoneuron pool and its input. B. Brookhart, V.B. Mountcastle, V.B. Brooks, and S.R. Geiger (eds.). *Handbook of Physiology. Section 1. The Nervous System. Vol. II. Motor Control. Part I.* Bethesda, MD: American Physiological Society, 1981, pp. 423–507.

87. Henneman, E., G. Somjen, and D.O. Carpenter. Functional significance of cell size in spinal motoneurons. *J. Neurophysiol.* 28:560–580, 1965.

88. Herbert, M.E., R.R. Roy, and V.R. Edgerton. Influence of one week of hindlimb suspension and intermittent high load exercise on rat muscles. *Exp. Neurol.* 102:190–198, 1988.

89. Hill, A.V. The heat of shortening and the dynamic constants of muscle. *Proc. R. Soc. Lond. Ser. B* 126:136–195, 1938.

90. Hnik, P., R. Vejsada, and E.V. Mackova. EMG activity in "compensatory" muscle hypertrophy. *Physiol. Bohemoslov.* 35:285–288, 1986.

91. Hodgson, J.A. The relationship between soleus and gastrocnemius muscle activity in conscious cats—a model for motor unit recruitment? *J. Physiol. (London)* 337:553–562, 1983.

92. Hoffmann, S.J., R.R. Roy, C.E. Blanco, and V.R. Edgerton. Enzyme profiles of single fibers never exposed to normal neuromuscular activity. *J. Appl. Physiol.* 69:1150–1158, 1990.

93. Hoh, J.F.Y., and C.J. Chow. The effect of the loss of weight-bearing function on the isomyosin profile and contractile properties of rat skeletal muscles. A.D. Kidman, J.K. Tomkins, C.A. Morris, and N.A. Cooper (eds.). *Molecular Pathology of Nerve and Muscle.* New Jersey: Humana Press, 1983, pp. 371–383.

94. Hoh, J.F.Y., B.T.S. Kwan, C. Dunlop, and B.H. Kim. Effects of nerve cross-union and cordotomy on myosin isoenzymes in fast-twitch and slow-twitch muscles of the rat. D. Pette (ed.). *Muscle Plasticity.* Berlin: de Gruyter, 1980, pp. 339–352.

95. Holloszy, J.O., and F.W. Booth. Biochemical adaptations to endurance exercise in muscle. *Ann. Rev. Physiol.* 38:273–291, 1976.

96. Hutchison, D.L., R.R. Roy, J.A. Hodgson, and V.R. Edgerton. EMG amplitude relationships between the rat soleus and medial gastrocnemius during various motor tasks. *Brain Res.* 502:233–244, 1989.

97. Hutchison, D.L., R.R. Roy, S. Bodine-Fowler, J.A. Hodgson, and V.R. Edgerton. Electromyographic (EMG) amplitude patterns in the proximal and distal compartments of the cat semitendinosus during various motor tasks. *Brain Res.* 479:56–64, 1989.

98. Ianuzzo, C.D., and V. Chen. Metabolic character of hypertrophied rat muscle. *J. Appl. Physiol.* 46:738–742, 1979.

99. Izumo, S., B. Nadal-Girard, and V. Mahdavi. All members of the MHC multigene family respond to thyroid hormone in a highly tissue-specific manner. *Science* 231:597–600, 1986.

100. Jiang, B., R.R. Roy, and V.R. Edgerton. Enzymatic plasticity of medial gastrocnemius fibers in the adult spinal cat. *Am. J. Physiol.* 259:C507–C514, 1990.

101. Jiang, B., R.R. Roy, and V.R. Edgerton. Expression of a fast fiber enzyme profile in the cat soleus after spinalization. *Muscle & Nerve.* 13:1037–1049, 1990.

102. Jiang, B., R.R. Roy, C. Navarro, Q. Nguyen, D. Pierotti, and V.R. Edgerton. Enzymatic responses of cat medial gastrocnemius fibers to chronic inactivity. *J. Appl. Physiol.* (In Press).

103. Johnson, D.L., L.A. Smith, E. Eldred, and V.R. Edgerton. Exercise-induced changes of biochemical, contractile and histochemical properties of muscle in cordotomized kittens. *Exp. Neurol.* 76:414–427, 1982.

104. Jolesz, F., and F.A. Sreter. Development, innervation, and activity-pattern induced changes in skeletal muscle. *Ann. Rev. Physiol.* 43:531–552, 1981.

105. Kandarian, S.C., and T.P. White. Force deficit during the onset of muscle hypertrophy. *J. Appl. Physiol.* 67:2600–2607, 1989.

106. Karpati G., and W.K. Engel. Correlative histochemical study of skeletal muscle after suprasegmental denervation, peripheral nerve section, and skeletal fixation. *Neurology* 18:681–692, 1968.

107. Kushmerick, M.J. Energetics of muscle contraction. S.R. Geiger, R.H. Adrian, and L.D. Peachey (eds.). *Handbook of Physiology.* Baltimore, MD: American Physiological Society, 1983, pp. 189–236.

108. Laufer, R., and J.P. Changeux. Calcitonin gene-related peptide elevates cyclic AMP levels in chick skeletal muscle: Possible neurotrophic role for a coexisting neuronal messenger. *EMBO J.* 6:901–906, 1987.

109. LeBlanc A, C. Marsh, H. Evans, P. Johnson, V. Schneider, and S. Jhingran. Bone and muscle atrophy with suspension of the rat. *J. Appl. Physiol.* 58:1669–1675, 1985.

110. Lestienne, F.G., and V.S. Gurfinkel. Postural control in weightlessness: a dual process underlying adaptation to an unusual environment. *TINS* 11:359–363, 1988.

111. Lestienne, F.G., and V.S. Gurfinkel. Posture as an organizational structure based on a dual process: a formal basis to interpret changes of posture in weightlessness. O. Pompeiano and J.H.J. Allum (eds.). *Progress in Brain Research, Vol. 76.* London: Elsevier Science Publishers B.V., 1988, pp. 307–313.

112. Lieber, R.L., J.O. Friden, A.R. Hargens, and E.R. Feringa. Long-term effects of spinal transection on fast and slow rat skeletal muscle. II. Morphometric properties. *Exp. Neurol.* 91:435–448, 1986.

113. Lieber, R.L., C.B. Johansson, H.L. Vahlsing, A.R. Hargens, and E.R. Feringa. Long-term effects of spinal cord transection on fast and slow rat skeletal muscle. I. Contractile properties. *Exp. Neurol.* 91:423–434, 1986.

114. Lomo, T., R.H. Westgaard, and H.A. Dahl. Contractile properties of muscle: control by pattern of muscle activity in the rat. *Proc. Roy. Soc. Med. B.* 187:99–103, 1974.

115. Lovely, R.G., R.J. Gregor, R.R. Roy, and V.R. Edgerton. Effects of training on the recovery of full weight bearing stepping in the adult spinal cat. *Exp. Neurol.* 92:421–435, 1986.

116. Lovely, R.G., R.J. Gregor, R.R. Roy, and V.R. Edgerton. Weight-bearing hindlimb stepping in treadmill-exercised adult spinal cats. *Brain Res.* 514:206–218, 1990.

117. Manchester, J.K., M. M.-Y. Chi, B. Norris, et al. Effect of microgravity on metabolic enzymes of individual muscle fibers. *FASEB J.* 4:55–63, 1990.

118. Martin, T.P., S. Bodine-Fowler, and V.R. Edgerton. Coordination of electromechanical and metabolic properties of cat soleus motor units. *Am. J. Physiol.* 255:C684–C693, 1988.

119. Martin, T.P., V.R. Edgerton, and R.E. Grindeland. Influence of spaceflight on rat skeletal muscle. *J. Appl. Physiol.* 65:2318–2325, 1988.

120. Martin, T.P., S. Bodine-Fowler, R.R. Roy, E. Eldred, and V.R. Edgerton. Metabolic and fiber size properties of cat tibialis anterior motor units. *Am. J. Physiol.* 255:C43–C50, 1988.

121. Martin, T.P., A.C. Vailas, J.B. Durivage, V.R. Edgerton, and K.R. Castleman. Quantitative histochemical determination of muscle enzymes: biochemical verification. *J. Histochem. Cytochem.* 33:1053–1059, 1985.

122. Mayer, R.F., R.E. Burke, J. Toop, B. Walmsley, and J.A. Hodgson. The effect of spinal cord transection on motor units in cat medial gastrocnemius muscles. *Muscle & Nerve* 7:23–31, 1984.

123. Meadows, I.D., R.R. Roy, P.L. Powell, and V.R. Edgerton. Contractile and fatigue properties of the compensatory overloaded cat plantaris. *Physiologist* 25:260, 1982.

124. Michel, R.N., A.E. Olha, and P.F. Gardiner. Influence of weight bearing on the

adaptations of rat plantaris to ablation of its synergists. *J. Appl. Physiol.* 67:636–642, 1989.

125. Midrio, M., D.D. Betto, R. Betto, D. Noventa, and F. Antico. Cordotomy-denervation interactions on contractile and myofibrillar properties of fast and slow muscles in the rat. *Exp. Neurol.* 100:216–236, 1988.

126. Miu, B., T.P. Martin, R.R. Roy, et al. Metabolic and morphologic properties of single fibers in the rat after space flight, Cosmos 1887. *FASEB J.* 4:64–72, 1990.

127. Morey, E.R. Spaceflight and bone turnover: correlation with a new rat model of weightlessness. *Bioscience* 29:168–172, 1979.

128. Munson, J.B., R.C. Foehring, S.A. Lofton, J.E. Zengel, and G.W. Sypert. Plasticity of medial gastrocnemius motor units following cordotomy in the cat. *J. Neurophysiol.* 55:619–633, 1986.

129. Musacchia, X.J., J.M. Steffen and R.D. Fell. Disuse atrophy of skeletal muscle: animal models. K.B. Pandolf (ed). *Exercise and Sport Science Reviews, Vo. 16.* New York: Macmillan Publishing, 1988, pp. 61–87.

130. Musacchia, X.J., J.M. Steffen, R.D. Fell, and M.J. Dombrowski. Comparative morphometry of fibers and capillaries in soleus following weightlessness (SL-3) and suspension. *Physiologist* 31:S28–S29, 1988.

131. Nesmeyanova, T.N. *Experimental Studies in the Regeneration of Spinal Neurons.* Washington, D.C.: V.H. Winston & Sons, 1977, pp. 61–64.

132. Nwoye, L., W.F.H.M. Mommaerts, D.R. Simpson, K. Seraydarian, and M. Marusich. Evidence for a direct action of thyroid hormone in specifying muscle properties. *Am. J. Physiol.* 242:R401–R408, 1982.

133. Offer, G., R. Starr, and J. Trinick. Phosphofructokinase: a component of the thick filament? *Adv. Exp. Med. Biol.* 226:61–73, 1988.

134. Olha, A.E., B.J. Jasmin, R.N. Michel, and P.F. Gardiner. Physiological responses of rat plantaris motor units to overload induced by surgical removal of its synergists. *J. Neurophysiol.* 60:2138–2151, 1988.

135. Pearson, J.K., and D.W. Sickles. Enzyme activity changes in rat soleus motoneurons and muscle after synergist ablation. *J. Appl. Physiol.* 63:2301–2308, 1987.

136. Perell, K.L., R.J. Gregor, E.G. Fowler, J.A. Hodgson, and R.R. Roy. Kinetic and kinematic analysis of locomotor capabilities of posturally trained adult spinal cats. *Soc. Neurosci. Abstr.* 15:394, 1989.

137. Peter, J.B., R.J. Barnard, V.R. Edgerton, C.A. Gillespie, and K.E. Stempel. Metabolic profiles of three fiber types of skeletal muscle in guinea pigs and rabbits. *Biochemistry* 11:2627–2633, 1972.

138. Pette, D., and G. Vrbova. Neural control of phenotypic expression in mammalian muscle fibres. *Muscle & Nerve* 8:676–689, 1985.

139. Pierotti, D.J., R.R. Roy, V. Flores, and V.R. Edgerton. Influence of 7 days of hindlimb suspension and intermittent weight support on rat muscle mechanical properties. *Aviat. Space Environ. Med.* 61:205–210, 1990.

140. Pierotti, D.J., R.R. Roy, R.J. Gregor, and V.R. Edgerton. Electromyographic activity of cat hindlimb flexors and extensors during locomotion at varying speeds and inclines. *Brain Res.* 481:57–66, 1989.

141. Pierotti, D.J., R.R. Roy, J.A. Hodgson, and V.R. Edgerton. Histochemical profiles of motor units of cat tibialis anterior after 6 months of electrical inactivity. *Soc. Neurosci. Abstr.* 16:329, 1990.

142. Pierotti, D.J., R.R. Roy, J.A. Hodgson, S. Bodine-Fowler, and V.R. Edgerton. Motor units of the cat tibialis anterior 6 months after spinal isolation. *Soc. Neurosci. Abstr.* 15:67, 1989.

143. Portugalov, V.V., and N.V. Petrova. LDH isoenzymes of skeletal muscles of rats after space flight and hypokinesia. *Aviat. Space Environ. Med.* 47:834–838, 1976.

144. Powell, P.L., R.R. Roy, P. Kanim, M.A. Bello, and V.R. Edgerton. Predictability of

skeletal muscle tension from architectural determinations in guinea pig hindlimbs. *J. Appl. Physiol.* 57:1715–1721, 1984.

145. Reiser, P.J., C.E. Kasper and R.L. Moss. Myosin subunits and contractile properties of single fibers from hypokinetic rat muscles. *J. Appl. Physiol.* 63:2293–2300, 1987.

146. Riedy, M., R.L. Moore, and P.D. Gollnick. Adaptive response of hypertrophied skeletal muscle to endurance training. *J. Appl. Physiol.* 59:127–131, 1985.

147. Riley, D.A., and S. Ellis. Research on the adaptation of skeletal muscle to hypogravity: past and future directions. *Adv. Space Res.* 3:191–197, 1983.

148. Riley, D.A., S. Ellis, G.R. Slocum, T. Satyanarayana, J.L. W. Bain, and F.R. Sedlak. Hypogravity-induced atrophy of rat soleus and extensor digitorum longus muscles. *Muscle & Nerve.* 10:560–568, 1987.

149. Riley, D.A., E.I. Ilyina-Kakueva, S. Ellis, J.L.W. Bain, G.R. Slocum, and F.R. Sedlak. Skeletal muscle fiber, nerve, and blood vessel breakdown in space-flown rats. *FASEB J.* 84–91, 1990.

150. Roy, R.R., and L. Acosta, Jr. Fiber type and fiber size changes in selected thigh muscles six months after low thoracic spinal cord transection in adult cats: exercise effects. *Exp. Neurol.* 92:675–685, 1986.

151. Roy, R.R., M.A. Bello, P. Boissou, and V.R. Edgerton. Size and metabolic properties of fibers in fast-twitch muscles after hindlimb suspension. *J. Appl. Physiol.* 62:2348–2357, 1987.

152. Roy, R.R., W.K. Hirota, M. Kuehl, and V.R. Edgerton. Recruitment patterns in the rat hindlimb muscle during swimming. *Brain Res.* 337:175–178, 1985.

153. Roy, R.R., D.L. Hutchison, J.A. Hodgson, and V.R. Edgerton. EMG amplitude patterns in rat soleus and medial gastrocnemius following seven days of hindlimb suspension. *IEEE Eng. Med. Biol.* 10:1710–1711, 1988.

154. Roy, R.R., I.D. Meadows, K.M. Baldwin, and V.R. Edgerton. Functional significance of compensatory overloaded rat fast muscle. *J. Appl. Physiol.* 52:473–478, 1982.

155. Roy, R.R., D.J. Pierotti, K.M. Baldwin, and V.R. Edgerton. Effects of cyclical passive stretch in maintaining cat soleus mechanical properties. *Soc. Neurosci. Abstr.* 14:948, 1988.

156. Roy, R.R., K.M. Baldwin, T.P. Martin, S.P. Chimarusti, and V.R. Edgerton. Biochemical and physiological changes in overloaded rat fast and slow ankle extensors. *J. Appl. Physiol.* 59:639–646, 1985.

157. Roy, R.R., K.M. Baldwin, R.D. Sacks, L. Eldridge, and V.R. Edgerton. Mechanical and metabolic properties after prolonged inactivation and/or cross-reinnervation of cat soleus. *Med. Sci. Sports Exerc.* 19:S50, 1987.

158. Roy, R.R., R.J. Gregor, R.G. Lovely, K.M. Baldwin, and V.R. Edgerton. Long-term exercise effects on the mechanical properties of the soleus muscle in adult spinal cats. *Soc. Neurosci. Abstr.* 11:1101, 1985.

159. Roy, R.R., R.D. Sacks, K.M. Baldwin, M. Short, and V.R. Edgerton. Interrelationships of contraction time, Vmax and myosin ATPase after spinal transection. *J. Appl. Physiol.* 56:1594–1601, 1984.

160. Roy, R.R., V. Flores, R.J. Gregor, R.G. Lovely, K.M. Baldwin, and V.R. Edgerton. Contractile and biochemical properties of hindlimb extensors and flexors from cats spinalized as adults and maintained for six months: exercise effects. *Soc. Neurosci. Abstr.* 12:685, 1986.

161. Roy, R.R., D.L. Hutchison, D.J. Pierotti, J.A. Hodgson, and V.R. Edgerton. EMG patterns of rat ankle extensors and flexors during treadmill locomotion and swimming. *J. Appl. Physiol.* (In Press).

162. Sacks, R.D., and R.R. Roy. Architecture of the hind limb muscles of cats: Functional significance. *J. Morphol.* 173:185–195, 1982.

163. Salmons, S., and J. Henriksson. The adaptive response of skeletal muscle to increased use. *Muscle & Nerve* 4:94–105, 1981.

164. Saltin, B., and P.D. Gollnick. Skeletal muscle adaptability: significance for metabolism

and performance. L.D. Peachey (ed.). *Handbook of Physiology. Section 10. Skeletal Muscle.* Baltimore: American Physiological Soceity, 1983, pp. 555–631.

165. Schiaffino, S., L. Gorza, G. Pitton, et al. Embryonic and neonatal myosin heavy chain in denervated and paralyzed rat skeletal muscle. *Dev. Biol.* 127:1–11, 1988.

166. Shaw, S.R., R.F. Zernicke, A.C. Vailas, D. DeLuna, D.B. Thomason, and K.M. Baldwin. Mechanical, morphological and biochemical adaptations of bone and muscle to hindlimb suspension and exercise. *J. Biomechanics* 20:225–234, 1987.

167. Sherif, M.H., R.J. Gregor, L.M. Liu, R.R. Roy, and C.L. Hager. Correlation of myoelectric activity and muscle force during selected cat treadmill locomotion. *J. Biomechanics* 16:691–701, 1983.

168. Smith, L.A., V.R. Edgerton, and E. Eldred. Fatigue properties of single motor units in exercised and non-exercised chronic spinal cats. *Soc. Neurosci. Abstr.* 7:683, 1981.

169. Steinbach, J.H., D. Schubert, and L. Eldridge. Changes in cat muscle contractile proteins after prolonged muscle inactivity. *Exp. Neurol.* 67:655–669, 1980.

170. Templeton, G.H., L. Sweeney, B.F. Timson, M. Padalino, and G.A. Dudenhoefter. Changes in slow fibers of the soleus muscle during rat hindlimb suspension. *J. Appl. Physiol.* 65:1191–1195, 1988.

171. Templeton, G.H., M. Padalino, J. Manton, T. LeConey, H. Hagler, and M. Glasberg. The influence of rat suspension-hypokinesia on the gastrocnemius muscle. *Aviat. Space Environ. Med.* 55:381–386, 1984.

172. Templeton, G.H., M. Padalino, J. Manton, et al. Influence of suspension hypokinesia on rat soleus muscle. *J. Appl. Physiol.* 56:278–286, 1984.

173. Thomason, D.B., and F.W. Booth. Atrophy of the soleus muscle by hindlimb unweighting, *J. Appl Physiol.* 68:1–12, 1990.

174. Thomason, D.B., K.M. Baldwin, and R.E. Herrick. Myosiin isozyme distribution in rodent hindlimb skeletal muscle. *J. Appl. Physiol.* 60:1923–1931, 1986.

175. Thomason, D.B., R.B. Biggs, and F.W. Booth. Altered protein metabolism and unchanged beta-myosing heavy chain mRNA in unweighted soleux muscle. *Am. J. Physiol.* 257:R300–R305, 1989.

176. Thomason, D.B., R.E. Herrick, and K.M. Baldwin. Activity influences on soleus muscle myosin during rodent hindlimb suspension. *J. Appl. Physiol.* 63:138–144, 1987.

177. Thomason, D.B., R.E. Herrick, D Surdyka, and K.M. Baldwin. Time course of soleus muscle myosin expression during hindlimb suspension and recovery. *J. Appl. Physiol.* 63:130–137, 1987.

178. Tower, S.S. Function and structure in the chonically isolated lumbo-sacral spinal cord of the dog. *J. Comp. Neurol.* 67:109–131, 1937.

179. Tsika, R.W., R.E. Herrick, and K.M. Baldwin. Interaction of compensatory overload and hindlimb suspension on myosin isoform expression. *J. Appl. Physiol.* 62:2180–2186, 1987.

180. Tsika, R.W., R.E. Herrick, and K.M. Baldwin. Subunit composition of rodent isomyosins and their distribution in hindlimb skeletal muscles. *J. Appl. Physiol.* 63:2101–2110, 1987.

181. Tsika, R.W., R.E. Herrick, and K.M. Baldwin. Time course of adaptations in rat skeletal muscle isomyosins during compensatory growth and regression. *J. Appl. Physiol.* 63:2111–2121, 1987.

182. Tsika, R.W., R.E. Herrick, and K.M. Baldwin. Effect of anabolic steroids on skeletal muscle mass during hindlimb suspension. *J. Appl. Physiol.* 63:2122–2127, 1987.

183. Tsika, R.W., R.E. Herrick, and K.M. Baldwin. Effect of anabolic steroids on overloaded and overloaded suspended skeletal muscle. *J. Appl. Physiol.* 63:2128–2133, 1987.

184. Vandenburgh, H.H., S. Hatfaludy, P. Karlisch, and J. Shansky. Skeletal muscle growth stimulated by intermittent stretch-relaxation in tissue culture. *Am. J. Physiol.* 256:C674–C682, 1989.

185. Vandenburgh, H.H., and S. Kaufman. An in vitro model for stretch-induced hypertrophy of skeletal muscle. *Science* 203:265–268, 1979.
186. Walmsley, B., J.A. Hodgson, and R.E. Burke. Forces produced by medial gastrocnemius and moving cats. *J. Neurophysiol.* 41:1203–1215, 1978.
187. Walsh, Jr., J.V., R.E. Burke, W.Z. Rymer, and P. Tsairis. Effect of compensatory hypertrophy studied in individual motor units in medial gastrocnemius muscle of the cat. *J. Neurophysiol.* 41:496–508, 1978.
188. West, S.P., R.R. Roy, and V.R. Edgerton. Fiber type and fiber size of cat ankle, knee and hip extensors and flexors following low thoracic spinal cord transection at an early age. *Exp. Neurol.* 91:174–182, 1986.
189. Wetzel, M.C., R.L. Gerlach, L.Z. Stern, and L.K. Hannapel. Behavior and histochemistry of functionally isolated cat ankle extensors. *Exp. Neurol.* 39:223–233, 1973.
190. Whiting, W.C., R.J. Gregor, R.R. Roy, and V.R. Edgerton. A technique for estimating mechanical work of individual muscles in the cat during treadmill locomotion. *J. Biomechanics* 17:685–694, 1984.
191. Winiarski, A.M., R.R. Roy, E.K. Alford, P.C. Chiang, and V.R. Edgerton. Mechanical properties of rat skeletal muscle after hindlimb suspension. *Exp. Neurol.* 96:650–660, 1987.
192. Young, B.C., R.J. Gregor, R.G. Lovely, and R.R. Roy. Hindlimb stepping in nonexercised adult spinal cats. *Soc. Neurosci. Abstr.* 12:685, 1986.

9
Regulation of Muscle Sympathetic Nerve Activity During Exercise in Humans

DOUGLAS R. SEALS, Ph.D.
RONALD G. VICTOR, M.D.

The sympathetic nervous system plays a crucial role in the regulation of arterial blood pressure and blood flow to active muscle in the exercising human. During vigorous exercise, increased sympathetic outflow to the heart contributes to the augmentation of cardiac output (systemic oxygen transport) by stimulating heart rate and ventricular contractility. Sympathetic neural activation to resistance vessels in non-active skeletal muscle, the viscera, and, under certain conditions, the skin mediates a vasoconstriction that is essential for redirecting the increase in oxygen (O_2) transport to the contracting skeletal muscles. These effects, as well as sympathetic stimulation of circulating hormone release (e.g., epinephrine, renin-angiotensin), act to maintain arterial pressure at an optimal level for organ perfusion.

The purpose of this chapter is to review what is currently known about the regulation of one part of this system during exercise in the human, viz., the control of sympathetic-vasoconstrictor nerve activity to resistance vessels in *non*active skeletal muscle (muscle sympathetic nerve activity or MSNA). The discussion is divided into five sections: 1) an overview of the measurement of MSNA during exercise in humans, 2) general features of the MSNA response to exercise, 3) control of MSNA by central command and contracting muscle afferent reflexes, 4) modulation of MSNA by arterial and cardiopulmonary baroreflexes, and 5) summary and conclusions.

MEASUREMENT OF MSNA DURING EXERCISE IN HUMANS

Indirect Methods

One approach to assessing MSNA during exercise is to measure the *end-organ response*. Typically, blood flow to a segment of a nonactive limb (calf or forearm) and arterial blood pressure are measured simultaneously, and the vascular resistance in that segment is calculated before and during exercise. Exercise-induced decreases in blood flow and increases in vascular resistance would indicate a vasoconstriction

313

presumably mediated by an increase in the activity of the sympathetic nerves in that region. Such measurements have provided important insight into the neural control of nonactive limb blood flow during exercise [5, 6, 15, 53, 74]. The interpretation of these data is limited, however, because local [74, 88], humoral [51, 74] and possibly other central neural (i.e., vasodilator nerves) [5, 74] factors can influence the blood flow responses to exercise independently of changes in MSNA. Furthermore, differences in adrenergic receptor function [49], blood vessel structure [22], and other factors can modulate these end-organ responses among subjects or groups of subjects. Finally, because whole limb blood flow is determined by flow to both skeletal muscle and skin, exercise-evoked changes in blood flow to skin also can confound interpretation of whole limb responses when the latter is used as an index of changes in MSNA [84].

A second approach to the estimation of MSNA is to measure plasma concentrations of norepinephrine, the primary neurotransmitter released from postganglionic, sympathetic nerve endings [25]. Increases in plasma norepinephrine levels from rest to exercise would suggest an increase in the activity of the sympathetic nerves [8, 23]. Such measurements are most often used as an index of overall ("whole body") sympathetic nervous system activity [25]. Determination of plasma norepinephrine concentrations from an antecubital vein blood sample (the most frequently used sample site), however, may actually provide a better estimation of exercise-induced changes in *MSNA* than whole body sympathetic activity, because up to 50% of the norepinephrine may be released from skeletal muscle nerves [29]. The main interpretive limitation of this measurement is that plasma levels are determined by norepinephrine clearance as well as release from sympathetic nerve endings. Assessment of plasma norepinephrine spillover from skeletal muscle [64] circumvents this particular limitation, but plasma concentrations as well as the rate of spillover are influenced by prejunctional modulation of norepinephrine release and reuptake of norephinephrine by the nerve endings [18]. In addition, because of the time involved for diffusion of neuronally released norepinephrine into plasma and the requirement for steady-state conditions with spillover measurements [18], these approaches cannot provide information on MSNA adjustments at the onset of exercise or during acute, transitional periods of sustained exercise. To satisfy these needs and to eliminate the numerous confounding factors involved with estimates of MSNA, direct measurement of sympathetic nerve activity to skeletal muscle is required.

Direct Method: Microneurography
Direct (intraneural), continuous measurements of MSNA in humans during exercise can be made using the microneurographic technique

developed by Hagbarth and colleagues in the late 1960s [extensive details of this procedure are discussed in previous reviews: 87, 96, 101]. In this technique, a thin (200 μm shaft, 1–5 μm tip) tungsten electrode is inserted percutaneously, and while stimulating (1–3 volts) through the tip, the electrode is slowly advanced and withdrawn in a systematic search for the nerve. When the tip enters a fascicle of the nerve containing fibers that innervate skeletal muscle, the motor neurons are stimulated and a muscle contraction is evoked. The electrode function is then switched to a recording mode and further, finer repositioning of the tip may be required until multiunit activity from the sympathetic axons within the fascicle can be obtained. In addition to the elicitation of the muscle contraction, at least two other criteria must be satisfied to document that the recording is MSNA: (1) tapping or stretching of the muscle or its tendons must evoke mechanoreceptor afferent discharge, and (2) the nerve activity must increase in response to a held end-expiration as well as during phases 2 and 3 of the Valsalva (strain) maneuver, two well-known stimuli for MSNA. Because measurements of sympathetic activity to skin also can be obtained using this technique, care is taken to ensure that the neural signals are not associated with any characteristics of skin activity. These include elicitation of paresthesias with electrical stimulation and afferent discharge by stroking the skin in the distribution of the nerve, and a nonpulse synchronous, irregular bursting pattern. The raw muscle sympathetic potentials are amplified, filtered (band width hrsp = 700–2000 Hz), full-wave rectified, and integrated (time constant hrsp = 100 ms) (Fig. 9.1). The MSNA can be quantitated from the integrated neurogram by determining the number of "bursts" (i.e., burst frequency) and the average amplitude (or area) of the bursts per unit time (usually 1 minute); "total minute activity" can then be calculated as the product of the burst frequency and average amplitude (area).

Recordings can be made from any peripheral nerve, but to date studies have been performed in either the arm (median, radial, or ulnar nerves) or the leg (peroneal or tibial nerves). Regardless of the particular recording site, the limb of the impaled nerve must remain relaxed; consequently, measurements of MSNA to *contracting* muscles are not possible. Adequate recordings can be obtained on 70–90% of all subjects, and most subjects experience no or only minor discomfort during the procedure. Local soreness or paresthesias are reported by 10–20% of the subjects for 1–3 days following an experiment; however, no permanent nerve damage has been reported in studies performed by investigators experienced in microneurography [2, 96].

General Characteristics of MSNA
The early work of Hagbarth, Wallin, and colleagues [9, 87, 96] demonstrated that sympathetic discharge in muscle nerve fascicles does not

FIGURE 9.1

Peroneal neurograms of MSNA (top) and brachial artery blood pressure tracings (below) from 2 subjects, one with low activity (**A**) *and one with high activity* (**B**). *Note that the rectified, integrated bursts of MSNA occur only intermittently, and only during spontaneous decreases in arterial pressure when arterial baroreceptor inhibition of sympathetic outflow is lessened. (Reprinted with permission from Sundölf, G., and B.G. Wallin. Human muscle nerve sympathetic activity at rest. Relationship to blood pressure and age. J. Physiol. (London) 274:621–637, 1978.)*

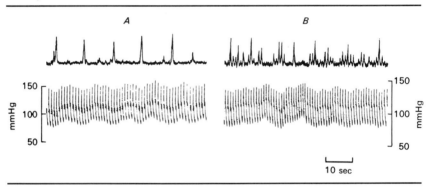

occur continuously, but rather shows an intermittent bursting pattern (Fig. 9.1). Although the fundamental central mechanisms responsible for this pattern are poorly understood, the discharge is coupled to the cardiac cycle by the arterial baroreflex. Thus, all of the activity is pulse-synchronous; i.e., bursts are generated only during diastole when the arterial baroreceptors are unloaded and their central inhibition of sympathetic outflow is removed. A respiratory rhythm to MSNA also occurs such that the activity is more frequent during expiration than inspiration [13, 28] because of the effects of breathing on arterial blood pressure, the stimulation of sympathoinhibitory lung inflation reflexes, or both [72]. Some evidence suggests that this intermittent pattern of discharge maximizes end-organ responsiveness (i.e., vasoconstriction) [36, 45].

Under resting conditions, MSNA burst frequency appears to be consistent over time in a particular person [81]. This bursting pattern at rest also is similar in simultaneous recordings of MSNA from nerves in the arm and leg, and in both legs [81], which suggests that (1) the activity represents "central" sympathetic outflow to nonactive skeletal muscle rather than regionally-determined activity, and (2) MSNA is uniform throughout the body (so that measurements made from any muscle nerve fascicle are assumed to be representative of those from all muscle nerves). In contrast, during supine rest there are striking differences in the burst frequency of MSNA among healthy individual subjects, ranging from 3 to 60 bursts per minute [81, 82]. Except for a positive correlation with age [82], the determinants of this interindividual variability in MSNA are unknown. At rest, MSNA is positively related to plasma norepinephrine concentrations [44, 98] and inversely related to acute changes in arterial blood pressure [10, 58, 80], but it is not correlated with chronic levels of arterial pressure [80, 99].

Finally, MSNA increases markedly in response to various forms of acute physical stress, including cold [19, 67, 90], hypoxia [52, 56], hypoglycemia [20], and orthostasis [7, 48, 80, 91] as well as exercise (see below). More modest, region-specific increases in MSNA also can occur during sustained mental stress [2]. In individual subjects, the nature of the MSNA response to these stressors is determined primarily by the characteristics of the stimulus.

GENERAL FEATURES OF THE MSNA RESPONSE TO EXERCISE

The direction, pattern and magnitude of the MSNA response to exercise is determined by the collective influence of some or all of a number of factors: exercise mode, intensity and duration, muscle fatigue, muscle mass, physical training, and environment. Other mitigating factors are its relationship to plasma norepinephrine concentrations and hemodynamic variables, regional homogeneity, and variability. Unless stated otherwise, the following discussion is based exclusively on information obtained from studies on *microneurographic* measurements of MSNA.

Mode. MSNA (recorded from either arm or leg nerves) increases in response to various types of exercise, including isometric [10, 35, 55, 68] and rhythmic [54, 93, 94] handgrip, isometric leg adduction [9], and arm cycling [93, 94]. To date, no data are available on the MSNA responses to large-muscle, dynamic exercise with the legs. In general, during exercise performed for the same duration and at the same percentage of maximal voluntary contraction force (MVC), the magnitude of the increase in MSNA is much greater with isometric than with dynamic muscle contractions [54, 93].

Intensity and duration. For a specific mode and duration of exercise, there appears to be a "threshold" *intensity* above which MSNA increases. During isometric exercise (primarily handgrip), MSNA generally does not increase at intensities ≤ 15% MVC (Fig. 9.2) [63, 68, 92], although a small increase in burst frequency has been reported at 10% MVC [55]. In contrast, isometric handgrip performed for a specific duration at levels above 20% MVC produces increases in MSNA proportional to the intensity of the contraction (Fig. 9.2) [55, 68]. However, this influence of intensity may not be present when isometric exercise is sustained to exhaustion. Preliminary evidence indicates that if isometric handgrip is

FIGURE 9.2

Average changes from baseline levels for peroneal MSNA in response to 2.5 minutes of isometric handgrip exercise performed at 15%, 25%, and 35% of MVC force in 8 subjects. Note that MSNA does not increase above baseline levels during handgrip at 15% MVC, but increases in a time- and intensity-dependent manner during the two highest levels of exercise. (Modified with permission from Seals, D.R., P.B. Chase, and J.A. Taylor. Autonomic mediation of the pressor responses to isometric exercise in humans. J. Appl. Physiol. *64:2190–2196, 1988.)*

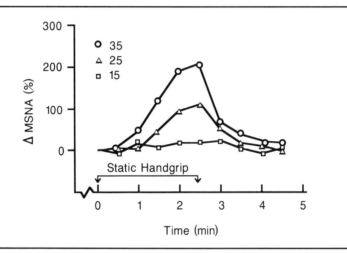

continued to the point at which the target force can no longer be maintained, the magnitudes of the increases in MSNA during strenuous efforts (i.e., >20% MVC) may be independent of the contraction intensity [71].

The threshold intensity for stimulating increases in MSNA during dynamic (rhythmic) exercise is higher than that for isometric contractions of the same duration. Rhythmic exercise of a small muscle mass (handgrip) for a brief duration (2 minutes) may not produce increases in MSNA at intensities as high as 50% MVC [93]. During brief periods of two-arm cycling exercise, MSNA does not increase at levels below ≈30% of a person's peak work load [93]; this threshold intensity corresponds to an increase in heart rate of 25–30 beats per minute (bt/min) above resting levels. Similarly, no load, one-arm cycling performed for up to 8 minutes fails to elicit an increase in MSNA, whereas even brief one-arm cycling at 30% of peak workload markedly stimulates MSNA [94]. Like isometric contractions, above this threshold level further increases in exercise intensity up to ≈60% of maximum produce correspondingly greater increases in MSNA during dynamic exercise

FIGURE 9.3

Peroneal MSNA in 1 subject at rest (control) and during the final 30 s of two-arm cycling exercise performed for 2 minutes each at 20, 40, and 60 watts. Note that MSNA does not increase above control levels during the lowest level of exercise (≈20% of peak workload), but increases somewhat at the middle level (≈35% of peak workload) and even more so at the highest level of cycling (≈50% of peak workload). (Reproduced with permission from Victor, R.G., D.R. Seals, and A.L. Mark. Differential control of heart rate and sympathetic nerve activity during dynamic exercise: insight from direct intraneural recordings in humans. J. Clin. Invest. 79:508–516, 1987, by copyright permission of the American Society for Clinical Investigation.)

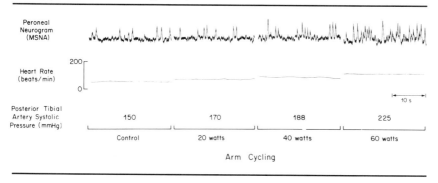

(Fig. 9.3) [93]. No microneurographic data are available at higher intensities of moderate- to large-muscle, dynamic exercise because excessive body movement results in the loss of the recording site; however, data from studies measuring antecubital venous norepinephrine concentrations indicate that MSNA may rise exponentially with increasing workrates above 60% of peak work rate [23].

The relationship between MSNA and exercise intensity is strongly influenced by the *duration* of the exercise. Typically, during exercise performed with small- (handgrip) or moderate- (arm cycling) sized muscle masses, MSNA does not increase during the initial 30–90 seconds of the bout (Figs. 9.2 and 9.4) [39, 68, 93]. This latency period is determined primarily by the exercise intensity, i.e., the greater the intensity, the sooner MSNA will increase after the onset of exercise (Fig. 9.2). It is not known, however, whether MSNA increases immediately with the onset of strenuous, large-muscle two-leg exercise.

Following this latency period, if the exercise is of sufficient intensity MSNA will increase in a duration-dependent manner throughout the exercise period (Figs. 9.2 and 9.4); this is true for both small-muscle, isometric exercise [36, 68] and for dynamic exercise performed with a moderate-size muscle mass (arm cycling) [93, 94]. For example, on average MSNA will increase approximately fivefold above resting levels

FIGURE 9.4

Peroneal MSNA (MSA) in one subject at rest (control), during 2 minutes of isometric handgrip exercise (30% MVC), and during 2 minutes of posthandgrip relaxation (recovery); corresponding values for heart rate (HR), total min MSNA, and mean arterial blood pressure (MAP) are shown below. Note that MSNA does not increase during the initial portion of the exercise period, but increases to a progressively greater degree with time until the contraction is terminated. (Reprinted with permission from Mark, A.L., R.G. Victor, C. Nerhed, and B.G. Wallin. Microneurographic studies of the mechanisms of sympathetic nerve responses to static exercise in humans. Circ. Res. 57:461–469, 1985, and by permission of the American Heart Association.)

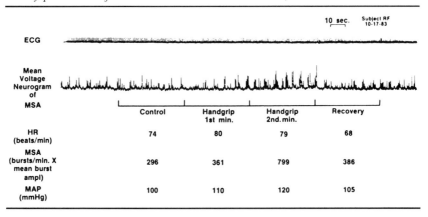

during sustained isometric contractions to exhaustion [57, 69]. No information is available on the MSNA responses to strenuous dynamic exercise performed longer than 6 minutes at the same workload. It is not known, therefore, whether MSNA continues to increase during prolonged exercise of this type, although antecubital venous norepinephrine responses suggest that this may be the case [23].

A good example of the interactive effects of exercise intensity and duration on MSNA is observed with rhythmic handgrip exercise. As mentioned previously, if the duration of the exercise is brief, one would conclude that the threshold intensity for eliciting increases in MSNA is >50% MVC [93]. If, however, exercise below this level (e.g., 40% MVC) is performed for a longer duration, MSNA will eventually rise well above resting levels [D. R. Seals and R. G. Victor, unpublished observations]. Thus, the "threshold" intensity at which an increase in MSNA is evoked is in part a function of the duration of the exercise.

Muscle fatigue. The stimulation of MSNA during isometric exercise appears to be related to the onset and development of muscle fatigue. During submaximal (30% MVC), isometric handgrip performed to exhaustion, heart rate and arterial blood pressure increase immediately,

FIGURE 9.5

Changes from baseline levels for peroneal MSNA (**A**), *heart rate (HR)* (**B**), *contracting forearm electromyographic (EMG) activity* (**C**), *and mean arterial blood pressure (MABP)* (**D**) *during three successive trials of isometric handgrip exercise (30% MVC) performed to exhaustion in one subject. The increase in the EMG was used as an objective measure of the onset and development of muscle fatigue. Note the tight coupling between increases in MSNA and EMG both within a specific trial and among the three trials, which suggests a link between the development of muscle fatigue and sympathetic neural activation. In contrast, changes in EMG were not clearly associated with exercise-induced increases in HR or MABP. (Reprinted with permission from Seals, D.R., and R.M. Enoka. Sympathetic activation is associated with increases in EMG during fatiguing exercise.* J. Appl. Physiol. *66:88–95, 1989.)*

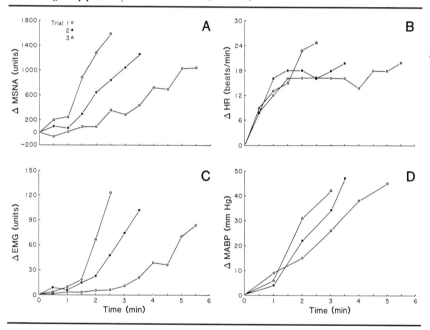

but neither MSNA nor the electromyographic (EMG) activity of the contracting forearm muscles increases above their respective baseline levels during the initial minute of exercise (Fig. 9.5) [69]. From the second minute on, MSNA and EMG activity increase in parallel [69]. During subsequent trials performed at the same exercise intensity, the increases in both MSNA and contracting muscle EMG activity are greater at the same absolute point in time. Thus, the increase in MSNA can be shifted with respect to time, but not with respect to the EMG response (i.e., to the index of fatigue). Recent evidence concerning the perception of fatigue supports this concept [57]. During isometric handgrip (25% MVC) performed to exhaustion, subjects' sensations of fatigue were exponentially related to increases in MSNA. No increase in MSNA was observed until the subjective rating reached a level described as "slightly fatiguing". This tight relationship between MSNA and the sensation of fatigue was quite reproducible. Taken together, these observations indicate that the MSNA response to isometric exercise is associated with the fatigue process, and that previous fatiguing muscle contractions can markedly influence this MSNA response. Whether there is a similar relationship between fatigue and MSNA during dynamic exercise performed with larger muscle groups has not been determined.

Muscle mass. As mentioned above, increases in MSNA have been observed during exercise performed with both moderate-size and small muscle groups. Concerning the latter, even sustained finger adduction evoked by contraction of a small hand muscle (the first dorsal interosseus) provides a sufficiently strong stimulus for increasing MSNA [D. R. Seals and R. M. Enoka, unpublished observations]. Moreover, recent evidence indicates that the size of the contracting muscle mass is an important determinant of the MSNA response to isometric exercise [64]. When submaximal, isometric handgrip exercise is performed by both arms simultaneously (i.e., with each arm exercising at 30% of its respective MVC) the increase in MSNA is 40–70% greater than during contractions of either arm alone (Fig. 9.6). Parenthetically, because the magnitude of the increase in MSNA during two-arm exercise is less than the simple sum of the responses to exercise with each arm alone, an inhibitory interaction is suggested.

These findings indicate that at a particular submaximal intensity and duration of isometric exercise, the degree of sympathetic neural activation to the nonactive skeletal muscle circulation is influenced by the size of the contracting muscle mass, but that the effect is not strictly proportional to the difference in mass. It is not known whether a similar relationship exists between MSNA and muscle mass during dynamic exercise, but data from antecubital venous plasma norepinephrine measurements are consistent with this concept [33].

Physical training. Little information exists on the possible effects of physical training on the MSNA responses to acute exercise. In young, healthy humans aerobic leg training does not influence MSNA at rest [66, 83], and recent findings indicate that physical conditioning has no effect on the MSNA responses to exercise performed with untrained muscle groups [66]. During submaximal, isometric handgrip exercise there was no significant difference in the MSNA response between young, untrained subjects and highly conditioned endurance athletes (primarily cyclists and runners) [66]. In contrast, two preliminary reports [78, 79] suggest that the MSNA response to handgrip exercise is

FIGURE 9.6

Average (±SE) changes in the minutes of burst frequency (top) and the total minutes of activity (bottom) of peroneal MSNA from baseline levels during 2.5 minutes of isometric handgrip exercise (30% MVC) performed with either the right or left arms alone, or with both arms simultaneously, in 9 subjects. After the first minute of exercise the magnitude of the increase in MSNA at any point in time was greater when handgrip was performed with both arms than with either arm alone. (Reprinted with permission from Seals, D.R. Influence of muscle mass on sympathetic neural activation during isometric exercise. J. Appl. Physiol. 67:1801–1806, 1989.)

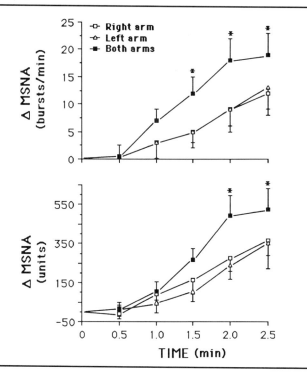

attenuated in subjects with physically-trained arms. It is therefore possible that physical training does influence the MSNA response to exercise, but only when the exercise is performed with the conditioned muscles (i.e., MSNA during exercise is influenced by the local, and not the systemic effects of training). This would be consistent with findings on the plasma norepinephrine responses to acute exercise following training [46, 102].

Environmental effects. Little is known about the possible modulatory effects of environmental factors (e.g., heat, cold, altitude) on the MSNA responses to exercise. Recent information suggests that exercise-induced increases in MSNA are augmented by hypoxia [70]. MSNA increased ≈100% above baseline levels in response to rhythmic handgrip exercise performed during room air breathing (normoxia) compared to an ≈250% increase when the same level of exercise was performed during systemic hypoxia (breathing 10% O_2 gas). MSNA did not increase with brief hypoxia at rest. The magnitude of the increase during hypoxic exercise therefore, was greater than the simple sums of the separate MSNA responses to normoxic exercise and hypoxic rest, which suggests a facilitatory interaction when the two stimuli are applied concurrently. Interestingly, when rhythmic exercise was performed under conditions of complete blood flow occlusion (i.e., local hypoxia), the magnitudes of the MSNA responses during room air breathing (systemic normoxia) and low O_2 breathing (systemic hypoxia) did not differ. This indicates that the mechanism for the potentiation of the response to normal exercise during hypoxia had its origin in the contracting muscles. No microneurographic data are available on the effects of hypoxia on MSNA during large-muscle, dynamic exercise, but studies measuring venous norepinephrine responses indicate that a similar potentiation is observed at intensities >40% of peak workload [17].

Relationship to plasma norepinephrine concentrations. In general, the MSNA and venous plasma norepinephrine responses to exercise appear to be similar, at least qualitatively. Neither MSNA nor plasma norepinephrine increases during mild arm-cycling exercise, but both variables increase above resting levels at the same submaximal (threshold) workload, and continue to increase in parallel fashion with further increases in exercise intensity (Fig. 9.7) [73]. The same qualitative relationship between the two variables is observed in response to isometric exercise [97]. In both cases, the relative (%) increase above baseline levels is 2- to 4-fold greater for MSNA compared to plasma norepinephrine. In addition, recent evidence indicates that rhythmic handgrip exercise of sufficient intensity and duration to elicit a 100% increase in MSNA does not necessarily produce an increase in plasma norepinephrine [70]. Thus, although in most cases the two variables exhibit directionally similar responses to exercise, plasma norepinephrine concentrations provide a less sensitive, less consistent measure of changes in sympathetic neural outflow to skeletal muscle.

Relationship to hemodynamic variables. One would expect that exercise-induced increases in postganglionic, sympathetic nerve activity would be directly related to certain regional and systemic hemodynamic adjustments, which accumulating evidence supports. During exercise, increases in MSNA are associated with decreases in blood flow in nonactive limbs [9]. Furthermore, simultaneous measurements of blood flow and MSNA in the nonactive limb, and systemic arterial blood pressure indicate that exercise-evoked changes in MSNA and limb vascular resistance are tightly coupled (Fig. 9.8) [65]. No change in

FIGURE 9.7

Average (±SE) percent changes from baseline levels for antecubital venous plasma norepinephrine concentrations, minutes of burst frequency of MSNA, and total minutes of activity of MSNA to the second minute of two-arm cycling exercise performed at 0, 10, 20, 40 and 60 watts in 6 subjects. Note that plasma nor-epinephrine levels and MSNA do not increase at the three lowest levels of cycling, but that both variables increase at the same threshold workload. The relative increases in MSNA are much greater than the corresponding changes in plasma norepinephrine. (Reprinted with permission from Seals, D.R., R.G. Victor, and A.L. Mark. Plasma norepinephrine and muscle sympathetic discharge during rhythmic exercise in humans. J. Appl. Physiol. 65:940–944, 1988.)

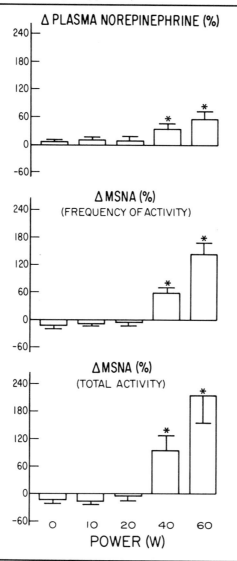

FIGURE 9.8

Average (± SE) changes from baseline levels for peroneal MSNA and calf vascular resistance during 2.5 minutes of isometric handgrip exercise (35% MVC) followed by 2 minutes of postexercise relaxation (recovery) in 9 subjects. Note that MSNA and calf vascular resistance increase during exercise and fall during postexercise relaxation in parallel. The average correlation coefficient (r) for this level of exercise was 0.94 ± 0.06. (Reprinted with permission from Seals, D.R. Sympathetic neural discharge and vascular resistance during exercise in humans. J. Appl. Physiol. *66:2472–2478, 1989.)*

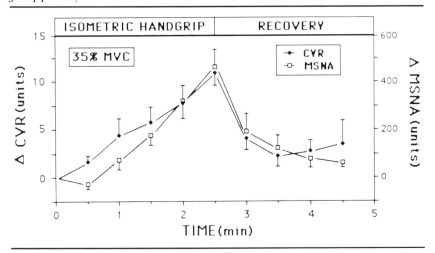

either lower leg MSNA or calf vascular resistance is observed during mild isometric handgrip exercise, nor do any changes occur in either variable during the initial phase of more strenuous contractions. Following this initial phase of strenuous exercise both MSNA and calf vascular resistance increase, and the changes in the two variables are strongly correlated.

MSNA responses to exercise also appear to be related to changes in arterial blood pressure. In general, increases in MSNA elicited during exercise always are associated with corresponding increases in arterial pressure [39, 68, 93]. During the latter phase of strenuous isometric exercise, when heart rate (and presumably cardiac output) is changing little or not at all, the average increases in MSNA and arterial pressure are highly correlated [68]. Taken together, these findings indicate that the stimulation of MSNA by muscular exercise has physiologically significant effects on both regional (nonactive skeletal muscle) and systemic hemodynamics.

Regional homogeneity. Tissue specificity is a well-documented property of the efferent sympathetic nervous system. During certain physiological perturbations (stress), sympathetic outflow can increase to one organ and decrease to another [76]. The regulation of MSNA during acute stress can show a similar degree of specificity. For example, it has been reported that MSNA is unchanged or decreases in the arm, but increases in the leg in response to sustained, strenuous mental arithmetic [2, 9]. In general, this type of regional diversity has not been observed in response to exercise. Increases in MSNA have been noted in the radial [100] and median [9] nerves in the arm in response to exercise with the contralateral arm or the leg, and in the tibial [55, 57] and peroneal [cf. 39, 93] nerves in the leg in response to arm exercise. Furthermore, during simultaneous recordings in the radial and peroneal nerves, the pattern and magnitude of the MSNA response during contralateral handgrip exercise is quite similar [100]. Taken together, these findings indicate that the MSNA responses to exercise, at least that performed with the arms, appear to be uniform throughout the body.

Variability. Little information exists on the reproducibility of the MSNA response to exercise within a person over time. In a recent study [57], the relationship between MSNA and subjective ratings of fatigue were similar in five subjects who performed submaximal, isometric handgrip exercise to exhaustion on 2 separate days. In these subjects the MSNA response was reproducible and could be estimated from the subjects' sensations of fatigue. In contrast to this observation on *within*-subject variability, the *inter*subject variability in the MSNA response to exercise is quite marked. During isometric exercise performed at a particular percentage of maximal force and sustained to exhaustion, the increase in MSNA above the control level can range from 1- to 7-fold among subjects [57, 66]. Striking differences among subjects also are observed during dynamic exercise performed at the same absolute, submaximal workloads [93, 94]. The MSNA response to exercise, therefore, cannot be predicted in individual subjects. This marked intersubject difference in MSNA reactivity is observed during other forms of acute stress as well [2, 9, 52, 91].

CONTROL OF MSNA BY CENTRAL COMMAND AND SKELETAL MUSCLE AFFERENT REFLEXES

Microneurographic studies of the MSNA responses to isometric and rhythmic arm exercise have provided some insight into the mechanisms that regulate sympathetic neural outflow during exercise. Two principal theories have been proposed. The first is that sympathetic activation is caused by the central neural drive, or central command, that accompanies volitional muscle contraction [16, 30, 42]. According to this theory, the motor command signal that emanates from the forebrain projects to autonomic circuits in the brainstem, producing a parallel activation of somatomotor and autonomic pathways.

The second theory is that sympathetic activation is caused by a reflex mechanism that arises in mechanoreceptor and metaboreceptor (chemosensitive) afferents in contracting skeletal muscle [42, 43, 51]. Mechanoreceptor endings are located in the connective tissue of the muscle interstitium and are activated by mechanical deformation of their receptive fields [4]. In contrast, metaboreceptor endings are located on the luminal surface of the microcirculation and are activated by local chemical products of muscle metabolism [3]. Although neurophysiologic studies in anesthetized animal preparations have provided abundant experimental support for both theories [16, 31, 40, 41, 43], the relative importance of muscle afferent reflexes and central command in causing sympathetic activation (and parasympathetic withdrawal to the heart) during exercise on conscious humans is an unsolved problem.

Before recent findings are discussed on these issues that have been obtained from microneurographic studies in humans, several important caveats must be emphasized. First, the new concepts arising from this work are based solely on the measurement of sympathetic discharge targeted specifically to inactive skeletal muscle, which may not be representative of sympathetic discharge to other regional circulations (e.g., heart, skin, and viscera). Second, as mentioned above, MSNA responses have been studied only during exercise with smaller or moderate-sized muscle masses and, thus, may not be representative of responses during larger muscle exercise (e.g., leg cycling, running). Third, without simultaneous measurements of end-organ responses, a linear relationship between sympathetic activity and vascular resistance cannot be assumed in every exercise condition.

With these caveats in mind, three new concepts will be presented in this section. First, during isometric handgrip exercise, the muscle metaboreceptor reflex is the main mechanism that increases MSNA. In contrast, central command and muscle mechanoreceptor feedback do not exert important influences on MSNA during this form of exercise. Second, the muscle metaboreflex plays an important role in the stimulation of MSNA during rhythmic (dynamic) arm exercise performed with small and moderate-sized muscle masses. This mechanism, however, is engaged during moderate and heavy submaximal exercise, but not during mild rhythmic muscle contractions. Third, muscle metaboreflex activation of MSNA is coupled, in part, to the breakdown of glycogen and the resultant cellular accumulation of hydrogen ions in contracting muscle.

Muscle Metaboreceptor Stimulation of MSNA During Isometric Exercise
Mark et al. [39] first demonstrated that isometric handgrip exercise performed for 2 minutes at 30% MVC markedly stimulates MSNA. Two characteristic features of the MSNA response to isometric handgrip suggested that this is a reflex response elicited by muscle metaborecep-

FIGURE 9.9

Peroneal neurogram of MSNA (MSA) at rest (control), during 2 minutes of isometric handgrip exercise (30% MVC) followed immediately by a 2 minutes muscle ischemic response (MIR-arrested perfusion of the previously exercising forearm), and during a period of nonischemic, postexercise relaxation (recovery) (see Figure 9.4 for other details). Note the slow pattern of activation and the maintenance of the exercise-evoked increase in MSNA during postexercise ischemia, both of which indicate muscle metaboreflex mediation. (Reprinted with permission from Mark, A.L., R.G. Victor, C. Nerhed, and B.G. Wallin. Microneurographic studies of the mechanisms of sympathetic nerve responses to static exercise in humans. Circ. Res. 57:461–469, 1985.)

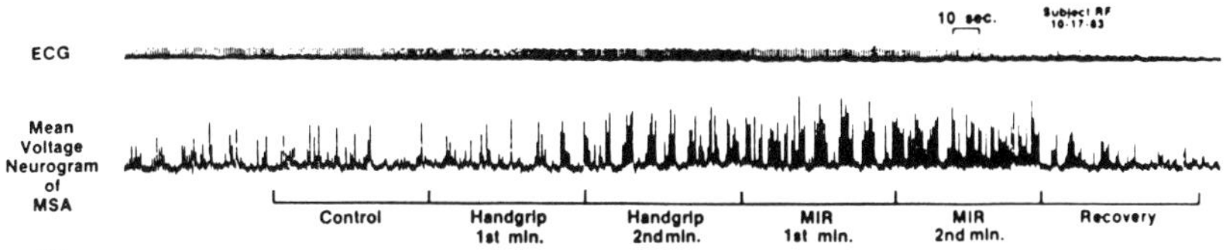

	Control	Handgrip 1st min.	Handgrip 2nd min.	MIR 1st min.	MIR 2nd min.	Recovery
HR (beats/min)	76	88	83	67	63	67
MSA (burst/min X mean burst ampl.)	476	410	1182	1473	1386	603
MAP (mmHg)	100	114	127	122	122	107

tors. First, in contrast to heart rate and arterial pressure, which increase almost immediately at the onset of voluntary exercise, MSNA shows a rather slow pattern of activation beginning about 45 s after the onset of handgrip (Fig. 9.4). When stimulated by sustained isometric muscle contraction in anesthetized cats, metaboreceptor muscle afferents also show a delayed pattern of neural activation [21, 41, 43]. Second, when isometric handgrip is followed by circulatory arrest of the previously contracting forearm muscles, which traps the reflex-activating metabolites and maintains the chemical stimulation of muscle afferents, the exercise-induced sympathoexcitation in the peroneal nerve is sustained even though muscular relaxation eliminates central command as well as the mechanical stimulation of muscle afferents (Fig. 9.9) [39, 68]. Radial and peroneal nerves show parallel MSNA responses to isometric handgrip and to posthandgrip circulatory arrest, which indicates that, when engaged, the muscle metaboreflex elicits a generalized activation of sympathetic outflow to all inactive skeletal muscle [100]. In contrast, the metaboreceptor reflex is thought to have little if any effect on autonomic outflow to the sinus node during isometric exercise, because handgrip-evoked increases in heart rate resolve promptly with the cessation of muscle contraction and are not maintained during posthandgrip forearm circulatory arrest [40, 68].

Previously, central command and muscle afferent feedback were thought to be highly redundant inputs that influence the same central neuronal pools and evoke the same efferent autonomic responses. In contrast, the present work suggested that the autonomic effects of central command and muscle afferent reflexes sometimes can be highly selective: during isometric handgrip exercise the muscle metaboreflex mainly increases MSNA, whereas central command increases heart rate but does not increase and may even decrease MSNA (see below).

INFLUENCE OF CENTRAL COMMAND ON MSNA The initial studies by Mark et al. [39] primarily isolated the autonomic effects of the muscle metaboreceptor reflex while eliminating central command. Subsequent studies by Victor et al. [92] isolated the autonomic effects of central command while controlling or minimizing the input from the muscle afferents. To determine if central command decreases or increases sympathetic activity to nonactive skeletal muscle, MSNA was recorded during attempted handgrip contraction with partial neuromuscular blockade produced by the systemic administration of curare. During curarization, subjects reported that they used near-maximal effort to attempt a sustained handgrip contraction (i.e., augmented central command) but they generated almost no force (i.e., attenuated muscle afferent input). Without sustained contraction, the intent to perform exercise alone (i.e., central command) caused statistically significant increases in MSNA (Fig. 9.10), arterial blood pressure, and heart rate. However, the increases in MSNA (56 ± 16% over control) and in mean arterial pressure (12 ± 2 mmHg) during the attempted handgrip were much smaller than the increases in MSNA (217 ± 37% over control) and in mean arterial pressure (25 ± 3 mmHg) during actual isometric handgrip at 30% MVC. In contrast, heart rate increased as much during the attempted handgrip (18 ± 2 bt/min) as during the actual handgrip (16 ± 4 bt/min). The heart rate response to attempted handgrip was mediated primarily by vagal withdrawal, rather than by sympathetic activation, because this response was greatly attenuated by atropine but unaffected by propranolol.

The principal new conclusion from this work was that central command and muscle afferent reflexes can have directionally similar but unequal effects on sympathetic neural outflow. During isometric handgrip, central command plays a major role in the withdrawal of parasympathetic outflow to the sinus node but only a minor role in the activation of MSNA.

Previously, Mark et al. [39] suggested that during isometric handgrip, central command tends to decrease rather than increase MSNA. This suggestion was based on three lines of evidence, each of which was indirect and subject to alternative explanations. First, MSNA did not increase but rather tended to decrease with the engagement of central command at the onset of isometric handgrip. Although this observation

FIGURE 9.10

Tracings of peroneal MSNA and handgrip force before and in response to iso-metric handgrip exercise performed at 15% (top) and 30% (middle) MVC prior to curare infusion, and attempted handgrip during curare infusion (i.e., neu-romuscular blockade) (bottom) in 1 subject. Note that MSNA increased during handgrip at 30% MVC, but not at 15% MVC. During curare (i.e., without the ability to sustain even the normal 15% MVC force level), MSNA increased only slightly, despite maximal effort (intent to perform exercise). (Reprinted with per-mission from Victor, R.G., S.L. Pryor, N.H. Secher, and J.H. Mitchell. Effects of partial neuromuscular blockade sympathetic nerve responses to static exercise in humans. Circ. Res. 65:468–476, 1989, and the American Heart Associa-tion.)

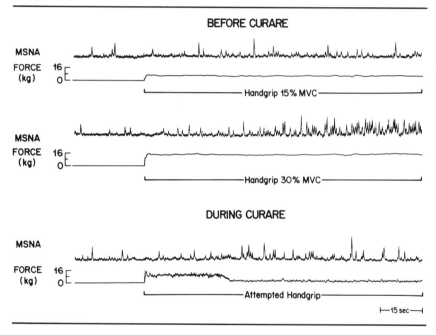

subsequently has been replicated, the precise mechanism remains unknown and may be related to arterial baroreflex activation (see below). Second, MSNA was higher when central command was elimi-nated during posthandgrip forearm vascular occlusion than when central command was engaged during handgrip exercise. The study by Victor et al. [92] replicated this finding but only when MSNA was expressed per 100 heart beats and not when MSNA was expressed as activity per unit time, the latter presumably reflecting the physiological stimulus for neurotransmitter release. Third, MSNA decreased during voluntary isometric biceps contraction but increased when central command was eliminated during electrically evoked biceps contraction. Although recorded force output was comparable with the voluntary and involuntary biceps contractions, it is unlikely that muscle afferent stimulation was equivalent because these two types of contraction cause very different patterns of motor unit activation.

Muscle Metaboreflex Effects on MSNA During Rhythmic Exercise
During isometric exercise, sustained increases in tissue pressure produce muscle hypoperfusion and cause the accumulation of ischemic (reflex-activating) metabolites in the vicinity of the metaboreceptor afferent endings [11, 34]. In contrast, with submaximal rhythmic exercise this hypoperfusion during the contraction phase is counteracted by a relatiive hyperperfusion during the relaxation phase. Consequently, the concentrations of these reflex-triggering metabolites might not increase to the same extent as during isometric exercise, and the metaboreflex may not be activated. Several studies were therefore conducted to determine if the muscle metaboreceptor reflex is important in the activation of MSNA during submaximal dynamic exercise (i.e., rhythmic handgrip and one- and two-arm cycling) [93, 94].

The new conclusions were twofold. First, in contrast to what had been previously assumed, the onset of dynamic exercise does not always cause an obligatory increase in sympathetic outflow to all regional circulations (i.e., mass sympathetic discharge). For example, brief periods of mild rhythmic arm exercise cause intensity-dependent increases in heart rate mediated by cardiac vagal withdrawal but, as stated earlier, have no effect on MSNA [93, 94]. MSNA remains unchanged during 2 minutes of rhythmic handgrip at levels $\leq 50\%$ MVC, during 2 minutes of two-arm cycling at loads $\leq 30\%$ of maximum, and during up to 8 minutes of no load one-arm cycling.

The second conclusion is that a metabolically generated reflex arising in presumably nonischemic working skeletal muscle plays an important role in the normal activation of MSNA during moderate but not during mild levels of rhythmic arm exercise. Thus, MSNA increases during rhythmic handgrip at levels $> 50\%$ MVC and during either one- or two-arm cycling at levels $> 30\%$ of maximum (Fig. 9.3) [93, 94]. During each of these exercise interventions, there is a slow onset of the MSNA response (latency of approximately 1 minute), which suggests metaboreflex mediation (Fig. 9.11). MSNA remains elevated when rhythmic handgrip at 60% MVC is followed by arrest of the forearm circulation, a maneuver that maintains muscle metaboreflex stimulation. Furthermore, complete ischemia (upper arm cuff inflated to 250 mmHg) is necessary to increase MSNA during mild one-arm cycling (Fig. 9.12a), whereas even partial ischemia (upper arm cuff inflated to 100 mmHg) greatly amplifies the stimulation of MSNA normally produced by a moderate level of one-arm cycling (Fig. 9.12b).

FIGURE 9.11

Average (±SE) levels of peroneal MSNA and heart rate before (time 0) and during 2 minutes of two-arm cycling exercise performed at 0 (left), 20 (middle) and 40 (right) watts in 6 subjects. Note that MSNA does not increase during the two lowest levels of exercise despite intensity-dependent increases in heart rate. MSNA does increase during the highest level of exercise, but only after some delay, whereas heart rate increases immediately. Both observations are consistent with the idea of muscle metaboreflex stimulation of MSNA, but not tachycardia. (Reproduced with permission from Victor, R.G., D.R. Seals, and A.L. Mark. Differential control of heart rate and sympathetic nerve activity during dynamic exercise: insight from direct intraneural recordings in humans. J. Clin. Invest. 79:508–516, 1987, by copyright permission of the American Society for Clinical Investigation.)

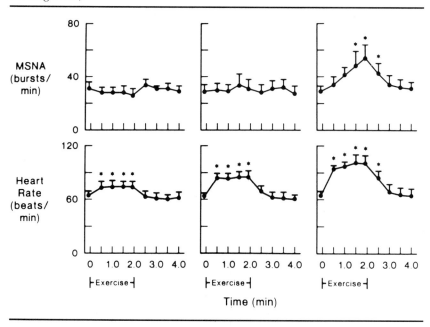

These microneurographic data in humans support recent hemodynamic findings in dogs, which have indicated that the reflex cardiovascular stimulation evoked by muscle metaboreceptor afferents is related to an interplay between muscle perfusion and exercise intensity [51, 75, 103]. In the human during mild rhythmic exercise, drastic reductions in muscle blood flow are required to generate a metabolic error signal and reflexly increase MSNA. In contrast, during moderately intense rhythmic exercise, the muscle contraction alone is sufficient to evoke a metabolic error signal which is readily exaggerated by artificial reductions in muscle perfusion. These recent findings suggest that during

FIGURE 9.12
(A) *Peroneal MSNA before (control) and during 8 minutes of no-load cycling (intrinsic ergometer resistance only) alone (A), and during the same level of exercise performed with graded inhibition of blood flow to the exercising arm produced by a cuff around the shoulder (B) in one subject. Note that MSNA did not increase during this mild level of cycling until blood flow to the exercising arm was completely arrested (cuff pressure of 250 mmHg).* (B) *Peroneal MSNA in the same subject during control and in response to cycling with a load equivalent to ⅓ of maximum, alone (A) and with graded blood flow occlusion (B). Load cycling alone increased MSNA above control levels, and, in contrast to no load cycling, this response was augmented by even partial occlusion of blood flow to the exercising arm (i.e., 100 mmHg cuff pressure). (Reprinted with permission from Victor, R.G., and D.R. Seals. Reflex stimulation of sympathetic outflow during rhythmic exercise in humans. Am. J. Physiol. 257 (Heart Circulation Physiology 26):H2017–H2024, 1989.)*

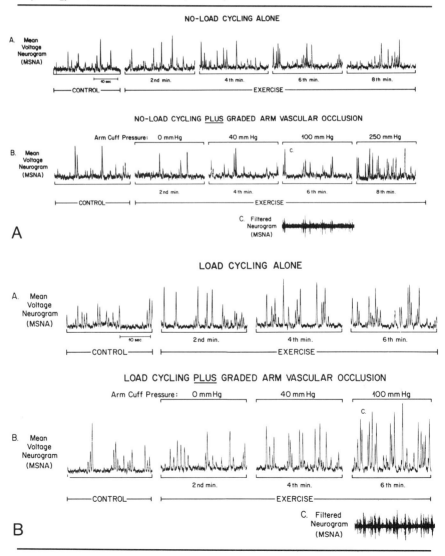

small- and moderate-sized muscle mass exercise, the threshold intensity for muscle metaboreflex-mediated activation of MSNA is at a submaximal level of exercise commonly performed during daily physical activity.

Nature of the Chemical Stimulus for Metaboreflex Activation of MSNA During Exercise

Although the discharge of metaboreceptor afferents is thought to signal the brain of a mismatch between muscle blood flow and metabolism, little is known about the specific metabolic pathways that are involved. In recent experiments, 31-phosphorus nuclear magnetic resonance spectroscopy (31P-NMR) was used to probe the cellular events in contracting muscle that initiate the reflex stimulation of MSNA [89]. Oxidative phosphorylation and glycolysis are the two primary pathways for the production of high-energy phosphates in mammalian skeletal muscle. These recent studies sought to determine if the reflex stimulation of MSNA during handgrip exercise is coupled either to the cellular accumulation of inorganic phosphate and adenosine diphosphate (ADP), which are important regulators of mitochondrial respiration, or to muscle cell pH, an index of glycolysis. Subjects performed rhythmic and isometric handgrip exercise with a surface coil placed over the active muscle mass and the forearm placed in a 30 cm-horizontal bore superconducting magnet which acquired phosphorus spectra every 60s. High energy phosphates and pH in active muscle forearm muscle cells were measured with 31P-NMR while MSNA was recorded simultaneously from the peroneal nerve (outside of the magnet). Experiments were performed first in normal humans and later in patients with myophosphorylase deficiency, a specific inborn error of skeletal muscle glycogenolysis.

During both isometric and rhythmic handgrip exercise in normal humans, the onset of sympathetic activation in the lower leg coincided with the onset of cellular acidification in the active forearm muscles. The increases in MSNA were closely correlated both in time course and magnitude to the exercise-induced decreases in intracellular pH but were dissociated from the changes in the cellular concentrations of inorganic phosphate and ADP (Fig. 9.13a and b). Sinoway et al. [77] recently found a similar relationship between handgrip-induced decreases in forearm muscle cell pH and increases in calf vascular resistance, the latter being the hemodynamic consequence of increased MSNA. These findings suggest that a specific metabolic process—the intracellular accumulation of hydrogen ion resulting from increased glycolytic flux—may be important in triggering metaboreflex activation of MSNA during exercise.

MSNA also was recorded during isometric handgrip in four patients with muscle phosphorylase deficiency (McArdle's Disease), a condition in which contraction is not accompanied by glycogen degradation and

FIGURE 9.13

(A) *Average (± SE) levels of exercising forearm muscle pH (as estimated by 3P-NMR) and peroneal MSNA during 4 minutes of rhythmic handgrip exercise (2 minutes at 30% MVC followed by 2 minutes at 50% MVC) in 7 subjects. Note the tight association between exercise-induced increases in MSNA and the development of intracellular acidosis.* **(B)** *Average MSNA and muscle pH responses to isometric vs. rhythmic handgrip exercise at comparable decreases in [PCr]/[Pi]* **(a–c)** *and estimated muscle pH* **(d–f)** *in the same subjects. Note that regardless of exercise mode the MSNA responses were always coupled to changes in muscle pH, but not to changes in [PCr]/[Pi]. (Reproduced with permission from Victor, R.G., L.A. Bertocci, S.L. Pryor, and Nunnally R.L. Sympathetic nerve discharge is coupled to muscle cell pH during exercise in humans. J. Clin. Invest. 82:1301–1305, 1988, by copyright permission of the American Society for Clinical Investigation.)*

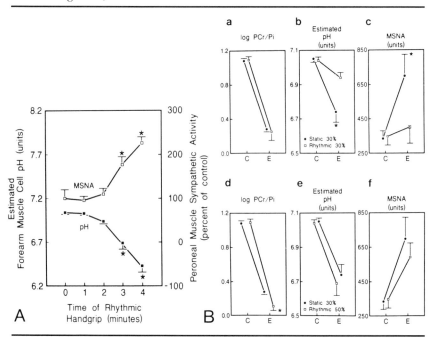

acidosis in exercising skeletal muscle [47]. A level of isometric handgrip (30% MVC for 90 s) that more than doubled MSNA in normal humans had no effect on MSNA and caused an attenuated rise in blood pressure in the patients with myophosphorylase deficiency (Fig. 9.14a and b). In contrast, two nonexercise stimuli, Valsalva's maneuver and hand immersion in ice water (i.e., a cold pressor test), evoked comparably large increases in MSNA in both patients and normals. Furthermore, heart rate increased comparably during isometric handgrip in normals and in myophosphorylase-deficient patients, which is consistent with the concept that heart rate, unlike MSNA, is governed mainly by central command rather than by the muscle metaboreflex (Fig. 9.14b).

These microneurographic findings in normal humans and in myophosphorylase-deficient patients are consistent with recent findings in experimental animals. In anesthetized cats, lactic acid stimulates metaboreceptor muscle afferents [50, 86] and reflexly increases arterial pressure [27]. In conscious dogs, the pressor response to progressive muscle ischemia during treadmill exercise is strongly correlated with venous effluent pH [75]. The findings in the myophosphorylase-deficient patients, however, do not exclude the possibility that in normal humans metabolic processes other than glycolysis are important in the reflex regulation of the autonomic nervous system during exercise. For example, reduced availability of substrate for mitochondrial respiration in myophosphorylase deficient muscle contributes to increases in cardiac output and resultant increases in blood pressure during dynamic leg exercise in patients with McArdle's Disease [32].

In summary, these human microneurographic experiments suggest that the activation of MSNA during isometric exercise is linked to specific metabolic events in contracting skeletal muscle associated with accelerated glycolysis and intracellular acidosis.

MODULATION OF MSNA BY CARDIOPULMONARY AND ARTERIAL REFLEXES

Numerous autonomic reflex pathways participate in the integrative control of arterial blood pressure and cardiovascular function in the human at rest. Several microneurographic studies have now been performed to determine if these reflexes also modulate the MSNA responses to acute exercise. To date, these investigations have all used isometric handgrip as the exercise model and recorded MSNA from the peroneal nerve in the leg.

Cardiopulmonary Baroreflexes
Studies in anesthetized animals have advanced the concept of a reflex interaction between the excitatory influence of the muscle afferent stimulation and the inhibitory influence of the activation of cardiopulmonary vagal afferents (i.e., cardiopulmonary baroreflexes) [1, 85]. The discharge of these afferents is stimulated by increases in ventricular preload, afterload, and contractility, in addition to tachycardia [1, 38]. Because acute exercise can evoke each of these changes in the human, it is possible that these reflexes would be activated and buffer increases in sympathetic outflow. This concept has been examined in conscious humans using isometric handgrip exercise to activate muscle afferents

FIGURE 9.14

(A) *Peroneal MSNA and handgrip force before and during 90 s of isometric handgrip exercise performed at 30% MVC in a normal subject (top) and a patient with myophosphorylase deficiency (below). The MSNA increased substantially during exercise in the normal subject but not in the patient.* **(B)** *Average (±SE) increases above baseline levels for total minutes of MSNA, mean arterial blood pressure* **(MAP)**, *and heart rate* **(HR)** *during isometric handgrip in 9 normal subjects and 4 patients. Handgrip evoked no increase in MSNA and a blunted blood pressure response in the patients compared to the normal subjects, but the exercise-induced tachycardia was similar in the two groups. (Reprinted with permission from Pryor, S.L., S.F. Lewis, R.G. Haller, L.A. Bertocci, and R.G. Victor. Impairment of sympathetic activation during static exercise in patients with muscle phosphorylase deficiency [McArdle's Disease]. J. Clin. Invest. 85:1444–1449, 1990, by copyright permission of the American Society for Clinical Investigation.)*

and lower body negative pressure (LBNP) to unload (deactivate) cardiopulmonary afferents. Because mild levels of LBNP (-5 to -15 mmHg) decrease central venous pressure (ventricular preload) without decreasing arterial pressure or increasing heart rate, nonhypotensive LBNP is though to reduce mainly the central sympathoinhibitory influence of cardiopulmonary baroreceptors without causing an important alteration in the discharge of arterial (sinoaortic) baroreceptor afferents [38].

In a nonmicroneurographic study, Walker et al. [95] found that LBNP at -5 mmHg augmented the forearm vasoconstrictor response to isometric handgrip performed at 10% and at 20% MVC, which suggests that the cardiopulmonary baroreflex normally restrains the reflex (sympathetic) vasoconstrictor response to exercise. This interpretation, however, has not been supported by three recent microneurographic investigations, all of which showed that decreased cardiopulmonary baroreflex stimulation with mild LBNP (-5 and -10 mmHg) has no detectable effect on the increases in MSNA produced by isometric handgrip exercise (Fig. 9.15) [58, 61, 63]. Handgrip-induced increases in MSNA also were unaffected during an intravenous infusion of normal saline, which increases ventricular preload, and, therefore, should increase cardiopulmonary baroreflex inhibition of sympathetic outflow [58].

These microneurographic studies fail to provide neurophysiological support for the hemodynamic findings of Walker et al. [95], and instead indicate that neither stimulation nor deactivation of cardiopulmonary baroreflexes modulates the MSNA responses to isometric exercise in humans.

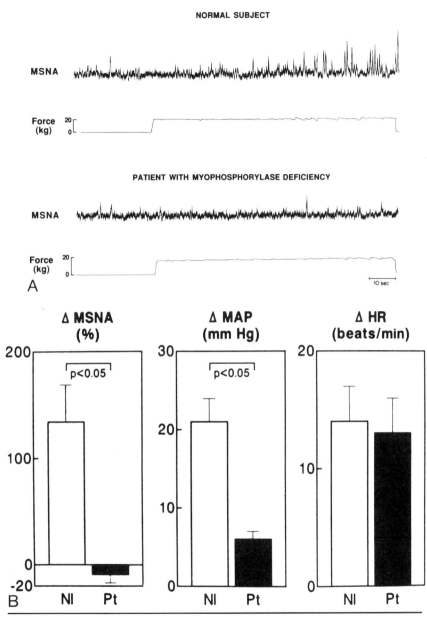

FIGURE 9.14

FIGURE 9.15

Peroneal MSNA and handgrip force before (−30 to 0s) and in response to 120 s of isometric handgrip exercise (30% MVC) performed alone (A) and during −5 mmHg of lower body negative pressure (LBNP) (i.e., decreased cardiopulmonary baroreceptor inhibition) (B) in the same subject. The time course and magnitude of the MSNA response was no different in the two conditions. (Reprinted with permission from Scherrer, U., S. Fløistrup Vissing, and R.G. Victor. Effects of lower body negative pressure on sympathetic nerve responses to static exercise in humans. Circ. 78:49–59, 1988, and by permission of the American Heart Association.)

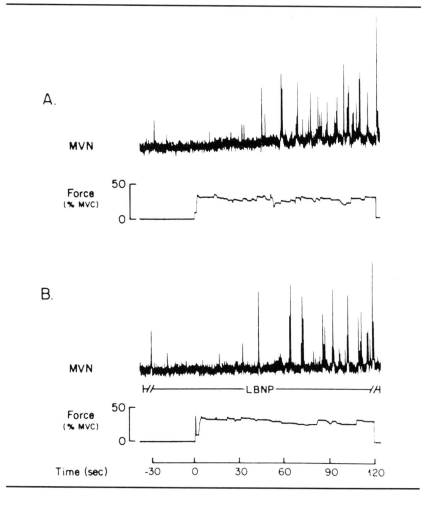

Lung Inflation Reflexes

In anesthetized animals, lung inflation activates vagal afferent nerve fibers, which reflexly decrease efferent sympathetic outflow [21, 23]. Similarly, within a breath cycle in conscious humans at rest, MSNA is inhibited during inspiration and is stimulated during expiration [13, 28, 72]. In the human, however, simulated exercise hyperpnea (i.e., isocapnic, high-frequency, deep breathing at rest) has no effect on either the minute burst frequency or the total minute activity of MSNA during muscle metaboreflex activation evoked by isometric handgrip or sustained with posthandgrip forearm muscle ischemia [72]. Hyperpneic stimulation of sympathoinhibitory pulmonary vagal afferents, therefore, does not appear to modulate the muscle metaboreflex-induced increase in MSNA evoked by isometric handgrip.

Arterial Baroreflexes

Arterial (sinoaortic) baroreflexes inhibit sympathetic outflow when stimulated by increases in systemic arterial pressure [1, 37]. Because acute exercise (particularly isometric contractions) produces increases in arterial blood pressure, one might postulate that the arterial baroreceptor reflex would act to buffer exercise-evoked increases in efferent sympathetic activity. Although the effects of exercise on arterial baroreflex function in humans are incompletely understood, the current thinking is that exercise causes the arterial baroreflex to operate at a higher-than-normal set point [12, 35]. This upward resetting might possibly attenuate arterial baroreflex buffering of MSNA during exercise. Recent microneurographic data indicate that this possibility is unlikely, however.

Eckberg and Wallin [14] found that the onset of isometric handgrip exerted rather small but directionally opposite effects on carotid baroreflex control of heart rate and MSNA. Compared to resting conditions, brief handgrip attenuated the transient decreases in heart rate, but did not attenuate, and actually slightly augmented, the transient decreases in MSNA evoked by carotid baroreflex activation (brief neck suction). These findings indicate that at the onset of isometric exercise the carotid baroreceptors retain their ability to evoke acute reflex decreases in MSNA. Whether the arterial baroreflex effectively buffers the sustained metaboreflex activation of MSNA that occurs during prolonged isometric exercise is, however, another question.

To address this, Scherrer et al. [62] recorded MSNA during 2 minutes of isometric handgrip (30% MVC), while attempting to manipulate the level of arterial baroreflex activation by controlling the exercise-induced rise in arterial pressure with pharmacological agents. They found that the increases in MSNA produced by a given level of handgrip are (a) augmented by > 300% when the exercise-evoked rise in arterial pressure is partially suppressed with an infusion of nitroprusside (i.e., with below

FIGURE 9.16

Representative data from one subject showing the **MSNA,** *heart rate* **(HR)**, *mean arterial pressure* **(MAP),** *and force responses to isometric handgrip exercise (33% MVC) for 2 minutes under normal conditions* **(A)**, *and during infusions of nitroprusside* **(B),** *or phenylephrine* **(C).** *Note that modest alterations in the level of blood pressure (stimulation of arterial baroreflexes) had profound effects on the exercise-induced increases in both heart rate and MSNA. (Reprinted with permission from Scherrer, U., S.L. Pryor, L.A. Bertocci, and R.G. Victor. Arterial baroreflex buffering of sympathetic activation during exercise-induced elevations.* J. Clin. Invest. 86:1855–1861, 1990, *and by copyright permission of the American Society for Clinical Investigation.)*

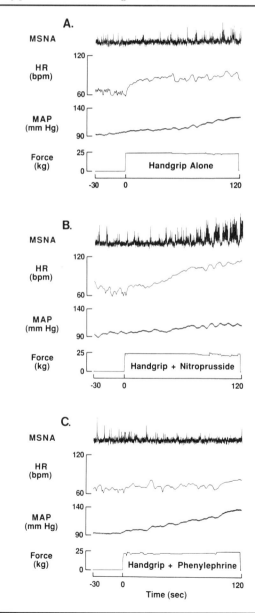

normal arterial baroreflex sympathoinhibition), and (b) attenuated by > 50% when the exercise-induced rise in arterial pressure is artificially accentuated with an infusion of phenylephrine (i.e., with greater than normal baroreflex inhibition of sympathetic outflow) (Fig. 9.16). These data suggest that the arterial baroreflex, when activated by the progressive increase in arterial pressure that accompanies isometric exercise, markedly buffers exercise-induced increases in MSNA. In contrast to cardiopulmonary baroreceptor and lung inflation reflexes, therefore, arterial baroreflexes appear to modulate the MSNA responses to isometric exercise in the human.

SUMMARY AND CONCLUSIONS

Recent investigations using direct (microneurographic) recordings of MSNA have provided a substantial amount of new information on the regulation of sympathetic nervous system control of nonactive skeletal muscle blood flow during exercise in humans. Some of the new conclusions from these studies discussed in this review include:

1. The direction, pattern and magnitude of the MSNA response to exercise depend on the collective influence of a number of factors, including the mode (isometric or rhythmic), intensity, and duration of the exercise, the size of the contracting muscle mass, and possibly the level of conditioning (physical training) of the exercising muscles. The MSNA response also appears to be tightly coupled with the onset and progression of muscle fatigue, at least during sustained, isometric contractions.
2. Increases in MSNA evoked during exercise with the arms are fairly uniform among different skeletal muscle nerves, and these responses correlate strongly with changes in venous plasma norepinephrine concentrations, limb vascular resistance and arterial blood pressure. Thus, increases in this neural activity during exercise are associated with the expected physiological responses.
3. The MSNA response to the same level of exercise varies markedly among healthy subjects but appears to be consistent over time within a particular subject.
4. The muscle metaboreflex (muscle chemoreflex) is the primary mechanism by which MSNA is stimulated during small-muscle, isometric exercise in humans. In contrast, central command has a relatively weak influence on MSNA during this type of exercise.
5. Muscle metaboreflex-stimulation of MSNA also occurs during dynamic exercise, but only at or above moderate, submaximal intensities (i.e., not during mild exercise).
6. Muscle metaboreflex-evoked increases in MSNA during exercise

are strongly associated with glycogenolysis and the consequent cellular accumulation of hydrogen ions in the contracting muscles.

7. Sympathoinhibitory cardiopulmonary reflexes do not appear to modulate the MSNA responses to isometric exercise in the healthy human. However, arterial baroreflexes exert a potent inhibitory effect on MSNA during this form of exercise.

The mechanisms involved in the regulation of MSNA during large-muscle, dynamic leg exercise is an important topic for future investigations, as is the relationship between MSNA and sympathetic outflow to other regional circulations (e.g., heart, viscera, skin) during various forms of exercise.

ACKNOWLEDGMENTS

The authors thank all their colleagues, especially Drs. Robin Callister and Kevin Kregel, for their comments and suggestions during the development of this review. Special thanks to Christine Coronado and Mary Jo Reiling for their assistance in the preparation of the text and graphics.

Dr. Seals's work was supported by grants HL-39966 from the National Heart, Lung and Blood Institute and AG-06537 from the National Institute on Aging, by a grant from the Arizona Heart Association, and by a Biomedical Research Support Grant from the University of Arizona. Dr. Seals was supported by Research Career Development Award AG-00423 from the National Institute on Aging during a portion of this work.

Dr. Victor's work was supported by the Lawson and Rogers Lacy Research Fund in Cardiovascular Diseases and by funding from the National Heart, Lung, and Blood Institute (Program Project Grant HL-06296; Clinical Investigator Award HL-01886), from the Ruby D. Hexter Estate, and from the American Heart Association National Center and Texas Affiliate. Dr. Victor is an Established Investigator of the American Heart Association.

REFERENCES

1. Abboud, F.M., and M.D. Thames. Interaction of cardiovascular reflexes in circulatory control. F.M. Abboud and J.T. Shepherd (eds.). *Handbook of Physiology: The Cardiovascular System. Peripheral Circulation and Organ Blood Flow, Vol. 3.* Bethesda, MD: American Physiological Society, 1983, pp. 675–753.

2. Anderson, E.A., C.A. Sinkey, M.P. Clary, J.S. Kempf, and A.L. Mark. Survey of symptoms experienced after microneurographic recording. *Circ.* 80(Suppl. 4):II-291, 1989.

3. Anderson, E.A., B.G. Wallin, and A.L. Mark. Dissociation of sympathetic nerve

activity in arm and leg muscle during mental stress. *Hypertension* 9(Suppl. III):114–119, 1987.

4. Andres, K.H., M. von Düring, and R.F. Schmidt. Sensory innervation of the achilles tendon by group III and IV afferent fibers. *Anat. Embryol.* 172:145–156, 1985.

5. Bevegard, S., and J.T. Shepherd. Regulation of the circulation during exercise in man. *Physiol. Rev.* 47:178–214, 1967.

6. Blair, D.A., W.E. Glover, and I.C. Roddie. Vasomotor responses in the human arm during leg exercise. *Circ. Res.* 9:264–274, 1961.

7. Burke, D., G. Sundlof, and B.G. Wallin. Postural effects on muscle nerve sympathetic activity in man. *J. Physiol.* 272:399–414, 1977.

8. Christensen, N.J., and H. Galbo. Sympathetic nervous activity during exercise. *Ann. Rev. Physiol.* 45:139–153, 1983.

9. Delius, W., K.-E. Hagbarth, A. Hongell, and B.G. Wallin. General characteristics of sympathetic activity in human muscle nerves. *Acta Physiol. Scand.* 84:65–81, 1972.

10. Delius, W., K.-E. Hagbarth, A. Hongell, and B.G. Wallin. Manoeuvres affecting sympathetic outflow in human muscle nerves. *Acta Physiol. Scand.* 84:82–94, 1972.

11. Donald, K.W., A.R. Lind, G.W. McNicol, P.W. Humphreys, S.H. Taylor, and H.P. Staunton. Cardiovascular responses to sustained (static) contractions. *Circ. Res.* 20, 21(Suppl):I-15–I-32, 1967.

12. Ebert, T. Baroreflex responsiveness is maintained during isometric exercise in humans. *J. Appl. Physiol.* 61:797–803, 1986.

13. Eckberg, D.L., C. Nerhed, and B.G. Wallin. Respiratory modulation of muscle sympathetic and vagal cardiac outflow in man. *J. Physiol.* (London) 365:181–196, 1985.

14. Eckberg, D.L., and B.G. Wallin. Isometric exercise modifies autonomic baroreflex responses in humans. *J. Appl. Physiol.* 63:2325–2330, 1987.

15. Eklund, B., L. Kaijser, and E. Knutsson. Blood flow in resting (contralateral) arm and leg during isometric contraction. *J. Physiol.* (London), 140:111–124, 1974.

16. Eldridge, F.L., D.E. Millhorn, J.P. Kiley, and T.G. Waldrop. Stimulation by central command of locomotion, respiration and circulation during exercise. *Respir. Physiol.* 59:313–337, 1985.

17. Escourrou, P., D.G. Johnson, and L.B. Rowell. Hypoxemia increases plasma catecholamine concentrations in exercising humans. *J. Appl. Physiol.* 57:1507–1511, 1984.

18. Esler, M., G. Jennings, P. Korner, et al. Assessment of human sympathetic nervous system activity from measurements of norepinephrine turnover. *Hypertension* (Dallas) 11:3–20, 1988.

19. Fagius, J., S. Karhuvaara, and G. Sundlöf. The cold pressor test: effects on sympathetic nerve activity in human muscle and skin nerve fascicles. *Acta Physiol. Scand.* 137:325–334, 1989.

20. Fagius, J., F. Niklasson, and C. Berne. Sympathetic outflow in human muscle nerves increases during hypoglycemia. *Diabetes* 35:1124–1129, 1986.

21. Folkow, B., G.F. Di Bona, P. Hjemdahl, P.H. Torén, and B.G. Wallin. Measurements of plasma norepinephrine concentrations in human primary hypertension. A word of caution on their applicability for assessing neurogenic contributions. *Hypertension* 5:399–403, 1983.

22. Folkow, B., Grimby, and O. Thulesius. Adaptive structural changes of the vascular walls in hypertension and their relation to the control of peripheral resistance. *Acta Physiol. Scand.* 44:255–267, 1958.

23. Galbo, H. *Hormonal and Metabolic Adaptation to Exercise.* New York: Thieme-Stratton, 1983.

24. Gerber, U., and C. Polosa. Effects of pulmonary stretch receptor afferent stimulation on sympathetic preganglionic neuron firing. *Can. J. Physiol. Pharmacol.* 56:191–198, 1978.

25. Goldstein, D.S., R. McCarty, R.J. Polinsky, and I.J. Kopin. Relationship between

plasma norepinephrine and sympathetic neural activity. *Hypertension* 5:552–559, 1983.

26. Gootman, P.M., J.L. Feldman, and M.I. Cohen. Pulmonary afferent influences on respiratory modulation of sympathetic discharge. H.P. Koepchen, S.M. Holton, and A. Trzebski (eds.). *Central Interaction Between Respiratory and Cardiovascular Control Systems*. Berlin: Springer-Verlag, 1980, pp. 172–178.

27. Gregory, J.E., P. Kenins, and V. Proske. Can lactate-evoked cardiovascular responses be used to identify muscle ergoreceptors? *Brain Res* 404:375–378, 1987.

28. Hagbarth, K.-E., and A.B. Valbo. Pulse and respiratory grouping of sympathetic impulses in human muscle nerves. *Acta Physiol. Scand.* 74:96–108, 1968.

29. Hjemdahl, P., U. Freyschuss, A. Juhlin-Dannfelt, and B. Linde. Differentiated sympathetic activation during mental stress evoked by the Stroop test. *Acta Physiol. Scand.* 527(Suppl.):25–29, 1984.

30. Hobbs, S.F. Central command during exercise: parallel activation of the cardiovascular and motor systems by descending command signals. O.A. Smith, R.A. Galosy, and S.M. Weiss (eds). *Circulation, Neurobiology, and Behavior*. New York: Elsevier, 1982, pp. 217–231.

31. Kaufman, M.P., J.C. Longhurst, K.J. Rybicki, J.H. Wallach, and J.H. Mitchell. Effects of static muscular contraction on impulse activity of groups III and IV afferents in cats. *J. Appl. Physiol.* 55:105–112, 1983.

32. Lewis, S.F., and R.G. Haller. The pathophysiology of McArdle's disease: clues to regulation in exercise and fatigue. *J. Appl. Physiol.* 65:391–401, 1986.

33. Lewis, S.F., W.F. Taylor, R.M. Graham, W.A. Pettinger, J.E. Schutte, and C.G. Blomqvist. Cardiovascular responses to exercise as functions of absolute and relative work load. *J. Appl. Physiol.* 54:1314–1323, 1983.

34. Lind, A.R. Cardiovascular adjustments to isometric contractions: static effort. F.M. Abboud and J.T. Shepherd (eds.). *Handbook of Physiology. The Cardiovascular System, Peripheral Circulation and Organ Blood Flow*, vol. III. Bethesda, MD: American Physiological Society, 1983, pp. 947–960.

35. Ludbrook, J., and W.F. Graham. Circulatory responses to onset of exercise: role of arterial and cardiac baroreflexes. *Am. J. Physiol.* 248:H457-H467, 1985.

36. Lundberg, J.M., A. Rudehill, A. Sollevi, E. Theodorsson-Norheim, and B. Hamberger. Frequency- and reserpine-dependent chemical coding of sympathetic transmission: differential release of noradrenaline and neuropeptide Y from pig spleen. *Neurosci. Lett.* 63:96–100, 1986.

37. Mancia, G., and A.L. Mark. Arterial baroreflexes in humans. F.M. Abboud and J.T. Shepherd (eds.). *Handbook of Physiology. The Cardiovascular System. Peripheral Circulation and Organ Blood Flow*, vol. III. Bethesda, MD: American Physiological Society, 1983, 755–793.

38. Mark, A.L., and G. Mancia. Cardiopulmonary baroreflexes in humans. F.M. Abboud and J.T. Shepherd (eds.). *Handbook of Physiology, The Cardiovascular System. Peripheral Circulation and Organ Blood Flow*, vol. III. Bethesda, MD: American Physiological Society, 1983, pp. 795–813.

39. Mark, A.L., R.G. Victor, C. Nerhed, and B.G. Wallin. Microneurographic studies of the mechanisms of sympathetic nerve responses to static exercise in humans. *Circ. Res.* 57:461–469, 1985.

40. McCloskey, D.I., and J.H. Mitchell. Reflex cardiovascular and respiratory responses originating in exercising muscle. *J. Physiol.* (London) 224:173–186, 1972.

41. Mense, S., and M. Stahnke. Responses in muscle afferent fibres of slow conduction velocity to contractions and ischaemia in the cat. *J. Physiol.* (London) 342:383–397, 1983.

42. Mitchell, J.H. Cardiovascular control during exercise: Central and reflex neural mechanisms. *Am. J. Cardiol.* 55:34D–41D, 1985.

43. Mitchell, J.H., M.P. Kaufman, and G.A. Iwamoto. The exercise pressor reflex: its

cardiovascular effects, afferent mechanism, and central pathways. *Ann. Rev. Physiol.* 45:229–242, 1983.

44. Morlin, C., B.G., Wallin, and B.M. Erikksson. Muscle sympathetic activity and plasma noradrenaline in normotensive and hypertensive man. *Acta Physiol. Scand.* 119:117–121, 1983.

45. Nilsson, H., B. Ljung, N. Sjoblom, and B.G. Wallin. The influence of the sympathetic impulse pattern on contractile responses of rat mesenteric arteries and veins. *Acta Physiol. Scand.* 123:303–309, 1983.

46. Peronnet, F., J. Cleroux, H. Perrault, D. Cousineau, J. de Champlain, and R. Nadeau. Plasma norepinephrine response to exercise before and after training in humans. *J. Appl. Physiol.* 51:812–815, 1981.

47. Pryor, S.L., S.F. Lewis, R.G. Haller, L.A. Bertocci, and R.G. Victor. Impairment of sympathetic activation during static exercise in patients with muscle phosphorylase deficiency (McArdle's Disease). *J. Clin. Invest.* 85:1444–1449, 1990.

48. Rea, R.F., and B.G. Wallin. Sympathetic nerve activity in arm and leg muscles during lower body negative pressure in humans. *J. Appl. Physiol.* 66:2778–2781, 1989.

49. Roberts, J., and G.M. Steinberg. Effects of aging on adrenergic receptors. *Federation Proc.* 45:40–41, 1986.

50. Rotto, D.M., and M.P. Kaufman. Effect of metabolic products of muscular contraction on discharge of group III and IV afferents. *J. Appl. Physiol.* 64:2306–2313, 1988.

51. Rowell, L.B. *Human Circulation Regulation During Physical Stress*, London: Oxford University Press, 1986.

52. Rowell, L.B., D.G. Johnson, P.B. Chase, K.A. Comess, and D.R. Seals. Hypoxemia raises muscle sympathetic activity but not norepinephrine in resting humans. *J. Appl. Physiol.* 66:1736–1743, 1989.

53. Rusch, N.J., J.T. Shepherd, R.G. Webb, and P.M. Vanhoutte. Different behavior of the resistance vessels of the human calf and forearm during contralateral isometric exercise, mental stress and abnormal respiratory movements. *Circ. Res.* 48(Suppl I):118–130, 1981.

54. Saito, M., S. Iwase, and T. Mano. Different responses of muscle sympathetic nerve activity to sustained and rhythmic handgrip exercises. *Japanese J. Physiol* 36:1053–1057, 1986.

55. Saito, M., T. Mano, H. Abe, and S. Iwase. Responses in muscle sympathetic nerve activity to sustained hand-grips of different tensions in humans. *European J. Appl. Physiol.* 55:493–498, 1986.

56. Saito, M., T. Mano, S. Iwase, K. Koga, H. Abe, and Y. Yamazaki. Responses in muscle sympathetic activity to acute hypoxia in humans. *J. Appl. Physiol.* 65:1548–1552, 1988.

57. Saito, M., T. Mano, and S. Iwase. Sympathetic nerve activity related to local fatigue sensation during static contraction. *J. Appl. Physiol.* 67:980–984, 1989.

58. Sanders, J.S., and D.W. Ferguson. Cardiopulmonary baroreflexes fail to modulate sympathetic responses during isometric exercise in humans: direct evidence from microneurographic studies. *J. Am. Coll. Cardiol.* 12:1241–1251, 1988.

59. Sanders, J.S., and D.W. Ferguson. Diastolic pressure determines autonomic responses to pressure perturbation in humans. *J. Appl. Physiol.* 66:800–807, 1989.

60. Savard, G., S. Strange, B. Kiens, E.A. Richter, N.J. Christensen, and B. Saltin. Noradrenaline spillover during exercise in active versus resting skeletal muscle in man. *Acta Physiol. Scand.* 131:507–515, 1987.

61. Scherrer, U., S. Fløistrup Vissing, and R.G. Victor. Effects of lower body negative pressure on sympathetic nerve responses to static exercise in humans. *Circ.* 78:49–59, 1988.

62. Scherrer, U., S.L. Pryor, L.A. Bertocci and R.G. Victor. Arterial baroreflex buffering

of sympathetic activation during exercise-induced elevations in arterial pressure. *J. Clin. Invest.* 86:1855–1861, 1990.

63. Seals, D.R. Cardiopulmonary baroreflexes do not modulate exercise-induced sympathoexcitation. *J. Appl. Physiol.* 64:2197–2203, 1988.

64. Seals, D.R. Influence of muscle mass on sympathetic neural activation during isometric exercise. *J. Appl. Physiol.* 67:1801–1806, 1989.

65. Seals, D.R. Sympathetic neural discharge and vascular resistance during exercise in humans. *J. Appl. Physiol.* 66:2472–2478, 1989.

66. Seals, D.R. Sympathetic neural adjustments to stress in physically trained and untrained humans. *Hypertension* (Dallas) 17:36–43, 1991.

67. Seals, D.R. Sympathetic activation during the cold pressor test: influence of stimulus areas. *Clin. Physiol.* 10:123–129, 1990.

68. Seals, D.R., P.B. Chase, and J.A. Taylor. Autonomic mediation of the pressor responses to isometric exercise in humans. *J. Appl. Physiol.* 64:2190–2196, 1988.

69. Seals, D.R., and R.M. Enoka. Sympathetic activation is associated with increases in EMG during fatiguing exercise. *J. Appl. Physiol.* 66:88–95, 1989.

70. Seals, D.R., D.G. Johnson, and R.F. Fregosi. Hypoxia potentiates exercise-induced sympathoexcitation in humans. *J. Appl. Physiol.* 1990.

71. Seals D.R., M.J. Reiling, D.G. Johnson. Peak sympathetic nerve activity during fatiguing isometric exercise in humans. *Soc. Neurosci. Abstr.* 16:862, 1990.

72. Seals, D.R., N.O. Suwarno, and J.A. Dempsey. Influence of lung volume on sympathetic nerve discharge in normal humans. *Circ. Res.* 67:130–141, 1990.

73. Seals, D.R., R.G. Victor, and A.L. Mark. Plasma norepinephrine and muscle sympathetic discharge during rhythmic exercise in humans. *J. Appl. Physiol.* 65:940–944, 1988.

74. Shepherd, J.T. Circulation to skeletal muscle. F.M. Abboud and J.T. Shepherd (eds.). *Handbook of Physiology, Section 2: The Cardiovascular System,* vol. III. Bethesda, MD: American Physiological Society 1983, pp. 319–370.

75. Sheriff, D.D., C.R. Wyss, L.B. Rowell, and A.M. Scher. Does inadequate oxygen delivery trigger pressor response to muscle hypoperfusion during exercise? *Am. J. Physiol.* 253 (Heart Circulation Physiology 21): H1199–H1207, 1987.

76. Simon, E., and W. Riedel. Diversity of regional sympathetic outflow in integrative cardiovascular control: patterns and mechanisms. *Brain Res* 87:323–333, 1975.

77. Sinoway, L., S. Prophet, I. Gorman, et al. Muscle acidosis during static exercise is associated with calf vasoconstriction. *J. Appl. Physiol.* 66:429–436, 1989.

78. Sinoway, L., R. Rea, M. Smith, and A. Mark. Physical training induces desensitization of the muscle metaboreflex. *Circ.* 80(Suppl):II 289, 1989.

79. Somers, V.K., K.C. Leo, M.P. Green, and A.L. Mark. Forearm training alters the sympathetic nerve response to isometric handgrip. *Circ.* 78(Suppl): II-177, 1988.

80. Sundlöf, G., and B.G. Wallin. Human muscle nerve sympathetic activity at rest. Relationship to blood pressure and age. *J. Physiol.* (London) 274:621–637, 1978.

81. Sundlöf, G., and B.G. Wallin. The variability of muscle nerve sympathetic activity in resting recumbent man. *J. Physiol.* (London) 272:383–397, 1977.

82. Sundlöf, G., and B.G. Wallin. Effect of lower body negative pressure on human muscle nerve sympathetic activity. *J. Physiol.* (London) 278:525–532, 1978.

83. Svendenhag, J., B.G. Wallin, G. Sundlöf, and J. Henriksson. Skeletal muscle sympathetic activity at rest in trained and untrained subjects. *Acta Physiol. Scand* 120:499–504, 1984.

84. Taylor, J.A., M.J. Joyner, P.B. Chase, and D.R. Seals. Differential control of forearm and calf vascular resistance during one-leg exercise. *J. Appl. Physiol.* 67:1791–1800, 1989.

85. Thames, M.D., and F.M. Abboud. Interaction of somatic and cardiopulmonary receptors in control of renal circulation. *Am. J. Physiol.* 237:560–565, 1979.

86. Thimm. F., and K. Baum. Response of chemosensitive nerve fibers of group III and IV to metabolic changes in rat muscles. *Pflügers Arch.* 410:143–152, 1987.

87. Vallbo, A.B., K.-E. Hagbarth, H.E. Torebjörk, and B.G. Wallin. Somatosensory, proprioceptive, and sympathetic activity in human peripheral nerves. *Physiol. Rev.* 59:919–957, 1979.

88. Vanhoutte, P.M., T.J. Verbeuren, and R.C. Webb. Local modulation of adrenergic neuroeffector interaction in the blood vessel wall. *Physiol. Rev.* 61:151–247, 1981.

89. Victor, R.G., L.A. Bertocci, S.L. Pryor, and Nunnally R.L. Sympathetic nerve discharge is coupled to muscle cell pH during exercise in humans. *J. Clin. Invest.* 82:1301–1305, 1988.

90. Victor, R.G., W.N. Leimbach, D.R. Seals, B.G. Wallin, and A.L. Mark. Effects of the cold pressor test on muscle sympathetic nerve activity in humans. *Hypertension* (Dallas) 9:429–436, 1987.

91. Victor, R.G., and W.N. Leimbach. Effects of lower body negative pressure on sympathetic discharge to leg muscles in humans. *J. Appl. Physiol.* 63:2558–2562, 1987.

92. Victor, R.G., S.L. Pryor, N.H. Secher, and J.H. Mitchell. Effects of partial neuro-muscular blockade on sympathetic nerve responses to static exercise in humans. *Circ. Res.* 65:468–476, 1989.

93. Victor, R.G., D.R. Seals, and A.L. Mark. Differential control of heart rate and sympathetic nerve activity during dynamic exercise: insight from direct intraneural recordings in humans. *J. Clin. Invest.* 79:508–516, 1987.

94. Victor, R.G., and D.R. Seals. Reflex stimulation of sympathetic outflow during rhythmic exercise in humans. *Am. J. Physiol.* 257 (Heart Circulation Physiology 26):H2017–H2024, 1989.

95. Walker, J.L., F.M. Abboud, A.L. Mark, and M.D. Thames. Interaction of cardio-pulmonary and somatic reflexes in humans. *J. Clin. Invest.* 65:14971–1497, 1980.

96. Wallin, B.G., and J. Fagius. Peripheral sympathetic neural activity in conscious humans. *Ann. Rev. Physiol.* 50:565–576, 1988.

97. Wallin, B.G., C. Morlin, and P. Hjemdahl. Muscle sympathetic activity and venous plasma noradrenaline concentrations during static exercise in normotensive and hypertensive subjects. *Acta Physiol. Scand.* 129:489–497, 1987.

98. Wallin, B.G., G. Sundlölf, B.M. Eriksson, P. Dominiak, H. Grobecker, and L.E. Lindblad. Plasma noradrenaline correlates to sympathetic muscle nerve activity in normotensive man. *Acta Physiol. Scand.* 111:69–73, 1981.

99. Wallin, B.G., and G. Sundlöf. A quantitative study of muscle nerve sympathetic activity in resting normotensive and hypertensive subjects. *Hypertension* 1:67–77, 1979.

100. Wallin, B.G., R.G. Victor, and A.L. Mark. Sympathetic outflow to resting muscles during static handgrip and postcontraction muscle ischemia. *Am. J. Physiol.* 256 (Heart Circulation Physiology 25): H105–H110, 1989.

101. Wallin, B.G. Intraneural recording and autonomic function in man. R. Bannister (ed.). *Autonomic Failure.* London: Oxford University Press, 1983, pp. 36–51.

102. Winder, W.W., R.C. Hickson, J.M. Hagberg, A.A. Ehsani, and J.A. McLane. Training-induced changes in hormonal and metabolic responses to submaximal exercise. *J. Appl. Physiol.* 46:766–771, 1979.

103. Wyss, C.R., J.L. Ardell, A.M. Scher, and L.B. Rowell. Cardiovascular responses to graded reductions in hindlimb perfusion in exercising dogs. *Am. J. Physiol.* 245 (Heart Circulation Physiology 14):H481–H486, 1983.

10
Exercise, Bone Mineral Density, and Osteoporosis

CHRISTINE SNOW-HARTER, Ph.D.
ROBERT MARCUS, M.D.

INTRODUCTION

The impact of exercise on skeletal dynamics and prevention of osteoporosis has provoked much interest and study. Loss of bone is an inevitable consequence of aging. This loss results in osteoporotic fractures in thousands of persons every year, constituting a major, growing public health problem for older women and men in Western society. It is probable that maintaining a higher bone mineral density (BMD) throughout life may help prevent many fractures associated with low bone density, and physical activity has gained attention as a method for improving BMD. The mechanisms by which the skeleton responds to activity are yet to be defined, but the evidence suggests that bone mineral increases in response to application of mechanical stress. Likewise, when the forces generated from stress are removed, BMD decreases.

In this chapter we review current issues related to bone strength, hypothesized mechanisms of bone loss, the influence of physical activity on bone mass accretion, and the role of exercise in preventing and treating osteoporosis. Before discussing these specific issues, however, we provide a brief overview of some fundamental aspects of skeletal organization, function, biomechanical properties, and assessment. For the purposes of our discussion, we will define **bone mineral** (synonymous with bone mass) as the absolute amount of hydroxyapatite (calcium phosphate crystal) present in measured bone and **bone mineral density** as relative value of bone mineral per measured bone area.

SKELETAL ORGANIZATION, FUNCTION, MECHANICAL PROPERTIES, AND ASSESSMENT

Organization of the Skeleton

The skeleton can be considered to be organized into two compartments, peripheral and central. The **peripheral** or cortical skeleton constitutes 80% of skeletal mass, and is composed primarily of compact plates, or

351

lamellae, organized about central nutrient canals. The shafts of long bones consist entirely of cortical bone that encloses the central marrow cavity. Trabecular, or cancellous bone, constitutes about 70% by volume of the **central** or axial skeleton. It consists of a honeycomb of vertical and horizontal bars called trabeculae which are filled with varying fractions of marrow and fat. The metaphyseal ends of long bones also contain trabecular bone but no marrow in the adult. Vertebral bodies contain about 35% trabecular bone by weight [87] and about 70% by surface area, which, although lower than previous estimates, greatly exceeds the trabecular component of peripheral bones. Although the surface prevalence of remodeling units is reasonably similar for cortical and trabecular bone, the greatly increased surface area of the latter accounts for the fact that changes in bone mass in response to altered turnover are earlier and more impressive in the trabecular skeleton [73].

Remodeling: The Basis of Skeletal Adaptation
The mechanisms by which bone responds to functional loading are poorly understood. There is little dispute, however, that bone adapts to imposed stress or lack of stress by forming or losing tissue. This process is mediated through remodeling, a continuous cycle of destruction and renewal of bone. Remodeling is performed by individual, independent bone remodeling units which comprise bone-resorbing osteoclasts and bone-forming osteoblasts (Figure 10.1). In a maintenance situation, remodeling may be somewhat inefficient, because small deficits appear to persist on completion of each cycle. Over the years, these accumulated deficits account for the bone loss associated with age [73]. The basis for this conclusion is the reported age-related decline in mean wall thickness of trabecular bone from iliac crest biopsies [57].

Bone hypertrophy occurs when stress is applied in excess of normal levels. Osteoblastic activity exceeds osteoclastic resorption, which leads to a net gain in bone. Net loss occurs when resorption is greater than formation. Carter [25] suggests that stress-related osteonal fatigue damage stimulates the remodeling process. Osteoclastic activity removes the damaged material so that osteoblasts can deposit matrix and mineral along the paths of imposed stress. When damage is gradual, bone mass increases. However, with a high rate of damage (from continuous repetitions), bone formation may not keep up with accumulation of fatigue damage, and fracture may result.

Biomechanical Properties
The skeleton is subjected on a daily basis to external ground reaction forces and forces generated by muscle contraction. These forces lead to alterations in bone shape, and, to a large degree, determine its strength. As a deformable object, bone has mechanical properties similar

FIGURE 10.1

The remodeling cycle: **(a)** *resting trabecular surface;* **(b)** *multinucleated osteo-clasts dig a cavity of approximately* 20 μm; **(c)** *completion of resorption to 60 μm by mononuclear phagocytes;* **(d)** *recruitment of osteoblast precursors to the base of the resorption cavity;* **(e)** *secretion of new matrix by osteoblasts:* **(f)** *con-tinued secretion of matrix, with initiation of calcification; and* **(g)** *completion of mineralization of new matrix. Bone has returned to quiescent state, but a small deficit in bone mass persists. (Reprinted with permission from Marcus, R. Normal and abnormal bone remodelling in man.* Adv. Int. Med. *38:129–141, 1987, and with copyright permission from Annual Reviews Inc.)*

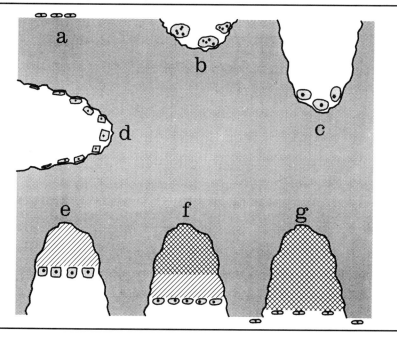

to any structural material [28]. All forces imposed on bone produce strain of some magnitude. The amount of strain a material is able to withstand determines the strength of that material. Loading creates stresses within a bone which may stimulate either external or internal remodeling, or both, and lead to a change in shape and possibly bone density. Strain is defined as the change in dimension produced by force divided by the original dimension. One "strain" is equivalent to a one percent change. Thus, one microstrain represents 10^{-6} "strain". The greater the strain, the higher the probability of damage and failure. If accumulated strain over time remains constant, bone will persist in an equilibrium state. If strain decreases, bone is lost until a new equilibrium is reached. This phenomenon has been observed in cases of immobilization and in space flight [32, 60, 68]. On the other end of the spectrum, application of repetitive strains beyond physiological limits could lead to damage and eventual fracture. Carter et al. [23] examined fatigue resistance of human femoral bone in vitro and predicted that repetitive loading at impacts equivalent to running would produce significant microfractures (small foci of structural failure) or fatigue damage after 100,000 cycles or 100 miles. In an in vivo study by Burr et al. [18] repetitive physiological loading of the dog ulna produced significant microdamage. It appears that remodeling serves a protective scavenger role in this regard. Although bone integrity is maintained in the short term, however, the remodeling inefficiency described above leads in the long term to bone loss.

Studies by Rubin and Lanyon [98] indicate that an optimal level of strain is necessary to maintain bone mass, and that bone mass is well correlated with functional loading. Using an avian model, they isolated the ulna in the left wing of turkeys and applied physiological loading at a constant rate over an 8-week period. The results, depicted in Figure 10.2, illustrate the increase in bone area with increasing microstrain.

Rubin and Lanyon [99] suggest that increasing the number of load cycles results in no additional increase in bone mass. Subsequent research by Whalen et al. [117] supports this conclusion. Using a mathematical model developed by Carter et al. [24], Whalen's group predicted that the magnitude of a load was a more important determinant of bone density than the number of repetitions. Applied to exercise training, this theory predicts that an exercise such as weight training, in which load is increased, would be more effective in improving bone mass than would jogging, in which repetitions are the primary training stimulus. Block et al. [12] compared very active men to age-matched sedentary men and found weight lifters to have the highest bone density values. Granhad and colleagues [46] found professional weight lifters to have much higher bone mineral content than controls. In fact, the bone mineral content of the third lumbar vertebra increased as annual weight lifted increased. Additional support for this model is discussed in the section on muscle mass, muscle strength, and bone density.

Assessment of Bone Mass
Initial assessments of bone mass and its changes with age were conducted using postmortem anatomic specimens and morphometric analyses of radiographs. During the past two decades, several noninvasive methods have been applied to this problem, including single and dual photon absorptiometry (SPA and DPA) and quantitative computed tomography (QCT). Iliac crest biopsy remains the primary invasive measurement.

Accurate, noninvasive measurement of bone mass emerged with the development of photon absorptiometry and QCT. Single photon absorptiometry is based on the attenuation of a collimated photon beam

FIGURE 10.2

Change in cross-sectional area of experimental turkey ulnae, loaded for 100 load reversals/day, to peak strains up to 4000 microstrain. These area changes are made by comparison between the left (experimental) and right (intact control) ulnae following an 8-week experimental period. (Reprinted with permission from Rubin, C.T., and L.E. Lanyon. Regulation of bone mass by mechanical strain magnitude. The effect of peak strain magnitude. Calcif. Tiss. Int. *37:411– 417, 1985.)*

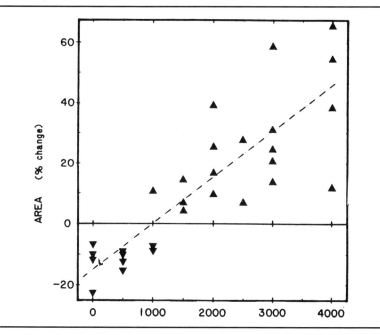

(usually iodine-125) by bone. The measurements are accurate, precise, and suited to regions of the body in which variations in soft tissue composition (fat vs. lean mass) are minimal, such as the forearm, leg, or heel, i.e., the cortical skeleton. Although estimates of cortical bone density in any region correlate reasonably well with whole body bone mineral, they give a very poor reflection of the central trabecular skeleton.

Isotopes that emit photons at two energies permit application of the photon absorptiometry principle to the central skeleton, most often the lumbar spine and proximal femur. Recent software modifications permit some models to measure whole body and regional skeletal mineral. Current DPA machines employ gadolinium-153, with energies of 44 and 100 keV; dual energy x-ray absorptiometry (DEXA) uses a dual energy x-ray beam. The person is recumbent while a photomultiplier tube records transmission from a narrowly collimated isotope or x-ray source located under the scanning table. The lumbar spine can be scanned in about 20 minutes with DPA and 5 minutes with DEXA. Radiation exposure from DPA and DEXA is approximately 10 millirem and 5 millirem, respectively. Because the detector recognizes all transmitted photons, estimates of bone density by this technique will include not only vertebral trabecular bone, but also such cortical elements as spinous and transverse processes. DPA is accurate and precise, with a coefficient of variation for replicate measurements of about 2.5%. The most advanced of the dual energy techniques, DEXA has lower precision error than DPA (<1.0%) with shorter examination time and less radiation exposure. With these techniques, mineral densities are reported as grams of mineral per square centimeter of bone area [77].

Quantitative computed tomography frequently has been used to determine trabecular bone density of the lumbar spine [20]. The person lies on the scanning table above a phantom of known densities. The operator selects a region of pure trabecular bone for analysis, and the mineral density, given as milligrams per cubic centimeter of bone volume, is computed. Although this technique can be modified for any region of the skeleton, most work has involved the lumbar spine, for which commercial software is available. For healthy, nonosteoporotic persons, the coefficient of variation of repeated measurements in the best hands may be as low as 1.6%. Radiation exposure, usually 500 to 1,000 millirem, is modest, but considerably greater than with photon and x-ray absorptiometry.

Trans-iliac bone biopsy is an invasive technique that provides a core sample of largely trabecular bone bordered by internal and external cortices. In most cases, transverse cylindrical cores are obtained approximately 2 cm posterior to the anterior superior iliac spine, just inferior to the iliac crest. Biochemical and histological analyses performed on these biopsies yield information regarding bone mass, adequacy of bone mineralization, and, when the bone has been previously labeled with tetracycline, dynamic aspects of bone turnover [17]. Recent applications of this technique also permit assessment of the degree to which trabecular elements are connected to each other, and the magnitude of spaces between adjacent trabeculae, i.e., the connectivity of trabecular bone [90].

BONE STRENGTH: MORE THAN BONE MINERAL DENSITY

Many patients with fractures of the vertebrae, wrist, and hip have low bone density. Consequently, the compressive strength of trabecular bone relative to bone mass has been studied by many investigators [38, 64, 75, 80–82, 113]. Results indicate that bone strength depends not

FIGURE 10.3

Effect of mass distribution on strength. Assume that the two cylinders have equal mass. The right one shows distribution of mass further away from the bending axis, resulting in substantially increased resistance to bending along this axis.

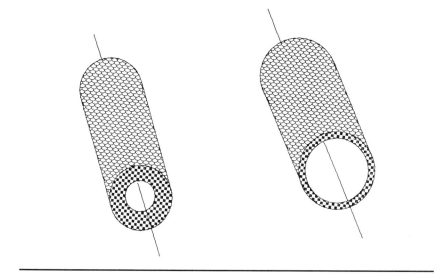

only upon bone mass, but also on its quality and architecture. Thus, bone mineral measurements provide only partial information regarding bone fragility, which means that substantial overlap in bone mineral content can exist between persons with and without fractures [52]. The qualitative and architectural contributions to bone differ for cortical and trabecular bone.

GEOMETRICAL PROPERTIES OF CORTICAL BONE. The distribution of bone mass around its bending axis constitutes an important geometrical determinant of the strength of cortical bone. This parameter, called the cross-sectional moment of inertia (CSMI), is illustrated in Figure 10.3. Two bones with the same mineral values have different strengths owing to differences in CSMI. Higher CSMI results in improved strength. Hui and colleagues [53] used SPA to measure forearm density in a longitudinal study of 268 Caucasian women ranging in age from 50 to 95. They observed the expected decline in forearm density beginning at age 50, but reported an increase in forearm bone mineral density after the age of 86 (Fig. 10.4). This augmentation was accompanied by an increase in bone width, which would result in an increase in CSMI and improved strength. The authors attributed this late, small increase to a gain in bone mass of the periosteal envelope in compensation for endosteal loss that occurred after age 50 and developed a

FIGURE 10.4

Relationship of age and forearm mineral density in normal women. Average bone mass has been normalized for body mass. (Reprinted with permission from Hui, S.L., P.S. Wiske, J.A. Norton, and C.C. Johnston. A prospective study of change in bone mass with age in postmenopausal women. J. Chronic Dis. *35:715–725, 1982, and with copyright permission from Pergammon Press plc.)*

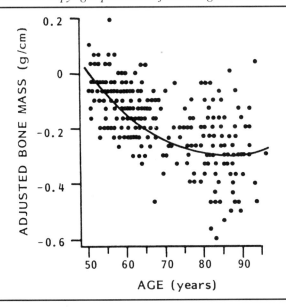

model of age-related bone loss in the radius (Fig. 10.5). Additional research using a large population of elderly individuals is necessary to substantiate this conclusion.

ARCHITECTURAL PROPERTIES OF TRABECULAR BONE. Orientation of vertical and horizontal trabeculae is critical to trabecular bone strength. Figure 10-6 illustrates the important contribution of the horizontal cross-linking to structural integrity of vertical struts. In a young person, the architecture of load-bearing trabecular bone is characterized by thick vertical plates and columns that are crossed by thinner horizontal trabeculae. Maximum strength is gained by the connection of all trabecular elements [89]. With age, trabecular connectivity is disrupted. The nature of this change is a topic of great research interest. Using iliac crest biopsies, Parfitt et al. [90] reported trabeculae to be progressively disconnected with age, reflecting disappearance of entire trabecular elements. Similarly, Weinstein and associates [116] found both decreased trabecular width and increased trabecular separation with age, and concluded that trabecular loss may occur after sufficient

FIGURE 10.5

A suggested model of age-related bone loss in the radius. (Reprinted with permission from Hui, S.L., P.S. Wiske, J.A. Norton, and C.C. Johnston. A prospective study of change in bone mass with age in postmenopausal women. J. Chronic Dis. *35:715–725, 1982, and with copyright permission from Pergammon Press plc.)*

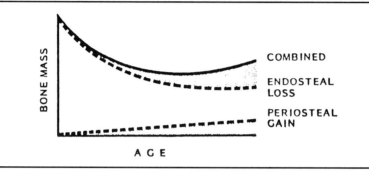

thinning to permit osteoclastic perforation. These changes in microarchitecture, in combination with a decline in overall bone mass, lead to extreme losses in bone strength. In support of this view are studies by Mosekilde and associates [81], who suggest that the loss of bone strength with age is much more pronounced than can be explained by loss of bone mass alone, and attribute this discrepancy to the loss in trabecular continuity.

In addition to iliac crest samples, vertebral trabecular specimens also exhibit age-related alterations in microarchitecture. Mosekilde [80] analyzed cylindrical trabecular specimens from the central third vertebral body of normal males and females and found a significant age-related decrease (r = −0.71) in mean horizontal trabecular thickness as well as significant increases between the horizontal and vertical trabeculae (r = 0.79 and r = 0.75, respectively). These changes are illustrated in Figure 10.7.

In conclusion, the loss in bone strength with age results from both trabecular thinning and disappearance. Although it is suggested that trabecular elements can be thickened but not replaced [116], further research is indicated to determine how various interventions can modify the microarchitecture of trabecular bone. Unfortunately, the methods to quantify microarchitecture require biopsy, a technique not accessible to many investigators and unacceptable to many persons. Until validated, noninvasive approaches to measuring bone strength become available, research in this area will be restricted.

FIGURE 10.6
*Effect of horizontal connections on resistance to buckling. The pillar on the left is not stabilized by any connecting elements and shows a critical buckling load (**Pcr**) of 1.0. The pillar on the right shows a single horizontal connection approximately halfway along its length. Buckling strength is 4-fold greater (Pcr = 4.0).*

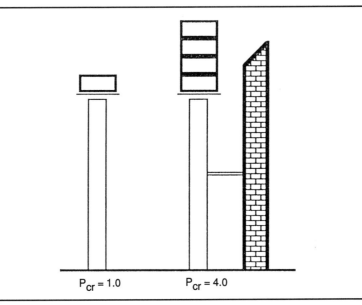

$P_{cr} = 1.0$ $P_{cr} = 4.0$

CHANGES IN BONE MASS

Aging

The traditional view of age-related bone loss was clearly enunciated by the landmark studies of Stanley Garn and associates [40]. Using careful measurements of metacarpal cortical thickness from hand radiographs, they described a characteristic trajectory of bone mass that was similar in men and women and was observed in virtually all ethnic groups. By this model, bone is gained during adolescence, reaches a plateau level sometime during the third decade, and remains stable until approximately age 50, after which progressive, gradual loss is observed. This model was confirmed by a number of independent laboratories, and was supplemented with the observation that the initial loss of bone at age 50 is temporarily more rapid in women, presumably because of the effects of menopause [78].

Experience with newer noninvasive methods, such as SPA, remain consistent with this model [53, 76, 107]. Although the age-related decline in bone mineral density of the radius provides an accurate

FIGURE 10.7

(a) *50-year-old man. An almost "perfect," continuous trabecular network.* **(b)** *58-year-old man. Discernible thinning of the horizontal trabeculae and some loss of continuity.* **(c)** *76-year-old man. Continued thinning of the horizontal trabeculae and wider separation of the vertical structures.* **(d)** *87-year-old woman. Advanced breakdown of the whole network, showing unsupported vertical trabeculae. Original magnification ×8. (Reprinted with permission from Mosekilde, Li. age-related changes in vertebral trabecular bone architecture—assessed by a new method. Bone 9:247–250, 1988 and with copyright permission from Pergammon Press plc.)*

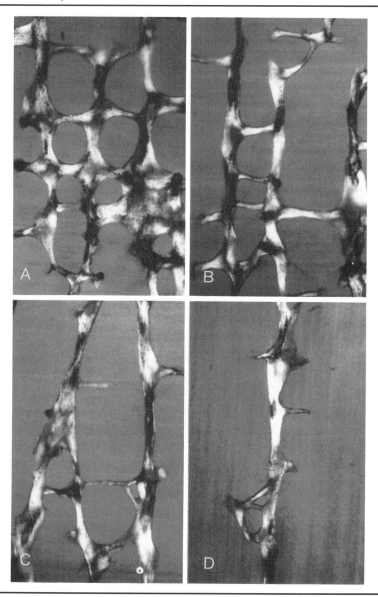

description of the trajectory of appendicular cortical bone mass, it was difficult for many years to validate its applicability to other areas of the cortical skeleton, such as the proximal femur, or to the axial or trabecular skeleton. In fact, pioneering studies with postmortem material [4, 33, 114] clearly indicated that loss of axial bone mass occurred earlier than one would have predicted from the forearm data. Subsequent analyses of iliac crest biopsy material confirm this view [11, 72, 79].

There is unanimous agreement, using multiple techniques, that trabecular bone is lost with age, and that axial density is substantially lower in older persons than in the young. Controversy today concerns the timing of the onset of axial loss and whether or not accelerated loss occurs at menopause.

Onset of Bone Loss
A decline in bone density has been reported to begin following the second [96], third [42], fourth [58] or fifth [2] decade of life. Measurements of anatomic specimens and results from biopsy studies both indicate that axial bone loss occurs as early as the third decade of life [5, 72, 115]. In particular, iliac crest biopsy data [11, 72, 79] have suggested that trabecular bone mass declines significantly in women prior to the menopause. Meunier et al. [79] showed an age-related loss of trabecular bone volume from iliac crest specimens that appeared to begin as early as the third decade. This study could be criticized, however, because the material was obtained from accident and sudden-death victims, and might not therefore be representative of a normal population. Marcus et al. [72] examined trabecular bone volume of iliac crest biopsy specimens taken from 62 active women with normal menstrual function, age 18–50 years. They found trabecular bone volume to be negatively correlated with age, with an annual predicted loss of 0.7% of the original bone volume (Fig. 10.8). The cumulative effect over a span of 30 years might amount to a loss of 25% of original trabecular bone volume before the age of menopause is reached. Once again, questions might be raised about the normalcy of this study group, because all subjects had undergone biopsy for preliminary staging of Hodgkin's disease. The great majority of women proved to have only limited disease, however, and all were active, normally menstruating women at the time of biopsy. More recently, Birkenhager-Frenkel and associates [11] conducted iliac crest biopsies on 94 healthy men and women aged 20–80 years, and reported a correlation of trabecular bone volume with age for premenopausal women that was the same as that observed by Marcus et al. [72]. Because their population included elderly persons, they also reported that the women had accelerated trabecular loss beginning at 50 years of age.

Trabecular vertebral specimens have been shown to follow the same pattern as iliac crest samples. Mosekilde and Mosekilde [82] examined

FIGURE 10.8

Trabecular bone volume (iliac crest biopsies) vs. age. Parallel lines indicate mean
± 1 and 2 SD. (Reprinted with permission from Marcus, R., J. Kosek, A.
Pfefferbaum, and S. Horning. Age-related loss of trabecular bone in premeno-
pausal women: a biopsy study. Calcif. Tiss. Int. 35:406–409, 1983.)

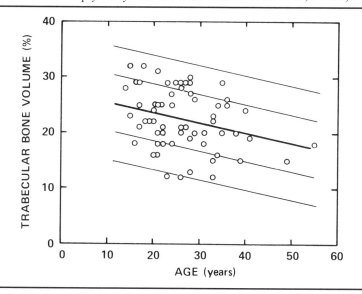

postmortem trabecular samples of the first lumbar vertebra from 42
normal persons, aged 15–87 years, and found a significant age-related
decrease in vertebral trabecular bone volume, beginning early in the
third decade. An accelerated loss at age 50 was not observed in the
women, but that may have been due to the small sample size. Thus,
although concerns remain about the limited nature of the data base,
postmortem and in vivo anatomic evidence both support the concept
that early loss of trabecular bone occurs in women.

The development of DPA and QCT as noninvasive measurements of
axial and trabecular bone mass has now permitted evaluation of this
question on a much larger scale. Measurements of spine density in both
normal and osteoporotic groups of patients have variably revealed
either a linear or an exponential loss of bone with age. One of the
major problems with these studies is the difficulty of predicting longitudinal changes from cross-sectional analyses. Depending on the number of subjects and measurement technique, some investigators have
reported constant loss of lumbar bone mineral from young adulthood,
whereas others have observed minimal or nonsignificant loss prior to
age 50 (or to menopause in women), followed by a linear decline
thereafter [58, 100].

Several groups have reported significant axial bone loss before age 50 [15, 49, 69, 94]. Madsen [69] suggested a linear loss with age. He reported lumbar spine densities on 41 women and 5 men from 20–93 years of age (mean = 61 years) and found a decrease of 0.5% per year. A similar pattern was later observed by Riggs and associates [94], who reported DPA spine densities for a large group of healthy women across the age range of 20 to 80 years. The best description of these data in women was a single negative correlation, the slope of which indicated a loss of axial bone mass over the entire adult age span of about 1% per year (Fig. 10-9). Similar measurements in normal men also gave a negative regression with age, although the slope was less than half of that observed with women. The authors concluded that there was no evidence of an increased rate of loss in axial bone mass in women after

FIGURE 10.9

Regression of bone mineral density of lumbar spine on age in normal women. (Reprinted with permission from Riggs, B.L., H.W. Wahner, W.L. Dann, R.B. Mazess, and K.P. Offord. Differential changes in bone mineral density of the appendicular and axial skeleton with aging. J. Clin. Invest. 67:328–335, 1981 and with copyright permission from the American Society for Clinical Investigation.)

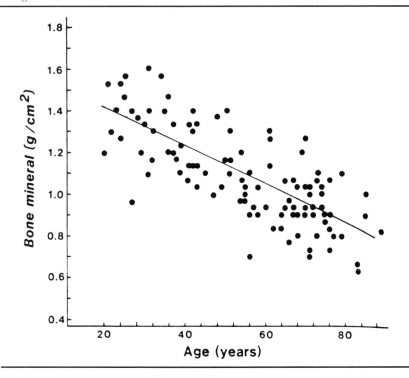

50 years of age. Buchanan et al. [15] measured vertebral trabecular bone density (QCT) in 74 healthy premenopausal women between the ages of 18 and 48. They found a linear regression with age (r = -0.39, p < 0.001) and concluded that vertebral trabecular bone loss begins during or prior to the third decade. In a cross-sectional study of 214 normal women between ages 35 and 80, Hansson and Roos [49] observed no age-related differences in the rate of vertebral bone loss, a pattern previously found by Riggs and associates [94]. They concluded that menopause does not have a direct effect on bone loss and that events occurring in the premenopausal years need to be considered in the prevention of osteoporosis.

Other studies fail to confirm a significant loss of bone prior to 50 years of age [2, 19, 37, 39, 42, 58, 85] but report the major loss to begin at the time of menopause. (These studies will be discussed in more detail in the next section.) The reasons for discrepancies among studies are not clear. The principal difficulty may arise from the fact that the vast majority of these studies are cross-sectional. Although such analysis may provide valid insights into population changes across time, they cannot distinguish secular trends, and are subject to multiple confounding factors. For example, the observation of a bone density at age 40 that is lower than that at age 20 could reflect loss of bone over this 20-year period, but also is consistent with an interpretation that peak bone mass is significantly higher in today's 20-year-old women than was true 20 years ago. Consequently, a number of important geographical, ethnic, dietary, and physical activity differences within and between study populations could account for the differences observed in this literature. Moreover, Sambrook and colleagues [100] recently have shown that the population size necessary to detect subtle changes in regression slope with certainty is far greater than that of any reported study. This is particularly relevant to detecting a menopausal acceleration of bone loss.

Menopause

Two issues arise when considering the changes in trabecular bone loss that occur at menopause. The first is whether bone loss begins around the time of menopause; second is whether menopausal loss subsides over time. All studies confirm that if bone loss has not started at an earlier age, it certainly is present during the menopausal years. The question remains, however, whether a transient increase in rate of loss, specifically due to the loss of endogenous estrogen, can be demonstrated.

The majority of studies confirm that trabecular bone loss accelerates at menopause [2, 19, 37, 39, 40, 58, 85]. Using DPA, Gallagher et al. [39] measured spine density on 392 normal women and reported the largest decrease in density to occur in the first 5 years following menopause. They found a decline of 3.4% per year in the second year,

1.7% per year in the fourth year and 0.8% per year in the ninth year. Cann et al. [19] used QCT to measure spine density and found stable values for trabecular bone mineral until menopause, followed by a rapid decline for 5–8 years, then a continued but slower decrease thereafter. The QCT measurements of spine density by Firooznia et al. [37] showed the same trend. Their results of 132 normal women demonstrated increased vertebral trabecular bone loss (from 2%/yr to 8%/yr) from ages 50 to 60 years. An accelerated loss of trabecular vertebral bone also has been demonstrated following surgical menopause [41].

A few cross-sectional studies using DPA have reported a linear decline in lumbar spine mineral beginning at age 50 [2, 58]. From a sample of 70 healthy women, Krolner and Pors Nielsen [58] observed a constant loss (1.4%/yr) in the rate of spine density from age 50 through 88 years (Fig. 10.10). Although they did observe a loss beginning at age 34, the authors reported that the slope in premenopausal women (triangles in the figure) did not differ significantly from zero. In the same report, Krolner and Pors Nielsen examined spine density of 59 normal women in a longitudinal study. These women had two spine density measurements within 3 to 19 months of follow-up. The premenopausal group (n = 27) showed no significant loss, whereas the postmenopausal women (n = 32) exhibited a decline of 1.6–7.1%/yr. The 12 women within 5 years of menopause demonstrated a mean decrease of 6.5%/yr, which supports the view that accelerated loss occurs in the first 5 years past menopause.

To summarize, bone loss is a result of both aging and menopause. From the published studies, it seems that trabecular bone loss begins prior to age 50 and increases at menopause in women. Although the linear loss reported by Riggs et al. [94] often is cited as the progression of bone loss in women, as suggested by the work of Sambrook et al. [100], the data may not be representative of the population of women-at-large. Resolution of this question will require additional longitudinal studies.

PEAK BONE DENSITY

Although considerable attention has been given to the onset of bone loss, little data exist concerning the time that peak bone density is achieved. It has been assumed that maximal bone mass is reached at some time during the third decade of life. In light of new data, however, it is likely that this assumption will need to be revised. Recent densitometric evidence [43] as well as previous anatomic and biopsy studies [4] permit the conclusion that peak bone density may occur in late adolescence. In addition, Gilsanz et al. [44] have reported significantly higher

FIGURE 10.10

Lumbar spine bone mineral content in 70 normal women in relation to age. Triangles represent premenopausal women and circles denote postmenopausal women. Note that significant bone loss does not occur in this group until the age of 50 years. (Reprinted with permission from Krolner, B., and S. Pors Nielsen. Bone mineral content of the lumbar spine in normal and osteoporotic women: cross-sectional and longitudinal studies. Clin. Sci. 62:329–336, 1982.)

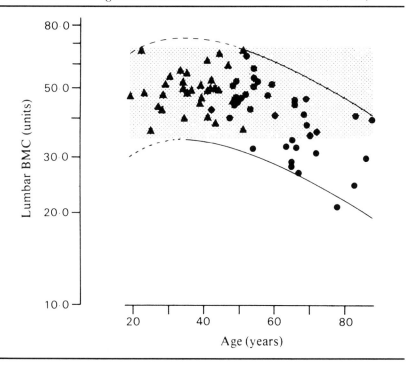

vertebral bone density following puberty in both girls and boys. The values measured at puberty remained stable through late adolescence, which indicates that the values had reached their peak directly after puberty. Unpublished observations from our laboratory support the notion that peak bone density is reached in adolescence. We measured spine density on 82 normal women from ages 12 to 30 and found a significant increase until the age of 17, after which no significant changes were observed. Although preliminary, these results indicate that peak bone density is reached much earlier than previously reported.

REGULATION OF BONE MINERAL DENSITY

Alteration in remodeling activity is the final common pathway to modifications in bone mineral density. Primary controllers of this process include physical activity, reproductive endocrine status, and calcium nutriture. In this section we discuss each of these factors, with emphasis on physical activity which is separated into the following five categories: (1) cross-sectional studies, (2) intervention studies, (3) muscle mass, muscle strength, and BMD, (4) cardiorespiratory fitness and BMD, and (5) reproductive endocrine status and physical training.

Physical Activity and Bone Mass

CROSS-SECTIONAL STUDIES. Examination of active and sedentary populations at single points in time generally supports a positive correlation between activity level and BMD. Although the type, duration, frequency, and intensity of the exercise have not been defined, these studies lend strong support to the notion that a positive relationship between activity and bone density does exist. Athletes have been observed to have higher bone density than nonathletes. Nilsson and Westlin [86] found 64 male athletes to have higher bone density of the distal femur than 39 sedentary controls. Comparing lifetime male tennis players to age-matched controls, Huddleston and colleagues [51] found the dominant radius to have significantly greater bone mineral than the nondominant radius. Pirnay et al. [91] observed similar results in professional tennis players. Compared to sedentary college students, the tennis players had 34% and 15% higher bone mineral in the dominant arm and nondominant arms, respectively.

Higher bone density also has been observed in experienced runners than in sedentary persons. Cross-country runners have exhibited 20% greater mineral content of the humeral head, calcaneus, radius, and ulna compared to controls. Axial sites at the neck of the femur and third lumbar vertebra have been found to be approximately 10% greater, which indicates that the response to running varies at different skeletal sites [29]. Brewer et al. [13] measured bone mineral densities of the radial midshaft, hand, and calcaneus in 80 women aged 30–49 years. Of these women, 42 were training for a marathon and had been running for 2 years; the remaining 38 women were not runners. Bone densities were significantly greater in the hands and at the radial midshaft of the running group. Yet the control group exhibited higher bone density of the calcaneus than the exercise group, which the authors concluded was likely a reflection of greater body weight in the sedentary controls.

Other studies have found runners to have higher axial bone density than nonrunners [1, 61, 71]. In a comparison of middle-aged runners whose lifelong running distance was 12,000 miles, Lane et al. [61] reported that density of the first lumbar vertebra was more than 30% higher than controls who were matched for age, sex, years of education, occupation, years past menopause, and hormone replacement. Additionally, some investigators have observed no differences in cortical bone density between the runners and nonrunners [1, 71]. Marcus et al. [71] observed higher lumbar spine density in elite women distance runners than in sedentary women of similar age. Radial densities of these women, however, were not significantly different.

Demonstrating specificity of bone mass accretion in relation to activity mode, Jacobson et al. [54] measured bone density in female intercollegiate athletes. Bone mineral content of the radius was higher in the tennis players and swimmers when compared to sedentary college students. Lumbar spine density was significantly higher only in the tennis players, which indicates the potential role of weight-bearing activities in bone mass accretion. Unfortunately in this study, body weight, a potential confounding variable, was not measured or discussed.

With regard to the importance of weight-bearing to the skeleton, recent studies suggest loads other than those generated by gravity, such as muscular pull, actively stimulate bone deposition. Davee and colleagues [31] found that young women who supplemented aerobic exercise with weight training of only 1 hour per week had higher spine densities than women who were sedentary or participating in aerobic exercise only. Additionally, Orwoll and colleagues [88] recently reported that radial and vertebral BMD were higher among men who swam regularly than in nonexercising men. Although swimming is considered a nonweight-bearing activity, its contributions to BMD may occur through loads created from high intensity muscular activity. Unfortunately, muscle strength was not measured in this study.

Not only is bone density higher in physically active people, but the literature also suggests that increased activity may be associated with a lower rate of age-related bone loss. Jacobson et al. [54] reported bone density values of the mid-radius and lumbar spine in older athletic women to be in the same range as for younger athletic women. Further, a 0.7% decrease per year in spine density was observed in a control population of women older than 50 years, which was not exhibited in a group of more active subjects. "Athletic" was used to describe adult women who exercised at least three times per week, eight or more months of the year for a minimum of three years. The type of exercise performed was not explained. Talmage et al. [112] found a negative correlation of bone density versus age in a group of nonathletic women, with apparent acceleration of loss between ages 45 and 55. An athletic group demonstrated weaker correlations of bone density with age and no accelerated loss from 45 to 55 years. Other recent literature suggests that muscle strength, physical fitness, and body weight, but not age, predict spine and hip BMD in premenopausal women [92]. Considering that bone loss parallels declines in muscle strength with age, physical activity may offset the age-related loss that has been defined in more sedentary populations.

INTERVENTION STUDIES. Intervention studies investigate the effects of an imposed exercise program on BMD. In limited numbers of intervention studies, the effects of exercise on bone density have been examined. Little attention has been given to understanding the type, intensity, frequency and duration of exercise most effective in improving bone mass. Other problems associated with many of these trials include nonrandomization, lack of adequate controls, poor subject compliance, and choice of measurement sites not stressed by the exercise protocol. Nonetheless, general results do indicate increased bone density following exercise training and tend to support site-specific responses.

In several studies postmenopausal women were trained with calisthenics and light aerobic activity [59, 108–110]. Women exercised three times a week for 30 to 50 minutes per session. The length of the exercise intervention varied between 8 and 48 months. Measurement sites for bone density were the lumbar spine, total body calcium, and the radius. In one study of less than 12 months [59], significant changes in total body calcium and lumbar spine density were found. No significant changes in the bone mineral of the radius was observed, however. Smith et al. [108–110] conducted two prospective studies. In one [108], elderly women (mean = 81 y) were placed into four groups: control, physical activity, calcium supplement, and combined activity/supplement. After 36 months, the activity and calcium groups increased radial bone mineral by 2.29% and 1.58%, respectively, whereas the combined exercise/calcium and control groups decreased radial bone mineral by 0.32% and 3.29%, respectively. In considering the reasons that the combination group failed to increase bone mass, the authors found that subjects randomized to that group were 2.6 years older than those in other groups and may have had a higher rate of overall decline in physical and mental function. In another study, Smith and colleagues [109] enrolled 200 women (80 exercisers, 120 controls), aged 35–65 years, in a similar exercise program over a 36-month period. Results demonstrated a significant decline in the exercise group during the first year, followed by increases in radial densities over the following 24 months. However, the observed increases did not make up for the loss during the first year. In a recent update of this study [110], which was extended to 48 months, the authors report that their first-year data were not valid because of equipment quality control problems. Results over the subsequent 3 years demonstrated that loss rates of the radius and ulna significantly decreased in the exercise group when compared to the controls. On examination of the exercise program, the first year consisted of weight-bearing activity, whereas additional emphasis was placed on upper body strength during successive years. From these results, the independent contributions of weight-bearing activity and strength training to bone mineral density cannot be determined.

In other prospective studies that have examined the effects of weight bearing on bone density, White et al. [119] observed no changes in the forearm bone density of postmenopausal women after 6 months of dancing. However, in a 9-month study of runners, Williams and colleagues [120] found a significant increase in bone density of the calcaneus. These data and those previously mentioned indicate that the site selected for measurement may be critical to the results obtained.

To demonstrate a proposed relationship between loading and bone density, Ayalon et al. [6] enrolled osteoporotic women in an exercise program designed to load the wrist and forearm. After performing a combination of bending, loading, compression, and torsion exercises three times a week for 5 months, the exercise group had a significant increase (3.8%) in forearm bone density. A group of osteoporotic controls demonstrated a 1.9% decrease at the radius. In a study examining the effects of back extension exercise on the rate of vertebral fracture, Sinaki and Mikkelson [103] found fewer additional fractures in osteoporotic women performing torso extension in comparison to flexion exercise. Because trunk extension exercises increase back strength and trunk flexion exercises do not, the type of loading to the bone may be very important.

The issue of bone density maintenance following exercise intervention has been addressed by Dalsky and colleagues [30]. After 9 months of weight-bearing and nonweight-bearing exercise with resistance, post-menopausal women had an increase of 5.2% in spinal bone mineral content. This value increased to 6.1% after an additional 13 months of exercise. A nonrandomized group of controls exhibited no change in spinal bone mineral content. Following a 13-month detraining period, bone mass was 1.1% above baseline. This return toward baseline exemplifies the dynamic nature of the skeletal system in response to functional load.

Cavanaugh and Cann [26] examined the effect of weight-bearing exercise (brisk walking) on spinal trabecular mineral density in post-menopausal women. The authors found that after 1 year the walkers (n = 9) actually lost trabecular bone—5.6% compared to the control group (n = 8) which lost 4%. These results are contradictory to those of Dalsky et al. [30], and may be related to small sample size and differences in experimental protocol. Dalsky's exercise group jogged in addition to walking, and performed exercises such as upright rowing, which specifically load the vertebrae. It appears, therefore, that resistance exercise may be more potent than brisk walking in promoting bone accretion.

As previously mentioned, the type of exercise that best promotes bone density is yet to be determined. Weight-bearing exercise, defined as walking, jogging, and running, has been the primary exercise therapy prescribed by physicians to arrest the bone loss associated with meno-pause. Recent evidence suggests, however, that exercise with higher loads at specific sites provides a more effective osteogenic stimulus than do lower loads that are generally distributed. For example, the forces produced at the lumbar vertebrae during fast walking and jogging are 1 times body weight (BW) and 1.75 times body weight, respectively [22]. On the other hand, during weight lifting activity (defined as a nonweight-bearing activity), loads on the lumbar vertebrae as much as 5–6 times body weight have been reported [46]. The specificity issue is supported by some of the literature, which suggests that the effects of exercise are not homogeneous but reflect the strains imposed at individual sites.

Although there is a paucity of data relative to the issue of the osteogenic response to exercise during the peak bone mass years, two recent longitudinal studies support a positive change in bone mineral density during this time period. Our laboratory investigated the effects of two different modes of exercise on BMD at the spine and proximal femur in women during their peak bone mass years (unpublished data). We randomly assigned a group of young women (mean = 19 y) to a running, weight-training, or control group. The exercise groups trained progressively for 8 months. During the last 2 months, the running group averaged 10 miles per week and the weight training group was lifting three sets of eight repetitions each at 85% of one repetition maximum. After 8 months of training, lumbar spine BMD increased significantly in the runners (1.32%) and the weight trainers (1.21%), but did not change in the controls. Results suggest that both modes of exercise elicited osteogenic benefits at the spine. A positive trend toward improved BMD at the hip was observed in the running group. In a study of young men, Leichter and colleagues [62] reported positive changes in tibial BMD following short-duration (14 weeks), very high intensity (eight hours per day) physical training. These data suggest that bone mineral density can be altered during the peak bone mass years.

In summary, although results from cross-sectional analysis support a positive effect of exercise on BMD, results from longitudinal studies provide mixed results. These results vary with the mode, duration, intensity, and frequency of exercise. Most studies have used weight-bearing activity (walking, jogging, running, dancing) as the exercise intervention. When the program, however, has been more intense, of longer duration, or included exercises which overload the muscular system, a better osteogenic stimulus has been observed. The interaction between muscle strength and BMD is a concept that is gaining much attention and will be discussed in the next section.

MUSCLE MASS, MUSCLE STRENGTH AND BONE MINERAL DENSITY. The effects of exercise on muscle are well documented [14]. Through training, functional adaptations occur that enable the muscular system to function at a higher level. Critical to the desired outcome however, is specificity of training. As a dynamic tissue aligned with the muscular system, it is not surprising that the skeleton exhibits changes similar to those observed in muscle. For example, the estimated loss of bone from its peak in young adulthood to 80 years of age is comparable to the reported 35–45% decline in muscle strength during the same life span [55].

The relationship between muscle strength and BMD has become an important research topic over the past few years as more investigators realize the logical interaction between the two systems. Doyle et al. [33] found a significant correlation between vertebral ash weight and psoas muscle weight from 46 routine autopsies. In a multiple regression analysis, psoas weight was the most robust predictor of vertebral ash weight. Aloia and colleagues [1] examined total body calcium, an index of bone mass, and total body potassium, an index of lean mass, in marathon runners and sedentary controls. Their results indicated a positive relationship between these indices of bone mass and muscle mass. In a muscle biopsy study, Aniansson et al. [3] found that hip fracture patients suffered a reduction in muscle fiber area, particularly in type II fibers.

Sinaki and Offord [104] found a significant positive correlation between bone density of the lumbar spine and back extensor strength in 68 healthy postmenopausal women. This correlation was constant even when bone density was corrected for age. In a similar study, Sinaki et al. [102] asked all the women to rate their level of physical activity on a questionnaire. Results revealed that women with higher physical activity had greater isometric back strength and higher spinal bone densities than those women with lower activity levels. These preliminary data suggest that a relationship does exist between strength of a specific muscle group and the corresponding bone. Unfortunately, because no additional groups of muscles were tested for strength, it is not known whether other strength contributions existed. In a recent longitudinal study, Sinaki et al. [106] imposed a 2-year program of nonweight-bearing back exercises on postmenopausal women and found that an increase in isometric back strength was not accompanied by a significant change in spine BMD. Absence of change in vertebral BMD may be explained by factors such as insufficient magnitude of loading (the amount of weight lifted was what would be used to increase local muscle endurance, not strength) and less than desirable compliance, a value not reported in the study.

The effect of muscular activity on bone mineral density has been assumed to be site-specific. Given this assumption, back strength would predict spine BMD, hip strength would predict hip BMD, and forearm strength would predict radial BMD. In a study by Bevier et al. [9], a significant correlation was found between grip strength and forearm density in 87 elderly men and women. Further, the men exhibited a significant relationship between back strength and lumbar spine density measured by dual photon absorptiometry. Sinaki et al. [105] recently reported similar results in 63 postmenopausal women. In a study of osteoporotic women, Simkin et al. [101] found a 3.8% increase in mid-radius BMD and after 5 months of exercises designed to create tension, torsion, compression, and bending forces on the forearm. Although muscle strength was not measured, one can assume that their exercise program led to some improvement in muscular performance. Beverly and colleagues [7] found that 6 weeks of brief (30 seconds), high-intensity forearm loading resulted in significant increases in grip strength (14.5%) and forearm mineral content (3.4%) in a group of 99 women, 30 of whom had fractured forearms. Moreover, the bone mass changes were more pronounced in the women with the best training response, and a detraining effect was noted on both variables in a 6-month follow-up visit.

Recent findings indicate that the relationship between strength and BMD is more complex than a simple consideration of muscle attachments to bone. Pocock et al. [92] evaluated pre- and postmenopausal women on muscle strength of the biceps brachii, quadriceps group, and BMD of the spine and proximal femur. They found biceps strength, but not quadriceps strength, to be a predictor of BMD at the spine and three regional sites on the proximal femur. For this population, muscle strength better explained the variance in BMD than age. Our group [111] recently had similar findings among a population of 59 young women (mean = 23 y). In stepwise multiple regression analysis, we found biceps strength the best predictor of hip density (Fig. 10.11), dominant grip strength the best predictor of spine density (Fig. 10.12), and nondominant grip strength the best predictor of nondominant mid-radius density (Fig. 10.13). At the femoral neck, back strength contributed significantly to bone mineral density. Additionally, we were able to measure hip strength in a subgroup of 32 women and found that hip adductor strength was an important predictor of total hip density. From these findings, we concluded that, in some cases, the relationship between strength and BMD were site-specific. In other cases, however, muscle groups more distant to the spine and proximal femur significantly contribute to bone density. These relationships may come about because arm activity is linked to the simultaneous contraction of trunk stabilizing muscles that directly exert forces on the hip and spine. Moreover, the length of the lever arm between arm muscles and the spine is considerably greater than that between back extensors and the spine, so that, when lifting the same weight, loads on axial bone generated by arm activity exceed those generated by back extensors [65].

CARDIORESPIRATORY FITNESS AND BONE MINERAL DENSITY. Cardiorespiratory fitness, often referred to as "physical fitness", recently has been related to bone density. Pocock et al. [93], using predicted maximal

FIGURE 10.11

Relationship between hip density and biceps strength in young women. (Reprinted with permission from Snow-Harter, C., M. Bouxsein, B. Lewis, S. Charette, P. Weinstein, and R. Marcus. Muscle strength as a predictor of bone mineral density in young women. J. Bone Min. Res. *5:589–595, 1990.)*

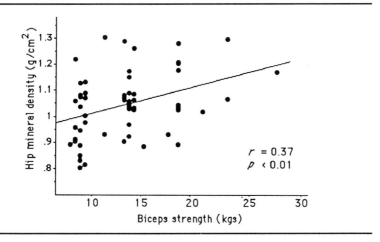

FIGURE 10.12

Relationship between lumbar spine density and grip strength in young women. (Reprinted with permission from Snow-Harter, C., M. Bouxsein, B. Lewis, S. Charette, P. Weinstein, and R. Marcus. Muscle strength as a predictor of bone mineral density in young women. J. Bone Min. Res. *5:589–595, 1990.)*

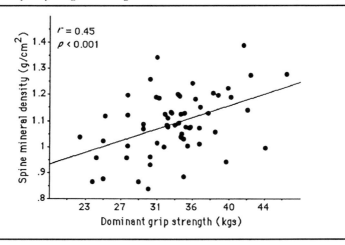

FIGURE 10.13

Midradius density (g/cm²) versus grip strength (kgs) of the nondominant arm in young women. (Reprinted with permission from Snow-Harter, C., M. Bouxsein, B. Lewis, S. Charette, P. Weinstein, and R. Marcus. Muscle strength as a predictor of bone mineral density in young women. J. Bone Min. Res. *5:589– 595, 1990.)*

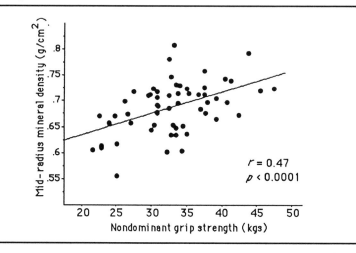

oxygen capacity (from submaximal tests) as a fitness index, found bone density of the femoral neck and lumbar spine significantly correlated with fitness, age, and weight in 84 women (aged 20–75 years). These authors expressed oxygen consumption in liters per minute rather than liters per kilogram body weight per minute, therefore, their measure was more a reflection of lean body mass than oxygen consumption. In a more recent report, Pocock et al. [92] reported maximal oxygen consumption (ml/kg/min) predicted BMD at the spine and femoral neck in an additive relationship with muscle strength and body weight. Chow et al. [27] reported similar findings when they estimated maximal oxygen consumption (ml/kg/min) and analyzed axial bone mineral by neutron activation. They found a significant correlation between these two variables in 31 healthy postmenopausal women. Contrary to the reports of Chow and Pocock, other studies have reported no significant correlation between maximal oxygen consumption and bone density [8, 9, 30, 84]. Bevier et al. [8] measured maximal oxygen consumption in 154 healthy men and women aged 25–50 years and observed no significant relationship with spinal bone density when the factor of body weight was removed. Likewise, in a study of 33 premenopausal women, Nelson and colleagues [84] found that bone density of the spine and hip were not different between the endurance-trained and sedentary groups. Dalsky et al. [30] found no significant correlation found between maximal oxygen consumption and lumbar spine bone mineral content. That these studies actually measured maximal oxygen consumption, rather than predicted it, lends more credibility to the reported results. As an independent predictor of bone density, therefore, cardiorespiratory fitness remains unreliable. Its relationship to BMD is likely through the weight-bearing stimulation that the activity itself provides the skeleton.

REPRODUCTIVE ENDOCRINE STATUS AND PHYSICAL TRAINING. It is now recognized that severe exercise training may interrupt menstrual function and lead to bone loss and increased fracture risk [21, 34, 71]. Although early reports by Cann et al. [21] reported reduced lumbar spine bone densities in exercising women with secondary amenorrhea compared to cyclic controls, the women were not well defined as a group with "athletic amenorrhea". That is, it was not clear whether they had amenorrhea as a result of exercise training or prior to that time.

Subsequent studies have been more rigorous in defining their populations. Drinkwater and colleagues [34] reported significantly lower lumbar spine density in a group of amenorrheic athletes when compared to controls who were matched for anthropometric indices. Forearm mineral content was similar in both groups. Marcus et al. [71] evaluated bone mass and metabolic status of elite distance runners. The amenorrheic athletes and controls were matched for aerobic capacity, body fat percent, exercise intensity and age of menarche. Mineral density in the amenorrheic group was 20% lower than in the cyclic group and 10% lower than that of nonathletic cyclic women of similar age. Cortical densities of the radius were similar in both groups (Fig. 10.14). Results reported by Nelson and colleagues [83] support these findings.

In each of the above studies circulating levels of estradiol were lower in the amenorrheic women. Although Drinkwater et al. [34] reported no significant correlation between serum estradiol and bone density, Nelson et al. [83] did find a significant relationship. In addition, all studies found potentially important nutritional contributions to bone loss in their subjects. These included extremely low total energy consumption and intakes of calcium that might be appropriate for young women with intact hypothalamic-gonadal axes, but grossly inadequate for women who are functionally menopausal.

An apparent contradiction to the aforementioned studies is a report by Linnel et al. [67] in which no significant differences were observed in bone mineral measured at two sites of the radius, distal and midshaft, in the nondominant arm of nonathletic controls, eumenorrheic runners, and amenorrheic runners. The authors concluded that amenorrhea was not related to reduced bone mineral content in their population. This conclusion was confounded by the fact that bone mineral density

FIGURE 10.14

Bone mineral density of cyclic (**cyc**) *and amenorrheic* (**amen**) *runners. Bars show mean ± SEM. Vertebral and radial mineral density for age-matched non-athletic controls is 166 ± 4 mg/cm³ and 0.71 ± 0.01 g/cm², respectively. (Reprinted with permission from Marcus, R., C. Cann, P. Madvig, et al. Menstrual function and bone mass in elite women distance runners: endocrine metabolic features.* Ann. Intern. Med. *102:158–163, 1985.)*

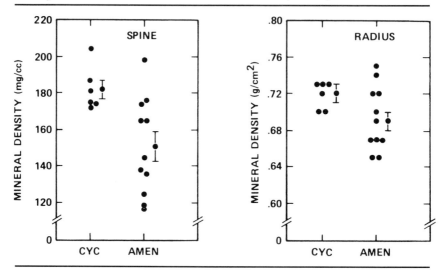

was determined only for the peripheral skeleton. Drinkwater et al., Marcus et al., and Nelson et al. [34, 71, 83] all reported normal values for cortical bone in their amenorrheic subjects, despite important reductions in trabecular bone mass. Notably, however, the site of cortical bone measurement in these studies was the forearm, and it remains possible that cortical deficits elsewhere went undetected. Nonetheless, loss of menstrual function has been clearly associated with a consistent decrease in trabecular bone despite apparent preservation of normal cortical bone density. Fortunately, reports indicate that although serious depletion of bone mass may occur in the amenorrheic athlete, a portion of this loss is potentially reversible [63].

Although an athletic amenorrheic analog has not been defined for men, recent findings suggest that high weekly mileage is associated with low vertebral BMD in male runners. Bilanin et al. [10] compared a group of runners who averaged 64 kilometers a week with sedentary men matched for age, height, and weight. The runners had higher oxygen uptake and lower body fat than the controls. Vertebral BMD was 9.7% lower in the runners than the controls. Tibial and radial BMD did not differ between groups. The authors concluded that, although not measured in this study, lower testosterone levels in the running group may explain the differences between groups. Other investigators [48, 118] have reported lower serum total and free testosterone levels in male long distance runners.

Calcium Nutritional State
It must be remembered that the skeleton is the repository for 99.5% of total body calcium, and it constitutes a source of mineral that can support plasma calcium levels at times of need. The published literature concerning the relationship between dietary calcium and skeletal integrity is complex and frequently ambiguous [50, 70, 74], and will not be detailed here. However, a few summary statements are in order.

The recommended dietary calcium intake for adolescent boys and girls is 1200 mg, a figure derived primarily from balance studies. Because the 2 or 3 years that constitute the pubertal growth spurt are accompanied by deposition of 60% of final bone mass, dietary inadequacy may impose far greater constraints on bone formation at this time of life than at other times. Consumption figures indicate that the calcium intake of American men corresponds reasonably well to recommended levels at most ages, but that median intakes for American girls are substantially below target levels by age 11, and never recover. It is likely, therefore, that calcium undernutrition has an important influence on peak bone mass in women.

During the third through fifth decades of life, growth has stopped, and robust compensatory mechanisms permit rapid adaptation to even severe dietary restriction. Consequently, it should not be surprising that calcium nutritional state appears not to be a major influence on the rate of bone loss at this time [95], and, as a corollary, it is unlikely that calcium supplementation will exert important beneficial effects on bone mass during this period. It is ironic that this population is the target for the greatest portion of calcium supplement advertising.

At menopause, the initial acceleration in bone loss reflects loss of endogenous estrogen and has little relationship to dietary calcium. Riis et al. [97] showed only modest effects on bone loss when early menopausal women were supplemented with calcium. However, the habitual dietary calcium of Danish women approximates 1100 mg, considerably higher than in the United States, so what may have been a marginal effect for Danish women might be more substantial for their American counterparts.

After age 60, the early effects of estrogen deficiency have subsided but the compensatory mechanisms for accommodating to dietary deficiency have become less efficient in both men and women. It is considered likely that disruption of these mechanisms leads to secondary hypersecretion of parathyroid hormone, which leads to support of plasma calcium at the expense of aggravated bone loss [35, 121]. At this time, proper attention to calcium nutritional state, be it from dietary calcium or from supplementation with calcium or vitamin D, is rational and has been shown to have beneficial effects on bone mass [50, 70].

Reproductive Endocrine Status
Formidable evidence supports an important role for gonadal function in the acquisition and maintenance of bone mass. Hypogonadal boys and girls have substantial deficits in both cortical and trabecular bone mineral. The loss of endogenous androgen or estrogen during adult life regularly leads to accelerated loss of bone mineral, an effect that is particularly striking when it occurs at an early age, such as after oophorectomy in a young woman.

In women, the loss of estrogen has dual effects. Decreased efficiency of intestinal and renal calcium homeostasis increases the level of calcium intake necessary to maintain calcium balance. In addition, recent evidence shows that estrogen directly affects bone cell function [36, 47, 56], and it is this interaction that is thought to underlie the accelerated bone loss of early estrogen deficiency. In terms of bone remodeling, estrogen deficiency permits osteoclasts to resorb bone with greater efficiency. This may lead to perforation of trabeculae, with no scaffold left for initiation of bone formation. Thus, entire trabecular elements may be eliminated. Replacement of estrogen at menopause protects bone mass and affords significant protection against risk for osteoporotic fractures [66]. Notably, estrogen deficiency may have an overwhelming influence on bone mass even when adequate attention is given to other important influences on bone health. For example, women athletes who experience interruption of menstrual function lose bone, despite regular exercise at high intensity [71].

The skeletal role of androgens is less well understood. Testosterone deficiency is an important contributor to osteoporosis in men, in whom replacement therapy restores bone mass. The mechanisms by which androgens interact with the skeleton are not known, however. One known action for androgens is to increase muscle mass, so it is possible that androgen effects on bone partly reflect the increased mechanical loading that would occur if muscle mass were to increase. Finally, recent evidence suggests that circulating androgens make a significant contribution to peak bone mass in women [16].

EXERCISE IN PREVENTION AND TREATMENT OF OSTEOPOROSIS

The focus of this chapter has been the regulation of bone *mass* and its loss throughout life. The clinical entity, *osteoporosis*, is considered to be the end result of this loss. It is currently fashionable to define osteoporosis as a critical reduction in bone mass to the point that fracture vulnerability increases. In this sense, osteoporosis is analogous to anemia defined as a low red blood cell mass. This definition is not strictly accurate, however. Osteoporosis consists not only of a reduction in bone mass but also of important changes in trabecular microarchitecture, such as trabecular perforation and loss of connectivity. In the large volume of data that we have discussed, the influence of exercise and physical activity on bone mass per se is considered, but the other material and geometrical properties of bone that are related to fragility are not addressed.

The efficacy of exercise in prevention and treatment of osteoporosis is unknown. Four primary questions are of general interest: (1) Can exercise maximize peak bone mass? (2) Can exercise forestall or minimize age-related losses? (3) Can exercise improve BMD in individuals with established osteoporosis? (4) Can exercise training replace estrogen replacement therapy during the early postmenopausal years? Information described earlier lends optimism to the first three of these questions. Certain caveats are warranted, however. First, although significant relationships do exist between activity, muscle strength, and peak bone mass, the fraction of the total variance in bone mineral attributable to differences in activity and strength is relatively low, approximately 20%, in comparison to the genetic contribution of about 75%. Consequently, although exercise can increase bone mineral significantly, there are probably fairly tight constraints on the magnitude of increase that can be expected. The limited base of experimental data appears to support this conclusion. Gleeson et al. [45] recently reported a 0.81% increase in spine BMD in a group of premenopausal women who ranged in age from 24–46 years and who engaged in a modest weight training over 12 months. Preliminary work from our laboratory shows that college-aged women randomly assigned to 3-days per week of running or weight training gain about 1.3% in lumbar spine BMD at 9 months. Although subjects in both studies might be expected to demonstrate larger increases over time, it is difficult to conceive that a woman whose bone mass is in the third percentile before exercise could ever achieve the 50th percentile for age from an exercise program, regardless of duration.

The second point follows from Wolff's law: Bone will accommodate the habitual stresses that are imposed upon it. If a person runs 5 miles per day, the equilibrium bone mass will be suited to that degree of loading. Once equilibrium is reached, bone mass should not increase over time, i.e. bone mass after running 5 miles a day for 20 years is probably no better than after 5 years. For added benefit, it should be necessary to increase the daily training schedule, i.e., the training must be progressive.

A third point is the phenomenon of initial values; i.e., the effect of training on bone mass should be greatest when exercise is imposed on a sedentary person rather than on a person who is already active. Further, once bone density has responded to increased mechanical loading, a point will be reached at which, even with increased training, bone mass may not improve at the initial rate and an augmentation in bone mass may not be detectable, i.e., the phenomenon of diminishing returns.

We consider the answer to question #4 to be more straightforward. There is powerful evidence that estrogen replacement maintains bone mass and reduces the fracture risk of postmenopausal women. It would be naive and inappropriate to consider exercise a replacement for hormonal therapy. To date, there is no basis for a claim that exercise would be superior to estrogen as a deterrent to bone loss, particularly during the first 5 years after menopause. Moreover, experience with the amenorrheic athlete makes it most unlikely that such a claim will be substantiable. The potential value of exercise for menopausal women is poorly understood, and future research should be directed at understanding the interactions of exercise interventions with hormone replacement in women of this age group.

The notion that resistance exercise provides a superior stimulus for bone, if validated, carries important therapeutic implications, because weight-bearing exercise, defined as walking, jogging, and running, has been the form of activity traditionally prescribed for skeletal benefit. Although it is clear that serious resistance training of frail elders could not safely be carried out, the results of Dalsky et al. [30] indicate that lower intensity resistance training can be successfully introduced to this population. The primary benefits of high-intensity, progressive resistance exercise would accrue to teenagers and young adults who are still acquiring bone mass, and whose spines could tolerate loading with minimal fracture risk. Based on published results, it seems reasonable to suggest that a combined program of weight-bearing and resistance activity, modified as necessary for frail persons, is a rational strategy to provide optimal cardiovascular and skeletal benefits for healthy men and women of all ages.

REFERENCES

1. Aloia, J.F., S.H. Cohn, T. Babu, et al. Skeletal mass and body composition in marathon runners. *Metabolism* 27:1793–1796, 1978.
2. Aloia, J.F., A. Vaswani, K. Ellis, K. Yuen, and S.H. Cohn. A model for involutional bone loss. *J. Lab. Clin. Med.* 106:630–637, 1985.
3. Aniansson, A., C. Zitterberg, M. Hedberg, et al. Impaired muscle function with aging. *Clin. Orthop. Rel. Res.* 191:193–210, 1984.
4. Arnold, J.S., M.H. Bartley, D.D.S. Bartley, S.A. Tont, and D.P. Henkins. Skeletal changes in aging and disease. *Clin. Orthop. Rel. Res.* 49:37, 1966.
5. Arnold, J.S. Amount and quality of trabecular bone in osteoporotic vertebral fractures. *Clin. Endocrinol. Metab.* 2:221–238, 1973.

6. Ayalon, J., A. Simkin, I. Leichter, et al. Dynamic bone loading exercises for postmenopausal women: effect on the density of the distal radius. *Arch. Phys. Med. Rehabil.* 68:280–283, 1987.

7. Beverly, M.C., T.A. Rider, M.J. Evans and R. Smith. Local bone mineral response to brief exercise that stresses the skeleton. *Br. Med. J.* 299:233–235, 1989.

8. Bevier, W.C., M.L. Stefanick, and P.D. Wood. Bone density, aerobic capacity and body composition of moderately overweight adults. *Med. Sci. Sports Exerc.* S60 (Abstract), 1988.

9. Bevier, W.C., R.A. Wiswell, G. Pyka, et al. Relationship of body composition, muscle strength and aerobic capacity to bone mineral density in older men and women. *J. Bone Min. Res.* 4:421–432, 1989.

10. Bilanin, J.E., M.S. Blanchard, and E. Rusek-Cohen. Lower vertebral bone density in male long distance runners. *Med. Sci. Sports Exerc.* 21:66–70, 1989.

11. Birkenhager-Frenkel, D.H., P. Courpron, E.A. Hupscher, et al. Age-related changes in cancellous bone structure. *Bone Mineral* 4:197–216, 1988.

12. Block, J.E., H.K. Genant, and D. Black. Greater vertebral bone mineral mass in exercising young men. *West. J. Med.* 145:39–42, 1986.

13. Brewer, V., B.M. Meyer, M.S. Keele, et al. Role of exercise in prevention of involutional bone loss. *Med. Sci. Sport Exerc.* 15:445–449, 1983.

14. Brooks, G.A., and T.D. Fahey. *Exercise Physiology: Human Bioenergetics and Its Applications.* New York: MacMillan Publishing Co., 1985, pp. 343–442.

15. Buchanan, J.R., C. Myers, T. Lloyd, and R.B. Greer III. Early vertebral trabecular bone loss in normal premenopausal women. *J. Bone Mineral Res.* 3:583–587, 1988.

16. Buchanan, J.R., C. Myers, R. Lloyd, P. Leuenberger, and L.M. Demers. Determinants of trabecular bone density in women: the role of androgens, estrogen and exercise. *J. Bone Mineral Res.* 3:673–680, 1988.

17. Burnell, J.M., D.J. Baylink, C.H. Chestnut III, M.W. Matthews, and E.J. Teubner. Bone matrix and mineral abnormalities in postmenopausal osteoporosis. *Metabolism* 31:1113–1120, 1982.

18. Burr, D.B., R.B. Martin, M.B. Schaffler, et al. Bone remodeling in response to in vivo fatigue damage. *J. Biomech.* 12:189–200, 1985.

19. Cann, C.E., H.K. Genant, F.O. Kolb, and B. Ettinger. Quantitative computed tomography for prediction of vertebral fracture risk. *Bone* 6:1–7, 1985.

20. Cann, C.E., and H.K. Genant. Precise measurement of vertebral mineral content using computed tomography. *J. Comput. Assist. Tomogr.* 4:493–500, 1980.

21. Cann, C.E., M.C. Martin, H.K. Genant, et al. Decreased spinal mineral content in amenorrheic women. *J.A.M.A.* 251:626–629, 1984.

22. Capozzo, A. Force actions in the human trunk during running. *J. Sports Med.* 23:14–22, 1983.

23. Carter, D.R., W.E. Caler, D.M. Spengler, et al. Fatigue behavior of adult cortical bone: the influence of mean strain and strain range. *Acta. Ortho. Scand.* 52:481–490, 1981.

24. Carter, D.R., D.P. Fyrie, and R.T. Whalen. Trabecular bone density and loading history: regulation of connective tissue biology by mechanical energy. *J. Biomech.* 20:785–794, 1987.

25. Carter, D.R. Mechanical loading histories and cortical bone remodeling. *Calcif. Tiss. Int.* 36(Suppl):19–24, 1984.

26. Cavanaugh, D.J., and C.E. Cann. Brisk walking does not stop bone loss in postmenopausal women. *Bone* 9:201–204, 1988.

27. Chow, R.K., J.E. Harrison, C.F. Brown, et al. Physical fitness effect on bone mass in postmenopausal women. *Arch. Phys. Med. Rehab.* 67:231–234, 1986.

28. Cornwall, M.W. Biomechanics of noncontractile tissue. *Phys. Ther.* 64:1869–1873, 1984.

29. Dalen, N., and K.E. Olsson. Bone mineral content and physical activity. *Acta. Ortho. Scand.* 45:170–174, 1974.

30. Dalsky, G., K.S. Stocke, and A.A. Ehsani. Weight-bearing exercise training and lumbar bone mineral content in postmenopausal women. *Ann. Int. Med.* 108:824–828, 1988.

31. Davee, A.M., C.J. Rosen, and R.A. Adler. Exercise patterns and trabecular bone density in college women. *J. Bone Mineral Res.* 5:245–250, 1990.

32. Donaldson, C.L., S.B. Hulley, J.M. Vogel, et al. Effect of prolonged bed rest on bone mineral. *Metabolism* 19:1071–1084, 1970.

33. Doyle, F., J. Brown, and C. LaChance. Relation between bone mass and muscle weight. *Lancet* 1:391–393, 1970.

34. Drinkwater, B.L., K. Milson, C.H. Chestnut III, et al. Bone mineral content of amenorrheic and eumenorrheic athletes. *N. Engl. J. Med.* 311:277–281, 1984.

35. Eastell R., H. Heath III, R. Kumar, and B.L. Riggs. Hormonal factors: PTH, vitamin D and calcitonin. B.L. Riggs and L.J. Melton (eds.). *Osteoporosis. Etiology, Diagnosis, and Management.* New York: Raven Press, 1988, pp. 373–388.

36. Eriksen, E.F., D.S. Colvard, N.J. Berg, et al. Evidence of estrogen receptors in normal human osteoblast-like cells. *Science* 241:84, 1988.

37. Firooznia, H., C. Golimbu, M. Rafii, M.S. Schwartz, and E.R. Alterman. Quantitative computed tomography assessment of spinal trabecular bone. Age-related regression in normal men and women. *J. Comput. Tomogr.* 8:91–97, 1984.

38. Galante, J., W. Rostoker, and R.D. Ray. Physical properties of trabecular bone. *Calcif. Tissue Res.* 5:236–246, 1970.

39. Gallagher, J.C., D. Goldgar, and D. Moy. Total bone calcium in normal women: effect of age and menopause status. *J. Bone Mineral Res.* 2:491–496, 1987.

40. Garn, S.M., C.G. Rohman, and P. Nolan, Jr. The developmental nature of bone changes during aging. J.E. Birren (ed.). *Relations of Development and Aging.* Springfield, CT: C.C. Thomas, 1966.

41. Genant, H.K., C.E. Cann, B. Ettinger, and G.S. Gordan. Spinal mineral loss in oophorectomized women. *J.A.M.A.* 244:2056–2059, 1980.

42. Geusens, P., A. Dequeker, A. Verstraeten, and J. Nijs. Age-, sex-, and menopause-related changes of vertebral and peripheral bone population study using dual and single photon absorptiometry and radiogrammetry. *J. Nucl. Med.* 27:1540–1549, 1986.

43. Gilsanz V., D.T. Gibbons, M. Carolson, et al. Peak vertebral density: A comparison of adolescent and adult females. *Calc. Tissue Int.* 43:260–262, 1988.

44. Gilsanz, D.T., T.F. Roe, M. Carlson, et al. Vertebral bone density in children: effect of puberty. *Radiology* 166:847–850, 1988.

45. Gleeson, P.B., E.J. Protas, A.D. LeBlanc, V.S. Schneider, and H.J. Evans. Effects of weight lifting on bone mineral density in premenopausal women. *J. Bone Mineral Res.* 5:153–158, 1990.

46. Granhad, H., R. Jonson, and T. Hansson. The loads on the lumbar spine during extreme weight lifting. *Spine* 12:146–149, 1987.

47. Gray, T.K., T.C. Flynn, K.M., Gray, and L.M. Nabell. 17b-estradiol acts directly on the clonal osteoblast cell line UMR 106. *Proc. Natl. Acad. Sci. USA* 84:6267, 1985.

48. Hackney, A.C., W.E. Sinning, and B.C. Bruot. Reproductive hormonal profiles of endurance-trained and untrained males. *Med. Sci. Sports Exerc.* 20:60–65, 1988.

49. Hansson, T., and B. Roos. Age changes in bone mineral of the lumbar spine in normal women. *Calc. Tiss. Intl.* 38:249–251, 1986.

50. Heaney, R.P. Nutritional factors in bone health. B.L. Riggs and L.J. Melton (eds.). *Osteoporosis, Etiology, Diagnosis, and Management.* New York: Raven Press, 1988, pp. 359–373.

51. Huddleston, A.L., D. Rockwell, D.N. Kulund, et al. Bone mass in lifetime tennis players. *J.A.M.A.* 244:1107–1109, 1980.

52. Hui, S.L., C.W. Slemenda, and C. Conrad Johnston, Jr. Age and bone mass as predictors of fracture in a prospective study. *J. Clin. Invest.* 81:1804–1809, 1988.

53. Hui, S.L., P.S. Wiske, J.A. Norton, and C.C. Johnston. A prospective study of change in bone mass with age in postmenopausal women. *J. Chronic Dis.* 35:715–725, 1982.

54. Jacobson, P.C., W. Beaver, S.A. Grubb, et al. Bone density in women: college athletes and older athletic women. *J. Orthop. Res.* 2:328–332, 1984.

55. Johnson, T. Age-related differences in isometric and dynamic strength and endurance. *Physical Therapy* 62:985–989, 1982.

56. Komm, B.S., C.M. Terpenening, D.J. Benz, et al. Estrogen binding, receptor mRNA, and biologic response in osteoblast-like osteosarcoma cells. *Science* 241:81–83, 1988.

57. Kragstrup, J., F. Melsen, and L. Mosekilde. Thickness of bone formed at remodeling sites in normal human iliac trabecular bone: variations with age and sex. *Metab. Bone Dis. Rel. Res.* 5:17–21, 1983.

58. Krolner, B., and S. Pors Nielsen. Bone mineral content of the lumbar spine in normal and osteoporotic women: cross-sectional and longitudinal studies. *Clin. Sci.* 62:329–336, 1982.

59. Krolner, B., B. Toft, S.P. Nielsen, et al. Physical exercise as prophylaxis against involutional bone loss: A controlled trial. *Clin. Sci.* 64:541–546, 1983.

60. Krolner, B. and B. Toft. Vertebral bone loss: an unheeded side effect of therapeutic bed rest. *Clin. Sci.* 64:537–540, 1983.

61. Lane, N.E., D. Block, H. Jones, et al. Long-distance running, osteoporosis and osteoarthritis. *J.A.M.A.* 255:1147–1151, 1986.

62. Leichter, I., A. Simkin, J.Y. Margulies, et al. Gain in mass density of bone following strenuous physical activity. *J. Orthop. Res.* 7:86–90, 1989.

63. Lindberg, J.S., M.R. Powell, M.M. Hunt, et al: Increased vertebral bone mineral in response to reduced exercise in amenorrheic runners. *West. J. Med.* 146:39–42, 1987.

64. Lindahl, O. Mechanical properties of dried defatted spongy bone. *Acta. Orthop. Scand.* 47:11–19, 1976.

65. Lindh, M. Biomechanics of the lumbar spine. V. Frankel and M. Nordin (eds.). *Basic Biomechanics of the Skeletal System.* Philadelphia: Lea & Febiger, 1980, pp. 255–290.

66. Lindsay, R. Sex steroids in the pathogenesis and prevention of osteoporosis. B.L. Riggs and L.J. Melton (eds.). *Osteoporosis, Etiology, Diagnosis, and Management.* New York: Raven Press, 1988, pp. 333–359.

67. Linnell, S.I., J.M. Stager, P.W. Blue, et al. Bone mineral content and menstrual regularity in female runners. *Med. Sci. Sport Exerc.* 16:343–348, 1984.

68. Mack, P.B., P.A. LaChance, G.P. Vose, et al. Bone demineralization of foot and hand of Gemini-Titan IV, V and VII astronauts during orbital flight. *Am. J. Roent: Rad. Ther. Nucl. Med.* 100:503–511, 1967.

69. Madsen, M. Vertebral and peripheral bone mineral content by photon absorptiometry. *Invest. Rad.* 12:185–188, 1977.

70. Marcus, R. Calcium intake and skeletal integrity: is there a critical relationship? *J. Nutrition* 117:631–635, 1986.

71. Marcus, R., C. Cann, P. Madvig, et al. Menstrual function and bone mass in elite women distance runners: endocrine metabolic features. *Ann. Intern. Med.* 102:158–163, 1985.

72. Marcus, R., J. Kosek, A. Pfefferbaum, and S. Horning. Age-related loss of trabecular bone in premenopausal women: a biopsy study. *Calcif. Tiss. Int.* 35:406–409, 1983.

73. Marcus, R. Normal and abnormal bone remodeling in man. *Adv. Int. Med.* 38:129–141, 1987.

74. Marcus, R. The relationship of dietary calcium to the maintenance of skeletal integrity in man—an interface of endocrinology and nutrition. *Metabolism* 31:93–101, 1982.

75. Martens, M., R. VanAudekercke, P. Delport, P. DeMeester, and J.C. Muller. The mechanical characteristics of cancellous bone of upper femoral region. *J. Biomech.* 16:971–983, 1983.

76. Mazess, R.B. On aging bone loss. *Clin. Orthop. Relat. Res.* 165:239–252, 1982.

77. Mazess, R.B. The noninvasive measurement of skeletal mass. Peck, W.A. (ed.). *Bone and Mineral Research Annual 1.* New York: Elsevier, 1981, pp. 223–279.

78. Meema, H.E., S. Meema. Cortical bone mineral density versus cortical thickness in the diagnosis of osteoporosis: a roentgenological-densitometric study. *J. Am. Geriatric Soc.* 17:120–141, 1969.

79. Meunier, P., P. Courpron, C. Edouard, J. Bernard, J. Bringuier, and G. Vignong. Physiological senile involution and pathological rarefaction of bone. *Clin. Endocrinol. Metab.* 2:239–256, 1973.

80. Mosekilde, Li. Age-related changes in vertebral trabecular bone architecture—assessed by a new method. *Bone* 9:247–250, 1988.

81. Mosekilde, Li., Le. Mosekilde, and C.C. Danielsen. Biomechanical competence of vertebral trabecular bone in relation to ash density and age in normal individuals. *Bone* 8:79–85, 1987.

82. Mosekilde, Li., and Le. Mosekilde. Iliac crest bone volume as a predictor for vertebral compressive strength, ash density and trabecular bone volume in normal individuals. *Bone* 9:195–199, 1988.

83. Nelson, M.E., E.C. Fisher, P.D. Castos, et al. Diet and bone status in amenorrheic runners. *Am. J. Clin. Nutr.* 43:910–916, 1986.

84. Nelson, M.E., C.N. Meredith, and B. Dawson-Hughes. Hormone and bone mineral status in endurance-trained and sedentary postmenopausal women. *J. Clin. Endocrin. Metab.* 66:927–933, 1988.

85. Nilas, L., A. Gotfredsen, A. Hadberg, and C. Christiansen. Age-related bone loss in women evaluated by the single and dual photon technique. *Bone and Mineral* 4:95–103, 1988.

86. Nilsson, B.E., and N.E. Westlin. Bone density in athletes. *Clin. Ortho.* 77:179–182, 1971.

87. Nottestad, S.Y., J.J. Baumel, D. Kimmel, R.R. Recker, and R.P. Heany. The proportion of trabecular bone in human vertebrae. *J. Bone Min. Res.* 2:221–229, 1987.

88. Orwoll, E.S., J. Ferar, S.K. Oviatt, M.R. McClung, and K. Huntington. The relationship of swimming exercise to bone mass in men and women. *Arch. Intern. Med* 149:2197–2200, 1989.

89. Parfitt, A.M. Age-related structural changes in trabecular and cortical bone: cellular mechanisms and biomechanical consequences. *Calcif. Tiss. Int.* 36:123–128, 1984.

90. Parfitt, A.M., H.E. Mathews, A.R. Villanueva, M. Kleerekoper, B. Frame, and D.S. Rao. Relationships between surface, volume and thickness of iliac trabecular bone in aging and in osteoporosis. *J. Clin. Invest.* 72:1396–1409, 1983.

91. Pirnay, F., M. Bodeux, J. M. Crielaard, et al. Bone mineral content and physical activity. *Int. J. Sport Med.* 8:331–335, 1987.

92. Pocock, N., J. Eisman, T. Gwinn, et al. Muscle strength, physical fitness and weight but not age predict femoral neck bone mass. *J. Bone Mineral Res.* 4:441–447, 1989.

93. Pocock, N.A., J.A. Eisman, M.G. Yeates, et al. Physical fitness as a major determinant of femoral neck and lumbar spine bone mineral density. *J. Clin. Invest.* 78:618–721, 1986.

94. Riggs, B.L., H.W. Wahner, W.L. Dann, R.B. Mazess, and K.P. Offord. Differential changes in bone mineral density of the appendicular and axial skeleton with aging. *J. Clin. Invest.* 67:328–335, 1981.

95. Riggs, B.L., H.W. Wahner, L.J. Melton III, L.S. Richelson, H.L. Judd, and W.M. O'Fallon. Dietary calcium intake and rates of bone loss in women. *J. Clin. Invest.* 80:979–982, 1987.

96. Riggs, B.L., H.W. Wahner, L.J. Melton III, L.S. Richelson, H.L. Judd, and K.P. Offord. Rates of bone loss in the appendicular and axial skeletons of women: evidence of substantial vertebral bone loss before menopause. *J. Clin. Invest.* 77:1487–1491, 1986.

97. Riis, B., K. Thomsen, and C. Christiansen. Does calcium supplementation prevent postmenopausal bone loss. A double-blind controlled clinical study. *New Eng. J. Med.* 316:173–177, 1987.

98. Rubin, C.T., and L.E. Lanyon. Regulation of bone mass by mechanical strain magnitude. The effect of peak strain magnitude. *Calcif. Tiss. Int.* 37:411–417, 1985.

99. Rubin, C.T., and C.E. Lanyon. Regulation of bone formation by applied dynamic loads. *J. Bone Joint Surg.* 66:397–402, 1984.

100. Sambrook, P.N., J.A. Eisman, S.M. Furler, and N.A. Pocock. Computer modeling and analysis of cross-sectional bone density studies with respect to age and the menopause. *J. Bone Mineral Res.* 2(2):109–114, 1987.

101. Simkin, A., J. Ayalon, and I. Leichter. Increased trabecular bone density due to bone-loading exercises on postmenopausal osteoporotic women. *Calcif. Tissue Int.* 40:59–63, 1987.

102. Sinaki, M., M.C. McPhee, S.F. Hodgson, et al. Relationship between bone mineral density of spine and strength of back extensors in healthy postmenopausal women. *Mayo Clin. Proc.* 61:116–122, 1986.

103. Sinaki, M., and B.A. Mikkelsen. Postmenopausal spinal osteoporosis: flexion versus extension exercises. *Arch. Phys. Med. Rehabil.* 65:593–596, 1984.

104. Sinaki, M., and K. Offord. Physical activity in postmenopausal women: effect on back muscle strength and bone mineral density of the spine. *Arch. Phys. Med. Rehabil.* 69:277–280, 1988.

105. Sinaki, M., H.W. Wahner, and K.P. Offord. Relationship between grip strength and related regional bone mineral content. *Arch. Phys. Med. Rehabil.* 70:823–826, 1988.

106. Sinaki, M., H.W. Wahner, K.P. Offord, and S.F. Hodgson. Efficacy of nonloading exercises in prevention of vertebral bone loss in postmenopausal women. *Mayo Clin. Proc.* 64:762–769, 1989.

107. Smith, D.M., M.R.A. Khairi, J. Norton, and C.C. Johnston. Age and activity effects on rate of bone mineral loss. *J. Clin. Invest.* 58:716–721, 1976.

108. Smith, E.L., W. Reddan, and P.E. Smith. Physical activity and calcium modalities for bone mineral increase in aged women. *Med. Sci. Sport Exerc.* 13:60–64, 1981.

109. Smith, E.L., P.E. Smith, C.J. Ensign, et al. Bone involution decrease in exercising middle-aged women. *Calc. Tiss. Int.* 36:S129–S138, 1984.

110. Smith, E.L., C. Gilligan, M. McAdam, C.P. Ensign, and P.E. Smith. Deterring bone loss by exercise intervention in premenopausal and postmenopausal women. *Calc. Tiss. Int.* 44:312–321, 1989.

111. Snow-Harter, C., M. Bouxsein, B. Lewis, S. Charette, P. Weinstein, and R. Marcus. Muscle strength as a predictor of bone mineral density in young women. *J. Bone Min. Res.* 5:589–595, 1990.

112. Talmage, R.V., S.S. Stinnett, J.T. Landwehr, L.M. Vincent, and W.H. McCartney. Age-related loss of bone mineral density in non-athletic and athletic women. *Bone Mineral* 1:115–125, 1986.

113. Townsend, P.R., P. Raux, R.M. Rose, R.E. Miegel, and E.L. Radin. The distribution and anisotropy of the stiffness of cancellous bone in the human patella. *J. Biomech.* 8;199–210, 1975.

114. Trotter, M., G.E. Broman, and R.P. Peterson. Densities of bones of white and negro skeletons. *J. Bone Joint Surg.* 42-A:58, 1960.

115. Weaver, J.K., and J. Chalmers. Cancellous bone: its strength and changes with aging and an evaluation of some methods for measuring its mineral content. *J. Bone Joint Surg.* 48-A:289–299, 1966.

116. Weinstein, R.S., and M.S. Hutson. Decreased trabecular width and increased trabecular spacing contribute to bone loss with aging. *Bone* 8:137–142, 1987.

117. Whalen, R.T., D.R. Carter, and C.R. Steele. The relationship between physical activity and bone density. *Trans. Orthop. Res. Soc. 33rd Mtg.* 12:464, 1987.

118. Wheeler, G.D., S.R. Wall, A.N. Belcastro, and D.C. Cumming. Reduced serum testosterone and prolactin levels in male distance runners. *J.A.M.A.* 252:514–516, 1984.

119. White, M.K., R.B. Martin, R.A. Yeater, et al. The effects of exercise on the bones of postmenopausal women. *Int. Orthop.* 7:209–214, 1984.

120. Williams, J.A., J. Wagner, R. Wasnich, et al. The effect of long-distance running upon appendicular bone mineral content. *Med. Sci. Sport Exerc.* 16:223–227, 1984.

121. Young, G., R. Marcus, J.R. Minkoff, L.Y. Kim, and G.V. Segre. Age-related rise in parathyroid hormone in man: the use of intact and midmolecule antisera to distinguish hormone secretion from retention. *J. Bone Min. Res.* 2:367–374, 1987.

11
Arm Movements in Three-dimensional Space: Computation, Theory, and Observation

JOHN F. SOECHTING, Ph.D.
MARTHA FLANDERS, Ph.D.

INTRODUCTION

Theories always have held a special place in the area of motor control. Perhaps because of our experience in designing and building devices that move, those theories also generally have been based on a popularization of the most current advances in engineering practice. So it is, then, that the emergence of control theory in the 1940s and 1950s led to the introduction of the follow-up length servo by Merton [87] as a postulate for how movements might be initiated and controlled on the basis of reflexes. In one fell swoop, Merton managed to introduce a great simplification into scientific thought about motor control. Posture and movement were equivalent; both were regulated by the stretch reflex, and movement was no more than a succession of postures.

Although it is now generally agreed that the idea of a follow-up length servo has no experimental support [59], the corollary that posture and movement are equivalent (from the point of view of the controller) has survived to this day, forming the basis of the equilibrium point hypothesis [11, 26, 53]. Other theories of movement control have been based on the idea that a particular parameter is optimized [19, 94]. A number of different parameters have been suggested. Among these are the energy expended for muscle activation [95, 97], the torque required to produce the movement [117], and the smoothness of the movement [52, 54].

Such theories all have had as their aim the discovery of the one unifying principle that would govern all movements. It is our opinion that although the aim may be laudable, it is unlikely to be satisfied. Biological systems have evolved subject to a variety of constraints, and the organization and control of movements is likely to reflect these constraints. Among such constraints are anatomical ones that derive from the musculoskeletal structure and physiological ones that derive from the contractile properties of muscles (i.e., the plant). Other

389

constraints are determined by the information sensory systems provided (e.g., proprioceptive, visual) as well as the limitations of that information and the rate at which it may be processed, as initially suggested by Fitts [27]. Still other constraints are evolutionary ones. In the process of encephalization, phylogenetically older structures are nevertheless retained and their functions are maintained to a certain degree, even as they are elaborated by phylogenetically newer structures [47, 116].

We therefore argue that the search for a single unifying theory of movement control is misguided. We do not wish to argue, however, that quantitative approaches, models (especially if they lead to testable predictions), and simulation have no place in the study of biological movements. In fact, our point of view is quite the opposite. In attempting to understand movement control, it is helpful to identify first the computational problems that need to be solved [82]. From this basis, an appropriate interplay between experimentation and simulation can be used to identify algorithms, that is, to identify the set of rules according to which a particular problem is solved. The ultimate goal is to uncover how a particular algorithm is implemented by the nervous system: to identify the anatomical structures involved in the implementation of the algorithm and to discover how information is encoded by neural activity in these structures.

This is not to suggest that this process is unidirectional, from computational problem to algorithm to implementation. Important clues to the nature of the algorithm can come as much from electrophysiological and anatomical studies as from behavioral studies and simulations. Regarding the latter, simulations based on neural nets [50, 77] hold much promise because they are closer approximations to the distributed and parallel processing characteristic of nervous systems. A number of such models have been presented recently [15, 67, 70, 84]. At this stage, these simulations appear to have as their primary aim the demonstration that neural networks can be trained successfully to generate limb movements—a necessary first step. The extent to which such models represent biological solutions and the extent to which they can yield testable predictions remain to be investigated.

In this review we focus on arm movements, that is, movements at the shoulder, elbow, and wrist joints. We attempt to outline some of the computational problems that must be solved by neural networks to produce such movements. We then discuss one hypothesis that has been proposed as a comprehensive theory for limb movements. Finally, referring back to some of the computational problems, we summarize the main experimental observations that have been made. In so doing, we hope to clarify some of the issues and unresolved questions regarding limb movements.

COMPUTATION

Why Study Multijoint Arm Movements?

It is unarguable that the computations required for many-degree-of-freedom movements are more complicated than the computations required for single-degree-of-freedom movements. Movements with many degrees of freedom also are more difficult to study. Simple means, such as goniometry, no longer suffice to measure motions, and the number of variables that must be measured (and kept track of) can become daunting. It is legitimate, then, to ask, Why create all these complications when even simple, one-degree-of-freedom movements are imperfectly understood?

The traditional approach has been to study simple, one-degree-of-freedom movements with the tacit assumption that the conclusions reached by studying simpler movements will generalize to multi-degree-of-freedom movements. This premise was stated by the authors of a recent target article in *Behavioral and Brain Sciences* on single-joint movements [39, p. 245]: "there is something to be learned from reducing a problem to its simplest meaningful components: for the problem of motor control, this occurs at the single joint." This point of view engendered a lively debate. Among those who disputed this view, Loeb [80, p. 227] stated that, "it is becoming clear that natural movements are not planned or controlled at the single-joint level and cannot be." We expand on this contention in the next few sections.

Certain concepts that seem clear in the context of simple movements become less so when one considers multijoint motions; the concepts need to be redefined rather than extended. Some questions that appear trivial in the context of simple movements suddenly become formidable for multijoint movements. Furthermore, distinctions that seem minor for single-joint movements, such as the distinction between kinematics and dynamics, are fundamental for multi-joint movements. By confronting complexity, therefore (experimentally and analytically), we may achieve a fundamentally different type of understanding of limb movements. This is not to argue that it is only legitimate to focus upon complex movements. Many questions can be addressed adequately at the level of the single joint (or a single muscle, motor unit, synapse, or molecule).

One such set of questions concerns the patterning of electromyographic (EMG) activity. It is well known that fast, unidirectional, one-joint movements are produced by a three-burst pattern of muscle activity [119], whereas slower movements may show a different patterning [37]. How does the pattern depend on movement speed, movement amplitude, movement time, or movement accuracy [39, 42, 51, 66]? These questions are still unresolved, as is the exact significance of the finding that more accurate movements require a longer time to execute [18, 27, 88, 100]. To state the problem another way, we still have not identified the neural commands that specify a movement of a particular extent, duration, and accuracy, even when that movement is restricted to a single joint.

Studies of simple movements can lead to the discovery of principles that may indeed generalize to more complicated movements. One noteworthy example is the recent work by Ghez and his colleagues [23, 48] concerning the processes by which movement amplitude and direction come to be specified. They studied the simplest motor task possible, the production of isometric force pulses, and required subjects to produce targeted force pulses at fixed latencies following the presentation of the target. Using this forced-reaction-time paradigm, they showed that the specification of response amplitude and response direction evolved gradually and that the processes specifying direction and amplitude were parallel. At latencies less than the usual reaction time, subjects sometimes produced forces in the wrong direction but with the correct amplitude. As we discuss in a following section, amplitude and direction information appear to be processed in separate channels for multidimensional arm movements as well.

Degrees of Freedom and Indeterminacy
The essential characteristic that differentiates the neural control of movement from engineering solutions is that the computational problems solved by neural networks involve many more degrees of freedom. To put it another way, biological systems are in principle indeterminate and an infinity of solutions is theoretically possible. Bernstein [10] in fact suggested that the central question of motor control was how does the central nervous system acquire a mastery of this large number of degrees of freedom? He also suggested the answer: as movements are learned, the ability to control a larger number of degrees of freedom increases by introducing constraints that decrease the number of degrees of freedom that are independent of each other. (We shall return to this suggestion in a later section.)

The problem of indeterminacy exists whether one studies multijoint movements or single-joint movements. Consider, for example, a simple movement such as flexion-extension at the elbow and assume that the task is to flex the arm by a certain amount in a given time, i.e., the amplitude and duration of the movement is specified. Even so, the velocity profile of the movement remains indeterminate. The movement could be performed at a constant speed, or the speed could vary in a variety of ways throughout the movement. Beginning with Woodworth [123] in 1899, a number of investigators have studied this problem [93], and it has been found that the velocity profile has a *roughly* symmetrical, bell-shaped appearance. This finding has been generalized also to hold for a variety of multijoint movements [52, 89, 90].

If the velocity profile is specified, then the torque profile required to produce the movement also is determinate. Because EMG activity has a reasonably simple relationship to the tension developed by a single muscle [2, 124, 125], the pattern of muscle activity needed to produce the torque might appear to be predictable. Another indeterminacy arises here, however: even for a simple movement such as flexion-extension at the elbow, there is more than one flexor (e.g., biceps, brachialis, and brachio-radialis) and more than one extensor (e.g., the three heads of triceps). Activity and tension could be distributed among the different muscles in a variety of ways. Furthermore, there is the possibility of agonist-antagonist coactivation, which produces no net torque and also provides for nonunique solutions for a desired force trajectory [25, 30, 43] (although the extent of redundancy is decreased if impedance is regulated along with force [53]).

One way to solve the indeterminacy for muscle activation is to assume that each of the agonists has similar activity [12, 85]. However, the moment arms of each of the agonists can vary in a different manner with joint angle and the muscles can be in different regions of their length-tension curve, depending on the joint angle [125]. Consequently, the effectiveness of each of the muscles in generating torque can vary in a different manner with joint angle. In fact, regarding the assumption that agonists are constrained to have similar activity, Hasan and Enoka [44] found that the pattern of activity in biceps and brachio-radialis can differ substantially during simple elbow flexion tasks, depending on the initial and final postures of the arm. The assumption, therefore, that a single constraint can define the activity of all muscles participating in a simple movement needs to be reexamined.

If we assume that a pattern of activity has been determined for a given muscle, the question now arises, How do individual motor units contribute to this overall pattern? The answer commonly given is that motor units are constrained to be recruited according to the size principle [16, 17, 49]. Yet some muscles are inhomogeneous in the following sense: if a muscle has more than one mechanical action (e.g., flexion and supination for biceps), the recruitment order of different motor units can depend on the force direction and not strictly on the size principle. For example, the threshold for recruitment of some biceps motoneurones depends only on the force in elbow flexion, whereas in others it depends on a linear combination of the forces in flexion and in supination [114, 115]. The recruitment order of all motoneurones in one muscle therefore need not be invariant, in apparent violation of the size principle. If one abandons the anatomical definition of muscle, however, and adopts a functionally based one (such as the idea of a task group [79]), then the size principle may yet hold as a constraint that ensures determinacy at the motoneurone level.

As should be clear from the above discussion, there is a large degree of indeterminacy even in single-joint motions that ultimately can be described by one degree of freedom (e.g., the angle of flexion-extension). These indeterminacies pertain to the temporal aspects of the movement and to the activation of muscles and motor units. A number of questions remain unresolved concerning each of these levels of description.

The indeterminacies hold true as well for multijoint movements. In addition, the spatial aspect of these movements is indeterminate. The skeletal system affords many more degrees of freedom than the three that are needed to specify the location of a point in space or the six that are needed to specify the location and orientation of an object in space [103]. Thus an object can be grasped with the arm assuming an infinite variety of postures, i.e., different joint angles at the shoulder, elbow, and wrist. Furthermore, if the object is grasped between the index finger and the thumb (for example), each of the joint angles of the thumb and index finger can take on a variety of values [20]. Finally, although the spatial location of the hand is specified by the task, the path taken by the hand as it moves from the initial position to the final position is not. Conceivably, the hand could move in a straight line or it could move along any number of curved trajectories.

By considering multijoint movements, we introduce a new question. In a single-degree-of-freedom movement (for example, elbow flexion), a unique relationship exists between muscle lengths and joint angle and between joint angle and the position of the hand. This is no longer the case for multijoint movements. How does the nervous system deal with indeterminacy at this level?

Space and Sensorimotor Transformations
In a typical experiment in which movement is restricted to a single joint, a target is displayed on a monitor and the subject is to make a flexion or extension movement of the arm to bring a cursor (with its position proportional to joint angle) to the target. The spatial demands of this task are simple. Once the scaling between cursor and joint has been learned, the relationship between target displacement and movement amplitude, measured in degrees of joint rotation, is straightforward. Even if movement amplitude is computationally specified by the required change in muscle length, the relationship between movement amplitude and target displacement, although nonlinear, would still be monotonic.

Consider now the situation in which the task is to grasp a target somewhere within the subject's reach [104, 105]. Suppose the location of the target is described in Cartesian coordinates (x, y, and z, where x

FIGURE 11.1

The angles used to describe the orientation of the arm and forearm. These angles are measured relative to the vertical axis and sagittal plane and were derived from psychophysical experiments [107] which revealed these as the angles involved in the perception of the arm orientation. Elevation is defined as the angle between the limb segment and the vertical axis, measured in the vertical plane. Yaw is measured in the horizontal plane and is the angle between the limb segment and the anterior axis. (Reprinted with permission from Soechting, J.F., and M. Flanders. Errors in pointing are due to approximations in sensorimotor transformations. J. Neurophysiol. *62:595–608, 1989.*

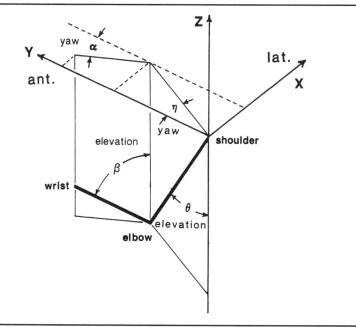

is in the lateral direction, y is anterior, and z is up), and the orientation of the arm is described by the angles illustrated in Figure 11.1. Suppose further, for the sake of simplicity, that there is no motion at the wrist. The relations between target location and arm orientation are then:

$$x = l_a \sin \theta \sin \eta + l_f \sin \beta \sin \alpha$$

$$y = l_a \sin \theta \cos \eta + l_f \sin \beta \cos \alpha \qquad [1]$$

$$z = l_a \cos \theta + l_f \cos \beta$$

where l_a is the length of the upper arm and l_f the length of the forearm.

The angles θ and η represent the elevation and yaw angles of the upper arm, β and α the elevation and yaw angles of the forearm [110].

The computational problem for an arm movement in three-dimensional space is the following: given x, y, and z, compute the values of η, θ, α, and β. First of all, it is clear that there is no unique solution because there are four unknowns and only three equations. Second, because x, y, and z depend in a nonlinear manner on the orientation angles, solving these equations exactly will probably not be easy. The problem becomes no simpler if we use a different set of coordinates to represent target location. For example, in spherical coordinates

$$R^2 = 2l^2 (1 - \cos\theta\cos\beta + 2\sin\theta\sin\beta\cos\gamma)$$

$$\tan\psi = (\cos\beta - \cos\theta)/(\sin^2\beta + \sin^2\theta + 2\sin\theta\sin\beta\cos\gamma) \quad [2]$$

$$\tan\chi = (\sin\theta\sin\eta + \sin\beta\sin\alpha)/(\sin\theta\cos\eta + \sin\beta\cos\alpha)$$

$$\gamma = \eta - \alpha$$

where the lengths of the upper arm and forearm are assumed to be equal to l, R is the distance from the shoulder to the target, ψ is the elevation of the target, and χ its azimuth, measured relative to the shoulder. The relationship between target location and joint angles also would be no simpler had we defined joint angles in a different way [101].

Obviously we are as adept at grasping objects within our reach as we are at moving a manipulandum to position a cursor. Yet, although the computational problem of sensorimotor transformations (muscle length to joint angle to cursor displacement) required to position the cursor appears trivial, the computational problem of solving equations [1] or [2] appears complicated. How is this problem solved by neural systems?

Kinematics and Dynamics
Another fundamental way in which multijoint arm movements differ from single-joint movements is in the manner in which movement kinematics and dynamics are related to each other. By kinematics, we mean displacements or their derivatives (velocity, acceleration), that is, a description of the movement. By dynamics (sometimes also referred to as kinetics), we mean the forces (or torques) that produce the movement.

If movement is restricted to a single joint, there is a simple relationship between kinematics and dynamics: angular acceleration is proportional to joint torque. This simple relationship does not hold when there is movement at more than one joint, as shown in Figure 11.2.

This illustrated example shows that elbow motion can induce shoulder motion in the absence of any actively produced shoulder torques. We

FIGURE 11.2

Schematic illustration of the dynamic coupling between forearm and upper arm motion. Rotation of the forearm into extension is accompanied by reaction forces at the elbow. The centripetal and the tangential forces on the forearm are produced by the upper arm; conversely, there are equal but opposite forces on the upper arm. These forces on the upper arm will lead to shoulder flexion. The broken arrow indicates that in addition to elbow extension causing shoulder flexion, shoulder flexion can cause elbow extension.

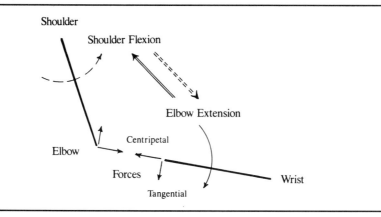

have taken a two-link system which consists of the upper arm and the forearm. Assume that the elbow is extending, as it would, for example, if we gave a gentle push to the forearm. Because the center of mass of the forearm follows a curved path, it is subject to a centripetal acceleration (equal to V^2/R) in the direction indicated in the figure. By Newton's second law, this acceleration is produced by a force acting on the forearm at the elbow joint. This force is exerted by the upper arm pulling the forearm back in the direction of the centripetal acceleration. By the same token, the forearm exerts the same force (but in the opposite direction) on the upper arm, as indicated by the arrow at the distal end of the upper arm in Figure 11.2. This centripetal force will set the upper arm into motion in the direction of shoulder flexion, even if none of the shoulder muscles are active. Similarly, shoulder flexion also can induce elbow extension, as indicated by the broken arrow in Figure 11.2.

For the sake of completeness, we also have indicated the tangential force at the elbow, that is, the force acting in the direction tangential to the motion of the center of mass of the forearm. This force will be present if there is an angular acceleration of the forearm. Thus, the initial angular acceleration of the forearm at the onset of a voluntary elbow extension also will induce shoulder flexion (the tangential force at the distal end of the upper arm pulls upward).

Angular acceleration at the shoulder joint will therefore depend not only on the torque exerted by shoulder muscles but also on the angular velocity (centripetal force) and acceleration (tangential force) at the elbow joint. The same conclusion holds true for the elbow joint—its angular acceleration does not depend only on the torque produced by elbow muscles. In multijoint motion, therefore, no proportionality exists between dynamics and kinematics of individual joints.

The mathematical derivation of the equations that relate kinematics to dynamics in the multijoint case has been presented in detail in a number of publications [58, 61, 125]; we do not repeat these derivations here. We do note one important consequence of the lack of a simple relationship between torque and angular acceleration. Activation of an elbow flexor, for example, will always contribute to the development of elbow torque in the flexor direction. However, the movement that results can be an elbow flexion, an elbow extension, or no motion at all at the elbow, depending on the actively produced torque at the shoulder (even when no other elbow muscles are active and no external loads are applied to the arm).

An example of this nonintuitive relationship between torque and movement is illustrated in Figure 11.3 [108]. In this instance, biceps and anterior deltoid (elbow or shoulder flexors) were active at the onset of the movement. The actively produced torques also were both in the flexor direction (upward deflection of the torque traces in Figure 11.3). Yet, there was flexion at the shoulder but extension at the elbow (upward and downward deflection of the angle traces in Figure 11.3).

Muscle Synergy

The concept of muscle synergy has been introduced as a constraint that may simplify the computational problems of motor control. This concept is different for single-joint and multijoint movements. If one considers only the elbow joint, all of the muscles have only one of two possible actions (i.e., flexion or extension). This is not true when more than one joint is considered. For example, biceps can act as a supinator at the wrist and as a flexor at the shoulder, as well as a flexor at the elbow; brachialis, on the other hand, is a pure elbow flexor. Some shoulder flexors tend to abduct the arm, others to adduct it. Few muscles have identical combinations of mechanical actions if one considers their effects in all of the degrees of freedom in which they can act.

The concept of "muscle synergy" founded on a biomechanical or anatomical basis suggests that muscles that have the same mechanical action are controlled as a unit. This concept becomes problematical in the case of multijoint motion. The concept of "muscle synergy" defined on a neurophysiological basis as a set of muscles that have a spatially and temporally coherent pattern of muscle activation but dissimilar

FIGURE 11.3

Nonintuitive relations between torque and motion. Data are from trials in which the subject pointed forward in the sagittal plane to a target at shoulder level. The movement required flexion at the shoulder but extension of the forearm, as shown by the angle traces. The agonists for this movement were shoulder and elbow flexors, however, as shown by the rectified EMG activity and shoulder and elbow joint torques which both changed in the flexor direction at the onset of the movement [modified from 108].

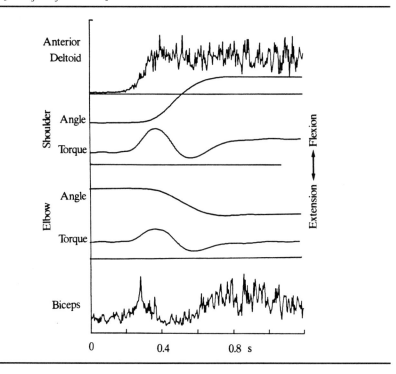

mechanical effects [76], remains as a possible simplification of complex computations.

THEORY

In the preceding sections we identified some of the computational problems with which the nervous system must deal in order to generate movements. We focused on multijoint movements and the new and different computational problems that arise in this situation.

We now take up the question, Is there a theory of movement that can provide a comprehensive explanation for the phenomenology of biological movements? If not, we are faced with the prospect of accepting the fact that there may be solutions that are task-specific, and that each of these solutions may be implemented in a distributed fashion, not amenable to being summarized succinctly.

One theory of movement control may appear to be able to account for single-joint and multijoint limb movements and cope with the computational problems described in the preceding sections, namely, the equilibrium point hypothesis. After describing it, we ask, Does the hypothesis actually lead to a simplification of the control problem? Does it have any validity for biological systems, i.e., is it in accord with experimental observations?

The Equilibrium Point Hypothesis

The hypothesis was originally formulated by Feldman [24, 26] and has since been modified by others [11, 53, 68]. According to this hypothesis, the nervous system takes advantage of the spring-like properties of muscles (and possibly their reflex circuitry), and a movement is achieved by changing the equilibrium point (the muscle length at which the muscle generates zero force) from a value appropriate for the initial posture to a value appropriate for the final posture. Movement, then, is no more than a succession of postures, and the speed of a movement could be regulated by an interplay between the rate at which the equilibrium point shifts and the mechanics of the limb.

A simple example illustrates the hypothesis. Suppose there is a mass, and a spring attached to it. If one displaces the other end of the spring, the mass will follow the displacement (with a lag that depends on the inertia of the mass, the stiffness of the spring, and the rate of displacement). Of course, for this model to work, the spring must be sufficiently stiff (to overcome the inertia of the mass) and there must also be appropriate damping (or else the mass will oscillate). The advantage of this mode of control is that the controller can ignore the dynamical laws of motion of the system, which can be quite complicated. The control signal could be completely kinematic, i.e., the desired endpoint or trajectory. Thus, if the equilibrium point of a muscle can be set by a simple neural signal to motoneurones, the control of movement could be simplified considerably.

Is the hypothesis valid? Is such a simplification achieved?

To answer these questions we must distinguish between the different formulations of the hypothesis. According to Feldman's formulation, the equilibrium point of a muscle is regulated by setting the threshold for the stretch reflex of each muscle by means of a central drive to alpha and gamma motoneurones. His model resembles the theory that the stretch reflex acts as a servo-assist device, introduced some time ago by Granit [41] and Matthews [86], among others, as a modification of Merton's hypothesis [87]. The validity of Feldman's hypothesis has been discussed extensively [cf. 113]. Hypothetical mechanisms involving the stretch reflex require that the gain of this reflex be appreciable. Although the reflex gain is difficult to measure, this supposition is questionable. Feldman [26] does not explicitly require a high-reflex gain, but at low gain his model becomes essentially indistinguishable from that of Bizzi et al. [11].

The second version of the equilibrium-point hypothesis [11, 52, 53, 98] also is based on the premise that muscles have spring-like properties. It does not invoke the stretch reflex, however, and consequently can overcome the need for a high-reflex gain. In fact, this later formulation of the hypothesis was based on findings in monkeys with deafferented limbs, in the absence of any reflex activity [11, 98].

According to the second version of the hypothesis, for a movement of the arm from one point in space to another there exists a virtual trajectory. This virtual trajectory consists of the straight line that connects the two points in space, and it has the property that a movement that followed exactly the virtual trajectory would be the smoothest possible [32, 52, 53]. The virtual trajectory defines the equilibrium muscle lengths of each of the muscles. Because it is assumed that the muscles act like springs, the force that produces the movement is proportional to the difference between the actual and the virtual position of the arm at each point in time. Because a force is required to produce movement, the actual movement does not follow exactly the virtual trajectory. That is, for a one-degree-of-freedom movement

$$I\ddot{\theta}_a + C\dot{\theta}_a + K\theta_a = K\theta_v \qquad [3]$$

where $\theta_a(t)$ is the actual trajectory and $\theta_v(t)$ is the virtual trajectory, and I, C, and K are constants that represent the inertia, viscous damping, and stiffness. Note that when $\theta_a = \theta_v$, acceleration and velocity terms are identically zero and the equation predicts a state of equilibrium.

According to this hypothesis, the equilibrium trajectory would be specified by neural drive to the alpha motoneurones. For multijoint movements, θ would be a vector, C and K would be matrices [31], as would the inertia (I), and nonlinear terms in velocity also would need to be included [58, 61, 125].

Bizzi and his collaborators [11, 98] have presented several lines of evidence consistent with the hypothesis. They initially found that they could train deafferented monkeys to make accurate elbow flexion-extension movements to random targets, even when these movements were perturbed by torque pulses [98]. They also found that when they clamped the monkey's arm at the initial position with a torque motor and then released it some time after the monkey had attempted to initiate the movement, the acceleration transient on release increased gradually, as would be predicted if the equilibrium point shifted gradually from the initial to the final position [11].

Other evidence comes from simulations. Flash [31] performed simulation studies showing that the hypothesis can yield movements that mimic closely measured trajectories of planar arm movements. To do so, she used measured values of the stiffness matrix K obtained under quasistatic conditions [91] and assumed a damping ratio (defined as $\sqrt{C^2/4IK}$) of 0.4 to 0.8. To fit the experimental trajectories, she needed to scale each of the coefficients of the stiffness matrix by different factors ranging from 1.0 to 3.0. Because the stiffness of the arm was not measured during movements, it is not clear whether her assumption that stiffness increases substantially and nonuniformly during movement is reasonable. Her simulations also suggest that arm impedance (stiffness and viscosity) is tuned differently for different movements. This prediction also awaits experimental confirmation.

In summary, the equilibrium-point hypothesis initially appeared to lead to a significant simplification of the computational problem of movement because it did not require a computation of joint torques. Simulation studies [31, 52] show, however, that dynamic parameters such as impedance do need to be controlled, along with kinematics, which detracts from the initial simplicity of the formulation. Some experimental data are in accord with the hypothesis [11, 98]; other experimental observations are not in accord with its predictions. According to the hypothesis, a viscous load applied to the arm should not affect the final posture. Nevertheless, viscous loads do lead to large errors in final position [22, 99]. Second, the hypothesis predicts that the path taken by the hand should be close to a straight line. Usually it is [36, 89, 108], but there are other instances when it clearly is not [5, 74]. Two such examples are shown in Figure 11.4.

Beyond the question of validity, an equally important question is whether this hypothesis actually leads to a simplification of the control problem. In this regard, we take up two points. First, how is motoneurone activity related to the equilibrium point of a muscle? Second, if a kinematic trajectory was a sufficient control signal, how could this hypothetical trajectory be computed by the nervous system?

Regarding the first point, little is known. Although one might suppose that a simple relationship exists between the equilibrium point of a muscle and that muscle's activity, this question has not been addressed to any extent [44]. If there is no such simple relationship, that is, if a muscle's activity were to depend in some complicated and nonunique fashion on its equilibrium point (and perhaps other parameters as well), then much of the simplicity of the hypothesis would be lost. The question is not, Can an equilibrium point be defined?, because any set of inputs to such a system necessarily defines an equilibrium posture. The question instead is, Does the nervous system implement a control

FIGURE 11.4

Not all trajectories of pointing movements follow straight paths. Illustrated are records of point to point arm movements, performed in approximately the sagittal plane, in which the hand followed a curvilinear path. (4A is modified from [5] and 4B is modified from [74]).

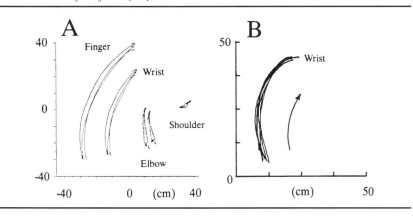

of this parameter? Another question of interest to the neurophysiologist might be, Is the hypothesis testable?

To compute the virtual trajectory, one needs to know the initial location of the hand in space and the location of the target in space. As Polit and Bizzi showed in their initial experiments [98], the specification of the initial position depends on proprioceptive information. When they displaced the arms of deafferented monkeys, the monkeys failed in the pointing task even when they could see their arm. The initial position of the arm, therefore, is derived from proprioceptive information that may be described in terms of joint angles (or muscle lengths); presumably the desired end position is specified in spatial coordinates. The computation of a virtual trajectory thus requires a coordinate transformation of the type given by equations [1] and [2]. To compute the equilibrium lengths of the muscles, the virtual trajectory as specified in hand coordinates must be transformed into joint coordinates. As we have already pointed out, this transformation is far from simple and is not unique. Although the equilibrium point hypothesis may avoid the problem of computing joint torques, it also avoids fundamental questions of coordinate transformations and the initial computation of control signals that specify the trajectory.

OBSERVATION

As we have tried to point out in the previous section, the equilibrium point hypothesis may be a useful analogy for the musculoskeletal system in a limited sense. Muscles do have a spring-like behavior, although their anatomical and mechanical characteristics are likely to be too complicated to be controlled in the simple manner proposed by the hypothesis. We find the hypothesis has two additional drawbacks. First, it deals with one part of the problem. Second, according to the Bizzi et al. formulation [11], it lacks predictive power. How would the scheme be implemented by a neural controller? What should the control signals look like?

The equilibrium-point hypothesis is the only theory that has attempted to provide a comprehensive explanation for how limb movements might be controlled. The tensor theory of Pellionisz and Llinas [96], which deals with the problem of coordinate transformations by neural systems, might be another candidate but at present it has limitations in predicting patterns of muscle activity for static arm postures [30] and has not been extended to movement.

In the absence of comprehensive theories, one faces the prospect of a piecemeal attack on the problem of how the nervous system generates limb movements. In the following sections we summarize observations that may be pertinent to the computational problems we have outlined and explain how these observations have been interpreted.

Approximations to Sensorimotor Transformations
As mentioned previously, pointing movements require that the initial posture of the arm be known as well as the location of the target in space. The information about arm position and target position is provided by two different sensory modalities (proprioceptive and visual) and in two different coordinate systems (e.g., joint angles and the coordinates of extrapersonal space). No unique relationship exists between these two sets of parameters and the equations relating them are complicated (see equations [1] and [2]). Although methods for achieving an exact solution have been presented [8, 9, 92], observations suggest that this problem is solved by means of approximations that (in the absence of feedback-mediated corrections) lead to errors in perform-ance. Because we have discussed our proposed algorithm for such coordinate transformations and the experimental evidence in support of it in detail elsewhere [28, 106], we shall provide only a short summary here.

The steps in the proposed algorithm are illustrated in Figure 11.5 in a model that incorporates elements of parallel as well as serial processing. One crucial element of the model is that there are several different levels of representation of the kinematics of a task. At the highest (most abstract) level are the requirements of the task. Several different tasks can be envisioned, each with its own demands of sensorimotor pro-cessing. Three examples are shown in Figure 11.5: move to a target, draw a circle, and move down.

FIGURE 11.5

A hypothesis for some of the early stages of the sensorimotor transformations required to move the arm to a target. Information about target position is provided by the visual system and about arm position by kinesthetic input. Information from the two sensory modalities is combined, after being transformed, to define the movement kinematics. (Reprinted with permission from Soechting, J.F., and M. Flanders. Deducing central algorithms of arm movement control from kinematics. D.R. Humphrey and H.-J. Freund (eds.). Motor Control: Concepts and Issues. *Dahlem Konferenzen Chichester: John Wiley & Sons Ltd. [in press].)*

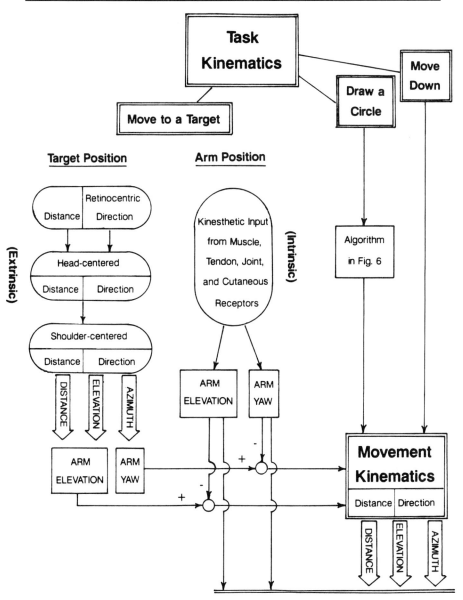

When the task is to move to a target, information about target position is provided by the visual system. We suggest that the retinocentric representation of target position is ultimately transformed into a shoulder-centered representation of the location of the target [107]. This shoulder-centered representation of target location is in a spherical coordinate system (equation [2]) and is used to compute the intended arm position that would bring the hand in contact with the target (Fig. 11.5, left). This computation involves an approximation. Intended final arm elevation angles are derived from a linear combination of target distance and elevation, whereas intended yaw angles are linearly related to target azimuth [28, 29, 105]. The difference between the present arm angles (derived from kinesthetic input, Fig. 11.5, middle) and the intended arm angles represents a "motor error" signal that specify the kinematics of the movement (Fig. 11.5, lower right).

The linear relationships between joint angles and target locations are only approximations to the mathematically exact nonlinear relationships. This hypothesis therefore predicts that subjects should make consistent errors in movement, a prediction that has been confirmed experimentally [104]. Subjects also make predictable errors when asked to produce figural motions, such as drawing circles and ellipses in free space [109, 111, 112]. The hypothesized algorithm that accounts for the kinematics of this task is shown in Figure 11.6. When drawing circles and ellipses, subjects produce joint rotations that are close to sinusoidal. They appear to use very simple rules to change the plane of motion and the figural slant of the ellipse. To adjust the plane of motion, they change only the phase between the forearm and upper arm yaw angles, and to adjust the slant of the figure they change the phase between the elevation and yaw angles. In each case, there is a simple linear relation between extrinsic and intrinsic parameters, subject to the constraint that modulation in forearm and upper arm elevations by 180° out of phase. This algorithm has one other consequence: the speed of the hand's movement and the curvature of the path traced by it are inversely related, in agreement with experimental observations [1, 75, 118]. This inverse relationship follows from the fact that the sinusoidal angular motion leads to approximately sinusoidal displacement of the hand.

Trajectory Planning

Given an arm movement to a target, the question has been raised: is the trajectory of the movement "planned"? As we discussed in the preceding section, there is good evidence that initial and final position are compared to determine a motor error signal. The question now is, Is this signal used to specify in detail the path that the hand takes in moving to the target and to specify the time course of the movement?

In one sense, the answer would appear to be obvious. If an obstacle

FIGURE 11.6

The transformations used to generate figural motion (drawing circles or ellipses).
The plane of wrist motion is defined by the phase between sinusoidal oscillations
of the yaw angles; the figural slant is related to the phase between elevation and
yaw angles. There is a constraint that forearm and upper arm elevation angles
be 180° out of phase. [Based on data presented in 111 and 112.] (Reprinted
with permission from Soechting, J.F., and M. Flanders. Deducing central al-
gorithms of arm movement control from kinematics. D.R. Humphrey and H.-J.
Freund (eds.). Motor Control: Concepts and Issues. *Dahlem Konferenzen*
Chichester: John Wiley & Sons Ltd. [in press].)

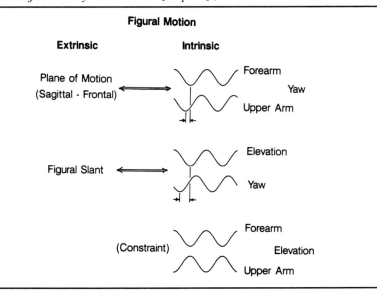

occurs along the way, we can adjust our movement to avoid it, which
implies some sense of the trajectory. This does not imply, however, that
unrestrained movements are performed in the same manner, or that
the presence of an obstacle does not lead to two movements performed
in succession. How the imposition of explicit path requirements (i.e.,
asking subjects to follow a specified trajectory) would affect arm
movements is not known.

A number of investigators have argued in favor of the idea that the
trajectory is planned, some arguing for hand coordinates [53, 89],
others for joint coordinates [56, 57, 65, 108]. The argument in favor
of trajectory planning in hand coordinates is that most point-to-point
arm movements follow paths that are close to straight. This idea is basic
to the equilibrium-point hypothesis advanced by Bizzi and Hogan.

The argument in favor of joint-based planning was originally based
on the observation that the angular motions at the shoulder and the

elbow were coupled in a fixed relationship as the hand approached the target [108]. It was later shown by Hollerbach and Atkeson [57] that for certain target locations, including those investigated by Soechting and Lacquaniti [108], one could not readily distinguish between joint-based and hand-based trajectory planning. They then proceeded to propose a modification of the idea, namely, staggered joint interpolation. According to their suggestion, the velocity profile at each joint is unimodal and invariant, but there can be an offset in the time. Motion would begin first at the joint at which the angular excursion is greatest.

Hogan and his colleagues [54] have argued against this interpretation, pointing to instances in which angular motion at one joint was found to reverse direction (a bimodal velocity profile). In these experiments, however, joint rotation was not measured directly but was computed from the measured movement of the hand. The displacement of the shoulder joint during the movement creates an uncertainty in the computation that is difficult to quantify. Hollerbach and Atkeson [57], who measured joint rotation, claim not to have seen such reversals in joint rotation.

So the argument continues. The idea that trajectories of point-to-point movements are planned explicitly is based in part on the finding that there is little variability in the trajectory from trial to trial, even for movements executed at different speeds and for movements in which there is an inertial load on the arm [5, 73, 108]. For arm movements, kinematics obey scaling laws. However, as Hollerbach and Atkeson [5, 55] have shown, this implies that movement dynamics also obey scaling laws (provided one separates the gravitational components of torque, which does not depend on speed) despite the nonlinear relation between kinematics and dynamics.

The finding that dynamics obey scaling laws implies that an invariant trajectory could result from an invariant torque profile. In other words, the trajectory need not be planned explicitly at all. Rather, the torque needed to bring the arm from the starting position to the final position could be computed on the basis of these two sets of position parameters. With some simple additional constraints, such as torque having one propulsive component and one decelerative component [74], the dynamic scaling law could conceivably suffice to account for the experimental results. Recent simulation studies by Uno and colleagues [117] are compatible with this suggestion. They found that an optimality criterion that minimized the rate of change of torque during the movement could better account for observed arm trajectories than could one that minimized jerk (the third derivative of position).

It also is possible that torque need not be computed explicitly, but rather a pattern of muscle activation could be derived directly from the desired movement kinematics. This possibility has not received much experimental attention. Hasan and Karst [45], who have begun to investigate two-joint arm movements from this perspective, have shown that simple rules can be devised to predict which muscles would be activated at the initiation of a movement. Whether such rules can be developed further to predict also the amplitude of muscle activity remains an open question.

In summary, the questions of whether and how trajectories are planned remain unanswered. In fact, exactly what is meant by "planning" remains to be defined precisely. In the sense of the model presented in Figure 11.5, neuronal representations and stages of processing subsequent to the representation of movement kinematics remain undefined. Whether there is a neuronal representation of joint torques and how this representation would be transformed into muscle activity are open questions.

Muscles
Although there have been extensive studies on the kinematics and the dynamics of multijoint movements, much less work has been done to characterize the patterns of muscle activity that produce the movements. A number of questions need to be addressed. What is the temporal pattern of muscle activity? How does the activity of a muscle depend on load direction or on movement direction (spatial tuning)? How different are the temporal and spatial patterns of different muscles? How is the pattern of activity in a muscle related to its mechanical action? To what extent does the mechanical action of a muscle depend on the posture and motion of the limb?

To begin with the last question, Zajac [124] and Zajac and Gordon [125], have dealt extensively with this issue in recent reviews. As they discuss, the lengths of the moment arm of muscles can depend significantly on the joint angle, as can the direction in which each muscle exerts force. The effectiveness of a muscle in generating torque also will depend on the length-tension characteristics of the muscle and on tendon elasticity. Detailed biomechanical studies of the musculature of the arm [3, 121, 122] and of the leg [60] should facilitate the development of better models of the musculoskeletal system to understand the mechanical constraints that shape the neural control of the musculature.

One can construct directional tuning curves to describe the relationship between mechanical action and the pattern of muscle activation, for example by asking subjects to produce isometric forces in different directions [13]. When one relates the force direction for which the muscle is most active to the direction in which the muscle produces the most force, one finds that these two directions do not coincide [13, 14, 30, 38, 97]. An extreme example of this lack of correspondence is shown in Figure 11.7, in which the directional tuning curve for activity in posterior deltoid is not centered around its mechanical action in either humeral rotation or shoulder abduction (arrows). The reason

FIGURE 11.7

Directional tuning curve for the EMG activity of the posterior deltoid. A woman stood with her upper arm vertical and forearm horizontal in a parasagittal plane, while the direction of a 31.4 Newton force was applied to the wrist in various directions in the frontal plane [30]. The distance from the origin to each data point represents the average EMG amplitude for two trials. Posterior deltoid was most active when the subject produced a lateral or downward force at the wrist. The mechanical effect of contracting only this muscle, however, was calculated [122] to be a downward, medial force at the wrist. The arrows show the mechanical effects as a result of the muscle's action in humeral rotation and abduction or adduction directions.

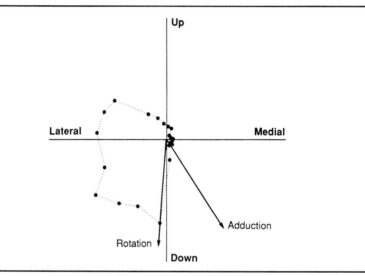

for this lack of correspondence is that the mechanical, pulling directions of all of the muscles at one joint must be considered to understand the pattern in one muscle, and that the pattern is shaped by neutral circuitry as well as by mechanical constraints [30, 96].

Because there are more muscles than there are degrees of freedom, and because there may be co-activation [30], there is no unique solution that would predict a pattern of muscle activity for a given pattern of force production. Theoretical predictions, based on energy minimization, have had some success in predicting neck muscle activation under isometric conditions [6, 7, 97, but see 69]. Eigenvectors, rather than energy minimization, also have been used to constrain the number of solutions [38]. Both energy minimization and techniques based on eigenvectors presume, however, that muscle activity (such as that shown in Fig. 11.7) should be symmetrically tuned around a single preferred direction. In a considerable number of cases [30], arm muscles are tuned around more than one direction (for example, when an antagonist muscle is involved in cocontraction).

During posture, the spatial tuning of each muscle can be different [14, 30, 81], reflecting (in part) the biomechanical action of each of the muscles. What are the temporal patterns of muscle activity and to what extent do the temporal features of motor patterns differ from muscle to muscle for multijoint movements? These questions have not been investigated extensively. The most exhaustive study in this regard was done by Wadman et al. [120]. They found that both the timing and the amplitude of the EMG activity depended on the direction of movement. They found three typical patterns of activity: "start" activity which was similar in structure to the pattern of agonist activity in single-joint movements, "stop" activity which corresponded to the antagonist burst in single-joint movements, and "support" activity which showed no clear bursts. Similar observations have been made by others, as well [35, 74]. It is possible, therefore, that despite the much greater complexity of multijoint movements, the motor patterns that produce them are in some respects very similar to those described for single-joint movements: an agonist burst–pause–burst and an antagonist burst.

The Arm as a Platform for the Hand
So far we have focussed our discussion on arm movements, that is, on the motion of the proximal, elbow, and shoulder joints. In many behaviors, this motion at the proximal joints is aimed at bringing the hand into contact with an object so that it can be graspect or manipulated in some way.

As a first approximation, it may be useful to distinguish between proximal and distal motions and to assume they are related to different aspects of the task. Thus, wrist trajectory produced by proximal arm motion would be related to the spatial location of the object, whereas hand orientation produced by distal joint motion would be related to the object's orientation texture [64], and to the nature of the task (grasping a cup *versus* pushing a button, for example). There is some experimental support for this distinction. The wrist trajectory did not differ when subjects were asked to grasp bars located at the same spot but oriented differently [72], or to push a button that required different amounts of wrist flexion or extension [102]. In other experiments, the wrist trajectory was found to depend on parameters such as target orientation, however. Marteniuk and colleagues [83] found that the velocity profile at the wrist was highly task-dependent as was the ratio of time spent in the acceleratory phase of the movement to the time in the deceleratory phase. They did not report the path taken by the wrist, so that the extent to which the spatial aspects of proximal motion are affected by factors other than target location is not known. Proximal and distal joint motions also may depend to a different extent on the amplitude of the movement [71].

One point is clear. Although the timing of elbow and shoulder motions is closely coupled, the timing of distal motion need not be closely coupled to proximal motion. The onset and termination of wrist flexion and supination can vary considerably compared to the movements of the proximal joints [72], although in other instances close coordination between distal and proximal motion has been reported [62, 63]. Considerable variations also can occur in the amplitude of each of the constituent components of hand movement. Cole and Abbs [20] found that in a grasping movement involving thumb and finger, the point of contact between thumb and finger was consistent, whereas the amplitude of the motion at the joints of the thumb and finger was variable. Similar invariances in the overall kinematics of the movement, despite large variability in the kinematic details, also have been found in speech [40].

The conclusions reached from the study of movements that involve primarily proximal muscles therefore may not hold true for movements that involve primarily distal muscles, and *vice versa*.

CONCLUSION

In this review we have focused on the kinematics, dynamics, and muscle patterns of multijoint limb movements. We have not addressed other aspects, such as the neural correlates of such behaviors [33, 34], their sensory feedback control [21, 46], and how they might be learned [4, 78]. We believe the study of such movements is useful, despite the increased complexity, and that new, interesting questions begin to arise with the inclusion of an additional joint and a third dimension in space. We have tried to frame some of these questions. It should be clear that most of them are far from being answered but that the work of the last decade has both clarified and changed the questions being asked. This appears to be a necessary prerequisite to arriving at answers. Such answers will most likely not point to a single underlying theory governing motor systems.

ACKNOWLEDGEMENT

The authors' work reviewed herein was supported by the U.S. Public Health Service, National Institute of Neurological Disorders and Stroke, grants #NS-15018 and #NS-27484.

REFERENCES

1. Abend, W., E. Bizzi, and P. Morasso. Human arm trajectory formation. *Brain* 105:331–348, 1982.

2. Agarwal, G.C., and G.L. Gottlieb. Mathematical modeling and simulation of the postural control loop. Part I. *Crit. Rev. Biomed. Eng.* 8:93–134, 1982.
3. An, K.N., K.R. Kaufman, and E.Y.S. Chao. Physiological considerations of muscle force through the elbow joint. *J. Biomech.* 22:1249–1256, 1989.
4. Atkeson, C.G. Learning arm movement kinematics and dynamics. *Ann. Rev. Neurosci.* 12:157–183, 1989.
5. Atkeson, C.G., and J.M. Hollerbach. Kinematic features of unrestrained vertical arm movements. *J. Neurosci.* 5:2318–2330, 1985.
6. Baker, J.F., J.M. Banovetz, and C.R. Wickland. Models of sensorimotor transformations and vestibular reflexes. *Can. J. Physiol. Pharmacol.* 66:532–539, 1988.
7. Baker, J., J. Goldberg, and B. Peterson. Spatial and temporal responses of the vestibulocollic reflex in decerebrate cats. *J. Neurophysiol.* 54:735–756, 1985.
8. Benati, M., S. Gaglio, P. Morasso, V. Tagliasco, and R. Zaccaria. Anthropomorphic robotics. I. Representing mechanical complexity. *Biol. Cybern.* 38:125–140, 1980.
9. Benati, M., S. Gaglio, P. Morasso, V. Tagliasco, and R. Zaccaria. Anthropomorphic robotics. II. Analysis of manipulator dynamics and the output motor impedance. *Biol. Cybern.* 38:141–150, 1980.
10. Bernstein, N. *The Coordination and Regulation of Movements.* Oxford: Pergamon, Oxford, 1967.
11. Bizzi, E., N. Accornero, W. Chapple, and N. Hogan. Posture control and trajectory formation during arm movement. *J. Neurosci.* 4:2738–2744, 1984.
12. Bouisset, S., F. Lestienne, and B. Maton. The stability of synergy in agonists during the execution of a simple movement. *EEG Clin. Neurophysiol.* 42:543–551, 1977.
13. Buchanan, T.S., D.P.J. Almdale, J.L. Lewis, and W.Z. Rymer. Characteristics of synergic relations during isometric contractions of human elbow muscles. *J. Neurophysiol.* 56:1225–1241, 1986.
14. Buchanan, T.S., G.P. Rovai, and W.Z. Rymer. Strategies for muscle activation during isometric torque generation at the human elbow. *J. Neurophysiol.* 62:1201–1212, 1989.
15. Bullock, D., and S. Grossberg. Neural dynamics of planned arm movements: emergent invariants and speed-accuracy properties during trajectory formation. *Psychol. Rev.* 95:49–90, 1988.
16. Burke, R.E. Motor units: anatomy, physiology and functional organization. V. Brooks (ed.). *Handbook of Physiology, Vol. 2, Motor Control.* Bethesda, MD: American Physiological Society, 1986, pp. 345–422.
17. Calancie, B., and P. Bawa. Motor unit recruitment in humans. M.D. Binder and L.M. Mendell (eds.). *The Segmental Motor System.* New York: Oxford University Press, 1990, pp. 75–95.
18. Carlton, L.G. Movement control characteristics of aiming responses. *Ergon.* 23:1019–1032, 1980.
19. Chow, C.K., and D.H. Jacobsen. Studies of human locomotion via optimal programming. *Math. Biosc.* 10:239–306, 1971.
20. Cole, K.J., and J.H. Abbs. Coordination of three-joint digit movements for rapid finger-thumb grasp. *J. Neurophysiol.* 55:1407–1423, 1986.
21. Cordo, P. and M. Flanders. Sensory control of target acquisition. *Trends in Neurosci.* 12:110–116, 1989.
22. Day, B.L., and C.D. Marsden. Accurate positioning of the human thumb against unpredictable dynamic loads is dependent upon peripheral feedback. *J. Physiol. (London)* 327:393–408, 1982.
23. Favilla, M., J. Gordon, W. Henning, and C. Ghez. Trajectory control in targeted force impulses. VII. Independent setting of amplitude and direction in response preparation. *Exp. Brain Res.* 79:530–538, 1990.
24. Feldman, A.G. The control of muscle length. *Biofiz.* 19:749–753, 1974.

25. Feldman, A.G. Superposition of motor programs—II. Rapid forearm flexion in man. *Neurosci.* 5:91–95, 1980.
26. Feldman, A.G. Once more on the equilibrium-point hypothesis (λ model) for motor control. *J. Motor Behav.* 18:17–54, 1986.
27. Fitts, P.M. The information capacity of the human motor system in controlling the amplitude of the movement. *J. Exp. Psychol.* 47:381–391, 1954.
28. Flanders, M., S.I. Helms Tillery, and J.F. Soechting. Early stages in a sensorimotor transformation. *Behav. Brain Sci.* (Submitted).
29. Flanders, M., and J.F. Soechting. Parcellation of sensorimotor transformations for arm movements. *J. Neurosci.* 10:2420–2427, 1990.
30. Flanders, M., and J.F. Soechting. Arm muscle activation for static forces in three-dimensional space. *J. Neurophysiol.* 64:1818–1837, 1990.
31. Flash, T. The control of hand equilibrium trajectories in multi-joint arm movements. *Biol. Cybern.* 57:257–274, 1987.
32. Flash, T. and N. Hogan. The coordination of arm movements: an experimentally confirmed model. *J. Neurosci.* 5:1688–1703, 1985.
33. Georgopoulos, A.P. On reaching. *Ann. Rev. Neurosci.* 9:147–170, 1986.
34. Georgopoulos, A.P. Spatial coding of visually guided arm movements in primate motor cortex. *Can. J. Physiol. Pharmacol.* 66:518–526, 1988.
35. Georgopoulos, A.P., J.F. Kalaska, M.D. Crutcher, R. Caminiti, and J.T. Massey. The representation of movement direction in the motor cortex: single cell and population studies. G.M. Edelman, W.F. Gall, and W.M. Cowan (eds.). Dynamical Aspects of Cortical Function. New York: John Wiley and Sons, 1984, pp. 453–473.
36. Georgopoulos, A.P., J.F. Kalaska, and J.T. Massey. Spatial trajectories and reaction times of aimed movements: effects of practice, uncertainty and change in target location. *J. Neurophysiol.* 46:725–743, 1981.
37. Ghez, C., and J.H. Martin. The control of rapid limb movement in the cat. III. Agonist-antagonist coupling. *Exp. Brain Res.* 45:115–125, 1982.
38. Gielen, C.C.A.M., and E.J. van Zuylen. Coordination of arm muscles during flexion and supination: application of tensor analysis approach. *Neurosci.* 17:527–539, 1986.
39. Gottlieb, G.L., D.M. Corcos, and G.C. Agarwal. Strategies for the control of voluntary movements with one mechanical degree of freedom. *Behav. Brain Sci.* 12:189–224, 1990.
40. Gracco, V.L., and J.H. Abbs. Variant and invariant characteristics of speech movements. *Exp. Brain Res.* 65:156–166, 1986.
41. Granit, R. The functional role of the muscle spindles—facts and hypotheses. *Brain* 98:531–556, 1975.
42. Hallet, M., B.T. Shahani, and R.R. Young. EMG analysis of stereotyped voluntary movements in man. *J. Neurol. Neurosurg. Psych.* 38:1154–1162, 1975.
43. Hasan, Z. Optimized movement trajectories and joint stiffness in unperturbed, inertially loaded movements. *Biol. Cybern.* 53:373–382, 1986.
44. Hasan, Z., and R.M. Enoka. Isometric torque-angle relationships and movement-related activity of human elbow flexors: implications for the equilibrium point hypothesis. *Exp. Brain Res.* 59:441–450, 1985.
45. Hasan, Z., and G.M. Karst. Muscle activity for initiation of planar, two-joint arm movements in different directions. *Exp. Brain Res.* 76:651–655, 1989.
46. Hasan, Z., and D.G. Stuart. Animal solutions to problems of movement control: the role of proprioceptors. *Ann. Rev. Neurosci.* 11:199–224, 1988.
47. Heiligenberg, W. Electrosensory maps form a substrate for the distributed and parallel control of behavioral responses in weakly electric fish. *Brain, Behav. Evol.* 31:6–16, 1988.
48. Hening, W. M. Favilla, and C. Ghez. Trajectory control in targeted force impulses. V. Gradual specification of response amplitude. *Exp. Brain Res.* 71:116–128, 1988.
49. Henneman, E., and L.M. Mendell. Functional organization of motoneuron pool and

its inputs. V.B. Brooks (ed.). *Handbook of Physiology, Vol. 2, Motor Control.* Bethesda, MD: American Physiological Society, 1981, pp. 423–507.

50. Hinton, G.E., J.L. McClelland, and D.E. Rumelhart. Distributed representations. D.E. Rumelhart and J.L. McClelland (eds.). *Parallel Distributed Processing, Vol. 1.* Cambridge, MA: MIT Press, 1986.

51. Hoffman, D.S., and P.L. Strick. Step-tracking movements of the wrist in humans. II. EMG analysis. *J. Neurosci.* 10:142–152, 1990.

52. Hogan, N. An organizing principle for a class of voluntary movements. *J. Neurosci.* 4:2745–2754, 1984.

53. Hogan, N., E. Bizzi, F.A. Mussa-Ivaldi, and T. Flash. Controlling multijoint motor behavior. *Exerc. Sports Sci. Rev.* 15:153–190, 1987.

54. Hogan, N., and T. Flash. Moving gracefully: quantitative theories of motor coordination. *Trends Neurosci.* 10:170–174, 1987.

55. Hollerbach, J.M. Dynamic scaling of manipulator trajectories. *J. Dyn. Syst. Meas. Contr.* 106:102–106, 1984.

56. Hollerbach, J.M., and C.G. Atkeson. Characterization of joint interpolated arm movements. *Exp. Brain Res. Ser.* 15:41–54, 1986.

57. Hollerbach, J.M., and C.G. Atkeson. Deducing planning variables from experimental arm trajectories: pitfalls and possibilities. *Biol. Cybern.* 56:279–292, 1987.

58. Hollerbach, J.M., and T. Flash. Dynamic interactions between limb segments during planar arm movement. *Biol. Cybern.* 44:67–77, 1982.

59. Houk, J.C., and W.Z. Rymer. Neural control of muscle length and tension. J.M. Brookhart and V.B. Mountcastle (eds.). *Handbook of Physiology, Vol. 1.* Bethesda, MD: American Physiological Society, 1981, pp. 257–324.

60. Hoy, M.G., F.E. Zajac, and M.E. Gordon. A musculoskeletal model of the human lower extremity: the effect of muscle, tendon, and moment arm on the moment-angle relationship of musculotendon actuators at hip, knee and ankle. *J. Biomech.* 23:157–169, 1990.

61. Hoy, M.G., and R.F. Zernicke. The role of intersegmental dynamics during rapid limb oscillations. *J. Biomech.* 19:867–877, 1986.

62. Jeannerod, M. The timing of natural prehension movements. *J. Mot. Behav.* 16:235–254, 1984.

63. Jeannerod, M. The formation of finger grip during prehension, a cortically mediated visuomotor pattern. *Behav. Brain Res.* 19:99–116, 1986.

64. Johansson, R.S., and G. Westling. Coordinated isometric muscle commands adequately and erroneously programmed for the weight during lifting task with precision grip. *Exp. Brain Res.* 71:72–86, 1988.

65. Kaminski, T., and A.M. Gentile. Joint control strategies and hand trajectories in multijoint pointing movements. *J. Mot. Behav.* 18:261–278, 1986.

66. Karst, G.M., and Z. Hasan. Antagonist muscle activity during human forearm movements under varying kinematic and loading conditions. *Exp. Brain Res.* 67:391–401, 1987.

67. Kawato, M., Y. Maeda, Y. Uno, and R. Suzuki. Trajectory formation of arm movement by cascade neural network model based on minimum torque-change criterion. *Biol. Cybern.* 62:275–288, 1990.

68. Kelso, J.S., K. Holt, and A.E. Flatt. The role of proprioception in the perception and control of human movement: toward a theoretical reassessment. *Percept. Psychophys.* 28:45–52, 1980.

69. Keshner, E.A., and B.W. Peterson. Motor control strategies underlying head stabilization and voluntary head movements in humans and cats. *Progr. Brain Res.* 76:77–81, 1988.

70. Kuperstein, M. Neural model of adaptive hand-eye coordination for simple postures. *Science* 239:1308–1310, 1988.

71. Lacquaniti, F., G. Ferrigno, A. Pedotti, J.F. Soechting, and C.A. Terzuolo. Changes

in spatial scale in drawing and handwriting: kinematic contribution by proximal and distal joints. *J. Neurosci.* 7:819–828, 1987.

72. Lacquaniti, F., and J.F. Soechting. Coordination of arm and wrist motion during a reaching task. *J. Neurosci.* 2:399–408, 1982.

73. Lacquaniti, F., J.F. Soechting, and C.A. Terzuolo. Some factors pertinent to the organization and control of arm movements. *Brain Res.* 252:394–397, 1982.

74. Lacquaniti, F., J.F. Soechting, and C.A. Terzuolo. Path constraints on point-to-point arm movements in three-dimensional space. *Neurosci.* 17:313–324, 1986.

75. Lacquaniti, F., C. Terzuolo, and P. Viviani. The law relating the kinematic and figural aspects of drawing movements. *Acta Psychol.* 54:115–130, 1983.

76. Lee, W.A. Neuromotor synergies as a basis for coordinated intentional action. *J. Motor Behav.* 16:135–170, 1984.

77. Linsker, R. Perceptual neural organization: some approaches based on network models and information theory. *Ann. Rev. Neurosci.* 13:257–281, 1990.

78. Loeb, G.E. Finding common ground between robotics and neurophysiology. *Trends Neurosci.* 6:203–204, 1983.

79. Loeb, G.E. Motoneurone task groups: coping with kinematic heterogeneity. *J. Exp. Biol.* 115:137–146, 1985.

80. Loeb, G.E. Strategies for the control of studies of voluntary movements with one mechanical degree of freedom. *Behav. Brain Sciences* 12:227, 1990.

81. Macpherson, J.M. Strategies that simplify the control of quadrupedal stance. II. Electromyographic activity. *J. Neurophysiol.* 60:218–231, 1988.

82. Marr, D. *Vision.* San Francisco: W.H. Freeman, 1982.

83. Marteniuk, R.G., C.L. MacKenzie, M. Jeannerod, S. Athenes, and C. Dugas. Constraints on human arm movement trajectories. *Can. J. Psychol.* 41:365–378, 1987.

84. Massone, L., and E. Bizzi. A neural network model for limb trajectory formation. *Biol. Cybern.* 61:417–425, 1989.

85. Maton, B., and S. Bouisset. The distribution of activity among the muscles of a single group during isometric contraction. *Eur. J. Appl. Physiol.* 37:101–110, 1977.

86. Matthews, P.B.C. Evolving views on the internal operation and functional role of the muscle spindle. *J. Physiol. (London)* 320:1–30, 1981.

87. Merton, P.A. Speculations on the servo-control of movement. G.E.W. Wolstenholme (ed.). *The Spinal Cord.* London: Churchill, 1953, pp. 247–255.

88. Meyer, D.E., J.E.K. Smith, and C.E. Wright. Models for the speed and accuracy of aimed movements. *Psychol. Rev.* 89:449–482, 1982.

89. Morasso, P. Spatial control of arm movements. *Exp. Brain Res.* 42:223–237, 1981.

90. Munhall, K.G., D.G. Ostry, and A. Parush. Characteristics of velocity profiles of speech movements. *J. Exp. Psych.: Hum. Percept. Perform.* 11:457–474, 1985.

91. Mussa-Ivaldi, F.A., N. Hogan, and E. Bizzi. Neural, mechanical and geometric factors subserving arm posture in humans. *J. Neurosci.* 5:2732–2743, 1985.

92. Mussa-Ivaldi, F.A., P. Morasso, and R. Zaccaria. Kinematic networks. A distributed model for representing and regularizing motor redundancy. *Biol. Cybern.* 60:1–16, 1988.

93. Nelson, W.L. Physical principle for economics of skilled movements. *Biol. Cybern.* 46:135–147, 1983.

94. Patriarco, A.G., R.W. Mann, S.R. Simon, and J.M. Mansour. An evaluation of the approaches of optimization models to the prediction of muscle forces during human gait. *J. Biomech.* 14:513–526, 1981.

95. Pedotti, A., V. V. Krishnan, and L. Stark. Optimization of muscle force sequencing in human locomotion. *Math. Biosc.* 38:57–76, 1978.

96. Pellionisz, A., and R. Llinas. Tensorial approach to the geometry of brain function: cerebellar coordination via a metric tensor. *Neurosci.* 5:1125–1136, 1980.

97. Pellionisz, A., and B.W. Peterson. A tensorial model of neck motor activation. B.W.

Peterson and F. Richmond (eds.). *Control of Head Movement*. Oxford: Oxford Univ. Press, 1988, pp. 178–186.

98. Polit, A., and E. Bizzi. Characteristics of motor programs underlying arm movements. *J. Neurophysiol.* 42:183–194, 1979.

99. Sanes, J.N. Kinematics and end-point control of arm movements are modified by unexpected changes in viscous loading. *J. Neurosci.* 6:3120–3127, 1986.

100. Schmidt, R.A., H. Zelaznik, B. Hawkins, J.S. Frank, and J.T. Quinn. Motor output variability: a theory for the accuracy of rapid motor acts. *Psychol. Rev.* 86:415–451, 1979.

101. Soechting, J.F. Kinematics and Dynamics of the Human Arm. Laboratory of Neurophysiology Report. Minneapolis, MN: University of Minnesota, 1983.

102. Soechting, J.F. Effect of target size on spatial and temporal characteristics of a pointing movement in man. *Exp. Brain Res.* 54:121–132, 1984.

103. Soechting, J.F. Elements of coordinated arm movements in three-dimensional space. S.A. Wallace (ed.). *Perspectives on the Coordination of Movement*. New York: North-Holland, 1989, pp. 47–83.

104. Soechting, J.F., and M. Flanders. Sensorimotor representations for pointing to targets in three-dimensional space. *J. Neurophysiol.* 62:582–594, 1989.

105. Soechting, J.F., and M. Flanders. Errors in pointing are due to approximations in sensorimotor transformation. *J. Neurophysiol.* 62:595–608, 1989.

106. Soechting, J.F., and M. Flanders. Deducing central algorithms of arm movement control from kinematics. D.R. Humphrey and H.-J. Freund (eds.). *Motor Control: Concepts and Issues*. Dahlem Konferenzen. Chichester: John Wiley & Sons Ltd. (In Press).

107. Soechting, J.F., S.I. Helms Tillery, and M. Flanders. Transformation from head- to shoulder-centered representation of target direction in arm movements. *J. Cogn. Neurosci.* 2:32–43, 1990.

108. Soechting, J.F., and F. Lacquaniti. Invariant characteristics of a pointing movement in man. *J. Neurosci.* 1:710–720, 1981.

109. Soechting, J.F., F. Lacquaniti, and C.A. Terzuolo. Coordination of arm movements in three-dimensional space. Sensorimotor mapping during drawing movement. *Neurosci.* 17:295–311, 1986.

110. Soechting, J.F., and B. Ross. Psychophysical determination of coordinate representation of human arm orientation. *Neurosci.* 13:595–604, 1984.

111. Soechting, J.F., and C.A. Terzuolo. An algorithm for the generation of curvilinear wrist motion in an arbitrary plane in three-dimensional space. *Neurosci.* 19:1395–1405, 1986.

112. Soechting, J.F., and C.A. Terzuolo. Sensorimotor transformations underlying the organization of arm movements in three-dimensional space. *Can. J. Physiol. Pharmacol.* 66:502–507, 1988.

113. Stein, R.B. What muscle variable(s) does the nervous system control in limb movements? *Behav. Brain Sci.* 5:535–540, 1982.

114. ter Haar Romeny, B.M., J.J. Denier van der Gon, and C.C. Gielen. Changes in recruitment order of motor units in the human biceps muscle. *Exp. Neurol.* 78:360–368, 1982.

115. ter Haar Romeny, B.M., J.J. Denier van der Gon, and C.C.A.M. Gielen. Relations between location of a motor unit in the human biceps brachii and its critical firing levels for different tasks. *Exp. Neurol.* 85:631–650, 1984.

116. Towe, A.L. Motor cortex and the pyramidal system. J.D. Masur (ed.). *Efferent Organization and the Integration of Behavior*. New York: Academic Press, 1973, pp. 67–97.

117. Uno, Y., M. Kawato, and R. Suzuki. Formation and control of optimal trajectory in human multijoint arm movement. Minimum torque change model. *Biol. Cybern.* 61:89–102, 1989.

118. Viviani, P., and C. Terzuolo. Trajectory determines movement dynamics. *Neurosci.* 7:431–437, 1982.
119. Wacholder, K. Willkurliche Haltung and Bewegung insbesondere im Licht elektro-physiologischer Untersuchungen. *Ergeb. Physiol.* 26:568–773, 1928.
120. Wadman, W.J., J.J. Denier van der Gon, and R.J.A. Derksen. Muscle activation patterns for fast goal-directed arm movements. *J. Hum. Movt. Stud.* 6:19–37, 1980.
121. Wood, J.E., S.G. Meek, and S.C. Jacobsen. Quantitation of human shoulder anatomy for prosthetic arm control. I. Surface modeling. *J. Biomech.* 22:273–292, 1989.
122. Wood, J.E., S.G. Meek, and S.C. Jacobsen. Quantitation of human shoulder anatomy for prosthetic arm control. II. Anatomy matrices. *J. Biomech.* 22:309–326, 1989.
123. Woodworth, R.S. The accuracy of voluntary movement. *Psychol. Re. Suppl.* 3 (Whole No. 13), 1899.
124. Zajac, F.E. Muscle and tendon: properties, models, scaling, and application to biomechanics and motor control. *Crit. Rev. Biomed. Eng.* 17:359–411, 1989.
125. Zajac, F.E., and M.E. Gordon. Determining muscle's force and action in multi-articular movement. *Exerc. Sports Sci. Rev.* 17:187–230, 1989.

12
Myotendinous Junction Injury in Relation to Junction Structure and Molecular Composition

JAMES G. TIDBALL, Ph.D.

INTRODUCTION

Each component of the musculoskeletal system can exhibit modifications in morphology and biochemical composition in response to chronic changes in mechanical use and to acute injuries associated with abnormal loading. In viewing the musculoskeletal system as a series of mechanical components specialized for force production and transmission, one would expect adaptations and perhaps mechanical failure to occur at the interfaces between the individual components of the system, as well as within the components themselves. Knowledge of the structure, adaptations, and mechanical failure of these interfaces has, however, lagged behind those of the separate musculoskeletal components, presumably because of the relative difficulty of biochemical, morphological, and mechanical analysis of these sites.

The purpose of this review is to summarize and analyze current knowledge of the structure, composition, and involvement in injury of one type of these important interfaces, myotendinous junctions (MTJs). These junctions are sites of force transmission between muscle and tendon that display structural and molecular specialization associated with force transmission. The specific questions to be addressed are, What is the evidence for MTJ involvement in musculoskeletal injury? How does the structure and biochemical composition of MTJs reflect their mechanical function? How well do experimental models resemble clinically encountered musculotendinous injuries? and, What variations in structure are present at MTJs that experience variations in mechanical loading?

MYOTENDINOUS JUNCTION INJURIES

Myotendinous Junctions Are Sites of Mechanical Failure During
Experimental Loading
Early investigation of sites of tears that occur in musculotendinous systems during loading in vitro (e.g., ref. [80], rabbit gastrocnemius)

showed that failure could occur at several sites, including, (1) within the muscle belly, (2) at tendinous insertions into bone or, (3) at myotendinous junctions. Although these investigations indicated that it was feasible for MTJs to be sites of muscle tears, loading conditions used were not easily related to in vivo conditions that would be experienced during musculoskeletal injury. However, subsequent loading experiments on musculotendinous units using controlled strain rates corroborated the involvement of MTJ tears in experimental injuries. Immediately following muscle loading (rabbit tibialis anterior, [84]) at 4% resting length per second (length/sec) to a stress anticipated to be ≈80% of breaking stress, histological and gross observations show an inflammatory reaction at MTJs. These preparations displayed some muscle fiber tearing at or near MTJs at the insertion end of the muscle but no tears reported at the muscle origin MTJs, muscle midbelly, or within the tendon.

Muscles loaded at strain rates from ≈0.4% to ≈90.0% resting length/sec until failure separated almost exclusively at or near the distal MTJ (rabbit hindlimb, [45]). These strain rates may be somewhat slower than those expected in normal locomotion or in sudden limb movements for these animals, but they do offer strong experimental support for the involvement of MTJs in strain injury. The MTJs are almost exclusively the site of separation in these experimental strain injuries, regardless of muscle type tested. Rabbit tibialis anterior, extensor digitorum longus, rectus femoris [45], and rat tibialis anterior [3] all fail at the MTJ during slow, controlled strain injuries. Although stress failure in these whole musculotendinous unit loading experiments was not measured, maximum strain was found to vary considerably between muscle types. Tibialis anterior failed at strains of ≈75%, whereas rectus femoris failed at strains of ≈225% [45]. No relationship between strain at failure and strain rate from ≈0.4–90% resting lengths/sec was observed.

In an attempt to measure breaking stress of MTJs, single frog skeletal muscle fibers and attached tendon collagen fibers have been tested to failure at strain rates that span those seen in locomotion in these animals (0.3 to 1.6 lengths/sec, [108]). These rates correspond to ≈0.5–2.5 times the strain rate experienced during swimming [109]. These single cell preparations failed at MTJs at a site called the lamina lucida which lies just external to the MTJ cell membrane. Breaking stress for MTJ failure in these preparations was ≈2.7×10^5 N/m^2, expressed relative to cell cross-sectioned area [108]. No relationship between breaking strength and strain rate or strain at failure were apparent.

Myotendinous Junctions Are Sites of Clinically Observed Muscle Tears
The MTJs are a primary site of lesion in many muscle tears [42]. The etiology of MTJ injuries is probably best known for "tennis leg" [6, 40, 81]. These injuries, initially misdiagnosed as plantaris tears, involve

avulsion of the medial head of the gastrocnemius and occur most commonly when the patient's foot is suddenly dorsiflexed while the knee is extended or knee suddenly extended while the foot is dorsiflexed [6, 81]. Tears at MTJs of the lateral head of the gastrocnemius have been reported less commonly [87], although the mechanism of injury is believed to be similar. A key factor in MTJ injury appears to be passive extension of active muscle (eccentric contraction). These injuries are exacerbated if the patient is not properly conditioned for the exercise undertaken or warmed up prior to exercise. MTJ injuries also are more common in biarticular muscles.

Although at first view, observations made of clinically observed injuries, whole muscle loading experiments, and single fiber loading experiments all appear consistent in indicating that MTJs are the common failure site during loading of myotendinous units, several inconsistencies between the experimental models and in vivo injuries apparently exist. First, strain at failure in whole muscle loading experiments exceeds that experienced by muscle in vivo. Muscle normally undergoes length changes of $\approx 20\%$ during locomotion, a value far less than that associated with muscle during experimental loading to failure (≈ 75–225%). Although the differences in maximum strain may relate to differences in strain rate between clinically encountered and experimentally induced injuries, site and maximum strain at failure are strain-rate independent, at least at strain rates tested thus far.

The single cell loading experiments also may have deficiencies in providing a model of MTJ failure in situ. Although single MTJs fail at $\approx 2.7 \times 10^5$ N/m^2 [108], this value is only about 20% greater than the average isometric stress these cells generate at the same sarcomere length (2.7 μm, [90]). This seems an unexpectedly small safety margin, especially in view of the additional stress that may be put on the MTJ by passive loading. This finding may indicate that some force during contraction is transmitted across lateral surfaces of the cell rather than solely at the MTJ. Experimental evidence supports this possibly additional site of force transmission at the muscle cell surface [97, 98], at least in injured muscle. Alternatively, the small safety margin may indicate that the single cell, myotendinous unit loading experiment is not a good model of in vivo loading conditions.

Observations also differ in the precise site of failure in whole muscle, myotendinous tears, and single cell, myotendinous tears. Whole muscle-tendon units loaded to failure display portions (≈ 0.5 mm) of at least some muscle fibers still attached to the tendon at which the tear occurred [45]. In single cell, myotendinous loading experiments, separation always occurred at the MTJ, external to the cell membrane, so that no portion of the cell was torn away to remain with the tendon [108]. Currently, the differences between these observations is unexplained. They may reflect differences in mode of failure of different fiber types;

perhaps some fiber types in whole muscle preparations divide within the fiber and other types divide between fiber and tendon. They also may reflect differences in loading conditions used or, perhaps, differences in the muscles' mechanical strength between the animals used for experimentation. Which of these failure sites is most representative of muscle tears encountered clinically is unknown. Currently, injuries identified clinically as MTJ tears are diagnosed by gross inspection or noninvasive methods (e.g., magnetic resonance imaging, computed tomography), which cannot resolve sites at the surface of the cell at the MTJ versus within the cell ≈ 0.5 mm from the MTJ. These noninvasive techniques do clearly show, however, that the MTJ region is the site of injury in at least some muscle strains (e.g., hamstring tears, [43]).

Delayed-Onset Muscle Soreness and Incomplete Muscle Tears May Involve Myotendinous Junctions

Delayed-onset muscle soreness (DOMS) is the condition associated with (1) tenderness encountered on palpation, (2) muscle weakness, and (3) restricted range of motion, that appear 24–48 hours after a period of intense or prolonged muscle activity. The condition may persist for 1 to 2 weeks in severe cases.

Available evidence indicates that DOMS may involve injury to MTJs. First, the etiology of DOMS and MTJ tears is similar; both occur primarily during eccentric contraction and are predisposed in inadequately conditioned individuals [7, 29, 33, 66]. Second, muscle tenderness associated with DOMS is most pronounced at sites where MTJs are most concentrated [61]. Finally, muscle loading during eccentric contraction at forces less than those leading to complete tears results in edema and inflammation at MTJs of experimental animals [3], which may be a tissue response associated with DOMS.

DOMS may therefore be a condition that represents incomplete tears at MTJs. This may not be testable in experimental animals, however, which cannot report the conditions associated with DOMS. Moreover, DOMS is difficult to dissociate clinically from other degradative changes related to intense exercise, such as elevated serum creatine kinase concentration (e.g., [83]), increased acid hydrolase activity [118], and increased urinary hydroxyproline concentration (e.g., [1]) or muscle spasm [32]. Partial MTJ injuries are likely, therefore, to remain a correlate rather than an established cause of DOMS.

Experimentally induced partial tears at MTJs can be caused by straining active or passive whole muscle until a decrease in stiffness is observed. Gross inspection of the loaded muscle shows hematoma overlying the distal MTJ of these preparations. Histological analysis of the healing process of partial tears at MTJs [3, 42] shows the initial hemorrhage followed by inflammatory reaction at the MTJ for the next 1–4 days. Muscle repair is observed at 4 days following injury [3], and connective tissue proliferation is apparent at the MTJ region about 1 week following injury [42]. The time course for histological repair of partial tears at MTJs is similar to that of recovery of normal muscle active tension and to the typical time course of DOMS resolution.

MYOTENDINOUS JUNCTION STRUCTURE AND COMPOSITION

The experimental and clinical observations reported above are adequate to implicate MTJs as primary sites of lesion in at least some physiological injuries of muscles. To understand the physiological bases for these injuries, one must know the structure and molecular composition of these sites and how MTJs may be modified in response to factors that predispose MTJs to injury. Current knowledge of MTJ structure, composition, and response to modified use is summarized in this section.

Myotendinous Junction Structure

Myotendinous junctions are located at each end of long, cylindrical skeletal muscle fibers (Figs. 12.1 and 12.2). Striking aspects of their morphology are the extensive membrane folding observed at these sites and the dense, subplasmalemmal material into which the terminal sarcomere of each myofibril extends (Fig. 12.3). It has been inferred from the crossbridge model of muscle contraction that force generated by crossbridge movement will be transmitted along the length of muscle fibers to ultimately act on the MTJ. This inference and the morphological and molecular specializations of MTJs are the basis for the assumption that MTJs are primarily specialized for force transmission at the muscle cell surface. This discussion of MTJ structure and injury will rely on that assumption, although the following limitations are noteworthy: (1) physiological and morphological observations indicate that contractile force can be transmitted across nonjunctional sites at the muscle cell surface [97, 98], and (2) MTJ specialization may relate to functions other than force transmission, such as myofibril growth, which occurs primarily at the ends of the muscle fiber [122].

This section of the review concerns those aspects of MTJ structure that relate to its role in force transmission. An analogy has been made previously between MTJs and adhesive joints [105] which provides a framework to begin analysis of the aspects of MTJ structure that are relevant to the MTJ role in joining muscle and tendon together. Several pertinent features appear in both theoretical and empirical treatments of adhesion between two mechanically nonidentical materials, such as muscle and tendon.

(1) Stress should be uniformly distributed at the interface, since non-uniformities lead to stress concentrations that greatly reduce adhesive strength [9].

FIGURE 12.1

Scanning electron micrograph of frog semitendinous muscle following dissection of epimysium. The tendon lies vertically in the center of the micrograph. Long, cylindrical muscle cell insert on the tendon from either side. Myotendinous junctions are located at the ends of the cells (arrowheads). Bar = 250 μm.

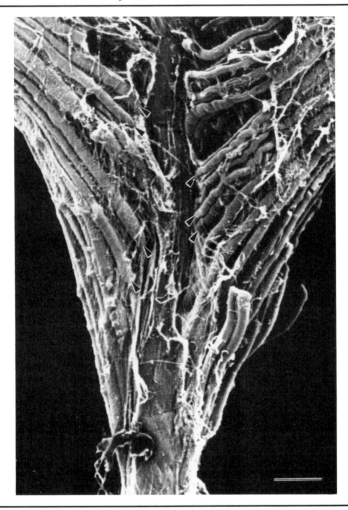

(2) The angle of loading of an adhesive joint can greatly influence adhesive strength [9, 75]. In general, if an interface between two adhesive materials lies at a low angle relative to the direction of loading (shear loading), adhesive strength is much greater than if loading is perpendicular to the interface (tensile loading). This is true even if

FIGURE 12.2

Transmission electron micrographs of myotendinous junction. Note that MTJ of cell is folded and appears to interdigitate with tendon **(arrowheads)**. *The connective tissue near the muscle cell is loose and contains fibroblasts* **(F)**. *The collagen fibers in the dense tendon* **(T)** *run at an oblique angle relative to the muscle fiber direction. Bar = 3.0 μm.*

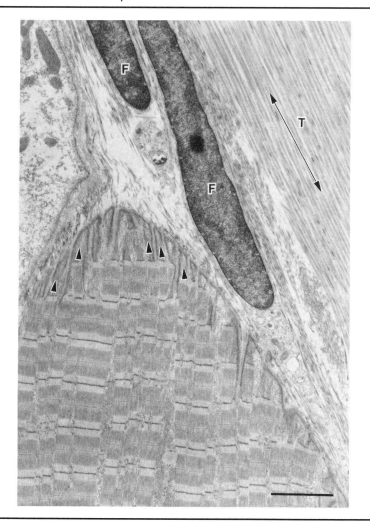

FIGURE 12.3
*Transmission electron micrograph of MTJ. Note that thin filaments extending toward folded cell membrane from terminal Z-disc (**arrowheads**) appear densely bundled. Also note collagen type I fiber (**arrow**) extending into folds in cell surface. Bar = 1.5 µm.*

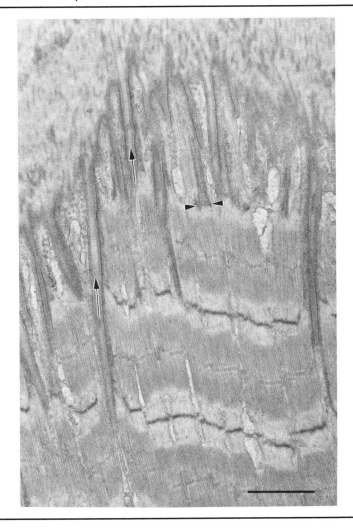

surface area and mechanical properties of structures that adhere together are the same in both shear and tensile loading.

(3) Adhesive strength can increase if the material at the interface (the adhesive) was less stiff than the structures it joined (the adherends) [9, 75].

TABLE 12.1
Myotendinous Junction Membrane Folding

Animal	Muscle	Fiber Type	Folding	Reference
Frog	semitendinosus (insertion)	fast twitch	22	110
Frog	semitendinous (insertion)	tonic	50	110
Frog	sartorius (origin)	fast twitch	24	34
Rat	semitendinosus (insertion)	mixed	13.5	106
Mouse	plantaris (insertion)	fast twitch	14.5	116
Mouse	plantaris (origin)	fast twitch	14.5	116
Mouse	soleus (insertion)	mixed	10.1	116
Mouse	soleus (origin)	mixed	12.7	116
Garter snake	costocutaneous	twitch	14	114
Garter snake	costocutaneous	tonic	16	114
Chicken	anterior latissimus dorsi	tonic	10	113
Chicken	posterior latissimus dorsi	twitch	14	113

In the following discussion, the structural specialization of MTJs that may relate to these mechanical aspects of their function and, therefore, to their possible tearing or injury during loading is presented.

MEMBRANE FOLDING. Scanning electron microscope observations first reported by Ishikawa et al. [62] show that membrane folding at MTJs can resemble anastomosing or nonanastomosing, digit-like extensions of the cell into the tendon or folds of the cell surface into which tendon extends. The functional significance of the differences in folding pattern is unknown and all folding is believed to serve similar mechanical functions. Ishikawa and co-workers [62] concluded that differences in the three-dimensional morphology of MTJs relate to differences between muscles and between species.

An important mechanical consequence of membrane folding at MTJs is an increase in junctional surface area which can reduce stress (force/unit area) placed on the junction during loading. Morphometric models have been developed specifically to quantify the amount of increase in junctional surface area attributable to folding, called the folding factor or surface amplification. Models based on the assumption that the processes at the MTJ were right cylinders were first used to analyze frog muscle [34], and later, mouse muscle [116]. An alternative model, based on the assumption that the processes were circular paraboloids [110], or digit-like, was later used to analyze frog MTJs. Notwithstanding these differences in assumptions concerning the shape of the processes, the values for folding factor are similar for twitch fibers, lying between $\approx 10-20$ times increase in surface area for a variety of vertebrate muscles. This means that for a typical muscle fiber 1 cm in length and 60 μm in diameter, $\approx 37\%$ of the cell's surface membrane lies at MTJs.

Although MTJ folding factors ($\overline{FF}_i$) are similar for a variety of muscles (Table 12.1), there are differences that correlate with fiber type. This was first noted in a comparison between folding of frog, semitendinosus tonic cells ($\overline{FF}_i = 50$), and frog semitendinous fast twitch ($\overline{FF}_i = 22$) [110]. Subsequent studies revealed that snake costocutaneous muscles [114] also show more folding in tonic fibers ($16\times$) than twitch fibers ($14\times$), but that twitch fibers from chicken display more folding ($14\times$) than chicken tonic fibers ($10\times$, [113]). The latter study of chicken muscle compared fibers from two different muscles, however, so that differences in muscle source also would correlate with differences in MTJ folding.

MYOTENDINOUS JUNCTION LOADING. In addition to reducing stress on the MTJ membrane during contraction, membrane folding also decreases the angle of loading of the junction interface [104, 105]. This lower angle of loading places the interface primarily under shear loading [105] which, as noted above, is a stronger configuration than loading in tension. This does not explain, however, why cells of different physiological types would have differences in membrane folding, especially in the tonic versus twitch fibers of frog semitendinosus where tonic folding is more than twice that of twitch folding [110]. The comparison of frog twitch and tonic cells also provides an apparent paradox in that tonic cells that generate less stress expressed relative to cell cross-sectional area ($\approx 1.7 \times 10^5$ N·m^{-2}) [72] have more extensively folded MTJ than twitch cells ($\approx 3 \times 10^5$ N·m^{-2}). A rationalization for these differences in tonic and twitch MTJ folding has been offered in terms of viscoelastic behavior of cell membranes [110]. The viscoelastic properties of membranes provide mechanical behavior that is a function of duration and rate of loading, as well as load magnitude. Time-dependent behavior may be especially important for tonic cells which, although contracting slowly, can maintain contractions for nearly 30 minutes [69]. Although the yield time of muscle cell membrane is unknown, data on other cell types (red blood cell, [91]) can provide values for speculation concerning muscle membrane behavior during loading. Calculations based on red cell membrane viscoelastic behavior [91] and stress applied to twitch and tonic MTJ membranes during contraction [110] show that if tonic cell MTJ membranes were not more folded than twitch cell MTJ membranes, they would tear during prolonged tonic contractions. Failure occurs because for any given stress, a viscoelastic material has a yield time when failure occurs, and that time limit would be exceeded if twitch cell membranes were loaded for tonic durations. By greatly increasing membrane folding, however, which occurs at tonic MTJs, stress is reduced resulting in longer yield time so that no failure occurs. Increased membrane folding, therefore, may relate to duration as well as magnitude of stress. This relies on the assumption that the mechanical properties, and therefore the molecular composition, of the twitch and tonic cell MTJs are identical. The other alternative by which MTJs can modify their breaking strength is through modification of their mechanical properties rather than modification of their membrane folding. This alternative may have the advantage of reducing the metabolic cost of producing the MTJ. For example, if changes in the molecular composition of a tonic cell MTJ could result in junctional material with longer yield time, less MTJ material would be needed for stress reduction.

The hypothesis that modifications in membrane folding can determine the breaking stress and yield time for MTJs suggests the possibility that pathological reductions in MTJ folding would result in mechanical failure at the MTJs. A morphometric analysis of muscle cells from frog semitendinosus displaying disuse-atrophic changes indicates that disuse atrophy can significantly reduce the breaking stress of atrophied MTJs (Fig. 12.4) [104]. The breaking stress of atrophied MTJs was less than maximum isometric stress for healthy fibers, although the exact values were not measured [104].

Limb immobilization can produce drastic decreases in MTJ breaking strength that may, perhaps, be attributable to reductions in MTJ folding or composition. Hind limb immobilization followed by loading myotendinous units to failure (rat tibialis anterior, [3]) showed that MTJ breaking strength declined to ≈55% control values after only 11 days immobilization. Tears in all cases occurred at the distal MTJ, as determined by gross inspection. These observations suggest that degenerative changes at MTJs that occur during prolonged bed rest or during joint immobilization after musculoskeletal injury may contribute significantly to predisposing muscle to injury following a return to activity.

Investigations concerning whether changes in MTJ structure also occur in response to increased muscle use or loading have focussed on electron microscopic evidence for increased anabolic activity near the MTJ [125]. Ultrastructural observations indicate increased fibroblastic activity near the MTJ of rat plantaris following removal of synergistic muscles and evidence of increased muscle membrane turnover in response to overloading for 1 to 2 weeks [125]. Findings concerning the possibility of increased MTJ surface area have not yet been published.

Myotendinous Junction Composition

THIN FILAMENT BUNDLING. In addition to membrane folding, MTJ structure appears morphologically distinct in that myofibrils terminate in dense material subjacent to the MTJ membrane (Figs. 12.3 and 12.5). Electron microscopic observations show that this material appears to crosslink or bundle thin filaments from the terminal sarcomere to one another and to the cell membrane. Based on structural observations, it appears, therefore, that these sites are enriched in proteins that may transmit force from myofibrils to the cell membrane.

The thin filaments that extend from the terminal Z-disc into the

FIGURE 12.4
Transmission electron micrograph of disuse-atrophied MTJ. Note that separation occurs between the cell membrane **(arrowheads)** *and the basement membrane* **(arrows)** *in disuse-atrophied fibers after loading. Digit-like processes of the cell are intact. Filamentous structures* **(double arrowheads)** *extend from cell membrane into zone of lesion. Bar = 1.5 μm. (Modified and reproduced with permission from Tidball, J.G. Morphological changes and mechanical failure associated with muscle cell atrophy.* Exp. Molec. Pathol. *40:1–12, 1984.)*

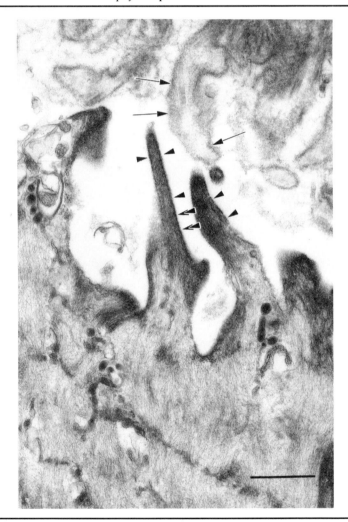

FIGURE 12.5

Transmission electron micrograph of components of MTJ which display in the extracellular space a collagen type I fiber (CO) and the basement membrane composed of lamina densa (LD) and lamina lucida (LL). Intracellularly, thin filaments (TF) are bundled and bound to the cell membrane. Bar = 100 nm. (Modified and reproduced with permission from Tidball, J.G. Morphological changes and mechanical failure associated with muscle cell atrophy. Exp. Molec. Pathol. *40:1–12, 1984.)*

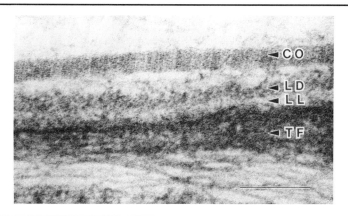

terminal processes of muscle cells were first shown to contain F-actin by Maruyama and Shimada [79] using heavy meromyosin labeling. Thus, it was expected that actin binding proteins would play important functional roles at MTJs. In view of the preceding discussion of design features that influence adhesive strength, it is predictable that variation in extent to which junctional actin is bound will modify its stiffness and thereby influence the breaking strength of the MTJ.

One of the earliest actin binding proteins identified was α-actinin, a Z-disc protein. Alpha-actinin has been shown to cause F-actin solutions to gel [126] which causes the formation of filamentous aggregates of F-actin that can be discerned by electron microscopy [88] and to form bridging structures between myofilaments [99]. These observations all suggest an actin bundling role for α-actinin.

Alpha-actinin has seemed, therefore, to be a likely candidate for thin filament bundling at MTJs, as well. Early electron microscopic studies noted structural similarities between Z-discs and subsarcolemmal densities in muscle [56, 120], and from this morphological similarity inferred homology. In addition, analogies between MTJs and fascia aderens of cardiac cells that contain α-actinin [73, 112] and focal contacts of cultured cells, also enriched in α-actinin [17], supported the supposition that MTJ thin filaments are bundled by α-actinin. It has been shown by electron microscope immunocytochemistry, however, that α-actinin is not present at MTJ subsarcolemmal densities or in the terminal Z-disc of each sarcomere [101]. This suggests some unique mechanism of thin filament bundling at the ends of the cells that may be important in determining the mechanical properties of these sites.

Dystrophin recently has been identified as a possible candidate for thin filament bundling protein at MTJs [93]. It is a 400,000 Dalton protein which is present subjacent to the muscle cell membrane and near some T-tubule membranes in healthy muscle [5, 11, 18, 121]. This protein is absent because of a genetic defect in Duchenne muscular dystrophy patients and in *mdx* mice [57]. It has been speculated that dystrophin may possibly serve this thin filament-crosslinking function at the MTJ for several reasons: (1) absence of dystrophin is associated with defects at the cell surface [82, 95], (2) dystrophin appears to be enriched at MTJs [93], and (3) dystrophin contains a domain that has a primary sequence similar to α-actinin [65]. Although this possible role of dystrophin at MTJs has not been tested, it could have important implications for understanding the pathophysiology of muscle in Duchenne's muscular dystrophy. Furthermore, the observation that the absence of this one structural protein enriched at MTJs can lead to the degenerative and ultimately lethal changes in muscle structure that occurs in Duchenne's muscular dystrophy accentuates the importance of normal organization of these sites in muscle function.

Dystrophin also contains a domain in which its primary structure is similar to another membrane-associated cytoskeletal protein, spectrin. Spectrin also is located subjacent to the muscle cell membrane [26, 92] and found at MTJ [106]. Spectrin can mediate actin attachment to the cell membrane (e.g., [49] for review) and can increase membrane elasticity and stiffness. Thus, it is feasible that dystrophin serves a role in thin filament crosslinkage and thin filament–membrane association at MTJs.

THIN FILAMENT ASSOCIATION WITH THE CELL MEMBRANE. An essential feature of MTJ structure is the presence of structural molecules that can attach thin filaments to the cell membrane and thereby transmit the contractile force. The identity of molecules that mediate thin filament-membrane association is important in numerous cell types, but has been especially well studied at specialized sites of cell adhesion to artificial substrata in vitro. These sites, called focal contacts, are locations where bundles of thin filaments terminate at the cell membrane. Vinculin, a 130,000 Dalton cytoskeletal protein, and talin, a 225,000 Dalton cytoskeletal protein, are concentrated at these sites and are likely to be involved in force transmission between thin filaments and the cell membrane. Talin and vinculin have an appreciable binding affinity for one another [17], and vinculin apparently interacts with actin through some poorly characterized structural protein [38]. It is hypothesized that actin filaments may interact with the cell membrane through a chain of structural proteins including talin and vinculin.

Immunofluorescent observations show that MTJs are enriched in both talin [111] and vinculin [14, 96], which indicates that these proteins also may be parts of a chain of force-transmitting proteins in vivo. Electron microscopic observations of antitalin-labeled muscle show talin present along the digit-like processes of the MTJ [111]. Vinculin has been demonstrated electron microscopically to lie within subsarcolemmal densities of muscle, although not specifically at MTJs [96]. Vinculin distribution does not always coincide with talin distribution in muscle, however. Although talin is largely restricted to the MTJ [111] and neuromuscular junction (NMJ), vinculin is found in chicken tonic cells to lie along nonjunctional regions of the cell surface [96]. This indicates that vinculin serves some unknown role at the surface of tonic cells in addition to thin filament-membrane attachment, or that it mediates these attachments without the presence of talin at nonjunctional sites.

Comparisons between focal contacts and MTJs show that mechanical similarities between membrane loading at these sites exist, in addition to similarities in molecular composition. The first estimates of stress placed on the MTJ, once corrected for membrane folding, indicated that these sites are loaded in shear at $\approx 2 \times 10^4$ N·m^{-2} during maximum isometric tension [104, 105, 110, 111]. Later work found that the same value is likely to be placed on snake MTJ membrane as well [114]. Calculations of the stress placed on the substratum by locomoting cells [111] that may utilize thin filament, vinculin, and talin assembles for force transmission to the cell membrane show similar stresses at the membrane ($\approx 10^4$ N·m^{-2}), assuming that fibroblasts exert shear stresses $\approx 10^{-2}$ N·m at the advancing edge of the cell [55] and adhere at sites 15 μm × 1 μm. Thus, the value $\approx 2 \times 10^4$ N·m^{-2} may represent a biologically important limit for membrane loading that could be important in determining if force is successfully transferred across the cell membrane or if injury occurs.

The preceding description provides evidence for an actin-vinculin-talin mediated system for force transmission at MTJs, but this does not mean that it is the exclusive mechanism at these sites. It also is feasible that parallel mechanisms that employ spectrin, dystrophin, or unidentified proteins may exist. In addition, there may be variations of assembly of these force-transmitting assemblages using actin, vinculin, and talin. For example, talin and vinculin are not always codistributed [47]. Talin and Vinculin are both located at many sites of cell-ECM adhesion, but vinculin without talin is commonly observed at sites of cell-cell adhesion [47].

TRANSMEMBRANE ASSOCIATION OF STRUCTURAL PROTEINS AT MTJs. An important requirement for force transmission for muscle cells to the extracellular matrix (ECM) is that the cells must adhere to ECM molecules. Fibronection, a ≈230,000 Dalton ECM glycoprotein, has long been a likely candidate to be a protein involved in this muscle cell adhesion to ECM. Fibronectin (FN) has been implicated in this role by several observations including that, (1) myogenic cell movements respond to differential distributions of FN and migrations cease when FN accumulates at the muscle cell surface [22, 117], (2) FN facilitates myogenic cell adhesion in vitro [22], and (3) structural rearrangement of the muscle cell surface to form MTJs follows the appearance of FN at the myogenic cell surface [107].

Those observations concerning the interactions of FN with the muscle cell surface implied the existence of some specific membrane protein that could bind FN. In pursuit of the receptor for FN, two groups of investigators [51, 59] made panels of monoclonal antibodies to membrane proteins and assayed for those that interfered with cell adhesion to FN-coated substrata. The protein thereby identified has been shown to be a member of a family of proteins, the integrin family, involved in cell adhesion.

The chick integrin protein that binds to FN (also called CSAT antigen, JG22, JG9, cell-substratum attachment antigen, avian fibronectin receptor) is a complex of three glycoproteins that are noncovalently associated [59]. Evidence supporting the role of integrin in cell adhesion to the ECM includes that it is located at focal contacts that contain FN [27], it binds to FN and laminin, another ECM glycoprotein [59], and antibodies to the receptor can block cell-substratum adhesion [19, 31, 51, 64].

The role of chick integrin in force transmission at MTJs is inferred from its enrichment at MTJs [14, 100] and at the ends of myotubes in vitro [27], and from the above cited examples of antibodies to integrin-disrupting, normal cell-substratum adhesion in vitro. However, integrin is not restricted to MTJs at the surface of adult skeletal muscle (14), however, which indicates that it may be involved in functions other than force transmission, or that force transmission also occurs at those non-MTJ sites of the muscle surface.

An additional, important observation that supports the role of integrin in force transmission at the muscle cell surface is the observation that the intracellular domain of the integrin molecule binds to talin [60]. Although this interaction may not be strong, it is believed to be adequate for force transmission across the cell membrane. Thus, a chain of mechanical links consisting of actin filaments, unknown protein, vinculin, talin, integrin, and fibronectin exists at MTJs and may be an important association for force transmission. However, other associations can also occur. For example, both integrin and vinculin are located at non-MTJ sites of fully differentiated muscle, in the absence of talin [14]. This may indicate that vinculin and integrin can interact directly at these sites or that some other protein mediates their association. Also, integrin may interact directly with α-actinin [85]. Because α-actinin can bind directly to actin, an actin–α-actinin–integrin assembly may be used for force transmisson at some sites. However, this association is not likely to be important for force transmission at MTJs, in view of the absence of α-actinin from those sites [101].

Although integrin appears likely to transmit force across adult MTJ membrane to FN bound to the ECM, its role in embryonic muscle in vivo is less clearly defined. MTJs first begin to assemble at the ends of chick myotubes at embryonic day 9 [103, 107, 119, 124]. Subsarcolemmal densities appear at the MTJ by embryonic day 12 to 13 and thin filaments insert into the subsarcolemmal material by day 15, at which time membrane folding begins [107] and continues through postnatal development [86]. Integrin distribution over this developmental time does not strictly coincide with the location of basement membrane or FN. Integrin is distributed in an apparently random and punctate pattern on the muscle cell surface at day 12. As development progresses, integrin distribution becomes more restricted, so that by 3 weeks posthatching integrin is most concentrated at MTJs and NMJs [14], whereas FN is located on the entire surface of the muscle cell. These observations suggest that some other protein may serve as a fibronectin receptor during the earliest stages of formation of MTJs.

A recently identified protein called myonexin [103] may serve as a fibronectin receptor in embryonic MTJs during their initial formation. Myonexin is an 80,000 Dalton membrane-associated protein found on the extracellular surface of skeletal but not cardiac muscle. The distribution of myonexin varies over developmental time in a pattern that is distinct from integrin. Myonexin is initially located at developing MTJs at sites where FN accumulation first occurs. In fully differentiated muscle, it is distributed more widely on the surface of the muscle and appears most concentrated at sites of close apposition between muscle cells [102]. Whether myonexin has an intracellular domain that can interact with cytoskeletal proteins in a manner similar to integrin has not yet been determined.

EXTRACELLULAR COMPONENTS OF MYOTENDINOUS JUNCTIONS. The complex associations formed between intracellular and extracellular structural proteins of MTJs is an important issue not only in understanding normal formation of these sites, but also for understanding the possible repair mechanisms that may follow injury of these structures. The mechanisms of formation and repair are made even more complex by the apparent, coordinated actions of both fibroblasts and muscle cells in junction formation.

The role of fibroblasts in myotendinous junction formation was first suggested in early histological studies [124] which described the accumulation of fibroblasts at the ends of myotubes where MTJs would form. Several subsequent findings indicated that a function of fibroblasts in MTJ formation could be the secretion of FN onto the surface of the incipient MTJs, thereby possibly initiating junction formation. The most significant of these findings include, (1) basement membranes, which contain FN, are not completely formed by myogenic cells in vitro unless fibroblasts are present [70, 71, 74, 94], (2) most FN in myogenic tissue is secreted by fibroblasts [22, 41], and (3) basement membrane first appears at the myogenic cell surface in vivo at sites at which fibroblasts and myotubes lie in close apposition [107]. Further observations also indicated that not only is FN apparently important in myogenic cell-substratum adhesion but myofibril association with the cell membrane also could require the presence of FN bound to the cell surface. For example, Puri and colleagues [89] found that myogenic cells grown in fibronectin-deficient media would not adhere to substrata, but normal myofibrillogenesis would occur within the nonadherent cells. The myofibrils did not attach to the cell membrane, however; rather, they appeared located more centrally in the cell.

These observations, together with observation that failure during loading of myotendinous units can occur between the cell membrane and the fibronectin-enriched basement membrane (108), suggest that MTJ failure may involve disruption of muscle interaction with FN, at least in part. This also suggests that repair at these injured sites would involve increased secretary activity by fibroblastic cells, a response that has been observed both clinically and experimentally [e.g., 3, 125].

The apparent importance of FN in MTJ formation and structure may reflect not only the functional significance of this molecule, but also the relatively intense interest in this protein by researchers. Other ECM proteins may have similarly essential, although less well-characterized, functions at MTJs. For example, cytotactin is another large ECM glycoprotein that is enriched at embryonic MTJs [21] and is secreted by fibroblasts [28, 37]. Cytotactin was independently identified in several labs and received several different names as a result, including myotendinous antigen [20, 21], hexabrachion [35], J1 [68], tenascin [23], glioma mesenchymal extracellular matrix protein [13], as well as cytotactin [52]. The early choice of the name myotendinous antigen [20, 21] resulted from the observation that antibodies to the protein bound preferentially to MTJ regions in embryonic tissues. However, many subsequent studies have shown, however, that the protein is a widely distributed ECM molecule [36], not an exclusive marker for MTJs.

The prominence of cytotactin at embryonic MTJs suggests a role in their formation or, perhaps, a role in early events in muscle-substratum attachment. Cell adhesion to substrata in vitro is enhanced by the presence of cytotactin [13, 23, 39], although cell adhesion to cytotactin does not appear to be as strong as cell adhesion to fibronectin. Cell binding to cytotactin also is mediated by an integrin protein, although the cytotactin-binding integrin complex is not identical to the integrin fibronectin receptor [13].

If cytotactin is a mechanical link at MTJs, it must bind to some other ECM protein as well as to the cell surface. The ability of cytotactin to bind to other ECM components is controversial, but FN is a possible ligand. Although cytotactin-FN binding has been reported [23, 58], binding in solution has not been shown, and FN-cytotactin binding may not be a strong interaction. Cytotactin does, however, appear to bind to chondroitin sulfate proteoglycan secreted in muscle culture [21] with an affinity that may be biologically significant.

In fully differentiated muscle, cytotactin is most concentrated at NMJs and within tendon near MTJs [28, 100]. Antibody staining of cytotactin by indirect immunofluorescence becomes more prominent at both the NMJ and MTJ following muscle denervation [28]. Denervation also leads to the appearance of cytotactin at nonjunctional regions of the muscle cell surface. This change in distribution following denervation is similar to that observed for the neural cell adhesion molecule (NCAM) [25] and may reflect regulation of cytotactin synthesis and distribution by synaptic interactions. These observations thereby introduce the possibility that MTJ structure and composition can be regulated not only by muscle-fibroblast interactions but also by muscle interactions with motor neurons.

Proteoglycans, especially heparan sulfate proteoglycan (HSP), may be of importance as force transmitting components at MTJs. Indirect immunofluorescence of MTJs using antisera to HSP show this glycoprotein greatly enriched at MTJs [100]. This potentially huge ($>10^7$ Daltons) proteoglycan is capable of binding to other ECM molecules also enriched at these sites. Laminin, an ECM glycoprotein also shown to be present [14] and perhaps enriched [100] at MTJs, can bind to HSP and to integrin [59] molecules enriched at the MTJ. Thus, a transmembrane association of structural proteins that does not involve FN may be present at MTJs. However, HSP also has a FN-binding domain (123), so that interactions between these possible force transmitting assemblies are not likely to involve distinct, extracellular mechanisms.

The possible enrichment of other ECM molecules at MTJs has been examined by indirect immunofluorescence with the goal of identifying proteins of possible importance in cell adhesion or force transmission at these sites. Collagen type I, III, IV, and VI are all present at or near MTJs, but not apparently concentrated at these sites relative to other nearby sites in the ECM [100]. Specializations in protein synthesis and distribution at sites of force transmission, therefore, seem to involve molecules that mediate cell interactions with collagens and not the collagens themselves.

RELATIONSHIP BETWEEN MTJ STRUCTURE AND INJURY

Previously noted studies have shown that there are at least two failure sites in myotendinous units: (1) sites near MTJs but within muscle cells of whole rabbit muscle loaded to failure [45], and (2) sites in a zone called the lamina lucida that lies immediately external to the MTJ membrane where failure occurs in whole, disuse-atrophied frog muscle [104, 105] or in single-cell, myotendinous preparations loaded to failure [108]. The different failure sites indicate different mechanisms for failure that may relate to the severity of the injury and vary with loading conditions and health of the muscle at time of injury.

Those injuries that occur by separation within the lamina lucida are expected to heal more rapidly because these injuries will not involve tearing and lysis of the cell itself. Electron microscopic observations suggest that separation is likely to occur within or between membrane receptors for ECM molecules and their associated ligands found in the basement membrane [108]. This injury, therefore, is a failure of adhesion between cell and ECM, and may be exacerbated by reduction in membrane folding and increase in angle of MTJ loading that occurs in disuse atrophy [104]. Repair of injuries within the lamina lucida may be facilitated by the presence of satellite cells within this zone, because satellite cells are mesenchymal cells that are of myogenic lineage and are involved in muscle repair following injury.

Muscle injuries that involve tears through the cells near the MTJ are expected to be slower to repair because they will lead to cell lysis and necrosis. The mechanism of injury and reason for occurrence near the MTJ are unknown. It has been noted previously that sarcomeres near MTJs are stiffer than elsewhere in the fiber [50] and that this may relate to determining site of injury in some way not yet understood [42]. This is a central, unanswered question in the mechanics of muscle injury.

CONCLUSION

In this review I have attempted to present current information concerning the structure of myotendinous junctions and their involvement in injuries. The hope has been that by reviewing our knowledge of MTJs from molecular structure to their involvement in injuries, the relationships between these levels of organization and defects in organization could be better seen. The MTJs are structurally complex, and as studies of their structure and involvement in injuries progress, more complexity will emerge. The past 10 years have produced the first information concerning how a chain of structural molecules can transmit force from myofibrils across the cell membrane to act on tendon. They also have shown that in some musculoskeletal injuries this chain of structural molecules can be disrupted so that lesions occur at the MTJs. The conditions leading to failure, however, can vary according to previous muscle use. This leads to one of the most interesting questions not only in exercise science but in biology and medicine as a whole: how is environmental information, in this case mechanical environment, transduced to the genome? In other words, how can factors such as stress, strain, frequency, and duration of use be translated by a cell into modifications in gene expression, protein structure, and cell organization? These questions are the most basic for understanding how MTJ structure relates to its use. The current state of knowledge of MTJ structure and involvement in injury provides only the names of the components involved in the adaptive processes that must occur at these sites. The most interesting work, showing how the interactions between these components is regulated in development and adaptation to use, is yet to come.

ACKNOWLEDGEMENTS

I thank Carol Bahnsen for critically reading this manuscript. This work was supported by grants from the National Institutes of Health (AR-40343), the National Science Foundation (DCB-841745), the Muscular Dystrophy Association, and the Academic Senate of the University of California.

REFERENCES

1. Abraham, W.M. Factors in delayed muscle soreness. *Med. Sci. Sports* 9:11–20, 1977.
2. Ajiri, T., T. Kimura, R. Ito, and S. Inokuchi. Microfibrils in the myotendon junction. *Acta. Anat.* 102:433–439, 1978.
3. Almekinders, L.C., and J.A. Gilbert. Healing of experimental muscle strains and the effects of nonsteroidal inflammatory medicine. *Amer. J. Sports Med.* 14:303–308, 1986.
4. Andreev, D.P., and W.A. Wassilev. Specialized contacts between sarcolemma and sarcoplasmic reticulum at the ends of muscle fibers in the diaphragm of the rat. *Cell Tiss. Res.* 243:415–420, 1986.
5. Arahata K., E. Ishiura, T. Ishiguro, et al. Immunostaining of skeletal and cardiac muscle surface membrane with antibody against Duchenne muscular dystrophy peptide. *Nature* 333:861–863, 1988.
6. Arner, O., and A. Lindholm, What is tennis leg? *Acta Chir. Scand.* 116:73–77, 1958.
7. Asmussen, E. Positive and negative muscular work. *Acta Physiol. Scand.* 28:364–382, 1953.
8. Baetsher, M., D.W. Pumplin, and R.J. Bloch. Vitronectin at sites of cell-substrate contact in cultures of rat myotubes. *J. Cell. Biol.* 103:369–378, 1986.
9. Bikerman, J.J. Stresses in proper adhints. *The Science of Adhesive Joints.* New York: Academic Press, Inc. 1968, pp. 192–263.
10. Bonilla, E. Ultrastructural study of the muscle cell surface. *J. Ultrastruc. Res.* 82:341–345, 1983.

11. Bonilla, E., C.E. Samitt, A.F. Miranda, et al. Duchenne muscular dystrophy: deficiency of dystrophin at the muscle cell surface. *Cell* 54:447–452, 1988.

12. Bourden, M.A., T.J. Matthews, S.V. Pizzo, and D.D. Bigner. Immunocytochemical and biochemical characterization of a glioma-associated extracellular matrix glyco-protein. *J. Cell Biochem.* 28:183–185, 1985.

13. Bourdon, M.A., and E. Ruoslahti. Tenascin mediates cell attachment through an RGD-dependent receptor. *J. Cell Biol.* 108:1149–1155, 1989.

14. Bozyczko, D., C. Decker, J. Muschler, and A.F. Horwitz. Integrin on developing and adult skeletal muscle. *Exp. Cell Res.* 183:72–91, 1989.

15. Burridge, K., and L. Connell. A new protein of adhesion plaques and ruffling membranes. *J. Cell Biol.* 97:359–367, 1983.

16. Burridge, K., and L. Connell. Talin: a cytoskeletal component concentrated in adhesion plaques and other sites of actin-membrane interaction. *Cell Motil.* 3:405–418, 1983.

17. Burridge, K., and P.H. Mangeat. An interaction between vinculin and talin. *Nature* (Lond.). 308:744–746, 1984.

18. Carpenter, S., G. Karpati, E. Zubrzycka-Gaarn, D.E. Bulman, P.N. Ray, and R.G. Worton. Dystrophin is localized to the plasma membrane of human skeletal muscle fibers by electron-microscope cytochemical study. *Muscle & Nerve* 13:376–380, 1990.

19. Chapman, A.E. Characterization of a 140 kD cell surface glycoprotein involved in myoblast adhesion. *J. Cell Biochem.* 25:109–121, 1984.

20. Chiquet, M., and D.M. Fambrough. Chick myotendinous antigen. I. A monoclonal antibody as a marker for tendon and muscle morphogenesis. *J. Cell Biol.* 98:1926–1936, 1984.

21. Chiquet, M., and D.M. Fambrough. Chick myotendinous antigen. II. A novel extracellular glycoprotein complex consisting of large disulfide-lined subunits. *J. Cell Biol.* 98:1937–1946, 1984.

22. Chiquet, M., H.M. Eppenberger, and D.C. Turner. Muscle morphogenesis: evidence for an organizing function of exogenous fibronectin. *Dev. Biol.* 88:220–235, 1981.

23. Chiquet-Ehrismann, R., E.J. Mackie, C.A. Pearson, and T. Sakakura. Tenascin: an extracellular matrix protein involved in tissue interactions during fetal development and oncogenesis. *Cell* 47:131–139, 1986.

24. Chiquet-Ehrismann, R., P. Kalla, C.A. Pearson, K. Beck, and M. Chiquet. Tenascin interferes with fibronectin action. *Cell* 53:383–390, 1988.

25. Covault, J., and J. Sanes. Neural cell adhesion molecule (NCAM) accumulates in denervated and paralyzed skeletal muscles. *Proc. Natl. Acad. Sci., USA.* 82:4544–4548, 1985.

26. Craig, S.W., and J.V. Pardo. Gamma actin, spectrin, and intermediate filament proteins colocalize with vinculin at costameres, myofibril-to-sarcolemma attachment sites. *Cell Motil.* 3:449–462, 1983.

27. Damsky, C.H., K.A. Knudsen, D. Bradley, C.A. Buck, and A.F. Horwitz. Distribution of the cell-substratum attachment (CSAT) antigen on myogenic and fibroblastic cells in culture. *J. Cell Biol.* 100:1527–1539, 1985.

28. Daniloff, J.K., K.L. Crossin, M. Pinçon-Raymond, M. Murawsky, F. Rieger, and G.M. Edelman. Expression of cytotactin in the normal and regenerating neuromus-cular system. *J. Cell Biol.* 108:625–635, 1989.

29. Davies, C.T.M., and C. Barnes. Negative (eccentric) work. I. The effects of repeated exercise. *Ergonomics* 15:3–14, 1972.

30. Davison, M.D., and D.R. Critchley. Alpha-actinins and the DMD protein contain spectrin-like repeats. *Cell* 52:159–160, 1988.

31. Decker, C., R. Greggs, K. Duggan, J. Stubbs, and A. Horwitz. Adhesive multiplicity in the interaction of embryonic fibroblasts and myoblasts with extracellular matrices. *J. Cell Biol.* 99:1398–1404, 1984.

32. deVries, H.A. EMG fatigue curves in postural muscles. A possible etiology for idiopathic low back pain. *Amer. J. Phys. Med.* 47:175–181, 1968.

33. Edwards, R.H.T., K.R. Mills, and D.J. Newham. Measurement of severity and distribution of experimental muscle tenderness. *J. Physiol.* 317:1P–2P, 1981.

34. Eisenberg, B.R., and R.L. Milton. Muscle fiber termination at the tendon in the frog sartorius: a stereological study. *Amer. J. Anat.* 171:273–284, 1984.

35. Erickson, H.P., and J.L. Iglesias. A six-armed oligomer isolated from cell surface fibronectin preparations. *Nature* 3111:267–269, 1984.

36. Erickson, H.P., and M.A. Bourdon. Tenascin: an extracellular matrix protein prominent in specialized embryonic tissue and tumors. *Ann. Rev. Cell Biol.* 5:71–92, 1989.

37. Erickson, H.P., and V.A. Lightner. Hexabrachion protein (tenascin, cytotactin, brachionectin) in connective tissues, embryonic brain, and tumors. *Adv. Cell Biol.* 2:55–90, 1988.

38. Evans, R.R., R.M. Robson, and M.H. Stromer. Properties of smooth muscle vinculin. *J. Biol. Chem.* 259:3916–3924, 1984.

39. Friedlander, D.R., S. Hoffman, and G.M. Edelman. Functional mapping of cytotacin: proteolytic fragments active in cell-substrate adhesion. *J. Cell Biol.* 107:2329–2340, 1988.

40. Froimson, A.I. Tennis leg. *J.A.M.A.* 209:415–416, 1969.

41. Gardner J.M., and D.M. Fambrough. Fibronectin expression in myogenesis. *J. Cell Biol.* 96:474–485, 1983.

42. Garret, W.E., Jr., and J.G. Tidball. Myotendinous junctions: structure, function and failure. S.L.-Y. Woo and J.A. Buckwalter (eds.). *Injury and Repair of the Musculoskeletal Soft Tissues.* Park Ridge, IL: American Academy of Orthopaedic Surgeons, 1988, pp. 171–207.

43. Garrett, W.E., Jr., F.R. Rich, P.K. Nikolaou, and J.B. Vogler. Computed tomography of hamstring muscle strains. *Med. Sci. Sports Exer.* 21:506–514, 1989.

44. Garrett, W.E., Jr., M.R. Safran, A.V. Seaber, R.R. Glisson, and B.M. Ribbeck. Biomechanical comparison of stimulated and nonstimulated skeletal muscle pulled to failure. *Am. J. Sports Med.* 15:448–454, 1987.

45. Garrett, W.E., Jr., P.K. Nikolaou, B.M. Ribbeck, R.R. Glisson, and A.V. Seaber. The effect of muscle architecture on the biomechanical failure properties of skeletal muscle under passive extension. *Am. J. Sports Med.* 16:7–12, 1988.

46. Geiger, B., K.T. Tokuyasu, A.H. Dutton, and S.J. Singer. Vinculin, an intracellular protein localized at specialized sites where microfilament bundles terminate at cell membrane. *Proc. Natl. Acad. Sci., USA.* 77:4127–4131, 1980.

47. Geiger, B., T. Volk, and T. Volberg. Molecular heterogeneity of adherens junctions. *J. Cell Biol.* 101:1523–1531, 1985.

48. Gelber, D., D.H. Moore, and H. Ruska. Observations of the myotendinous junction in mammalian skeletal muscle. *Zeitschrift fur Zellfurschung.* 52:396–400, 1960.

49. Goodman, S.R., and K. Shiffer. The spectrin membrane skeleton of normal and abnormal human erythrocytes: a review. *Amer. J. Physiol.* 244:C121–C141, 1983.

50. Gordon, A.M., Huxley, A.F., and F.J. Julian. Tension development in highly stretched vertebrate muscle fibers. *J. Physiol.* 184:143–169, 1966.

51. Greven, J.M., and D.J. Gottlieb. Monoclonal antibodies which alter the morphology of cultured myogenic cells. *J. Cell. Biochem.* 18:221–229, 1982.

52. Grumet, M., S. Hoffman, K.L. Crossin, and G.M. Edelman. Cytotactin, an extracellular matrix protein of neural and non-neural tissues that mediates glia-neuron interactions. *Proc. Nat. Acad. Sci., USA* 82:8075–8079, 1985.

53. Hammond, R.G., Jr. Protein sequence of DMD gene is related to actin binding domain of a α-actinin. *Cell* 51:1, 1987.

54. Hammond, R.G., Jr. Protein sequence of DMD gene is related to actin binding domain of α-actinin. *Cell* 51:1, 1987.

55. Harris, A.K., P. Wild, and D. Stopak. Silicon rubber substrata: a new wrinkle in the study of locomotion. *Science* 208:177–179, 1980.

56. Heuson-Stiennon, J.A. Morphogenèse de la cellular musculaire striée etudiée au microscope electronique. *J. Microsc.* 4:657, 1965.

57. Hoffman, E.P., R.H. Brown, Jr., and L.M. Kunkel. Dystrophin: the protein product of the Duchenne muscular dystrophy locus. *Cell*: 51:919–928, 1987.

58. Hoffman, S., K.L. Crossin, and G.M. Edelman. Molecular forms, binding functions, and developmental expression patterns of cytotactin and cytotactin-binding proteoglycan, an interactive pair of extracellular matrix molecules. *J. Cell Biol.* 106:519–522, 1988.

59. Horwitz, A.F., K. Duggan, R. Greggs, C. Decker, and C. Buck. The cell substrate attachment (CSAT) antigen has properties of a receptor for laminin and fibronectin. *J. Cell Biol.* 101:2134–2144, 1985.

60. Horwitz, A.K., K. Duggan, C. Buck, M.C. Beckerle, and K. Burridge. Interaction of plasma membrane fibronectin receptor with talin—a transmembrane linkage. *Nature* (Lond.). 320:531–533, 1986.

61. Hough, T. Ergographic studies in muscular soreness. *Amer. J. Physiol.* 7:76–92, 1902.

62. Ishikawa, H., H. Sawada, and E. Yamada. Surface and internal morphology of skeletal muscle. *Handbook of Physiology*. Section 10. 1983, pp. 1–21.

63. Kieny, M., and A. Mauger. Immunofluorescent localization of extracellular matrix components during muscle morphogenesis. I. In normal chick embryos. *J. Exp. Biol.* 232:327–341, 1984.

64. Knudsen, K.A., P. Rao, C.H. Damsky, and C.A. Buck. Membrane glycoproteins involved in cell substratum adhesion. *Proc. Natl. Acad. Sci. USA.* 78:6071–6078, 1981.

65. Koenig, M., A.P. Monaco, and L.M. Kunkel. The complete sequence of dystrophin predicts a rod-shaped cytoskeletal protein. *Cell* 53:219–228, 1988.

66. Komi, P.V., and E.R. Buskirk. Effect of eccentric and concentric muscle conditioning on tension and electrical activity of human muscle. *Ergonomics* 15:417–434, 1972.

67. Korneliussen, H. Ultrastructure of myotendinous junctions in *Myxine* and rat. Specializations between the plasma membrane and the lamina densa. *Z. Anat. Entwickl.-Gesch.* 142:91–100, 1973.

68. Kruse, J., G. Keilhauer, A. Faissner, R. Timpl, and M. Schachner. The J1 glycoprotein—a novel nervous system cell adhesion molecule of the L2/HNK-1 family. *Nature* 316:146–148, 1985.

69. Kuffler, S.W., and E.M. Vaughan-Williams. Properties of the "slow" skeletal muscle fibers of the frog. *J. Physiol.* 121:318–340, 1953.

70. Kühl, U., M. Öcalan, R. Timpl, R. Mayne, E. Hay, and K. von der Mark. Role of muscle fibroblasts in the deposition of type-IV collagen in the basal lamina of myotubes. *Differentiation* 28:164–172, 1984.

71. Kühl, U., R. Timpl, and K. von der Mark. Synthesis of Type IV collagen and laminin in cultures of skeletal muscle cells and their assembly on the surface of myotubes. *Develop. Biol.* 93:344–354, 1982.

72. Lannergren, J., and R.S. Smith. Types of muscle fibers in toad skeletal muscle. *Acta Physiol. Scand.* 68:263–274, 1966.

73. Lemanski, L.F., D.J. Paulson, C.S. Hill, L.A. Davis, L.C. Riles, and S.S. Lim. Immunoelectron microscopic localization of α-actinin on Lowicryl-embedded thin sectioned tissues. *J. Histochem. Cytochem.* 33:515–522, 1985.

74. Lipton, B.H. Collagen synthesis by normal and bromodeoxyuridine modulated cells in myogenic cultures. *Dev. Biol.* 61:153–165, 1977.

75. Lubkin, J.L. The theory of adhesive scarf joints. *J. Appl. Mech.* 24:255–260, 1957.

76. Mackay, B., T.J. Harrop, and A.R. Muir. The fine structure of the muscle tendon junction in the rat. *Acta Anat.* 73:588–604, 1969.

77. Mackay, P., and T.J. Harrop. An experimental study of the longitudinal growth of skeletal muscle in the rat. *Acta Anat.* 72:38–49 1969.

78. Mair, W.G.P., and F.M.S. Tomé. The ultrastructure of the adult and developing human myotendinous junction. *Acta Neuropathol* (Berlin). 21:239–252, 1972.

79. Maruyama, K., and Y. Shimada. Fine structure of the myotendinous junction of lathyritic muscle with special reference to connectin, a muscle elastic protein. *Tiss. Cell.* 10:741–748, 1978.

80. McMaster, P.E. Tendon and muscle ruptures: clinical and experimental studies on the causes and location of subcutaneous ruptures. *J. Bone and Joint Surg.* 15:705–722, 1933.

81. Miller, W.A. Rupture of the musculotendinous juncture of the medial head of the gastrocnemius muscle. *Amer. J. Sports Med.* 5:191–193, 1977.

82. Mokri, B., and A.G. Engel. Duchenne dystrophy: electron microscope findings pointing to a basic or early abnormality in the plasma membrane of the muscle fiber. *Neurol.* 25:1111–1120, 1975.

83. Newham, D.J., D.A. Jones, and R.H.T. Edwards. Large delayed plasma creatine kinase changes after stepping exercise. *Muscle & Nerve* 6:380–385, 1983.

84. Nikolaou, P.K., B.L. Macdonald, R.R. Glisson, A.V. Seaber, and W.E. Garrett, Jr. Biomechanical and histological evaluation of muscle after controlled strain injury. *Am. J. Sports Med.* 15:9–14, 1987.

85. Otey, C.A., F.M. Pavalko, and K. Burridge. An interaction between α-actinin and β-integrin subunit *in vitro. J. Cell Biol.* 111:721–729, 1990.

86. Ovalle, W.K. The human muscle-tendon junction: a morphological study during normal growth and at maturity. *Anat. Embryol.* 176:281–294, 1987.

87. Patton, G.W., and R.J. Parker. Rupture of the lateral head of the gastrocnemius muscle at the musculotendinous junction mimicking a compartment syndrome. *J. Foot Surg.* 28:433–437, 1989.

88. Podlubnaya, Z.A., L.A. Tskhovrebova, M.M. Zaalishvilli, and G.A. Stefanenko. Electron microscope study of a α-actinin. *J. Molec. Biol.* 92:357–359, 1975.

89. Puri, E.C., M. Caravatti, J-C. Perriard, D.C. Turner, and H.M. Eppenberger. Anchorage independent muscle cell differentiation. *Proc. Natl. Acad. Sci. USA* 77:5297–5301, 1980.

90. Ramsey, R.W., and S.F. Street. The isometric length-tension diagram of isolated skeletal muscle fibres of the frog. *J. Cell Comp. Physiol.* 15:11–34, 1940.

91. Rand, R.P. Mechanical properties of the red cell membrane. II. Viscoelastic breakdown of the membrane. *Biophys. J.* 42:303–316, 1964.

92. Repasky, E.A., B.L. Granger, and E. Lazarides. Widespread occurrence of avian spectrin in non-erythroid cells. *Cell* 29:821–833, 1982.

93. Samitt, C.E., and E. Bonilla. Immunocytochemical study of dystrophin at the myotendinous junction. *Muscle & Nerve* 13:493–500, 1990.

94. Sanderson, R.D., J.M. Fitch, T.R. Linsenmayer, and R. Mayne. Fibroblasts promote the formation of a continuous basal lamina during myogenesis in vitro. *J. Cell Biol.* 102:740–747, 1986.

95. Schmalbruch, H. Segmental fiber breakdown and defects of the plasmalemma in diseased human muscles. *Acta Neuropath.* 33:129–141, 1975.

96. Shear, C.R., and R.J. Bloch. Vinculin in subsarcolemmal densities in chicken skeletal muscle: localization and relationship to intracellular and extracellular structures. *J. Cell Biol.* 101:240–256, 1985.

97. Street, S.F. Lateral transmission of tension in frog myofibrils: a myofibrillar network and transverse cytoskeletal connections are possible transmitters. *J. Cell. Physiol.* 114:346–364, 1983.

98. Street, S.F., and R.W. Ramsey. Sarcolemma: transmitter of active tension in frog skeletal muscle. *Science* 149:1379–1380, 1965.

99. Stromer, M.H., and D.E. Goll. Studies on purified α-actinin. II. Electron microscopic studies on the competitive binding of α-actinin and tropomyosin to Z-line extracted myofibrils. *J. Molec. Biol.* 67:489–494, 1972.

100. Swasdison, S., and R. Mayne. Location of the integrin complex and extracellular matrix molecules at the chicken myotendinous junction. *Cell Tiss. Res.* 257:537–543, 1989.

101. Tidball, J.G. Alpha-actinin is absent from the terminal segments of myofibrils and from subsarcolemmal densities in frog skeletal muscle. *Exper. Cell Res.* 170:469–482, 1987.

102. Tidball, J.G. Identification of an 80-kD glycoprotein enriched at sites of close apposition between skeletal muscle cells. *Eur. J. Cell Biol.* 46:161–167, 1988.

103. Tidball, J.G. Myonexin: and 80 kD glycoprotein that binds fibronectin and is located at embryonic myotendinous junctions. *Devel. Biol.* 142:103–114, 1991.

104. Tidball, J.G. Myotendinous junction: morphological changes and mechanical failure associated with muscle cell atrophy. *Exper. Molec. Pathol.* 40:1–12, 1984.

105. Tidball, J.G. The geometry of actin filament-membrane interactions can modify adhesive strength of the myotendinous junction. *Cell Motility.* 3:439–447, 1983.

106. Tidball, J.G. Unpublished observation.

107. Tidball, J.G., and C. Lin. Structural changes at the myogenic cell surface during formation of myotendinous junctions. *Cell Tiss Res.* 257:77–84, 1989.

108. Tidball, J.G., and M. Chan. Adhesive strength of single muscle cells to basement membrane at myotendinous junctions. *J. Appl. Physiol.* 67:1063–1069, 1989.

109. Tidball, J.G., and T.L. Daniel. Elastic energy storage in rigored skeletal muscle cells under physiological loading conditions. *Amer. J. Physiol.* 150:R56–R64, 1986.

110. Tidball, J.G., and T.L. Daniel. Myotendinous junctions of tonic muscle cells: structure and loading. *Cell Tiss. Res.* 245:315–322, 1986.

111. Tidball, J.G., T.O'Halloran, and K. Burridge. Talin at myotendinous junctions. *J. Cell Biol.* 103:1465–1472, 1986.

112. Tokuyasu, K.T., A.H. Dutton, B. Geiger, and S.J. Singer. Ultrastructure of chicken cardiac muscle as studied by double immunolabeling in electron microscopy. *Proc. Natl. Acad. Sci. USA.* 78:7619–7623, 1981.

113. Trotter, J.A., and J.M. Baca. A stereological comparison of the muscle-tendon junctions of fast and slow fibers in the chicken. *Anta. Rec.* 218:256–266, 1987.

114. Trotter, J.A., and J.M. Baca. The muscle-tendon junctions of fast and slow fibres in the garter snake: ultrastructural and stereological analysis and comparison with other species. *J. Mus. Res. Cell Motil.* 8:517–526, 1987.

115. Trotter, J.A., K. Corbett, and B. Avner. Structure and function of the murine muscle-tendon junction. *Anat. Rec.* 201:293–302, 1981.

116. Trotter, J.A., K. Hsi, A. Samora, and C. Wofsy. A morphometric analysis of the muscle-tendon junction. *Anat. Rec.* 213:26–32, 1985.

117. Turner, D.C., J. Lawton, P. Dollenmeier, R. Ehrismann, and M. Chiquet. Guidance of myogenic cell migration by oriented deposits of fibronectin. *Dev. Biol.* 95:497–504, 1983.

118. Vihko, V., A. Salminen, and J. Rantamäki. Exhaustive exercise, endurance training and acid hydrolase activity in skeletal muscle. *J. Appl. Physiol.* 47:43–50, 1979.

119. Wake, K. Formation of myoneural and myotendinous junctions in the chick embryo. *Cell Tiss. Res.* 173:383–400, 1976.

120. Warren, R.H., and K.R. Porter. An electron microscope study of differentiation of the molting muscles of *Rhodnius prolixus*. *Amer. J. Anat.* 124:1–30, 1969.

121. Watkins, S.C., E.P. Hoffman, H.S. Slayter, and L.M. Kunkel. Immunoelectron microscopic localization of dystrophin in myofibers. *Nature* 333:863–866, 1988.

122. Williams, P., and G. Goldspink. Changes in sarcomere length and physiological properties in immobilized muscle. *J. Anat.* 127:459–468, 1978.

123. Woods, A., M. Hook, L. Kjellan, C.G. Smith, and D.A. Rees. Relationship of heparan sulfate proteoglycans to the cytoskeleton and extracellular matrix of cultured fibroblasts. *J. Cell Biol.* 99:1743–1753, 1984.

124. Wortham, R.A. The development of the muscles and tendons in the lower leg and foot of chick embryos. *J. Morphol.* 83:105–148, 1948.

125. Zamora, A.J., and J.F. Marini. Tendon and myotendinous junction in an overloaded skeletal muscle of the rat. *Anat. Embryol.* 179:89–96, 1988.

126. Zeece, M.G., R.M. Robson, and P.J. Bechtel. Interaction of α-actinin, filamin and tropomyosin with F-actin. *Biochem. Biophys. Acta.* 581:365–370, 1979.

13
Exercise, Training and Hypertension: An Update

CHARLES M. TIPTON, Ph.D.

INTRODUCTION

The purpose of this review is to describe and integrate the findings from my 1984 review [179] with current results on the acute and chronic effects of exercise on hypertension. To help accomplish this goal, only those pre-1984 studies are included that are necessary in providing the foundation for concepts presented.

Despite advances made in recent years [77, 78], hypertension remains a disease and a risk factor [77, 78, 169]. Hypertensive populations face the prospect of shorter life spans as well as heart failure, renal failure, vascular lesions in the central nervous system, brain, or kidney, and myocardial infarctions. As noted by Horan and Mockrin [78], hypertension is "a serious public health problem."

Hypertension has been classified into two types: primary (benign, essential) and secondary [179]. More than 90% of the cases are classified as primary in nature. Secondary hypertension includes renal hypertension, pheochromocytoma, corticoid hypersecretion and primary aldosteronism [179]. Unfortunately, the responsible mechanisms for 80–90% of the individuals with primary hypertension are unknown.

In recent years, attempts have been made (Table 13.1) to reclassify the disease into more precise categories for diagnostic and treatment purposes. Most investigators do not follow these recommendations, however, when they describe and explain their study populations. In this review, the terminology of the authors is used whenever their results are discussed. Otherwise, the term *hypertension* is used to denote resting arterial systolic and diastolic pressures in adults that exceed 140 and 90 mmHg, respectively.

The exact number of individuals who are hypertensive is unknown. In 1988, it was estimated that 58 million Americans had arterial pressures that classified them as being hypertensive [85], a prevalence rate that was higher than reported earlier [179] and one that is likely to increase if more effective intervention programs are not implemented. One positive change in recent years has been the decrease in the number of persons who have experienced cerebrovascular lesions

447

TABLE 13.1
Recommended Nomenclature for Resting Arterial Blood Pressure

I. Adults

    A. Systolic (when the diastolic blood pressure in less than 90 mmHg).
      Normal = Less than 140 mmHg.
      Borderline isolated = 140–159 mmHg systolic hypertension.
      Isolated systolic hypertension = 160 mmHg and higher.

    B. Diastolic
      Normal = Less than 85 mmHg.
      High Normal = 85–89 mmHg.
      Mild Hypertension = 90–104 mmHg.
      Moderate Hypertension = 105–114 mmHg.

II. Children

Age	Significant (mmHg)	Severe (mmHg)
3–5	116/76	124/84
6–9	122/78	130/86
10–12	126/82	134/90
13–15	136/86	144/92
16–18	142/92	150/98

Recommendations for adults [85] were from a joint national committee, for children they originated from the second task force on blood pressure control [133].

or strokes [182], although the explanation for this change is not evident from existing data.

According to Horan and Lenfant [77], the primary risk factors for hypertension are genetic predisposition, age, body weight, excessive sodium intake, increased alcohol consumption, and lack of exercise. These same authorities incorporate the concept of risk factors to identify the predictors of hypertension which include ventricular mass, plasma hormonal and catecholamine concentrations, mental and emotional stressors, and the response to acute exercise. In subsequent sections, these risk factors and predictors are discussed in more detail. In the earlier analysis (179), I concluded that the most viable interventions for hypertensive populations are those that singularly or in combination result in:

1. a reduction in fat mass,
2. a reduction in caloric intake,
3. a reduction in sodium intake,
4. a reduction in plasma volume,
5. the use of antihypertensive pharmacological agents,
6. the practice of aerobic exercise.

To reduce morbidity and mortality from elevated resting arterial pressures, one or more of these interventions must be instituted. Moreover, health practitioners must realize that the possibilities of these two consequences can be reduced even if the interventions will not normalize the pressures [173, 179]. In this review, the use of pharmacological agents to normalize pressures will not be extensively discussed because the topic is sufficiently complex and comprehensive to deserve a separate review.

Implicit in any discussion of hypertension is that a change in arterial pressure will occur because of the interrelationships between pressure, resistance, and flow as defined by Poiseuille's Law [46]. The intrinsic and extrinsic factors that modify cardiac output and alter peripheral vascular resistance also will influence the resultant arterial pressure. Although autoregulatory mechanisms are important and involved in the control of blood pressure [46], this aspect will not be covered because it is seldom measured in exercising or trained populations.

THE ACUTE EFFECTS OF EXERCISE

For reference purposes, exercise is defined as the disruption of homeostasis caused by physical movements [150]. The anatomical, neural, humoral, and local factors that would influence the regulation of arterial blood pressure have been discussed previously [179] and will not be repeated here. Equally important is the awareness that dynamic exercise relates to patterns of muscle activation that requires concentric and eccentric contractions, whereas static exercise refers to conditions in which the muscles are contracting isometrically. In most complex movements, both dynamic and static components are present.

More than 70 years ago, it was suggested [16] that persons with a propensity for hypertension would exhibit an excessive response to stressors such as cold and mental tests. In recent years, acute exercise has been included as a stressor and used with children and adults as a possible predictor of hypertension [77]. Lauer and associates [103] recently reviewed this relationship in children and noted that hypertensive youngsters with elevated pressures at rest and during exercise had a greater risk in the subsequent 5 years of becoming hypertensive than their normotensive controls. In a study of 264 adolescents from Muscatine, Iowa Schieken et al. [151], found that those with the highest arterial pressures at rest had the highest pressures during both static and dynamic exercise. Molineux and Steptoe [116] tested 64 teenaged boys between the ages of 14 and 16 years of whom 24 had a positive parental history of hypertension; the authors found consistently higher systolic pressure responses in the boys with the hypertensive parents by approximately 7 mmHg during cycling at 100 to 150 watts. Dlin [29] attempted to develop guidelines on the importance of the exercise testing of normotensive and hypertensive children and young adults (ages 6–33) by summarizing the results of 16 separate studies of which five pertained to persons with elevated pressures. Not unexpectedly, he concluded that during exercise, hypertensive youths had higher systolic blood pressures than normotensive persons.

Drory and associates [30] reported on their results from 900 border-line hypertensive young males (mean age 19 years) and 336 normotensive controls of similar ages. The authors concluded that routine exercise testing should be advocated for youths classified as borderline hypertensive, although it was not evident that the pressures obtained during exercise provided more information about the disease state or the incidence of hypertension than the values obtained at rest. Because their previous results pertained to males, the 1990 Drory et al. [31] investigation is of interest. They reported the blood pressure findings from 157 borderline females with a mean age of 19 years who were compared to the results from 105 normotensive controls of similar ages. Although the pre-exercise pressures for the hypertensive females were higher than for the normotensive group, the pressure responses during exercise were similar, which indicated that the exercise test had not further differentiated or characterized the two populations.

To evaluate the role of exercise testing as a predictor of hypertension, Benbassat and Froom [8] evaluated 11 studies on this topic. Reporting on the sensitivity and the specificity of an exaggerated blood pressure response to exercise, they defined sensitivity as "among persons with hypertension, the proportion of those with a previous normotensive response to exercise" and specificity as "among persons with hypertension, the proportion of those with a previous normotensive response to exercise." Their results for sensitivity ranged from 16–60% whereas the specificity values varied from 53–95%. The prevalence of hypertension among normotensive subjects who exhibited exaggerated pressor responses was 2.1 to 3.4 times higher than among subjects with normal responses. The authors believed, however, that the value of exercise testing as a predictor of hypertension was limited because between 38 and 89% of the persons with an exaggerated response to exercise did not exhibit evidence for hypertension on subsequent follow-ups, which occurred from 0.5 to 15 years. They concluded that more research was needed and better standardization was required before exercise testing could be endorsed as a routine procedure to predict the development of hypertension.

There have been a limited number of longitudinal studies on this topic. Fixler and co-workers [43] selected 131 individuals from a population sample of 10,641 students. They were 16 years old and had resting pressures equal to or above the 95th percentile of the norms developed by the Dallas Independent School District from 25,000 students. Dynamic and static exercise tests were performed on three separate occasions and step-wise regression analyses were performed to determine the best model for predicting blood pressure levels 2 years later. The results showed that systolic blood pressure and heart rates measured during and following peak dynamic exercise and during isometric contractions (25% maximal voluntary contraction [MVC]) were not significantly correlated with the systolic blood pressures determined 2 years later on three separate occasions. At that time, 32% of the 131 students had resting pressures that remained in the 95th percentile, and 26% had consistently normal pressures. The authors concluded that exercise testing was not a valid or useful procedure to identify persons whose resting blood pressures would remain elevated for the next 2 years. They did recommend exercise testing, however, to determine whether hypertensive persons could participate in competitive athletics. Chaney and Eyman [16] also used the longitudinal approach, but with older subjects between the ages of 28 and 79 years. They identified 100 normotensive persons and measured their blood pressures at rest, during a hand grip dynamometer test, and during a graded treadmill procedure. Fourteen years later, 16% had resting pressures in excess of 140/90 mmHg. Using statistical procedures, they determined which measurements were the best predictors of hypertension and concluded that resting diastolic blood pressure was the most important single measurement because it predicted 88% of the hypertensives and 69% of the normotensives. The diastolic blood pressure measurement with the hand grip was the next most valuable, followed by the diastolic blood pressure value recorded during the treadmill run.

When step test procedures have been used to predict the future occurrence of hypertension, positive relationships have been reported. Jette and co-workers [82] used the 9-minute step test within the Canadian Aerobic Fitness Test, which is standardized for age, sex, and fitness levels, for 15,519 males and females between the ages of 7 and 69 years. Using postexercise blood pressure data (30 seconds after stopping) from subjects who were told to stop the test because their heart rates had exceeded the established criterion, they analyzed the pressure results from those subjects whose recovery values were two standard deviation above the norms established for sex, age, and stage of the test. The authors predicted that if they had tested during the previous 5 years all Canadians between the ages of 20–69, as many as 176,198 adults would now be classified as hypertensive. Tanji et al. [176] employed the step test with 26 normotensive college men and found that 11 (43%) had exaggerated systolic blood pressures immediately after exercise (>200 mmHg) and after 3 minutes of recovery (>135 mmHg). Ten years later, 10 of the 11 men had resting pressures that would classify them as hypertensive. In the same time period, only one of 15 subjects who were normotensive became hypertensive.

In all the studies cited above, the exercise procedures used would be described as an aerobic test. Spence et al. [164] have proposed the use, however, of an anaerobic threshold test to evaluate the blood pressure responses of hypertensives. Although they showed that hypertensive subjects had a disproportionate blood pressure response just after the threshold was reached, they presented no evidence that this acute exercise test would be an advantage in the prediction of the prevalence of hypertension in future years.

ACUTE EXERCISE AND HEMODYNAMIC RESPONSES

To better understand the disease process and its effects on myocardial and whole body functioning, Fagard et al. [40] studied 50 untreated hypertensive men (aged 32 years) with limited organ damage (World Health Organization [WHO] stages I and II) who exercised to exhaustion on a bicylce ergometer in a graded exercise test. They measured cardiac output, brachial and pulmonary wedge pressures, as well as $\dot{V}o_2$max, heart rate, and a-v O_2 differences and evaluated their interrelationships through regression analysis statistical approaches. They concluded that high blood pressure was associated with a reduction in maximum oxygen consumption because of a reduction in stroke volume during peak exercise conditions. When they compared the relationships between pulmonary wedge pressures and stroke volumes at different experimental conditions, they concluded that left ventricle function was impaired because of a possible reduction in left ventricle compliance. Iskandrian and Heo [80] conducted an extensive invasive study to evaluate the hemodynamic responses of three different populations to acute exercise. One subgroup was normotensive, a second subgroup was normotensive at rest but had exaggerated systolic blood pressure responses when exercising, and a third subgroup was hypertensive at rest with no evidence for coronary heart disease. The primary purpose was to compare left ventricular function during exercise as evaluated by radionuclide angiography. The exercise responses of the two normotensive populations were similar in total vascular resistance, left ventricular ejection fraction, and end-systolic volume. Cardiac index and systolic blood pressure were significantly higher in the second group, however. When they compared the responses between groups 2 and 3, the normotensive subjects with the exaggerated exercise responses had significantly higher systolic blood pressure, cardiac index, and left ventricular ejection fraction and significantly lower total vascular resistance and end-systolic volume than the hypertensive subjects. After comparing and discussing their results, the authors [80, p. 215] stated that, "based on our current knowledge, subjects with exaggerated systolic blood pressure response to exercise represent more closely a supernormal group of subjects. They should not be treated with antihypertensive agents and should be allowed to pursue a normal (and competitive) life style."

Melin et al. [115] also used radionuclide angiography to study left ventricular responses to exercise in 10 normal and nine mild hypertensive individuals with no evidence for coronary heart disease. Five of the hypertensive subjects had abnormal responses as judged by a reduction in their ejection fraction responses. After comparing the ratio between systolic blood pressure and end systolic volume, they concluded that the reduction in ejection fraction was not related to an increased afterload, rather it was due to intrinsic factors which had altered myocardial contractility. Montain and associates [117] followed the hemodynamic changes in older normotensive and hypertensive men and women during graded treadmill exercise. They noted that the older subjects had elevated pressures and higher peripheral vascular resistances at rest, whereas during submaximal exercise these same subjects had lower cardiac outputs, reduced stroke volumes, and higher total peripheral resistances than their age-matched normal controls.

Insights on the progression of hypertension and on the hemodynamics of the acute response to exercise can be gained from the study of Lund-Johansen [106]. He followed the hemodynamic changes of 48 normotensive and 93 hypertensive (WHO, stage I) of various ages over a 20-year period. The acute results were obtained when the subjects performed periods of 50, 100, and 150 watt steady-state exercise. When he compared the resting data from a cross-sectional perspective, the younger hypertensive (<40 years) had a profile of higher cardiac outputs with normal peripheral vascular resistances, unlike the older hypertensives who had higher cardiac outputs and higher peripheral vascular resistances. During exercise, the younger hypertensives exhibited lower cardiac outputs than their normotensive controls, which they attributed to a reduced stroke volume caused by decreased ventricular compliance. When he examined these same subjects after 10 years, the resting and exercise blood pressures had changed slightly for the hypertensive group while their indices for stroke volume and cardiac output had decreased by approximately 15 percent as their peripheral vascular resistance values increased by 20 percent. Because most of his hypertensive patients over 40 years of age were on medication, the investigator withdrew the drugs for 1 week before securing measurements after the 20-year period. At that time, there was an immediate increase in peripheral vascular resistance that persisted at rest and during steady-state exercise. Resting and exercise heart rate, cardiac index, and stroke index were markedly reduced, with the latter two indices being reduced by approximately 20% when compared to previous results. Lund-Johansen's data allowed for longitudinal and cross-sectional comparisons between younger and older hypertensive subjects. He reported that aging would significantly increase systolic blood pressure and peripheral vascular resistance and markedly reduce cardiac output. Moreover, he was able to follow the progression of untreated hypertension over a 20-year period and he concluded that hypertensive persons will progress from a "high output low resistance" phase to a "low output high resistance" phase with time.

Because the lifting of weights in free-exercise routine or in circuit training is being advocated as well as practiced by cardiac and hypertensive patients [44, 57, 90, 163, 168], the hemodynamic results of MacDougall et al. [108] are of interest. They obtained direct measurements of arterial blood pressure from five normotensive body builders who performed single arm curls, overhead presses, and single and double leg presses at 80–100% of their maximums. They also measured the effect of the Valsalva maneuver on blood pressure because weight lifters use this maneuver when performing. The results were striking because the peak systolic blood pressures for any of the lifts exceeded 200 mmHg (one reached 480/350 mmHg) and the Valsalva procedure alone could raise blood pressure by 60 mmHg. These investigators also demonstrated that the smaller the active muscle mass, the lower the pressure response.

POSTEXERCISE HYPOTENSION

The postexercise hypotension observed by Kral et al. [97] more than 2 decades ago has been confirmed by other investigators using humans and animals. Although the response is best associated with dynamic and aerobic exercises, it has been observed after weight lifting activities which can cause systolic blood pressures to exceed 400 mmHg [180]. Kaufman and associates [89] investigated this topic in three distinctive normotensive and hypertensive groups ranging in age from 19 to 62 years. The subjects exercised at 67% of their age-predicted heart rates for five 10-minute bouts which were followed by a 60-minute seated recovery period. Postexercise results demonstrated that all groups exhibited lower resting systolic (10–12 mmHg) and diastolic (5–7 mmHg) blood pressures with no marked differences between the normotensive and hypertensive subjects. Hagberg et al. [63] measured hemodynamic changes in older normotensive and hypertensive men and women who exercised for 45 minutes between 50–70% $\dot{V}o_2$max and followed their cardiovascular changes from 1–3 hours postexercise. Mean blood pressure and cardiac output were significantly decreased, whereas peripheral vascular resistance was increased. Stroke volume was decreased, a change attributed to a reduction in preload caused by a possible decrease in plasma volume. Paulev et al. [129] followed the recovery blood pressure values of 10 hypertensive females with a median age of 50 years (165/95 mmHg) who served as their own controls. They exercised for 20 minutes at a mean heart rate of 130 beats per minute and had blood pressures and constituents measured during a 4-hour recovery period. Compared to pre-exercise conditions, blood pressure was lowered by approximately 25 mmHg and remained reduced throughout the postexercise period. They also measured catecholamine concentrations and a select number of hormones and reported that the levels of epinephrine, dopamine, and cortisol were the most reduced during the recovery process.

The involvement of the sympathetic nervous system in postexercise hypotension was studied by Floras and coworkers [45]. They used the microneurographic technique to measure muscle sympathetic nerve traffic in three normotensive and 12 borderline hypertensive subjects. The subjects exercised on a treadmill for 45 minutes at a heart rate calculated to be 70% of their resting heart rate reserve. Mean systolic blood pressure was significantly reduced (10 mmHg), and muscle sympathetic nerve traffic was reduced by more than 40% in those subjects who exhibited lowered pressures after exercise. From other procedures used at that time (hand grip, cold pressor test, and nitro-prusside infusions), they concluded that the mechanisms that reflexly increased blood pressure and muscle sympathetic activity were not attenuated after a single bout of exercise and that inhibition of sym-pathetic nerve traffic appeared to be the most viable mechanism for postexercise hypotension.

A preliminary report on this subject was made by Boone and associates [12] who gave a bolus injection of naloxone to subjects after a 30-minute submaximal exercise bout. They observed several minutes after the injection that the postexercise blood pressures increased and ap-proached the pre-exercise levels. The authors attributed this effect to the nonspecific actions of naloxone on enkephalin receptors which augment sympathetic responses. Whether a change in central command is associated with postexercise hypotension is unknown. Secher and associates [154] conducted an interesting exercise study on the role of central command in the blood pressure and heart rate responses with the onset of exercise. Using normotensive subjects who had partial neuromuscular blockage with tubocurarine who exercised on a bicycle ergometer, they observed that with tubocurarine, blood pressure first fell before it subsequently increased. They attributed this change to the effect of central command and its effect on muscle arterioles.

The human experiments on postexercise hypotension have been confirmed and extended in animals [71, 72–74, 121, 124, 146, 159] who have been measured before and after running on treadmills [124], running in activity wheel [73, 146], or swimming [121, 146]. In addition, hypotensive results have been reported in rats where sciatic nerves were electrically stimulated [74]. From their previous and current research efforts, Thoren and associates [71, 72, 74, 159] have proposed that central and peripheral mechanisms were responsible that involved the activation of endogenous opioids, serotonergic pathways, and their receptors which inhibited the sympathetic nervous system.

Other possibilities for the occurrence of postexercise hypotension include the peptides released from atrium and ventricle [25, 49, 156], the endothelium-relaxing factors [52, 60] and the hypotensive effects of calcium on the nucleus tractus solitarious (NTS) [70].

SUMMARY

The concept that acute exercise could be used as a predictor for future hypertension is an attractive one. The evidence accumulated in recent years has not been overwhelmingly convincing, however, and routine treadmill or bicycle testing is not warranted at this time. Although the use of the step test appears to be more successful than conventional exercise tests in identifying future hypertension, the number of studies have been too few to render an objective judgement.

As noted previously [179], numerous reports have indicated that many, but not all, hypertensive subjects will exhibit exaggerated increases in blood pressure when performing acute exercise. Unfortunately, researchers have not systematically quantified what constitutes an exaggerated response in relative or absolute units. To Attina et al. [2] an exaggerated pressure response is one that exceeds 230 mmHg for systolic blood pressure and 110 mmHg for diastolic blood pressure. However, the response continues to be documented even though the mechanisms are uncertain. Possible explanations include the central and peripheral actions of catecholamines [179], autonomic dysfunction [139, 179], reduced myocardial compliance [106], impaired muscle vasodilatory capacity [13], altered baroreceptor function [6], or the local effects of endothelin [120]. Unfortunately, the evidence for any one of these possibilities has not been substantiated; hence, we are left with an observation that does not give an adequate or complete explanation.

The collective information from previous [179] and current studies involving both humans and animals indicates that postexercise hypotension is an expected physiological effect of moderate to severe exercise that can prevail for several hours. The responsible mechanisms include central inhibition of efferent sympathetic traffic with possible involvements with opioid and serotonergic pathways and receptors, the vasodilating effects of the atrial natriuretic peptides, and the actions of the factors released from the endothelium. The limited data available [64, our unpublished data] on hemodynamic changes with postexercise hypotension favors a reduction in cardiac output with peripheral vascular resistance remaining close to its pre-exercise values. Future research on the acute effects of exercise is necessary to remove the uncertainties and speculation about these mechanisms.

THE CHRONIC EFFECT OF EXERCISE

Relevant Epidemiological Studies

Although the results of acute exercise have importance in the diagnosis and management of hypertension, chronic exercise will likely have more impact on the prevention and management aspects of the disease. Insights can be obtained from both epidemiological and longitudinal investigations.

The basic approach in epidemiological studies is to establish a relationship between an index of physical fitness and the presence of the future development of hypertension. In children and young adolescents, an inverse relationship between physical activity and resting blood pressure has not been well established. Fraser and co-workers [48] compared fitness scores from a treadmill test with the blood pressure results of 270 caucasian boys and girls between the ages of 7 and 17 years and reported that both systolic and diastolic pressures were lower in the individuals who had above average fitness scores. In addition, higher blood pressure levels were associated with lower fitness scores. Panico et al. [128] studied this relationship in 1341 school children in Naples, Italy aged 7 to 14 years; more than 700 boys and almost 600 girls participated in the study. The Harvard Step Test was used to denote physical fitness. They found that resting systolic blood pressure was more strongly associated with physical fitness than diastolic blood pressure and that this relationship was significant in the boys and was independent of age, height, and body mass. These trends were not found in the girls. It was interesting to observe that the systolic pressure difference between the lowest and the highest fitness group was 7 mmHg. Hofmann et al. [75] examined the association between physical fitness scores and resting blood pressure in 2061 fourth grade students in the New York City area over one year. A modified Harvard Step Test was used to classify students into various fitness categories. As a group, the children with the lowest fitness scores had the highest resting systolic and diastolic pressures. Moreover, the authors observed that the students who exhibited a decrease in physical fitness over a 1-year period had the highest increases in resting pressures. Fripp and associates [50] selected 37 students from 289 tenth graders to evaluate the relationships between fitness levels, as determined from the Cooper run-walk test, and the risk factors for atherosclerosis which include high blood pressure. With respect to hypertension, their statistical analysis revealed that the students assigned a low fitness score had the highest systolic and diastolic blood pressures. As a group, they also had the highest body mass index value. The mean difference between the low and the moderately fit group for both systolic and diastolic blood pressure was approximately 9 mmHg.

Because race is an important consideration in the etiology of hypertension, the Harshfield et al. [67] investigation is of interest. They evaluated the fitness levels of a biracial normotensive population of 80 boys and 95 girls between the ages of 10 and 18 years using the results of a $\dot{V}O_2$max text. Subsequently, the adolescents were assigned by sex and race into "less fit" and "more fit" categories. In addition, ambulatory blood pressure measurements were secured to examine the effects of day, night, and diurnal rhythms. Using this approach, they found that race and fitness were important considerations to explain blood pressure differences between populations. For example, there were no significant differences between "less fit" and "more fit" white boys and girls in their resting blood pressures whether awake or asleep. This was not the situation for black adolescents. Specifically, less fit black males had significantly higher systolic blood pressures than the more fit subjects whether awake or asleep. Moreover, this same pattern existed when the "less fit" black students were compared with the "less fit" white subjects; namely, the blacks had significantly higher pressures under any condition. These same differences prevailed when similar comparisons were made with "less fit" and "more fit" black females. Because black Americans between the ages of 18 and 74 have a prevalence of essential hypertension that is 1.4 times higher than found for white Americans [85], these results have important implications for the managment of hypertension in black populations.

Earlier, Kral et al. [97] published results that indicated that 1% or less of the athletes studied had blood pressures in excess of 160/100 mmHg. In the age group evaluated, they anticipated an incidence percentage between 5 and 10%. Lehmann and Keul [104] presented the blood pressure results from 810 sportsmen who included 125 cyclists, 109 "game players," 29 swimmers, and 25 weight-lifters between the ages of 14–69 years. After statistical calculations and adjustments, they concluded that the incidence of borderline hypertension (11%) and hypertension (5%) was half of what would be expected for this age group. The two populations that exhibited the highest resting blood pressures were the swimmers and the weight lifters.

One of the most impressive and quoted epidemiological investigations of the last decade is by Paffenbarger et al. [126]. Their research, discussed previously [179], reported on the resting blood pressure findings from approximately 15,000 males who were alumni from Harvard University. The most interesting conclusion for this review was that alumni who did not participate in "vigorous" athletics as students had a greater risk (35%) to be hypertensive than those who did.

An equally important contribution was the study by Blair et al. [10] at the Cooper Clinic in Dallas, Texas. They used a treadmill and heart rate test to assess and assign fitness scores to more than 6,000 normotensive persons aged 20–65 years, 1219 of whom were females. In a follow-up period ranging from 1–12 years (median was four years), 240 new cases of hypertension were identified. After adjusting for age, sex, baseline values, and body mass, the individuals assigned low fitness scores had a relative risk of 1.52 for becoming hypertensive than those with high fitness ratings. The racial and socioeconomic characteristics of the population studied were not provided.

A recent survey by Darga et al. [24] on this subject involved 1269 members of the American Medical Joggers Association and 683 members of the American Medical Association who were nonrunners. In contrast, the joggers averaged approximately 10 miles per week. Attempts were made to equate the groups with regard to age, sex, socioeconomic status, and professional speciality. The authors reported that normal resting blood pressures were present in 93% of the joggers and 81% of the nonrunners. One additional, interesting statistic was that approximately five times as many nonrunners as runners had been or were taking antihypertensive medication.

Stamler and her numerous coworkers [165] recently published their results of a 5-year nutritional-hygienic trial with 102 subjects in an intervention group and 99 in a monitored control group. The ages were between 30–40 years, and 86% of the subjects in both groups were males. Selection into the study was determined by the person's diastolic blood pressure results (85–89 mmHg) or by diastolic blood pressures (80–84 mmHg) and being between 10–49% over desirable weight. At the end of the trial, the changes in resting pressures ranged from 2–4 mmHg, which, although not excessive, were statistically significant. According to the authors, the incidence of hypertension was 9% in the intervention and 19% in the control group. Although an increase in daily physical activity was cited as one of the reasons for the change, little objective data supported this view. During this time (5 years) the intervention group experienced a 2.7 kg loss in weight, a 25% reduction in sodium intake, and a 30% reduction in alcohol consumption; therefore, it is likely that these changes were more important than chronic exercise in explaining the difference in the incidence of hypertension.

Buck and Donner [14] examined the evidence on the prevalence of hypertension in occupations that required isometric contractions at the work site. Companies were selected from the Canadian Dictionary of Occupations and involved 4,273 individuals. They were evaluated on age, body mass index, social class, alcohol consumption, and whether they performed either low or high amounts of daily isometric exercise. The authors concluded that the daily performance of isometric activity prevented rather than induced hypertension. This unexpected finding emphasized the need for medical authorities to re-examine the issue of the chronic effects of isometric exercise on resting blood pressure. This topic is discussed in more detail in the section on longitudinal studies.

Summary

The collective effect of the epidemiological studies reviewed before and after 1984 provides a solid foundation for the concept that chronic exercise is beneficial for improving physical fitness levels that will be associated with lower resting blood pressures in younger and older populations. There does not appear a need for more studies that show the majority of sportsmen will have lower resting pressures than nonsportsmen as this same conclusion was reached by Steinhaus in his classic review of 1933 [167]. The populations that could benefit from these investigations in the future would be females, minorities and children.

LONGITUDINAL STUDIES

Summarized in Tables 13.2–13.5 are 35 human and 25 animal longitudinal studies on the chronic effects of exercise. With limited exceptions, most were conducted in 1980 and only a few were discussed in detail in the 1984 review [179]. In the sections that follow, these results are integrated with previous investigations and discussed with a concern for their biological significance, responsible mechanisms, and potential for future studies. Unknown to most, investigations were initiated in 1974 in Japan by Shindo et al. [158] on the relationship between the intensity of exercise and the change in resting blood pressure. Emerging from this early study have been investigations [92, 95, 188] that have used an exercise intensity between 40–70% $\dot{V}o_2$max, with most following a level of between 50–60%. It is convenient, therefore, to speculate that the longitudinal investigations and their subgroups in Tables 13.2 and 13.3, which did not report a significant lowering effect or trend with aerobic training [55, 84, 145], occurred because the exercise intensities being prescribed were too high for the hypertensive subjects who participated in the studies. In the investigation reported by Roman and associates [145] and shown in Table 13.2, they increased the intensity of exercise to be higher than 70% of the maximum heart rate and no longer observed the 20/16 mmHg declines in resting systolic and diastolic blood pressures, respectively, that had been observed with the prescription of low-intensity exercise.

This point is noteworthy because most of the subjects had been previously trained at a lower intensity. Insights on this topic can be obtained from the Tipton et al. [180] spontaneously hypertensive rats (SHR) study in which rats were exercised-trained at an intensity exceeding 90% $\dot{V}o_2$max. In these animals, there was no evidence of a blood pressure-lowering effect even though other indices of a training effect were reported. Moreover, when the training intensity was reduced to 40–70% $\dot{V}o_2$max, the trained rats had resting pressures that were

10–15 mmHg lower than their controls. When other investigators [69, 100, 187] exercised their hypertensive rats on treadmills or had rats in activity wheels running at speeds suggesting an intensity higher than 80% $\dot{V}o_2$max, the trained rats also exhibited higher, rather than lower, pressures than the nontrained animals. Consequently, one of the reasons why aerobic exercise training per se is not universally associated with lowered resting pressures could be that the exercise intensity being prescribed has been too high. There are other considerations such as duration. Exercise designs that require animals to exercise from 3–6 hours per day are not likely to enhance our understanding of the mechanisms responsible for a lower resting blood pressure with training.

It is surprising that none of the longitudinal studies listed in Tables 13.2 and 13.3 used swimming as the exercise modality. In Lehmann and Keul's [104] cross-sectional study, swimmers and weight lifters had higher resting pressures than the other sportsmen, a finding similar to that reported by Cureton et al. for swimmers at the Rome Olympics [23, 179]. One explanation for this observation was that the swimmers were "overtrained." When highly conditioned, normotensive collegiate swimmers participated in a 10-day program designed to double the daily distance covered while maintaining the intensity level of 95% $\dot{V}o_2$max [94], resting heart rates and systolic blood pressures did not change significantly, whereas resting diastolic blood pressure exhibited an increase of approximately 6 mmHg after 8 days of intense training. On the other hand, the majority of swimming studies with hypertensive rats show significant reductions in pressures when the animals were exercised for 180 minutes or less per day. Careful observational studies by Sturek and coworkers [172] with swimming hypertensive rats indicated the swimmers spent more than 50% of their time being submerged. In addition, after 30 minutes of swimming, they exhibited signs of hypoxia, hypercapnia, acidosis, and diving bradycardia. Because blood gas measurements in running hypertensive rats did not demonstrate such significant changes [53, 172], it was speculated that the reductions in resting pressure associated with swimming were primarily a result of changes in chemoreceptor mechanisms, which was not the situation with running rats. When the cardiovascular differences between running and swimming were studied in rats, Geenan et al. [53] concluded that swimming had more of sympathoadrenal effect on the myocardium than running. Clearly, more research on this topic is needed because these two exercise modalities will continue to be used in hypertension research.

Although Kasch and coworkers [88] have impressive longitudinal results on the benefits of 20 years of endurance training (Table 13.2), the results of Nomura et al. [122], Jennings et al. [81], Urata et al. [188], and Roman et al. [145] suggested that the blood pressure-lowering effects associated with endurance training would likely occur after 3

TABLE 13.2
Recent Longitudinal Studies on the Effects of Aerobic Training on the Resting Blood Pressures of Humans

Investigator	Ref	Group	Duration of Study (weeks)	N	Age (yrs)	Sex	Mode of Training	Frequency (weeks)	Session Duration (min)	Intensity
Rogers et al.	144	E-H	1	9	53	M	Combinations	6	56	68% $\dot{V}O_2$ max 50% HR max
Weber et al.	193	E-H	4	70	60–80	M,F	Walking, jogging	15	140	70–80% predicted HR
Tanabe et al.	175	E-H	10	13	51	M	Cycle ergometer	3	70	50% $\dot{V}O_2$ max
		E-H	10	11	51	F	Cycle ergometer	3	70	50% $\dot{V}O_2$ max
Kiyonaga et al.	96	E-H	10	12	46	M,F	Cycle ergometer	3	60	50% $\dot{V}O_2$ max
Westheim et al.	196	E-H	12	34	41	M,F	Combinations	3	Not listed	70% work
Roman et al.	145	E-H	12	27	NA	F	Combinations	3	30	70% HR max
Cade et al.	15	E-H	12	58	39	M,F	Walking	3	40	1 mile/20 min
		E-HM	12	23	44	M,F	Walking	3	40	1 mile/20 min
		E-HM	12	16	NA	M,F	Walking	3	40	1 mile/20 min
		E-HM	12	7	35	M,F	Walking	3	40	1 mile/20 min
		E-HD	12	15	NA	NA	Detrained			
Adranaga et al.	1	C-N+H	12	26	34	M				70–85% of
		E-N+H	12	34	34	M	Combinations	3 to 5	30–45	Karvonen's Formula
Baglivo et al.	4	C-H	12	17	51	M,F				
		E-H	12	15	49	M,F	Combinations	3	50	NA
Jo et al.	83	E-N	12	14	42	M	Combinations	2	60	50% $\dot{V}O_2$ max
		E-H	12	14	43	M	Combinations	2	60	50% $\dot{V}O_2$ max
Van Hoof et al.	189	E-N	16	26			Combinations	3	60	Not stated
Duncan et al.	34	C-H	16	12	21–37	M				
		E-H	16	44	21–37	M	Walking & jogging	3	60	70–80% HR max
		E-HNA	16	26	21–37	M	Walking & jogging	3	60	70–80% HR max
		E-HHA	16	18	21–37	M	Walking & jogging	3	60	70–80% HR max
Kukkonen et al.	99	C-N	16	17	35–50	M				
		E-N	16	17	35–50	M	Cycle ergometer	3	50	66% of HR max
		C-H	16	12	35–50	M				
		E-H	16	13	35–50	M	Cycle ergometer	3	50	66% of HR max
Kiyonaga et al.	96	E-H	20	9	46	M,F	Cycle ergometer	3	60	50% $\dot{V}O_2$ max
Cleroux et al.	17	C	20	7	33	M,F				
		E-	20	7	37	M,F	Cycle ergometer	3	20–45	60% $\dot{V}O_2$ max
		E	20	5	32	M	Jogging	3	20–45	60% $\dot{V}O_2$ max
Painter et al.	127	C-N	24	6	42	M,F				
		E-H	24	13	42	M,F	Cycle ergometer	3 to 4	30–45	75–85% $\dot{V}O_2$ max
Attina et al.	2	E-H	52	14	36	M	Combinations	3	NA	NA
		E-H	52	12	36	M	Combinations	3	NA	NA
Roman et al.	145	E-HD	52	24	NA	F	Combinations	3	NA	
Gleichmann et al.	56	E-H	56	29	43–73	NA	Combinations	Not listed	180–210 min/wk	NA
Kasch et al.	88	E-N	1040	15	45–60	M	Combinations	4	45–61	77–84% HR

Table organized according to the duration of the study, means and standard deviations listed, * denotes difference listed in text that was statistically significant; C = Control; E = Exercised; N = Normotensive; H = Hypertensive; HD = Hypertensive detrained; HM = Hypertensive on medication; E-HNA = Exercised hypertensive who was normal adrenergic; E-HHA = Exercised hypertensive who was hyper adrenergic; NA = Not available.

Initial Measurements			Final Measurements			
SBP (mmHg)	*MBP* (mmHg)	*DBP* (mmHg)	*SBP* (mmHg)	*MBP* (mmHg)	*DBP* (mmHg)	*Comments*
No change reported for either SBP or DBP						Only exercise BP changed
144 ± 20		77 ± 11	132 ± 25*		73 ± 11	Had physician- supervised exercises; fat, carbohydrate, and fiber changed in diet; no controls
147 ± 15	115 ± 9	99 ± 9	139 ± 18*	110 ± 115*	95 ± 15	
156 ± 15	117 ± 9	98 ± 9	139 ± 15*	107 ± 12*	91 ± 12	
153 ± 13	120 ± 6	103 ± 3	139 ± 16*	109 ± 10*	94 ± 11*	
182 ± 16		113 ± 10	161 ± 18*		97 ± 4* 95 ± 7*	Most were E-H subjects; When detrained for 12 weeks the SBP and DBP increased by 18 and 16 mmHg
150 ± 6		95 ± 3	135 ± 6*		83 ± 4*	Data extrapolated from figures and calculated from tables
165 ± 14		110 ± 9	135 ± 10*		89 ± 7*	
163 ± 10	126 ± 14	108 ± 4	131 ± 14*	98 ± 11*	84 ± 10*	
172 ± 14	136 ± 8	114 ± 5	141 ± 26*	111 ± 22*	95 ± 20*	
130 ± 9		80 ± 7	147 ± 9*			
130 ± 11		85 ± 11	No change reported; NA			Assigned both normotensive and hypertensive subjects into either control or exercise groups, no evidence for a BP effect
127 ± 11		85 ± 11	No change reported; NA			
155 ± 4		99 ± 2	142 ± 6		101 ± 2	Training associated with decrease in LV mass
155 ± 10		101 ± 3	136 ± 8*		87 ± 7*	
121 ± 9		76 ± 6	120 ± 9		72 ± 4*	
147 ± 17		98 ± 7	136 ± 5*		90 ± 5*	
131 ± 11		89 ± 8	129 ± 13		84 ± 9	Subjects assigned to 2 groups, served as their own controls, only values recorded during day were changed because night and 24 hour measurements were not significant
145 ± 5		93 ± 3	139 ± 7		96 ±	Assigned 44 E-H into normoadrenergic or hyperadrenergic on plasma catecholamine concentration; mmHg, Reductions reflect this classification
148 ± 6		94 ± 6	134 ± 6		87 ± 4*	
			− 10		− 6	
			− 15		− 8	
136 ± 12		94 ± 8	128 ± 8*		83 ± 8*	Control normotensive subjects exhibited significant decreases
134 ± 16		93 ± 12	130 ± 12		83 ± 4*	
142 ±		104 ± 7	138 ± 10		96 ± 7	
142 ± 10		103 ± 7	146 ± 14		99 ± 7	
157 ± 12	122 ± 6	104 ± 3	136 ± 12*	105 ± 9*	90 ± 9	Most were studied at 10 weeks
130 ±		90 ±	145 ±		90 ±	Standing measurements listed; supine data did not exhibit these trends
145 ±		98 ±	135 ± *		90 ± *	
140 ±		95 ±	135 ±		90 ±	
124 ± 15			124 ± 17			Renal patients on hemodialysis; At 90 days, SBP of E-H group was 143 ± 27 mmHg
152 ± 34			138 ± 29*			
141 ± 10		87 ± 6	136 ± 12*		80 ± 8*	Medication decreased in 10% and increased in 26% of subjects
143 ± 8		87 ± 5	144 ± 14		92 ± 6	
179 ± 22		113 ± 9	159 ± 12*		95 ± 7	Same subjects as above
153 ± 18		93 ± 11	139 ± 17*		87 ± 11*	Subjects in program 5–28 months; medication decreased in 10% and increased in 26%
120		79	120		77	Data on sedentary subjects not listed

TABLE 13.3
The Influence of Chronic Exercise on Select Hemodynamic Measurements

Investigator	Ref	Group	N	Duration of Study (weeks)	Invasive	Sex	Age (yrs)	Mode of Training	Frequency (weeks)	Exer. Duration (min)	Intensity	Before SBP (mmHg)	Before MBP (mmHg)
Nomura et al.	122	E-H	7	3	Partially	M	25–52	Cycle ergometer	20	9	75% V̇O₂ max	141 ± 6	
		E-H	14	3		M,F	25–52	Cycle ergometer	20	9	75% V̇O₂ max	141 ± 18	
Ressel et al.	140	E-H	10	4	Yes	M	38–53	Cycle ergometer	5	36	70% V̇O₂ max	182 ± 15	130 ± 9
Jennings et al.	81	C	12	4	No	M,F	19–27	Below sedentary				117	86
		C	12	4	No	M,F	19–27	Sedentary				112	86
		E	12	4	No	M,F	19–27	Cycle ergometer	3	40	60–70% W max		
		E	12	4	No	M,F	19–27	Cycle ergometer	7	40	120–150 HR		
Sannerstedt et al.	148	E-H	5	6	Yes	M	26–38	Cycle ergometer	3	60	150–160 HR		108 ± 6
Urata et al.	188	C-H	10	10	Partially	M,F	32–60				40–60% V̇O₂ max	154 ± 12	118 ± 12
		E-H	10	10		M,F	32–60	Cycle ergometer	3	65	Lactate threshold	153 ± 12	121 ± 9
Kinoshita et al.	92	E-R	12	10	No	M,F	32–60	Cycle ergometer	3	70	40–60% V̇O₂ max	153 ± 15	116 ± 9
		E-NR	9	10	No	M,F	32–60	Cycle ergometer	3	70	40–60% V̇O₂ max	157 ± 7	122 ± 11
Johnson & Grover	84	E-H	4	10	Yes	NA	NA	Treadmill	3	35	160 HR	188	134
DePlaen & Detry	28	C-H	4	12	Yes	M,F	47					158 ± 22	
		E-H	5	12		M,F	47	Combinations	3	60	50–70% V̇O₂ max	162 ± 26	128 ± 17
Gilders et al.	55	C		16		M,F	43					123 ± 18	93 ± 9
		E-N	10	16	No	M,F	43	Cycle ergometer	3	30	80% HR max	114 ± 6	90 ± 6
		E-H	7	16	No	M,F	43	Cycle ergometer	3	30	80% HR max	125 ± 7	100 ± 2
Hagberg et al.	62	C		20	No	M,F	17					136 ± 4	
		E		20	No	M,F	16	PE classes, jogging	5	30–40	70–80% V̇O₂ max	137 ± 5	
Reiling et al.	137	C	12	24	No	M,F	61					131 ± 7	100 ± 3
		E	14	24	No	M,F	61	Combinations	3,4	30–50	50% HR max	137 ± 13	103 ± 4
Hanson & Nedde	65	E	5	28	Yes	M	30–54	Combinations	3	60	NA	120	108
Hagberg et al.	64	C	11	37	No	M,F	64					152 ± 9	110 ± 7
		E	11	37	No	M,F	65	Combinations	3	60	50% V̇O₂ max	158 ± 18	113 ± 11
		E	11	37	No	M,F	64	Combinations	3	60	70–85% V̇O₂ max	160 ± 21	120 ± 13
Reiling et al.	138	C	12	52	No	M,F	61					131 ± 7	100 ± 3
		E	14	52	No	M,F	61	Combinations	3,4	30–50	50% HR max	137 ± 1	103 ± 4

Table organized according to the duration of the study, means and standard deviations listed; * denotes a text designated statistical difference; E = Exercised; C = Nonexercised controls; H = Hypertensive; R = Responders; NR = Nonresponders; partially refers to the use of the ear lobe densiometer to measure cardiac output (Q); CI = Cardiac index; TPR = Total peripheral resistance; HR = Heart rate.

	Training			After Training					
DBP (mmHg)	*Q or CI units*	*TPR Units*	*SBP (mmHg)*	*MBP (mmHg)*	*DBP (mmHg)*	*Q or CI Units*	*TPR units*		*Comments*
98±10	3.4±1.3	2800±280	135±7	104	89±7	3.0±.3	2650±360		Subjects' diet contained 170 mEq NaCl/day;
93±14	3.2±2.6	3000±600	130±13*	93	85±8*	3.0±.6	2800±160		E-H subjects consumed a diet containing 34 mEq of NaCl/day
99±5	3.0±.4			129±9	98±4	2.7±.4	33		
74	3.5	24	117	86	74	3.5*	24		Latin square statistical design; values extrapolated from figures
74	3.2	27	112	86	74	3.2	27		
			105*	82*	70	3.8*	22*		
			103*	78*	70	3.9*	21*		
	9.4±.2	15±7		107±10		8.0±.2	16±6		
97±6	4.0±.7	19±6	158	121	99	3.5±.9	22±6		Blood and plasma volume were significantly decreased in exercise group; plasma norepinephrine also was significantly decreased
103±12	3.7±.9	22±6	144±15*	113±15*	98±15	3.3±.6	23±6		
97±6	4.0±.7	19±4	134±12*	102±9*	85±6*	2.8±.5	20±5		Nonresponders were labelled because they did not change 10 mmHg in MBP
105±11	3.2±.6	26±6	150±11*	119±14	105±14	2.8±.5	26±5		
103	5.1	2136	195	136	105	6	1924		
113±12			154±12		107±3				No Q or TPR data reported for controls
104±14	5.5±.7	1841±135	158±29	124±18	104±14	4.6±1.0	2149±98*		
81±6			114±8	90±6	79±6				Only 24-hour data listed, no day or night trends; 8 weeks of deconditioning had no significant effect on resting values
79±6	4.8±1.6	1796±837	114±6	93±6	82±6	4.6±1.5	1759±591		
88±5	4.6±1.0	1862±580	121±7	98±5	87±5	5.0±1.4	1799±590		
75±8	4.0±.8	562±164	138±8		73±6	3.9±.8	581±212		After 9 months of inactivity, SBP and DBP increased 10/3 mmHg, respectively
78±10	4.3±1.0	551±155							
89±3			136±11	100±3	91±3	3.3±0.4	33±12		Results were from 24-hour data; night results exhibited no significant intragroup differences; hemodynamic results from a sitting position
89±4			132±14*	101±4*	88±4	3.3±0.4*	32±6		
87	7	16	135	95	75	5.8	16.4		
90±7	4.7±.8	1957±417	151±11	110±6	89±4	5.4±1.8	1805±623		
90±10	4.2±1.0	2263±546	151±7	108±9*	87±7	3.7±0.9*	2516±844		
100±10	4.5±1.0	2223±546	154±16	112±9*	91±7*	4.7±0.8	1944±325*		
89±3	3.4±1.0	34±11	131±9	100±9	40±7	3.3±0.6	33±10		Results were from 24-hour data, night results exhibited no significant intragroup differences; hemodynamic results were from a sitting position
88±4	4.0±1.1	29±9	131±9*	99±4*	88±4	3.4±0.7*	31±6		

TABLE 13.4
Recent Longitudinal Studies on the Effect of Training on the Resting Blood Pressure of Rats

Investigator	Ref	Group	Duration of Study (weeks)	N	Initial Age (weeks)	Sex	Mode of Training	Frequency (weeks)	Duration Day (min)	Intensity	Direct or Indirect	Initial SBP (mmHg)	Initial MBP (mmHg)	Final SBP (mmHg)	Final MBP (mmHg)	Comments
A. Normotensive Rats																
Ghaemma-ghami et al.	54	C-LL	5	9	5	F	Swim	5	360		I	95		118		
		E-LL	5	9	5	F					NA	—	97		125	
		C-NL	5	9	5	F					I	103		122		
		E-NL	5	9	5	F				NA	I	94		120		
Rakusan et al.	135	C-WKY	6	14	6	F	Swim	5	120	NA	D				110 ± 7	
		E-WKY	6	14	6	F					D				109 ± 7	
Geenen et al.	53	C	8	8	15	F	Run	10	60	20 m.min^{-1} 0 grade	D		NA		115 ± 2 to 14	Data extrapolated from figures; no evaluation of statistical significance
		E	8	8	15	F	Run	10	60	NA	D		140 ± 7		114 ± 2 to 14	
		E	8	7	15	F	Swim		60		D		143 ± 4		113 ± 2 to 14	
Marcus & Tipton	110	C	12	11	6	M	Run	4 to 6	45–75	50–70% $\dot{V}O_2$ max	I	112 ± 5		132 ± 4		
		E	12	9	6	M					I	114 ± 4		132 ± 3		
Tipton et al.	184	C-SR	12	9	6	F	Run	5	55	40–70% $\dot{V}O_2$ max	I	108 ± 17		117 ± 11		
		E-SR	12	9	6	F					I	100 ± 11		115 ± 11		
Tomanek et al.	187	C-WKY	12	8	16	M	Run	5	80	70–90% $\dot{V}O_2$ max	D	NA		133 ± 25		
		C-WKY	12	4	16	M					D	NA		137 ± 16		
Savage et al.	149	C	12	20	7	M	Run	5	115	26.4 m.min^{-1} on 5% grade	D	NA	NA		121 ± 27	Animals on normal NaCl diet; no initial measurement from femoral artery; after 4 weeks of training, C = 100 ± 11, **E = 89 ± 6* mmHg**
		E	12	19	7	M					D	NA	NA		$97 \pm 7^*$	
Edwards et al.	36	C	16	17	4	M	Run	5	70	5–70% $\dot{V}O_2$ max	I	92 ± 24		133 ± 20		
		E	16	14	4	M					I	94 ± 6		125 ± 20		
		C-WKY	16	7	4	M	Run	5	60	40–60% $\dot{V}O_2$ max	I	110 ± 7		143 ± 17		
		E-WKY	16	7	4	M					I	113 ± 9		148 ± 10		

Reference		Group				Sex	Type			Intensity					Comments
Lutgemeier et al.	107	C-WKY	22	20	1.5	M	Swim	12	90	NA	I	NA		132 ± 20	Used ether to measure resting BP; data extrapolated from figure
		E-WKY	22	20	1.5							NA		125 ± 20	
B. Normotensive Rats on High Fat Diet															
Drummond et al.	32	C	16	9	4	M	Run	5	60	60–90% $\dot{V}O_2$ max	I	156 ± 8		188 ± 11	Differences existed by 8 weeks, diet consisted of 40% fat, 45% sucrose and 15% protein
		C-WM	16	8	4	M					I	155 ± 8		158 ± 11*	
		E	16	6	4	M					I	154 ± 7		154 ± 9*	
C. Normotensive Rats Made Hypertensive by Renal Artery Constriction (two kidney–1 clip)															
Rakusan et al.	135	C	6	14	6	F	Swim	5	120	NA	D	NA		177 ± 18	Swimming did not improve the reduced capillarization with hypertension
		E	6	14	6	F					D	NA		172 ± 25	
Marcus & Tipton	110	C-MOD	8	19	6	M	Run	5	75	50–70% $\dot{V}O_2$ max	I	130 ± 6		160 ± 4	Swimming with severely constricted arteries decreased myocardial capillarization
		E-MOD	8	19	6	M	Run					135 ± 7		158 ± 4	
		C-SEV	12	9	6	M	Run	5	75	50–70% $\dot{V}O_2$ max	I	170 ± 35		189 ± 24*	
		E-SEV	12	11	6	M	Run					170 ± 32		210 ± 19	
Hoffman et al.	73	C	6	8	9	M	Vol. wheel	7	NA	NA	I	211 ± 18		200 ± 14	Data extrapolated from figures; unusual for younger SHR rats to have higher initial means than older rats
		E-YNG	6	8	9	M	Vol. wheel	7			I	196 ± 24		173 ± 10*	
		C	6	10	13	M	Vol. wheel				I	180 ± 22		200 ± ?	
		E-OLD	6	10	13	M	Vol. wheel				I	185 ± 11		213 ± ?	
D. Genetic Borderline Hypertensive Rats															
Lutgemeier et al.	107	C	21	12	1.5	M	Swim	12	90	NA	I	NA		167 ± 20	Used ether measure blood pressure; data evaluated from figure
		E	21	12	1.5	M	Swim				I	NA		147 ± 20*	
E. Genetic Borderline Hypertensive Rats Receiving Electrical Shocks															
Cox et al.	21	C	12	7	11	M	Swim	7	120	NA	D	160 ± 15	NA	98 ± 10	No initial pressures taken; swim-trained were significantly lower than the two control groups; they also had lower plasma norepinephrine concentrations
		C-S	12	8	11	M	Swim				D	180 ± 8	NA	118 ± 8	
		E	12	8	11	M	Swim				D	166 ± 11	NA	108 ± 5	

(continued)

TABLE 13.4 *(continued)*

Investigator	Ref	Group	Duration of Study (weeks)	N	Initial Age (weeks)	Sex	Mode of Training	Frequency (weeks)	Duration Day (min)	Intensity	Direct or Indirect	Initial Measurements SBP (mmHg)	Initial Measurements MBP (mmHg)	Final Measurements SBP (mmHg)	Final Measurements MBP (mmHg)	Comments
F. Genetic Hypertensive Rats (SHR, LH)																
Noma et al.	121	C	3	9	16	M	Swim	5	180	NA	I	193 ± 12		225 ± 16		Swam twice a day for 90 min/session; data extrapolated from figures
		E	3	9	16	M	Swim	5	180	NA	I	193 ± 16		181 ± 12		
		C	3	8	44	M	Swim	5	180	NA	I	225 ± 12		217 ± 12		
		E	3	8	44	M	Swim	5	180	NA	I	217 ± 25		173 ± 4*		
Ghaemma-ghami et al.	54	C	5	9	5	F	Swim	5	360	NA	I	122		144		Lipoproteins were reduced in the trained
		E	5	9	5	F	Swim	5	360	NA	I	117		144		
Higuchi et al.	69	C	8	10	10	M	Vol. wheel	7	NA	NA	I	177 ± 5		198 ± 16		Rats running on treadmill exhibited largest changes in resting pressures
		E	8	10	10	M	Vol. wheel	5	60	26.8 m.min-1 on 0% grade	I	176 ± 5		202 ± 13		
		E	8	10	10	M	Run				I	172 ± 7		206 ± 11		
Sharma et al.	155	C	9	25	4	M	Swim	7	180	NA	I			198 ± 10		Swam twice daily, data extrapolated from figures
		E	9	25	4	M	Swim	7	180	NA	I			198 ± 10		
Overton et al.	125	C	11	8	5	F	Vol. wheel	7	NA	80–90% HR max	I	110 ± 3		185 ± 11		
		E	11	8	5	F	Vol. wheel	7	NA	80–90% HR max	I	105 ± 4		165 ± 15*		
Tomanek et al.	187	C	12	13	16	M	Run	5	80	70–90% $\dot{V}O_2$ max	D	NA		187 ± 24*		Training did not reverse the 12% decrease in myocardial capillarity
		E	12	11	16	M	Run	5	80	70–90% $\dot{V}O_2$ max	D	NA		201 ± 28		
Edwards & Tipton	35	C	16	18	4	M	Swim	5	60	2% BW on tail	I	140 ± 12		218 ± 21		
		E	16	9	4	M	Swim	5	60	2% BW on tail	I	137 ± 8		196 ± 28*		
		E	16	18	4	M	Run	5	60	40–60% $\dot{V}O_2$ max	I	137 ± 12		204 ± 21*		
Lutgemeier et al.	107	C	21	12	1.5	M	Swim	12	90	NA	D	NA		194 ± 3		Used ether to secure BP; data extrapolated from figures
		E	21	12	1.5	M	Swim	12	90	NA	D	NA		180 ± 5*		
G. Genetic Hypertensive Rats Receiving Either a High or Low Calcium Diet																
Drummond et al.	33	C-low	13	10	5	M	Run	5	60	40–70% $\dot{V}O_2$ max	I	157 ± 5		238 ± 20		Low Ca^{2+} diet contained 0.6% whereas the high diet had 2.5%; Ca^{2+}/PO_4 ratio maintained at 3:2
		E-low	13	8	5	M	Run	5	60	40–70% $\dot{V}O_2$ max	I	159 ± 7		222 ± 14*		
		C-High	13	10	5	M	Run	5	60		I	157 ± 6		238 ± 19		
		E-High	13	8	5	M	Run	5	60		I	157 ± 6		238 ± 19		

H. Genetic Hypertensive Rats that are Self Sensitive Consuming a High Salt Diet

Study	Dur.	Group	n			Sex	Exercise	#	Intensity	Code				Comments
Savage et al.	149	C	12	19	7	M	Run	115	26.4 m·min-1 on	D	NA	NA	166 ± 24	Animals consumed 1.9% sodium in chow, data extrapolated from figures
		E	12	18	9	M				D			134 ± 16*	
Tipton et al.	184	C	12	8	6	F	Run	55	40–70% V̇O₂ max	I	124 ± 11	NA	205 ± 24	Animals consumed 8.0% sodium diet, had similar sodium excretions and blood volume
		E	12	8	6	F				I	118 ± 18		206 ± 22	

I. Genetic Hypertensive Rats that are Stroke Prone

Study	Dur.	Group	n			Sex	Exercise	#	Intensity	Code				Comments
Overton et al.	125	C	5	6	4	F	Vol. wheel	>50 session	65–74 m·min-1. session-1	I	120 ± 16	NA	178 ± 16	Animals consumed high salt diet and consumed 1% NaCl drinking solution; life span was less than 100 days
		E-YNG	5	8	4	F				I	124 ± 16		198 ± 24*	
Tipton et al.	182	C	33	10	19	M,F	Run	55	40–70% V̇O₂ max	I	160 ± 13	NA	238 ± 6	Trained were significantly lower after 4 weeks; thereafter pressures increased and animals died
		E-OLD	33	12	19	M,F				I	164 ± 15		257 ± 50	

J. Genetic, Stroke Prone, Hypertensive Rats Performing Static Isometric Exercise

Study	Dur.	Group	n			Sex	Exercise	#	Intensity	Code				Comments
Tipton et al.	183	C-SHAM	21	8	7	M	Sham hang		Rats performed 2–3 sets with 6–10 repetitions/set.	I	138 ± 11	NA	221 ± 10	Five animals had histological evidence for strokes, 1 was trained; acute hanging caused MBP to increase 70 mmHg and HR by 115/min
		E	21	8	7	M	Hang w/wt.	7–10 sec		I	129 ± 5		221 ± 16	
			21	8	7	M				I	128 ± 13		228 ± 10	
		C-SHAM	21	8	7	F	Sham hang	7–10 sec		I	131 ± 8		222 ± 11	
		E	21	8		F	Hang w/wt.				121 ± 8		220 ± 11	

Table organized according to duration of study, means and SD listed; * denotes a statistical difference listed in text; C = Nonexercised; WKY = Wistar Kyoto rats; LL = Lyon lower pressures; LN = Lyon normotensive; SR = Salt resistant rat; S = Electrical shocking; MOD = Moderate constriction; SEV = Severe constriction.

TABLE 13.5
Influence of Isometric, Circuit-Training, Weight-Lifting and Resistive Exercises on Resting Blood Pressure of Humans

Investigator	Ref	Group	N	Duration of Study (weeks)	Invasive	Sex	Age (yrs)	Type	Training Details	Before Training SBP (mmHg)	Before Training DBP (mmHg)	After Training SBP (mmHg)	After Training DBP (mmHg)	Comments
Kiveloff & Huber	95	E	8	5 to 8	No	M,F	64	Isometric	6 second contractions for all large muscle groups, three times daily; 5 days/week			157	87	According to authors, changes ranged from 2 mmHg to 42 mmHg, no control data shown
Harris & Holly	66	C E	16 10	9 9	No No	M M	32 32	Circuit training	3 sets on 10 CT stations, 20–25 repetitions, 3/1 exercise-rest ratio, 40% RM for intensity, three times/week	146 ± 32 142 ± 24	95 ± 15 96 ± 19	146 ± 27 142 ± 22	93 ± 13 91 ± 24*	Total weight lifted increased by 57%, strength increased by 12–53%
Kelemen	90	E	51	10	No	M	25–59	Circuit training, walking	Subjects on placebo, diltiazem, or propranolol; exercised 1 hr/day, 3 times/wk on 8 variable resistance units	145	97	131*	84*	No controls listed, placebo group exhibited reductions similar to others. All increased in total strength by 20%
Hagberg et al.	62	C E	17 5	32 20	No No	M,F M,F	16 15	Weight training	Trained 3 times/wk free weights with 3 sets of 5–8 repetitions with 6 exercises or machines that allowed 14 exercises with 12–15 repetitions	136 ± 4 141	75 ± 8 63	138 ± 10 115	75 ± 8 63	Weight lifting lowered resting pressures after previous endurance training

Table organized according to the duration of the study; means and standard deviations listed; * denotes a text-designated significant difference; C = Control; E = Exercisee.

weeks and before 12 weeks of training had been completed. Our unpublished and published [180] data on SHR groups add credence to this impression. Hence, it is possible that the time course of the responsible mechanism(s) will be different depending on the time intervals between measurements.

The results of Roman et al. [145] and Cade et al. [15] (Table 13.2) showed that resting blood pressure will increase with the cessation of aerobic training. In the former study, increases of 18/16 mmHg occurred with 3 months of inactivity, whereas in the latter investigation, the same period of time was associated with increases of 17/20 mmHg in systolic and diastolic pressures, respectively. This trend generally did not occur in the Gilders et al. [55] study, although the authors did report a 13 mmHg increase in systolic blood pressure levels in the data collected at night. When a detraining experiment was conducted with trained hypertensive rats (SHR) [159], the resting pressures returned to non-trained values within 3–4 weeks.

Inspection of the age range of the subjects included in Tables 13.2 and 13.3, as well as those included in the 1984 review [179] revealed that the beneficial effect of exercise was best demonstrated in the older subjects. The Kasch et al. interesting 20-year longitudinal study [88] would have been more convincing about the long-term benefits of endurance exercise in the aging process if they had had complete blood pressure data from their sedentary controls. The research by Hagberg et al. [64] on older subjects (Table 13.3) and his recent review [61] favors the concept that moderate exercise will be very beneficial for lowering resting pressures in elderly populations. When older SHR populations were exercise-trained, the runners maintained their pressures near their starting values, unlike the nonrunners whose pressures increased with time [180]. This pattern did not occur with swimming rats [121] because the older SHR groups demonstrated significant reductions in their resting systolic blood pressures. This result reinforced the concept in rats that different mechanisms were responsible to explain the chronic effects of swimming or running on resting blood pressures.

Although mechanisms will be discussed in a subsequent section, investigations during the last decade have provided insights as to why exercise training by certain populations will not be associated with lowered resting pressures. As Hagberg noted in his meta-analysis of 25 endurance training studies [61], subsets of hypertensive subjects did not exhibit changes in their resting pressures after participating in an exercise program. Besides aspects related to genetics, exercise prescription, and program compliance, explanations included hypertensive individuals who had (a) demonstrated an "exaggerated" pressor response to acute exercise [2], (b) evidence for increased resting adrenergic tone [34], (c) altered myocardial compliance [106], (d) or cardiac enlargement [42, 51, 103]. Specifically, Attina et al. [2] exercise-trained hypertensive subjects (Table 13.3) for 1 year who were classified as "normal responders or abnormal responders" to a stress test. An abnormal response was an elevation of systolic blood pressure over 230 mmHg or diastolic blood pressure over 110 mmHg. After 1 year, the normal-responders group demonstrated a significant reduction of 5 (systolic) and 7 (diastolic) mmHg, respectively, whereas the abnormal responders had a 1 mmHg increase in systolic blood pessure and a 5 mmHg elevation in diastolic pressure. This same type of differentiation occurred when submaximal exercise tests were conducted. Unfortunately, they had no control subjects for comparative purposes. Kinoshita and coworkers [92] evaluated the effects of 10 weeks of training (Table 13.3) on 21 hypertensive subjects, who were classified into groups of responders and nonresponders and whose changes were compared with 10 control subjects. Classification was determined by whether the subjects demonstrated a 10 mmHg decrease in resting mean pressure, a procedure used by Japanese pharmacological companies to ascertain the effectiveness of an antihypertensive compound. Besides failing to demonstrate a decrease in mean blood pressure, the nonresponders did not exhibit significant changes in plasma catecholamine concentrations, plasma volume, blood volume, cardiac index, or in the serum sodium:potassium ratio. Most of the responders were women (9/12) and the sex of the nonresponders was not listed. Moreover, they were approximately 12 kg lighter in body mass when the experiments were initiated. Consequently, one must be cautious in accepting their description as to what truly characterizes a responder. When Duncan et al. [34] compared the resting blood pressure changes of 44 hypertensive subjects who exercise-trained with the pressure reductions of 12 subjects who did not, significant differences existed only with the diastolic pressure results. After classifying subjects by their resting plasma catecholamine concentrations, however, the 18 trained subjects considered to be hyperadrenergic demonstrated greater changes in systolic and diastolic blood pressure than the 26 trained individuals with normoadrenergic concentrations, although the differences between them in diastolic pressures was approximately 2 mmHg. From their experiences from testing normal and hypertensive children in the Muscatine, Iowa, study, Lauer et al. [103, personal communication] indicate that hypertensive individuals with evidence for cardiac enlargement may not be responders to an exercise training program because of the changes in cardiac mechanics that could alter cardiac output. As discussed in the acute exercise section, this possibility has some experimental support from studies with hypertensive patients [106]. Although more research is needed to determine the characteristics of a responder versus a nonresponder, it would be advantageous for current and future investigators to consider these possibilities before and after conducting an exercise training study.

ISOMETRIC, WEIGHT-LIFTING, AND RESISTIVE EXERCISES

For many years, health organizations and medical authorities have advised hypertensive-prone or hypertensive populations not to perform static or weight-lifting activities [179]. This has been a prudent recommendation because direct blood pressure measurements in humans have demonstrated that weight-lifting activities can elicit systolic blood pressures in excess of 200 mmHg [108] in nonhypertensive subjects. Moreover, it is well documented in animals [179, 183] and in humans [179] that isometric contractions will elicit high pressor responses that are related to the intensity of the contraction and to the mass of the muscles involved [108, 179]. Despite these facts, an increasing number of investigators have been advocating weight-lifting or circuit-training principles for either cardiac or hypertensive patients [57, 66, 90, 168] (Table 13.5). Kiveloff and Huber [95] prescribed isometric exercises for their elderly population (Table 13.5) and reported changes ranging from 2–42 mmHg. Even though the study left much to be desired in all respects, it is interesting that it was conducted approximately 20 years ago when exercise, much less static exercise, was not seriously considered for the management of hypertension. In the last decade, three studies (Table 13.5) were conducted that are relevant to this topic. Hagberg et al. [62] had 6 hypertensive adolescents who had been previously trained by aerobic activities use free weights for 20 weeks and found a 17 mmHg reduction in resting systolic blood pressure and a 7 mmHg decrease in diastolic blood pressure. Harris and Holly [66] had 10 subjects with borderline hypertension follow circuit-training procedures for 9 weeks. At the end of the program, the subjects were stronger and had an increase of 1 mmHg in systolic and a 5 mmHg decrease in diastolic blood pressure. There were 16 controls who exhibited no significant mean changes in resting blood pressures during this time. Circuit training was combined with running and jogging by Kelemen [90] with 50 borderline hypertensive patients for 10 weeks. As a group, they exhibited a decline of 14 mmHg in systolic and a reduction of 13 mmHg in diastolic blood pressure. Unfortunately, there were no reports on the changes noted in their controls. These preliminary studies demonstrate that supervised weight-resistive programs have been used successfully despite the inherent potential for eliciting elevated pressures. The circuit-training principles developed by others [66, 90, 163] that should be considered are to prescribe loads that are between 40 and 50% of one's maximum repetition, avoid elevating blood pressures with exercise higher than 150 mmHg systolic and 100 mmHg diastolic, start with 8–10 repetitions per exercise, and perform one set per specific exercise. It is interesting to note that when stroke-prone hypertensive rats performed 16 weeks of static exercises [182] (Table 13.4), the trained rats did not have more cerebrovascular lesions and did not demonstrate higher resting pressures. Even though these human and animal results would have to be labelled as "preliminary", they do suggest that it is time for health and medical groups to reconsider their guidelines on the exercise programs for hypertensive persons.

MEASUREMENT CONSIDERATIONS

The respective tables cannot summarize all the various ramifications of the experimental designs and methodologies associated with the studies cited. Although myriad circumstances favor the use of the laboratory or the office for the measurement of blood pressure, the use of ambulatory equipment to secure daily recordings provides more information on the clinical significance of the results. Harshfield et al. [67] used this approach with adolescents in a cross-sectional design with 80 boys and 95 girls of which 36 boys and 58 girls were black. The teens were assigned to "more fit" or "less fit" categories according to their maximum oxygen consumption scores. The less fit black males had higher systolic pressures than the more fit black males when either awake or asleep. Moreover, the less fit black males had higher systolic blood pressures than the less fit white males when either awake or asleep and had pressures that were elevated more the fit black males when asleep. Less fit black females had similar trends with both systolic and diastolic pressures. The authors concluded that fitness levels would influence blood pressure profiles in black adolescents when obtained by ambulatory methods. In addition, it was apparent that time of day and sex also had to be considered.

In the longitudinal studies conducted by Gilders et al. [55], Reiling et al. [137, 138, unpublished data from Dr. Seals's laboratory] and Van Hoof [189] (Tables 13.2 and 13.3), both Van Hoof and Seals reported that training was associated with lower pressure values during the day but not at night. Gilders et al. [55] found no statistically meaningful results during the day or night. In fact, some authorities consider elevated blood pressures during the sleeping hours abnormal and suggestive of organ damage, atherosclerosis, or autonomic dysfunction [67].

The position of the subject at the time of the resting measurement also is a factor to consider when evaluating the results of a training program. Cleroux et al. [17] concluded that exercise training had no statistical effect on the resting blood pressures of "labile" hypertensive subjects who participated in either a jogging or a bicycle ergometer exercise program. When measured in the standing position, however, the subjects who trained on the ergometer had significantly lower systolic and diastolic blood pressures, whereas the subjects who jogged and who were measured in the supine position had significantly lower systolic blood pressure values. Although the magnitude of the changes were not large (7–10 mmHg), they were of the order that consistently has been reported with moderate exercise.

MECHANISTIC CONSIDERATIONS

As noted by others [179], it is unlikely that a change in a physical measurement can be explained by a single or simple physiological mechanism. Included within Table 13.3 are the results from most of the longitudinal training studies that contained hemodynamic data pertaining to cardic output and total peripheral vascular resistance. It is noteworthy that of the 14 separate investigations listed, only the Johnson and Grover study [84] showed an increase (1%) in resting mean pressure. On the other hand, it was not evident from Table 13.3 whether the nonsignificant or significant reductions in the other studies were due to a change in cardiac output or total peripheral vascular resistance, or both. When direct catheterization methods were used, four of the five studies [28, 65, 84, 148] exhibited a decline in cardiac output and three [28, 140, 148] showed an increase in total peripheral vascular resistance. In the 1984 review [179], we wondered whether the process of direct catheterization had an effect on the resting blood pressure measurement, given that most of the significant effects of training on resting blood pressure were demonstrated with indirect measurements. During the last decade, I have found no longitudinal training study concerned with blood pressure changes that include direct arterial catheterizations within the experimental design. We are left, therefore, with the problem of determining whether the methodology used can help explain why certain investigators report significant changes in total peripheral resistance while others observe significant reductions in cardiac output. Both Jennings et al. [81] and Hagberg and associates [64] had subgroups that showed an increase in cardiac output which accompanied the decline in resting blood pressures. Because Hagberg et al. had one elderly subgroup that exhibited an increase and one subgroup that demonstrated a decrease in cardiac output with training, the age of the subjects was an unlikely explanation for these contrasting results. Disappointingly, limited hemodynamic data are available from anesthetized [132, 185] and unanesthetized hypertensive animals [185] on the effects of training. Preliminary results from nontrained and trained SHR populations [185] indicated that trained rats had significantly lower absolute resting cardiac output values which became insignificant when corrected for surface area and body mass. When peripheral vascular resistance comparisons were made in these rats, there were no trends that favored the viewpoint that mechanisms associated with peripheral vascular resistance were responsible for the training effect. Obviously, more human and animal studies are necessary to resolve this matter.

ADRENERGIC MECHANISMS

Of all the mechanisms mentioned by investigators, ones pertaining to the sympathetic nervous system are the most frequently cited. In the longitudinal studies listed in Tables 13.2 and 13.3, ten investigators found reductions in adrenergic indices [17, 34, 64, 81, 84, 92, 95, 122, 138, 188], although Cleroux and coworkers [17] found inconsistent trends. Plasma catecholamine concentrations have been used by most investigators as an index of sympathetic nervous system activity; however, more direct techniques are being used as measuring norepinephrine spillover rate in the plasma [39] or monitoring peripheral sympathetic nerve traffic [45, 138, 190]. Jennings et al. [81] found that 10 of their 12 subjects who exercised 7 days per week experienced a 65% reduction in the norepinephrine spillover rate [39]. These same subjects did not demonstrate this effect when they exercised 3 times a week, however. When plasma norepinephrine concentrations were evaluated, exercising 7 days/week significantly decreased this measurement by 52%, whereas exercising 3 days/week lowered the plasma concentration by 12%. Because norepinephrine spillover rate in the plasma represented a measure of average sympathetic neural activity, the issue becomes complex when trying to determine whether central, peripheral, or local mechanisms were primarily or secondarily responsible for the changes noted. Whole body spillover rate is most influenced by sympathetic activity in muscle, lung, and skin [39, 81]; thus, Jennings and co-workers [81] believe that the decrease in resting peripheral vascular resistance noted in their trained subjects was best explained by the decrease in the norepinephrine spillover rate in these tissues. Other investigators listed in Table 13.3, however, found a decrease in plasma catecholamines with either no change or an increase in peripheral vascular resistance [64, 92, 122, 138]. To date, careful studies on the possibility of down regulation of adrenergic receptors of trained and nontrained hypertensive subjects participating in a well-designed, longitudinal experiment have not been reported. As reviewed previously [186], SHR populations that were chemically sympathectomized at birth exhibited a 10–12 mmHg reduction in resting systolic blood pressure with endurance training. When chemically sympathectomized rats were also demedullated, however, the training program had no significant influence on resting systolic blood pressure [186]. These findings suggest an intact and functioning adrenal medulla is necessary for a reduction in resting blood pressure to occur with training. The perfection of the microneurographic technique to directly record sympathetic nerve activity to skeletal muscles [45, 190] has introduced a new dimension for research on the select functions of the sympathetic nervous system. Using this technique with normotensive and hypertensive subjects, Wallin and co-workers [190] found no significant differences between the two populations in sympathetic nerve traffic when they were measured at rest and performed an isometric test at 30% MVC. To date, this technique has not been employed with hypertensive subjects participating in a training study. It is hoped that these data will be in the scientific literature within the near future. A similar statement can be made for hypertensive rats.

Heistad and co-workers [5, 22, 41] have proposed that the sympathetic nervous system has a protective influence on the cerebral vascular vessels against the disruption of the blood-brain barrier and against the subsequent incidence of strokes. Besides an intact sympathetic nervous system, the vascular smooth muscle of cerebral vessel must be hypertrophied to achieve a maximum protective effect. Heistad's experimental results in adult animals convincingly demonstrated that a decrease in cerebral sympathetic activity was associated with an increase in cerebral lesions. When stroke-prone, spontaneously hypertensive rats (SP-SHR) were trained, we found that exercise training initially attenuated the rise in systolic blood pressure; however, this effect was not maintained as the exercise training continued. Because the intent was to determine whether training would delay the onset of a stroke and increase the longevity of the rat, a diet high in sodium was provided. Contrary to our expectations, the trained rats had cerebrovascular lesions earlier and died sooner than their nontrained controls, a finding similar to that reported by Kunii et al. [100] almost a decade ago. Indirect evidence from animals suggests that resting sympathetic nervous activity will be decreased with endurance training [131]; therefore, we are using this concept to explain the SP-SHR results. More research will be necessary to resolve this matter.

METABOLIC MECHANISMS

Since 1923, body weight has been recognized as a contributing factor for the development of hypertension [178]. It is not surprising, then, that in the nonpharmacological control of resting blood pressure, a reduction in body weight is universally advised [87, 161, 165, 179]. Inherent with this advise is that the change in fat mass is the most important aspect of the recommendation. Although the muscle fiber type distributions of hypertensive individuals have been reported to be different than for normotensive individuals with hypertensives having a higher percentage of fast twitch or Type II fibers [86], a weight-loss program is not designed to lose muscle mass or to alter its fiber type composition. The association, however, between a change in body weight with a change in blood pressure is not a cause and effect relationship [179], because not all individuals who have lost weight experienced a reduction in blood pressure [38, 87], and not everyone who has exhibited a decrease in blood pressure has lost weight [161].

In my last review [179], I felt that it was the 1979 exercise and metabolic experiments of Krotkiewski et al. [98] that provided the experimental foundation for the insulin hypothesis [105] as it pertained to the effects of endurance training on obese or overweight hypertensive subjects [79]; namely, inactive and obese hypertensive individuals will have higher plasma insulin concentrations that will increase the activity of the sympathetic nervous system and, at the same time, will facilitate an increased reabsorption of sodium by the kidney tubules. The net effect would be an increase in resting pressure caused, in part, by the increased plasma volume and by the increased activity of the sympathetic nervous system.

As documented for normotensive populations [177, 179], endurance-trained subjects have been associated with lower plasma concentrations of insulin and an increased sensitivity to the peripheral actions of insulin. Studies by Fournier et al. [47] and by Weinsier and associates [195] with sedentary and obese nonhypertensive or nondiabetic subjects have shown that plasma insulin concentrations will be significantly correlated with resting blood pressure, although it is not clear whether the relationship is a direct or indirect one. When obese hypertensive and normotensive subjects were compared by Manicardi and others in a multiple regression model [109], the hypertensives not only had a greater tissue resistance to insulin, but their plasma insulin concentration and the degree of obesity also accounted for 65% of the variance associated with systolic blood pressure. Because it is known that a reduction in body weight is associated with a reduction in the release of catecholamines [101], the remaining 35% of their unaccountable variance could have been a sympathetic component. Insights on the relationships between insulin and the sympathetic nervous system can be found with the nontrained animal studies conducted by Edwards et al. [36]. They infused insulin into normotensive rats maintained with a euglycemic clamp, and observed significant increases in resting blood pressure. When the animals were sympathectomized, the pressor responses were abolished. Mondon and Reaven [119] recently reported that hyperinsulinemia and insulin resistance are present in hypertensive rats (SHR). When they examined this relationship, the hypertensive rats were different than the normotensive rats in their clearance of insulin because of a decreased removal by skeletal muscles and kidneys. Rocchini et al. [142] experimentally examined the effects of weight reduction, behavior modification, and exercise training on the resting blood pressure of obese adolescents during a 20-week period. Using statistical procedures to correct for the effects of each intervention, the authors concluded that the reductions in blood pressure and in insulin concentrations during weight loss were facilitated by exercise training. There were no measures of catecholamines reported that would provide a link between these results and changes in the sympathetic nervous system.

It is well recognized that many individuals consuming a diet high in fat have higher plasma insulin concentrations, especially if they become obese. In a preliminary report several years ago [181] with normotensive rats fed a diet high in fat and sucrose, we observed that the trained animals exhibited less weight gain, lower plasma insulin concentrations, and lower resting systolic blood pressures than their nontrained controls who were significantly heavier. We recently repeated this study but included weight-matched controls [32]. As shown in Table 13.4, the trained rats not only had lower resting pressures and reduced body weights, they also had lower plasma insulin concentrations. The study by Rocchini et al. [143] with animals may help explain these observations. They fed dogs either a high or a low fat diet and observed that the significant gain in weight over a 6-week period was associated with an increase in blood pressure, sodium retention, elevated plasma insulin, aldosterone, and norepinephrine concentrations as well as with an increase in plasma volume. Because the catecholamine concentration increased before changes were noted for insulin and aldosterone levels, they felt that sodium retention was the primary mechanism for the elevation in blood pressure that initially was stimulated by the norepinephrine changes and later by the actions of insulin and aldosterone. Because decreases in resting pressures with endurance training range from 5–25 mmHg, the insulin hypothesis is an attractive one for advocating chronic exercise for the management of individuals with a proneness for hypertension and obesity.

ELECTROLYTE AND RENAL MECHANISMS

Although a reduction in salt intake has been advocated [179] and debated [141] for many years to lower resting pressures, there has been a paucity of well-controlled dietary studies that would indicate the contributions of chronic exercise. Stamler and her associates [165] reported that subjects who lowered their blood pressure by nonpharmacological methods would accomplish this result by a combination of exercise, weight loss, and reduced sodium intake. However, their evidence was not very helpful in understanding the relationships between exercise and sodium intake. Almost two decades ago, Heistad et al. [68] demonstrated that vascular reactivity was enhanced when the sodium concentration was increased. Block and co-workers subsequently (11) have shown that high salt concentration will diminish the catecholamine responses and their plasma levels. When normotensive and borderline hypertensive subjects were provided a diet that was increased from 10 mEq. of sodium per day to 170 mEq./day [11], acute exercise by the hypertensive subjects was associated with a significant reduction in the plasma concentrations of norepinephrine, epinephrine, and renin as well as with an increased pressor response. Although interesting, and confirming the earlier study by Heistad et al. [68], these results provide minimal insights as to the effects of chronic exercise on sodium metabolism. Nomura et al. [122] reported that hypertensive subjects provided a diet that contained 170 mEq./day of sodium experienced a significant reduction in resting diastolic blood pressure after only 3 weeks of physical activity (Table 13.3). They also noted a reduction in the plasma concentrations of aldosterone and norepinephrine and a decrease in the urinary excretion of renin. Plasma volume was increased slightly. In another group, they restricted dietary sodium to 34 mEq./ day and followed a similar training program for 3 weeks (Table 13.3). Systolic, mean, and diastolic pressures as well as the cardiac index were significantly reduced. Associated with the sodium restriction, plasma volume was significantly reduced before the exercise program commenced and was significantly increased at the end of the training period. Plasma concentrations of aldosterone at rest were significantly decreased while the urinary excretion of norepinephrine and renin also were significantly reduced when compared to control conditions. Unfortunately, the study had no control subjects. Kiyonaga and his colleagues [96] conducted a 20-week training program with 9 hypertensive subjects (Table 13.2). Like Nomura et al. [122], a control group was not included. After 10 weeks, they observed a significant reduction in resting pressure, and a significant increase in the urinary excretion of sodium, which remained elevated during the next 10 weeks of training. Plasma insulin was not measured, so it is unknown whether this hormone had any influence on their results. In addition, the plasma concentration of angiotensin II was significantly increased after 20 weeks, whereas the concentration of norepinephrine was significantly reduced when compared to pretraining values. Plasma renin activity was essentially unchanged throughout the training program. Urine kallikrein excretion decreased by approximately 38% during the experimental period, but this difference had no statistical significance. Although Jo and co-workers [83] reported that 12 weeks of exercise training reduced resting pressures (Table 13.2) in their hypertensive subjects, they had negative results concerning the effects of training on urinary sodium excretion. Unfortunately, they did not measure changes in plasma volume. Urata et al. [188] measured changes in resting pressures, resting hemodynamics, plasma, and urinary concentrations of hormones and electrolytes, plus the blood volumes of hypertensive subjects assigned to control or experimental groups (Table 13.3). Measurements were taken before and after 10 weeks of endurance training, with resting pressures and cardiac index values being significantly reduced during this time internal. Plasma concentrations of norepinephrine were significantly lowered, although renin and aldosterone levels were similar to pretraining values. The group serum sodium concentration significantly decreased from 142.5 to 140.2 mEq./L; however, this small change was considered to be biologically important. Urinary sodium excretion values were not significantly altered in these subjects at any time. When blood and plasma volumes were measured, both parameters were associated with a significant 11% decrease. Because the daily sodium intakes of these subjects were not stated, it was unknown whether their plasma volume results were a result of a dietary or exercise mechanism. This fact is important because the Japanese citizen can consume up to 25 grams of sodium chloride per day [194], which is approximately two to five times the amount consumed by the average American adult. Kinoshita et al. [92] (Table 13.3) also reported that 10 weeks of endurance training was associated with significant reductions in blood pressure and plasma volume, but they provided no data on their subjects' daily dietary sodium intakes. These collective findings were difficult to reconcile with existing information because there are data that favor an increase in blood and plasma volume with endurance training [18, 19, 150], which is associated, in part, with the increase in the circulating concentration of aldosterone. In their study on responders and nonresponders to endurance training, Kinoshita et al. [92] observed that the serum sodium/potassium ratio was significantly lower with the responders. The meaning and significance of this difference were not discussed.

Studies with normotensive and hypertensive individuals have demonstrated that differences exist between the two populations in cation transport across red cell membranes [1, 103]. This finding has prompted numerous studies to determine whether this difference could be used as a predictor for hypertension in normotensive populations. Adragna and associates [1] investigated this matter in normotensive and hypertensive subjects (Table 13.2) who participated in a 12-week training program and found that sodium-lithium countertransport was statistically reduced in the trained groups. The significance of this finding was unclear because the trained individuals exhibited no statistical evidence for a lowered resting blood pressure.

Animal results on the effects of exercise on electrolyte balance are conflicting. In 1984 we were impressed by the results of Shepherd and co-workers [157] who reported that training was associated with as much as 50 mmHg difference in the resting systolic blood pressures of the salt sensitive hypertensive rat. Since that time, Shepherd's conclusions have been confirmed by Savage et al. [149] (Table 13.4). Using the Dahl salt-sensitive rat, they found that 12 weeks of treadmill running was associated with mean pressures that were 20–25 mmHg lower than their nontrained controls. This difference could not be explained by food intake because the trained rats consumed more chow containing 1.90% sodium than the nontrained animals. On the other hand, our laboratory [184] (Table 13.4) did not confirm these findings with Dahl salt-sensitive rats. We found that chronic exercise slightly attenuated the rise in pressure during the early weeks of training, after which this effect was lost. We also reported that trained rats did not consume significantly more food than controls or excrete more sodium in the urine than the nontrained controls. Because these rats were provided a higher concentration of salt to the rat (8% sodium in the diet, 1% saline solution as the drinking solution), it is quite possible that the expected training effects were masked because the recommended salt concentrations for these animals [174] were too high. Obviously, a dose-response training study with Dahl rats will be necessary to reconcile these differences.

CALCIUM

In 1984, McCarron and his associates [113] analyzed the results of the HANES I survey with regard to nutrient intake and hypertension. Blood pressure results from 10,372 persons aged 18–74 years were analyzed as they pertained to 17 different nutrients. Of the six conclusions made, the following are germane to this review.

1. Nutritional deficiencies rather than excesses will characterize the hypertensive person in America.
2. The primary nutritional markers of hypertension were reduced consumptions of calcium and potassium.
3. Hypertensive populations had reduced consumptions of calcium, potassium, Vitamin A, and Vitamin C when compared to normotensive individuals.
4. The observations concerning calcium were largely independent of age, race, sex, body mass index, and alcohol consumption.

Excluded from the debate on the importance of calcium and sodium in the etiology and management of hypertension [102, 112] is the role of exercise training. Because calcium supplementation to humans [7] and to hypertensive rats (SHR) [3, 114] has been shown to reduce resting pressures, Drummond et al. [33] consulted McCarron and designed an exercise training study using SHR groups that received high (2.5%) or low (0.6%) concentrations of calcium in their specially prepared diets. After 13 weeks of training (Table 13.4), both exercising groups had significantly lower resting systolic blood pressures than their nontrained controls, but chronic exercise and a high calcium diet had no additive effects. In addition, the nontrained groups had similar pressures regardless of the calcium concentrations in their food. Our unpublished measurements of total and ionized calcium concentrations, calcitonin, or parathyroid hormone levels were not helpful in explaining these findings. One factor that needs to be considered in future research studies is the constancy of the calcium/phosphate ratio. In the Drummond et al. investigation [33], this ratio was constant for both diets whereas this has not always been the case in other studies that were not concerned with training.

KIDNEY

In addition to its key role in the regulation of electrolyte metabolism [199], the kidney is of importance to the incidence of secondary hypertension [179]. As noted in the earlier review [179], the training studies with the renal hypertensive rat (Two-kidney-1 clip, Goldblatt) have been consistently negative with respect to the benefits of endurance running or swimming on resting blood pressures. This trend continued with recent publications by Rakusan et al. [135] and by Marcus and Tipton [110] (Table 13.4). Rakusan et al. swam their renal hypertensive rats 2 hours per day for 6 weeks and found that the swimmers had slightly higher mean pressures than the nonswimmers. They also noted an increase in left ventricular mass and a decrease in a number of indices associated with capillary density. In the Marcus and Tipton experiment, moderate and severe constrictions of the renal artery were performed. Although the exercise program was effective in producing a training state, the trained animals with severely constricted arteries had significantly higher resting pressures and significantly lower indices for myocardial capillarization. As a result of these studies, we have concluded that the rat model for renal hypertension will not exhibit a lower resting blood pressure with endurance training. It is Zambraski's opinion [personal communication] that the miniature pig would be a better animal model than the rat to study the effects of exercise training on renal hypertension, a point that should be kept in mind when planning future investigations on this topic.

Recent exercise training studies [58, 127] involving patients with kidney diseases on hemodialysis have confirmed previous investigations [179] which demonstrated that resting blood pressures were lowered when physical activity was included in the process. In the Goldberg et al. report [58], a 52-week exercise program for 14 individuals on a training schedule (70% V̇o₂max) resulted in the elimination or reduction of the antihypertensive medication for eight of the hypertensive subjects (data not known), with no significant changes in their plasma volumes. Painter and associates [127] exercised 14 patients, three times per week for 24 weeks at an intensity level that was progressively increased to 85% V̇o₂max. The exercise was performed during hemodialysis. The study lasted 24 weeks and included seven controls. Improvement in V̇o₂max indicated that the training schedule had altered the functional capacity of the subjects. At the start of the study, resting systolic blood pressure was 152 mmHg whereas it was reduced to 143 mmHg after 12 weeks and to 138 mmHg after 24 weeks had elapsed. The controls resting pressures remained at 124 mmHg throughout the experimental period. Eight of the patients were on medication, and 50% were able to eliminate this requirement after 6 months of training. Unfortunately, the authors had no measures of plasma volume or of electrolyte balance from any of the subjects. Even so, the data supported the conclusion that many patients with kidney diseases on hemodialysis will benefit from an exercise training program.

NEURAL AND BAROREFLEX MECHANISMS

Since my last review, several exciting developments pertaining to the central nervous system and its reflex actions have occurred. The most notable is the involvement of central opioid and serotonergic mechanism in the post exercise hypotension response [71]. Whether these systems are involved in the resting blood pressure adaptations with chronic exercise remains to be determined. The hypertension literature is replete with reports on the involvement of the central nervous system in the regulation and control of blood pressure that include the importance of the C-1 area of the brain stem [139], the area postrema [162], the nucleus tractus solitarius (70), or the paraventricular hypothalamic nucleus (134). None, however, were directly concerned with exercise training as it affects resting blood pressures or were by scientists interested in exercise mechanisms. Until such individuals appear or are encouraged to consider central contributions, our neural explanations will be focused primarily on peripheral mechanisms.

Whether endurance training will increase, decrease, or have no effect on the sensitivity and functioning of the arterial baroreceptors is being debated in scientific circles [20, 136] because of their importance to blood pressure regulation in prolonged space flight. Proponents of the various viewpoints have substantial evidence to favor their position, with most of the data emerging from human investigations. Responsible investigators have started to resolve this dilemma, and it is likely that a better standardization of subject selection, methodology, and data analysis will have emerged by the time the next review on hypertension is published. Until then, we will rely on animal results to provide insights on the role of the arterial baroreceptor in establishing a lower resting pressure in trained populations.

Our previous data [179] from anesthetized nontrained and trained animal preparations that were exposed to conditions of lower body negative pressure favored the attenuation hypothesis. Bedford and Tipton [6] exercised trained normotensive rats and used a carotid sinus preparation to further test this possibility. Static pressures and regional blood flows were measured in nontrained and trained animals. Compared to the nontrained animals, the baroreflex control of blood pressure and calculated regional vascular resistances of the trained rats were less responsive to changes in carotid sinus pressures. We concluded that the arterial baroreflex control of blood pressure was attenuated by exercise training and postulated that this change would decrease the sympathetic traffic associated with the baroreflex. Whether this change was due to baroreceptor resetting, central integration, or end organ adaptations was unknown.

In recent years, Bishop's laboratory in Texas has taken an active role in studying this problem. When they deafferented the aortic barore-ceptors in the baboon [9], they found that resting blood pressure increased because of the increased activity of the sympathetic nervous system and the inability of the carotid sinus baroreceptor to buffer the changes. DiCarlo and Bishop [26] subsequently instrumented rabbits for measurements of pressure, renal nerve sympathetic nervous system activity, and cardiac output before blocking cardiac afferent nerve activity before and after endurance training. Before training, afferent blocking had no significant effect on resting pressure, vascular peripheral resistance, or renal nerve sympathetic activity. This was not the situation with trained rabbits as they found after afferent blockage that arterial blood pressure was elevated and that there was an increase in the range and gain of the arterial baroreflex regulation of renal nerve sympathetic activity. From these results, the authors concluded that the attenuated effect of training on the arterial baroreflex was the result of an enhanced inhibitory effect by the cardiac afferents and not by a change in the arterial baroreflex per se. The mechanism responsible for this result was not described. In a related experiment, these two investigators [27] reported that training had altered the vascular resistances of the renal and mesenteric vascular beds because of its effect on the functioning of cardiac afferents. Whether the change is peripheral or central in nature remains unknown and will require the attention of individuals trained in the neurosciences and in exercise physiology.

MYOCARDIAL AND VESSEL STRUCTURAL MECHANISMS

As mentioned previously, myocardial hypertrophy has been suggested as one possibility to explain why some hypertensive subjects do not exhibit a blood pressure-lowering effect with endurance training. Although interesting, the critical evidence is lacking. There is considerable documentation, however, that cardiac enlargement occurs early in hypertension [51, 77, 103, 192]. It is essential, therefore, that the exercise being prescribed not accelerate the process, because for the hypertensive person the degree of enlargement becomes an important consideration not only for a possible reduction in resting pressure but also for changes in myocardial compliance, function, and capillarization.

Baglivo et al. [4] recently addressed this subject by prescribing exercise for hypertensive individuals (resting pressures of 155/101 mmHg) who also were placed on a low sodium diet (2 gram/day) for 12 weeks. The exercise program was varied, not well quantified, and likely to be classified as moderate in nature. Echocardiographic measurements of left ventricular mass and shortening exhibited insignificant changes. Resting blood pressure significantly decreased by 19/14 mmHg for systolic and diastolic blood pressures, respectively. A control group that performed no exercise demonstrated a 13 mmHg decrease in systolic blood pressure and a 2 mmHg increase in diastolic blood pressure. In addition, they also demonstrated a nonsignificant increase in left ventricular mass with training. The authors concluded that it would be prudent to recommend "physical training to mild hypertensive patients" because it did not induce increases in left ventricular mass.

Ferrara et al. [42] statistically evaluated the relationships between resting or exercise blood pressures and left ventricular mass in 45 patients with uncomplicated hypertension and concluded that blood pressure alone accounted for only 20% of the increase in the mass of the left ventricle. The significance of this finding was that other factors must be considered to avoid prescribing an exercise program that would significantly increase myocardial mass in hypertensive subjects. One of the other factors mentioned by the authors was increased activity of the sympathetic nervous system.

Although cardiac patients and hypertensive subjects are currently participating in a variety of weight resistive programs [57, 90, 163], the inherent problem is the degree of enlargement. Using circuit training [90], an increase of 15% in left ventricular mass was reported, with no significant changes in measures of myocardial functioning. As noted earlier, cardiac enlargement in the hypertensive individual can be associated with a decrease in myocardial compliance which could alter stroke volume, cardiac output, and blood pressure. According to Lund-Johansen [106], hypertensive subjects of all ages will exhibit subnormal stroke volumes during submaximal exercise. One practical significance of this information for future blood pressure studies is to perform cardiac echocardiographic measurements before and after a training program and to consider cardiac enlargement when determining whether an individual will be or has been a responder or a nonresponder. If no enlargment is found in a nonresponder, then other mechanisms for a lack of a training effect have to be considered. Therefore, in prescribing exercise for the hypertensive to reduce resting blood pressure and to prevent further cardiac enlargement, it would be prudent to exercise at an intensity lower than 70% $\dot{V}o_2max$ (Tables 13.2 and 13.3), while establishing an upper limit of 40–50% for maximum repetitions or for maximum voluntary contractions [37, 44, 90, 141, 163].

Sufficient animal information is available from nontrained and trained hypertensive animals [110, 135, 187] to expect a decrease in myocardial capillarization with high-intensity exercise of long duration. Although the mechanism is elusive, it is evident that cardiac enlargement, reductions in myocardial capillarization, and elevations in resting pressures will not be functionally beneficial for trained hypertensive rats. Although there are detailed investigations on the myocardial functions of trained hypertensive rats [132, 155, 187], it is difficult to extrapolate this information to humans because of the intensity of exercise prescribed and the different methods employed.

The importance of the heart as an endocrine organ should not be ignored, especially as it pertains to the synthesis and release of the arterial natriuretic peptides (ANP) [25, 94, 147, 166, 191] which have diuretic, natriuretic, and hypotensive effects [25, 156, 197] by a myriad of actions which includes the inhibition of the sympathetic nervous system [76]. Because trained humans and rats have elevated blood volumes [150, 179], it is possible they also would have higher densities of atrial and ventricular (ANP) granules. No published data are available, however, to support this speculation, and the limited results on plasma ANP concentrations [49, 171] indicate that training has no significant effect on this parameter.

Studies by Folkow [46] have been responsible for the concept that vessel structural changes will precede the functional changes that result in an increase in peripheral vascular resistance, which in turn will facilitate the elevated pressures associated with hypertension. Inherent in this concept is that the increase in vessel vascular resistance occurs because there is an increase in arteriolar wall thickness, which is coupled with a decrease in lumen diameter causing an increase in the wall/lumen ratio. Although numerous wall/lumen ratio studies have been conducted with experimental hypertensive animals [46], this topic has not been extensively investigated in trained WKY or SHR populations. Oppliger and associates [123, 186, unpublished data] conducted a detailed histological investigation on this topic with a wide assortment

FIGURE 13.1

The relationship between endurance training and wall:lumen ratios of select arteries from adult hypertensive (SHR) male rats when compared to mean values of WKY normotenise controls. Seven to twelve rats per group. Perfusion details can be found in references 123 and 186.

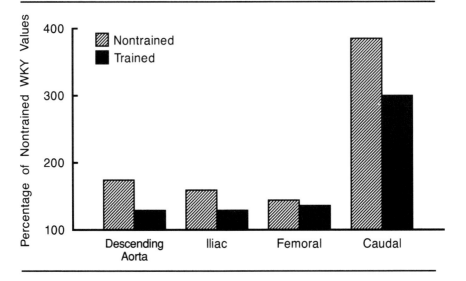

of experimental groups. Summarized in Figure 13.1 are group differences between adult nontrained and trained male hypertensive rats (SHR) and their WKY nontrained controls. Endurance training was associated with lower vessel wall/lumen ratios because the runners had wall thickness values that were similar to the nontrained hypertensive rats; but, had significantly larger lumen diameters. This was not surprising as other investigators have reported for animals that training will result in larger lumen diameters, especially in the coronary arteries [198], although no studies, including our own can explain the responsible mechanism. With a larger lumen, one would anticipate a decrease in resting vascular resistance in trained hypertensive rats. This effect has not been observed in hemodynamic measurements in unanesthetized trained rats [185] which suggests that other extrinsic and intrinsic factors were involved. Because microvessel rarefaction (reduction in the number of terminal arterioles in select vascular beds) has been cited as a possible contributor to the increase in vascular resistance present in adult hypertensive rats [59], this topic would be of interest to pursue in future training studies with SHR populations.

MISCELLANEOUS MECHANISMS

Several reports [130, 170, 179] indicate that hypertensive populations, especially borderline hypertensives or persons with hypertensive parents, have exaggerated blood pressure responses to mental and emotional stressors when compared to normotensive controls. The mechanism is obscure, but central nervous system activation and adrenergic responsiveness have been cited [130, 170]. If exercise training could decrease the central nervous system activation and diminish the adrenergic responsiveness, then this could be another argument for the inclusion of exercise training in the management of hypertension.

To determine whether trained subjects respond differently than nontrained populations to a mental stress, Perkins et al. [130] had borderline hypertensive subjects react to a video game stressor before and after a 10-week aerobic conditioning program (details not provided). When compared to their nonexercised controls, the "trained" exhibited a 33% reduction in resting systolic blood pressure and a 50% decrease in their resting diastolic blood pressure. Cox et al. [21] (Table 13.4), used a genetic model for borderline hypertension (SHR-bred with a WKY) and swam-trained one group that also received daily tail shocks and compared their resting blood pressures with animals that did not swim and/or did not receive electrical stimulation. After 12 weeks, the animals that were sedentary and free from daily shocking had systolic and diastolic pressures of 160/90 mmHg, respectively, whereas those who were only shocked had values of 180/118 mmHg. In contrast, the trained and shocked rats had means of 166/108 mmHg. Because the latter group had significantly lower plasma norepinephrine concentrations than the shocked animals, the authors felt that changes in the responsiveness of the autonomic nervous system were responsible for the observed differences in resting blood pressure.

This last decade has experienced an increased awareness of the physiological importance of the endothelium in vascular smooth muscles. It is well accepted that the endothelium will synthesize and release compounds (paracrine hormones) that have vasorelaxant and vasoconstrictor properties [52, 60, 120, 160]. How they are effected by acute and chronic exercise remains to be investigated. The changes in the release and actions of the peptides of the endothelin family could be useful to explain why blood pressures recorded during submaximal exercise are attenuated with endurance training and may help explain the lower pressures at rest. This speculation will, however, have to be tested by future researchers and summarized in forthcoming reviews.

SUMMARY

In 1984, I concluded [179, p. 284] that "there was sufficient experimental evidence to justify including exercise training as a separate countermeasure in any program designed to lower resting blood pressure in hypertensive populations." This conclusion was obtained after reviewing more than 50 longitudinal investigations from humans and animals. In updating the topic in this review by summarizing the findings listed in Tables 13.2–13.5 from 24 human and 25 animal studies, the conclusion is confirmed. Earlier, it was stated that exercise training would be associated with a 5–25 mmHg reduction in systolic blood pressure and a 3–15 mmHg decline in diastolic blood. The additional studies did not significantly alter the ranges or the conclusion. Hagberg [61] recently published the results of a meta-analysis of 25 chronic exercise studies of which 15 were reviewed previously [179] and 10 have been included in this review (Tables 13.2–13.5 [1, 15, 28, 34, 64, 66, 81, 99, 188, 193]). He reported that the average reduction with training for systolic blood pressure was 10.8 mmHg and for diastolic blood pressure it was 8.2 mmHg. Whether these mean values would be changed if his next analysis considered the results from studies 2, 17, 56, 57, 83, 88, 92, 122, 137, 138, 175, 189, 196 remains to be determined.

The end result is that it is no longer good scholarship or grantsmanship to state that exercise training will result in increases, decreases, or no changes in resting arterial blood pressure [152]. It is disappointing to observe in the more recent investigations that many researchers failed to include normotensive or hypertensive control groups, a point also made several years ago [91, 153, 179].

Either by chance or by design [158], it appears that most investigators studying hypertensive humans are prescribing aerobic endurance exercises between 40–70% O_2max. This approach has strong support from animal studies [179, 183, 187] because when the exercise intensities were increased to levels characterized as heavy or severe, blood pressures were usually higher than lower. Why swimming is so seldom used by researchers in human experiments is not clear. It is evident from the animal data summarized in Table 13.4 that the swimming of SHR groups was generally identified with marked reductions in resting pressures despite the fact that rats who swam for 35 minutes or longer usually were associated with acidosis, hypoxia, and hypercapnia [172]. We interpret this result as being a chemoreceptor-mediated response which is unique to swimming rats because running rats do not experience these types of blood changes [53, 172]. It is an interesting physiological question, however, and one that should be investigated in the future.

In 1984, I felt that resistive training that included free weights, circuit training, or isometric activities had no place in an exercise program designed for hypertensive populations because of their potential to elicit exaggerated pressor responses. I now favor a cautious approach because the preliminary results in Table 13.5 indicate that these fears are not justified when prudent guidelines are followed [44, 57, 66, 90, 163].

The research of the last decade has been important in identifying individuals who do not respond to an exercise training program [2, 92]. Factors to consider besides the intensity of the prescribed program are exercise systolic pressures over 230 mmHg and diastolic pressures higher than 110 mmHg, significantly elevated plasma catecholamine concentrations [34], and echocardiographic evidence for cardiac enlargement [103]. This latter point may be the most important guideline for children or young adolescents. Although not explained, the Kinoshita et al. [92] data on this matter included sex and the plasma sodium/potassium ratio.

Although I deliberately avoided discussing the role and importance of pharmacological agents in managing blood pressure in exercising subjects, this topic is deserving of a review article and detailed research in the future. A nonpharmacological approach for the management of hypertension is an admirable goal but inadequate for a population of 60 million hypertensives. Adequate human [15, 179] and animal studies [180] exist, however, to show that medication for hypertension can be reduced in some individuals or eliminated in others when combined with a moderate endurance training program.

As summarized in Table 13.3, most studies with hemodynamic measurements have demonstrated that chronic exercise is associated with lower resting pressures. The evidence is far from equivocal, however, as to whether reductions in cardiac output or total peripheral vascular resistance, or both, are responsible for this change. Because a variety of noninvasive methods and experimental designs were used to secure the hemodynamic data listed in Table 13.3, this must be taken into consideration in future studies before the experiments are planned and when the results are analyzed. Better standardization and understanding of methodology must occur before we will be able to determine which components of Poiseuille's Law [46] are responsible for the blood pressure-lowering effect associated with endurance training. We favor the explanation that a reduction in cardiac output has occurred [185]; however, more data are required before this possibility can be regarded as a viable concept.

Of the numerous mechanisms that could be responsible for the lowered resting blood pressure in responders, the ones that included reduced functions of the autonomic nervous system had the greatest experimental support [21, 34, 64, 81, 84, 92, 95, 122, 138, 146, 179, 186, 188]. Plasma norepinephrine spillover rate [81] and microneurographic recordings [45, 190] provide new approaches to investigate the contributions of the sympathetic nervous system in the training process and should be used more in the next decade.

The insulin hypothesis [105], especially as it pertains to borderline hypertension, have experimental support [36, 47, 98, 101, 118, 142, 161, 177, 195], to explain why resting blood pressures are elevated with an increase in fat mass and why they are reduced with training or when training and weight loss are combined. It would be advisable, therefore, for researchers to secure plasma insulin concentrations in studies that address the role of exercise training on resting blood pressure.

To date, it has been primarily the Japanese investigators [95, 122, 188] who have provided the most information on the relationship between training, electrolyte intake, and changes in resting blood pressure. Unfortunately, the results were difficult for extrapolation purposes because not all the studies had control groups [95, 122], or regulated electrolyte intakes [95, 188], or demonstrated a significant increase in the urinary excretion of sodium [188]. Some Japanese investigators [92, 188] have been reporting reductions in plasma volume with their training programs, presumably because of increases in sodium excretion or decreases in sodium intake, or both. Because training will increase plasma volume in normotensive [18] and hypertensive [122] humans as well as in hypertensive rats [179], it is difficult to reconcile these findings and to conclude that the reduction of resting blood pressure with training is directly related to electrolyte mechanisms. Unfortunately, the situation has not been helped by animal training studies with genetic models for salt sensitivity [110, 149, 157] because conflicting results have been reported and dose-response studies have not been conducted. The calcium hypothesis is intriguing [112, 113, 114], but the data have been too preliminary [33] for extrapolation purposes.

While it is well accepted that baroreceptor structure and function will change with the disease of hypertension [179], too much uncertainty currently prevails concerning how they are altered by chronic exercise to conclude that they have a primary role in the reduction of resting blood pressure with endurance training. This statement reflects a disappointment in expectations, because in 1984 we felt future research would demonstrate their contributions to the lowered resting pressures of trained populations. In fact, the role of the central nervous system in producing a trained state is virtually unknown. Until this situation changes, our explanations will be governed by peripheral mechanisms. The data summarized in Figure 13.1 are important because they show that the wall/lumen ratio of select arteries would change with endurance training of hypertensive rat populations by mechanisms that affect the lumen but not the wall areas [123, 186, our unpublished data]. On either a local, segmental, or regional basis, this change could alter vascular resistance provided that vascular smooth muscle tone remained constant or decreased. However, the impact of any structural changes by endurance training on whole body total peripheral resistance is not evident from the limited animal data available [185], or consistent when evaluating the hemodynamic results obtained from human subjects (Table 13.3). The importance of ventricular mass as a primary mechanism to explain the lowered resting blood pressure of trained population is debatable because changes in myocardial compliance must precede myocardial contractility alterations before modifications in stroke volume and cardiac output can occur. Thus, information about myocardial mass appears to be more useful for predicting hypertension in individuals than for identifying nonresponders who are participating in a training program.

The peptides and factors located in the myocardium [25, 94] and the endothelium [52, 63, 120, 160] are of interest and likely play a secondary role in lowering resting blood pressure with training because of their vasodilating influences and because ANP can promote diuresis and have an inhibitory effect on the sympathetic nervous system [76]. To date, however, the evidence that they are altered by endurance training is limited [49, 171].

Finally, there has been no convincing evidence from experimental animals published since 1984 to demonstrate that endurance training would lower resting blood pressure in renal hypertensive populations. Whether positive results would be obtained with a different specie is unknown and deserving of investigation, before we can convincingly conclude that the resting blood pressures of individuals with secondary hypertension will not benefit from chronic exercise.

RECOMMENDATIONS AND FUTURE DIRECTIONS

From the integrated information presented in the text, tables, and summaries, the following general recommendations and research directions are proposed for future human and animal research.

Acute Exercise
1. The role of acute exercise as a predictor of future hypertension deserves further investigation, especially in children whose parents have a history of hypertension, and in adults who exhibit various risk factors for hypertension. Experimental designs must consider not only the absolute value of the blood pressure response, but also the magnitude of the change in blood pressure at each established work load and attempt to establish norms that include race, sex, body mass, heart mass, and fitness levels. One primary objective of these research studies should be to replace the words "an exaggerated blood pressure response" with a more meaningful descriptive term. Statistical prediction studies are needed with school children that would relate the future blood pressure value to the organizational structure of the school (e.g., grades 3–6, 7–

9, 10–12). Although the step test has practical appeal, we favor the use of the bicycle ergometer for testing purposes because it is better for standardization purposes.

2. More studies are needed on the acute blood pressure responses of women.
3. Careful as well as additional studies are needed on the specific blood pressure responses of individuals who are either hypertensive or prone to become hypertensive who are performing various exercises associated with weight-lifting and circuit-training programs. In these investigations, concern must be given to the percentage of maximum weight being lifted. Emerging from these investigations should be data that will reinforce and modify existing medical guidelines and practices on the subject.
4. The elucidation of the mechanisms responsible for postexercise hypotension will require additional human and animal experiments, and should include experimental designs that consider the central and peripheral actions of exogenous opioids, sympathetic and serotonergic pathways, and the actions of the peptides and related factors released from the myocardium and the endothelium during exercise.
5. Postexercise hypotension investigations are required that will measure hemodynamic changes and will be concerned with the ethnic and fitness backgrounds of the subjects.

Epidemiological and Methodological Studies
1. There is little need for more investigations on the relationship between resting blood pressure and white sportsmen. There is justification, however, for more epidemiological studies on the relationship between fitness levels and resting blood pressures in younger and older females and with "minority" populations.
2. There is a need for ambulatory investigations that will determine the relationships between resting blood pressures and race, sex, time of day, posture when testing, and/or fitness classification.

Chronic Exercise
1. Investigators planning future studies on the chronic effects of exercise must include control groups within their experimental designs if they expect to make a contribution to the scientific literature.
2. Researchers planning future studies on the chronic effects of exercise with hypertensive populations must realize that many individuals will not respond to the training programs with a reduction in resting blood pressure. Investigations that attempt to identify and characterize those individuals who are responders and nonresponders are needed. It is recommended that in the

experimental design aspects related to the hyperresponsiveness of emotional and mental stimuli be considered, as well as the body mass and sex of the person, the magnitude of the resting plasma catecholamine concentration, the degree of cardiac hypertrophy, and the proposed intensity level of the prescribed exercise program.

3. It is recommended that well-supervised and monitored weight-lifting or circuit-training programs be initiated for hypertensive populations. Inherent in this recommendation is that the programs not be implemented until the acute pressor effects of the various lifting events have been quantified.

4. It is recommended that more hemodynamic investigations be undertaken with humans and animals to determine whether changes in cardiac output and/or total peripheral resistance are responsible for the lowered resting arterial blood pressure with training. To help resolve the current controversy on the topic, different methodologies should be compared in the same subjects.

5. It is recommended that the microneurographic technique to record sympathetic nerve traffic be utilized with hypertensive populations to study the longitudinal effects of chronic exercise.

6. Studies with trained and nontrained, stroke-prone hypertensive rats are needed to determine whether a reduction in resting or basal sympathetic tone is associated with an increase in the incidence of cerebrovascular lesions.

7. Investigators planning to conduct chronic exercise studies with obese or overweight hypertensive animals or humans should consider including within the experimental design the effects of insulin on sympathetic nervous system activity and on sodium reabsorption.

8. Investigators planning to conduct chronic exercise and electrolyte studies with hypertensive populations should consider within their experimental designs the measurements of electrolyte intakes, electrolyte excretions, plasma volumes, and the plasma concentrations of insulin and aldosterone. To advance our current knowledge on this topic, control subjects are essential.

9. Animal and human studies are needed to test the hypothesis that chronic exercise and the supplement of exogenous calcium will result in significantly lower resting blood pressures in hypertensive populations when compared to their nontrained controls.

10. Animal and human studies are needed to resolve the controversy over whether chronic exercise can significantly change the functions of baroreceptors that would be associated with lower resting blood pressures.

11. Experimental studies are needed to explore the role of the central

nervous system in the regulation of resting blood pressure in trained normotensive and hypertensive humans and rats.
12. Experimental studies are needed to examine the relationships between chronic exercise and the influences from the endothelium on the resting blood pressures of hypertensive populations.

ACKNOWLEDGEMENT

This review was supported in part by funds from NIH grant HL 37782-04. The author thanks Dr. Douglas R. Seals for his critical comments and helpful suggestions associated with the preparation of this manuscript.

REFERENCES

1. Adragna, N.C., J.L. Chang, M.C. Morey, and R.S. Williams. Effect of exercise on cation transport in human red cells. *Hypertension* 7:132–139, 1985.
2. Attina, D.A., G. Guiliano, G. Arcangeli, R. Musante and V. Cupelli. Effects of one year of physical training on borderline hypertension: an evaluation by bicycle ergometer exercise testing. *J. Cardiovasc. Pharmacol.* 8(Suppl. 5):S145–S147, 1986.
3. Ayachi, S. Increased dietary calcium lowers blood pressure in spontaneously hypertensive rat. *Metabolism* 28:1234–1238, 1979.
4. Baglivo, H.P., G. Fabreques, H. Burrieza, R.C. Esper, M. Talarico, and R.J. Esper. Effect of moderate physical training on left ventricular mass in mild hypertensive persons. *Hypertension* 15(Suppl. 1):I153–I156, 1990.
5. Baumbach, G.L., P.B. Dorbrin, M.N. Hart, and D.D. Heistad. Mechanics of cerebral arterioles in hypertensive rats. *Circ. Res.* 62:56–64, 1988.
6. Bedford, T.G., and C.M. Tipton. Exercise training and the arterial baroreflex. *J. Appl. Physiol.* 63:1926–1932, 1987.
7. Belizan, J.M., J. Vilar, O. Pineda, et al. Reductions of blood pressure with calcium supplementation in young adults. *J.A.M.A.* 249:1161–1165, 1983.
8. Benbassat, J., and P.F. Froom. Blood pressure response to exercise as a predictor of hypertension. *Arch. Intern. Med.* 146:2053–2055, 1986.
9. Bishop, V.S., J.R. Haywood, R.E. Shade, M. Siegel, and C. Hamm. Aortic baroreceptor deafferentation in the baboon. *J. Appl. Physiol.* 60:798–801, 1986.
10. Blair, S.N., N.N. Goodyear, L.W. Gibbons, and K.H. Cooper. Physical fitness and incidence of hypertension in healthy normotensive men and women. *J.A.M.A.* 252:487–490, 1984.
11. Block, L.H., B.E. Lutold, P. Bolli, W. Kiowski, and F.R. Buhler. High salt intake blunts plasma catecholamine and renin responses to exercise: less suppressive epinephrine in borderline essential hypertension. *J. Cardiovasc. Pharmacol.* 6(Suppl. 1):S95–S100, 1984.
12. Boone, J.B., M. Levine, M.G. Flynn, F.X. Pizza, G.R. Kubitz, and F.F. Andres. Opioid receptor modulation of post exercise hypotension. *Med. Sci. Sports Exerc.* 22(Suppl. II):S106, 1990 (Abstract).
13. Borghi, C., F. Costa, S. Boschi, and E. Ambrosioni. Impaired vasodilator capacity and exaggerated pressor response to isometric exercise in subjects with family history of hypertension. *Am. J. Hypertens.* 1:1065–1095, 1988.
14. Buck, C., and A.P. Donner. Isometric occupational exercise and the incidence of hypertension. *J. Occup. Med.* 27:370–372, 1985.

15. Cade, R., R. Mars, H. Wagemaker, et al. Effect of aerobic exercise training on patients with systemic arterial hypertension. *Am. J. Med.* 77:785–790, 1984.

16. Chaney, R.H., and R.K. Eyman. Blood pressure at rest and during maximal dynamic and isometric exercise as predictors of systemic hypertension. *Am. J. Cardiol.* 62:1058–1061, 1988.

17. Cleroux, J., F. Peronnet, and J. de Champlain. Effects of exercise training on plasma catecholamines and blood pressure in labile hypertensive subjects. *Eur. J. Appl. Physiol.* 56:550–554, 1987.

18. Convertino, V.A., J.E. Greenleaf, and E.M. Bernauer. Role of thermal and exercise factors in the mechanism of hypervolemia. *J. Appl. Physiol.* 48:657–664, 1980.

19. Convertino, V.A., L.C. Keil, and J.E. Greenleaf. Plasma volume, renin and vasopressin responses to graded exercise after training. *J. Appl. Physiol.* 54:508–514, 1983.

20. Convertino, V.A., C.A. Thompson, D.L. Eckberg, J.M. Fritsch, G.W. Mack, and E.R. Nadel. Baroreflex responses and LBNP tolerance following exercise training. *Physiologist* 33:(Suppl. 1):S40–S44, 1990.

21. Cox, R.H., J.W. Hubbard, J.E. Lawler, B.J. Sanders, and V.P. Mitchell. Exercise training attenuates stress-induced hypertension in the rat. *Hypertension* 7:747–751, 1985.

22. Coyle, P., and D.D. Heistad. Blood flow through cerebral collateral vessels in hypertensive and normotensive rats. *Hypertension* 8(Suppl. II):II67–II71, 1986.

23. Cureton, T.K. Jr. *Physical Fitness Appraisal and Guidance.* St. Louis: C.V. Mosby, 1947, pp. 218–219.

24. Darga, L.L., C.P. Lucas, T.R. Spafford, M.A. Schork, W.R. Illis, and N. Holden. Endurance training in middle-aged physicians. *Phys. Sportsmed.* 17:(7)85–101, 1989.

25. de Bold, A.J., H.B. Borenstin, A.T. Veress, and H.A. Sonnenberg. A rapid and potent natriuretic response to intravenous injections of atrial myocardial extract in rats. *Life Sci.* 28:89–94, 1981.

26. DiCarlo, S.E., and V.S. Bishop. Exercise training enhances cardiac afferent inhibition of baroreflex function. *Am. J. Physiol.* 258:H212–H220, 1990.

27. DiCarlo, S.E., and V.S. Bishop. Regional vascular resistance during exercise: role of cardiac afferents and exercise training. *Am. J. Physiol.* 258:H842–H847, 1990.

28. De Plaen, J.E., and J.M. Detry. Hemodynamic effects of physical training in established hypertension. *Acta Cardiol.* 35:179–188, 1980.

29. Dlin, R. Blood pressure response to dynamic exercise in healthy and hypertensive youths. *Pediatrician* 13:34–43, 1986.

30. Drory, Y., A. Pines, E.Z. Fisman, et al. Exercise testing in juvenile borderline hypertension. *Isr. J. Med. Sci.* 23:807–810, 1987.

31. Drory, Y., A. Pines, E.Z. Fisman, and J.J. Kellermann. Exercise responses in young women with borderline hypertension. *Chest* 97:298–301, 1990.

32. Drummond, H.A., L.A. Sebastian, P.E. Edwards, R.K. Coomes, and C.M. Tipton. Influence of training on the resting blood pressure of normotensive rats consuming a diet high in fat and sucrose. *Physiologist* 33:A75, 1990 (Abstract).

33. Drummond, H., L.A. Sebastian, P.K. Edwards, R.K. Coomes, and C.M. Tipton. The influence of exercise training and calcium diets on the resting blood pressures of hypertensive rats (SHR) *Med. Sci. Sports Exerc.* 22(Suppl. II):S608, 1990 (Abstract).

34. Duncan, J.J., J.E. Farr, S.J. Upton, R.D. Hagan, M.E. Oglesby, and S.N. Blair. The effects of aerobic exercise on plasma catecholamines and blood pressure in patients with mild essential hypertension. *J.A.M.A.* 254:2609–2613, 1985.

35. Edwards, J.G., and C.M. Tipton. Influences of exogenous insulin on arterial blood pressure measurements of the rat. *J. Appl. Physiol.* 67:2335–2342, 1989.

36. Edwards, J.G., C.M. Tipton, and R.D. Matthes. Influence of exercise training on reactivity and contractility of arterial strips from hypertensive rats. *J. Appl. Physiol.* 58:1683–1688, 1985.

37. Effron, M.B. Effects of resistive training on left ventricular function. *Med. Sci. Sports Exerc.* 21:694–697, 1989.

38. Eliahou, H.E., A. Iaina, T. Gaon, J. Scochar, and M. Modan. Body weight reduction necessary to attain normotension in overweight hypertensive patient. *Int. J. Obes.* 5(Suppl. 1):157–163, 1981.

39. Esler, M., G. Jennings, P. Korner, et al. Assessment of human sympathetic nervous system from measurements of norepinephrine turnover. *Hypertension* 11:3–20, 1988.

40. Fagard, R., J. Staessen, and A. Amery. Maximal aerobic power in essential hypertension. *J. Hypertens.* 6:859–865, 1988.

41. Faraci, F.M., W.G. Mayhan, W.H. Werber, and D.D. Heistad. Cerebral circulation: effects of sympathetic nerves and protective mechanisms during hypertension. *Circ. Res.* 61(Suppl II):II102–II106, 1987.

42. Ferrara, L.A., M. Mancini, G. De Simone, M.L. Fasano, and M. Mancini. Left ventricular mass and blood pressure during ergometric exercise in primary hypertension. *Jpn. Heart J.* 28:349–355, 1987.

43. Fixler, D., W.P. Laird, and K. Dana. Usefulness of exercise stress testing for prediction of blood pressure trends. *Pediatrics* 75:1071–1075, 1985.

44. Fleck, S.J. Cardiovascular adaptations to resistance training. *Med. Sci. Sports Exerc.* 20:(5)Suppl S146–S151, 1988.

45. Floras, J.S., C.A. Sinkey, P.E. Aylward, D.R. Seals, P.N. Thoren, and A.L. Mark. Postexercise hypotension and sympathoinhibition in borderline hypertensive men. *Hypertension* 14:28–35, 1989.

46. Folkow, B. Physiological aspects of primary hypertension. *Physiol. Rev.* 62:347–503, 1982.

47. Fournier, A.M., M.T. Gadia, D.B. Kubrusly, J.S. Skyler, and J.M. Sosenko. Blood pressure, insulin and glycemia in nondiabetic subjects. *Am. J. Med.* 80:861–864, 1986.

48. Fraser, G.E., R.L. Phillips, and R. Harris. Physical fitness and blood pressure in children. *Circulation* 67:405–412, 1983.

49. Freud, B.J., C.E. Wade, and J.R. Claybaugh. Effect of exercise on atrial natriuetic factor. *Sports Med.* 6:346–364, 1988.

50. Fripp, R.R., J.L. Hodgson, P.O. Kwiterovich, M.C. Werner, H.G. Schuler, and V. Whitman. Aerobic capacity, obesity and atherosclerotic risk factors in adolescents. *Pediatrics* 75:813–818, 1985.

51. Frohlich, E.G. The heart in hypertension: unresolved conceptual challenges. *Hypertension* 11(Suppl I):I-19–I-24, 1988.

52. Furchgott, R.F. The role of the endothelium in responses of vascular smooth muscle. *Circ. Res.* 53:557–573, 1983.

53. Geenen, D., P. Buttrick, and J. Scheuer. Cardiovascular and hormonal responses to swimming and running in the rat. *J. Appl. Physiol.* 65:116–123, 1988.

54. Ghaemmaghami, F., A. Sassolas, G. Gauquelin, et al. Swim training in genetically hypertensive rats of the Lyon strain: effects on plasma lipids and lipoproteins. *J. Hypertens.* 4:319–324, 1986.

55. Gilders, R.M., C. Voner, and G.A. Dudley. Endurance training and blood pressure in normotensive and hypertensive adults. *Med. Sci. Sports Exerc.* 21:629–636, 1989.

56. Gleichmann, U.M., H-H Philippi, S.I. Gleichmann, et al. Group exercise improves patient compliance in mild to moderate hypertension. *J. Hypertens.* 7(Suppl. 3):S77–S80, 1989.

57. Goldberg, A.P. Aerobic and resistive exercise modify risk factors for coronary heart disease. *Med. Sci. Sports Exerc.* 21:669–674, 1989.

58. Goldberg, A.P., E.M. Geltman, J.R. Gavin III, et al. Exercise training reduces coronary risk and effectively rehabilitates hemodialysis patients. *Nephron* 42:311–316, 1986.

59. Gray, S.D. Histochemical analysis of capillary and fiber-type distributions in skeletal muscles of spontaneously hypertensive rats. *Microvas. Res.* 36:228–238, 1988.
60. Gryglewski, R.J., R.M. Botting, and J.R. Vane. Mediators produced by the endothelial cell. *Hypertension* 12:530–548, 1988.
61. Hagberg, J.M. Exercise, fitness and hypertension. *Exercise, Fitness and Health.* C. Bouchard, R.J. Shephard, T. Stephens, J.R. Sutton, and B.D. McPherson (eds.). Champaign, IL: Human Kinetics, 1990, pp. 455–456.
62. Hagberg. J.M., A.A. Ehsani, D. Goldring, A. Hernandez, D.R. Sinacore, and J.O. Holloszy. Effect of weight training on blood pressure and hemodynamics in hypertensive adolescents. *J. Pediat.* 104:147–151, 1984.
63. Hagberg, J.M., S.J. Montain, and W.H. Martin. Blood pressure and hemodynamic responses after exercise in older hypertensives. *J. Appl. Physiol.* 63:270–276, 1987.
64. Hagberg, J.M., S.J. Montain, W.H. Martin, and A.A. Ehsani. Effect of exercise training in 60–69 year-old persons with essential hypertension. *Am. J. Cardiol.* 64:348–353, 1989.
65. Hanson, J.S., and W.H. Nedde. Preliminary observations on physical training for hypertensive males. *Cir. Res.* 26(Suppl. 1):I49–I53, 1970.
66. Harris, K.A., and R.G. Holly. Physiological responses to circuit weight training in borderline hypertensive subjects *Med. Sci. Sports Exerc.* 19:246–252, 1987.
67. Harshfield, G.A., L.M. Dupaul, B.S. Alpert, et al. Aerobic fitness and the diurnal rhythm of blood pressure in adolescents. *Hypertension* 15:810–814, 1990.
68. Heistad, D.D., F.M. Abboud, and D.R. Ballard. Relationship between plasma sodium concentration and vascular reactivity in man. *J. Clin. Invest.* 50:2022–2032, 1971.
69. Higuchi, H., I. Hashimoto, and K. Yamakawa. Effect of exercise training on aortic collagen content spontaneously hypertensive rats (SHR). *Eur. J. Appl. Physiol.* 53:330–333, 1985.
70. Higuchi, S., A. Takeshita, H. Higashi, et al. Lowering calcium in the nucleus tractus solitarius causes hypotension and bradycardia. *Am. J. Physiol.* 250:H226–H230, 1986.
71. Hoffmann, P. Endogenous Opiod Effects Elicited by Muscle Activity. An Attempt to Explain Cardiovascular, Analgesic and Behavioral Mechanisms of Exercise. Ph.D. Thesis, Univ. Goteborg, 1–59, 1990.
72. Hoffmann, P., S. Carlsson, J.O. Skarphedinsson, and P. Thoren. Role of different serotonergic receptors in the long-lasting blood pressure depression following muscle stimulation in the spontaneously hypertensive rat. *Acta Physiol. Scand.* 139:305–310, 1990.
73. Hoffmann, P., P. Friberg, D. Ely, and P. Thoren. Effects of spontaneous running on blood pressure, heart rate and cardiac dimensions in developing and established spontaneous hypertension in rats. *Acta Physiol. Scand.* 129:535–542, 1987.
74. Hoffmann, P., and P. Thoren. Long-lasting cardiovascular depression induced by acupuncture-like stimulation of the sciatic nerve in unanaesthetized rats. Effects of arousal and type of hypertension. *Acta Physiol. Scand.* 127:119–126, 1986.
75. Hofman, A., H.A. Walter, P.A. Connelly, and R.D. Vaughan. Blood pressure and physical fitness in children. *Hypertension* 9:188–191, 1987.
76. Holtz, J., O. Sommer, and E. Bassenge. Inhibition of sympathoadrenal activity by atrial natriuretic factor in dogs. *Hypertension* 9:350–354, 1987.
77. Horan, M.J., and C. Lenfant. Epidemiology of blood pressure and predictors of hypertension. *Hypertension* 15(Suppl I):I-20–I-24, 1990.
78. Horan, M.J., and S.C. Mockrin. Hypertension research: the next five years. *Hypertension* 15(Suppl I):I-25–I-28, 1990.
79. Horton, E.S. The role of exercise in the treatment of hypertension in obesity. *Int. J. Obes.* 5(Suppl 1):165–171, 1981.
80. Iskandrian, A.S., and J. Heo. Exaggerated systolic blood pressure response to exercise: a normal variant or a hyperdynamic phase of essential hypertension? *Int. J. Cardiol.* 18:207–217, 1988.

81. Jennings, G., L. Nelson, P. Nestel, et al. The effects of changes in physical activity on major cardiovascular risk factors, hemodynamics, sympathetic function, and glucose utilization in man: a controlled study of four levels of activity. *Circulation* 73:30–40, 1986.

82. Jette, M., F. Landry, K. Sidney, and G. Blumchen. Exaggerated blood pressure response to exercise in the detection of hypertension. *J. Cardiopulm. Rehab.* 8:171–177, 1988.

83. Jo, Y., M. Arita, A. Baba, et al. Blood pressure and sympathetic activity following responses to aerobic exercise in patients with essential hypertension. *Clin. Exp. Theory Pract.* A 11(Suppl. 1):411–417, 1989.

84. Johnson, W.P., and J.A. Grover. Hemodynamic and metabolic effects of physical training in four patients with essential hypertension. *Can. Med. Assoc. J.* 96:842–846, 1967.

85. Joint National Committee on Detection, Evaluation, and Treatment of High Blood Pressure. The 1988 report of the Joint National Committee on Detection, Evaluation, and Treatment of High Blood Pressure. *Arch. Int. Med.* 148:1023–1038, 1988.

86. Juhlin-Dannfelt, A., M. Frisk-Holmberg, J. Karlsson, and P. Tesch. Central and peripheral circulation in relation to muscle-fiber composition in normo- and hypertensive man. *Clin. Sci.* 56:335–340, 1979.

87. Kaplan, N.M. *Clinical Hypertension*. Baltimore: Williams and Wilkins, 1978, pp. 94–159.

88. Kasch, F.W., J.L. Boyer, S.P. Van Camp, L.S. Verity, and J.P. Wallace. The effect of physical activity and inactivity on aerobic power in older men (a longitudinal study). *Phys. Sportsmed.* 16(4):73–83, 1990.

89. Kaufman, F.L., R.L. Hughson, and J.P. Schaman. Effect of exercise on recovery blood pressure in normotensive and hypertensive subjects. *Med. Sci. Sports Exerc.* 19:17–20, 1987.

90. Kelemen, M.H. Resistive training safety and assessment guidelines for cardiac and coronary prone patients. *Med. Sci. Sports Exerc.* 21:675–677, 1989.

91. Kenney, W.L., and E.J. Zambraski. Physical activity in human hypertension: a mechanisms approach. *Sports Med.* 1:459–473, 1984.

92. Kinoshita, A., H. Urata, Y. Tanabe, et al. What types of hypertensives respond better to mild exercise therapy. *J. Hpertens.* 6:(Suppl. 4):S631–S633, 1988.

93. Kish, B. Electron microscopy of the atrium of the heart. I. The guinea pig. *Exp. Med. Surg.* 14:99–112, 1956.

94. Kirwan, J., D.L. Costill, M.G. Flynn, et al. Physiological responses to successive days of intensive training in competitive swimmers. *Med. Sci. Sports Exerc.* 208:255–259, 1988.

95. Kiveloff, B., and O. Huber. Brief maximal isometric exercise in hypertension. *J. Am. Geriatr. Soc.* 19:1006–1012, 1971.

96. Kiyonaga, A., K. Arakawa, H. Tanaka, and M. Shindo. Blood pressure and hormonal responses to aerobic exercise. *Hypertension* 7:125–131, 1985.

97. Kral, J., J. Chrastek, and J. Adamirova. The hypotensive effect of physical activity. W. Raab (ed). *Prevention of Ischemic Heart Disease: Principles and Practice*. Springfield, IL: Charles C. Thomas, 1966.

98. Krotkiewski, M., K. Mandroukas, L. Sjostrom, L. Sullivan, H. Wetterquist, and P. Bjorntorp. Effects of long-term physical training on body fat, metabolism and blood pressure in obesity. *Metabolism* 28:650–658, 1979.

99. Kukkonen, R. Rauramaa, E. Voutilainen, and E. Lansimies. Physical training of middle-aged men with borderline hypertension. *Ann. Clin. Res.* 14(Suppl 34) 139–145, 1982.

100. Kunii, S., Y. Fukuda, K. Wakabayashi, H. Fumino, K. Hirota, and H. Kita. Effect of exercise on blood pressure and attack of cerebrovascular lesions of stroke-prone spontaneously hypertensive rats (SHRSP). *Jpn. J. Phys. Educ.* 27:35–46, 1982.

101. Landsberg, L., and J.B. Young. Diet and the sympathetic nervous system relationship to hypertension. *Int. J. Obes.* 5:79–92, 1981.
102. Lau, K., and B. Eby. The role of calcium in genetic hypertension. *Hypertension* 7:657–667, 1985.
103. Lauer, R.M., T.L. Burns, L.T. Mahoney, and C.M. Tipton. Blood pressure in children. C.V. Gisolfi and D.R. Lamb (eds.). *Perspectives in Exercise Science and Sports Medicine.* Indianapolis: Benchmark Press, 2:431–463, 1989.
104. Lehmann, M., and J. Keul. Haufigkeit der hypertonie bei 810 Mannlichen Sportlern. *Zeits. Kardiol.* 73:137–141, 1984.
105. Lucas, C.P., J.A. Estigarribia, L.L. Darga, and G.M. Reaven. Insulin and blood pressure in obesity. *Hypertension* 7:702–706, 1985.
106. Lund-Johansen, P. Central haemodynamics in essential hypertension at rest and during exercise—a 20 year follow-up study. *J. Hypertens.* 7:(Suppl 6):S52–S55, 1989.
107. Lutgemeier, I., F.C. Luft, T. Unger, et al. Blood pressure, electrolyte and adrenal responses in swim-trained hypertensive rats. *J. Hypertens.* 5:241–247, 1987.
108. MacDougall, J.D., D. Tuxen, D.G. Sale, J.R. Moroz, and J.R. Sutton. Arterial blood pressure response to heavy resistance exercise. *J. Appl. Physiol.* 58:785–790, 1985.
109. Manicardi, V., L. Camellini, G. Bellodi, C. Coscelli, and E. Ferrannini. Evidence for an association of high blood pressure and hyperinsulinemia in obese man. *J. Clin. Endocrinol. Metab.* 62:1302–1304, 1986.
110. Marcus, K.D., and C.M. Tipton. Exercise training and its effects with renal hypertensive rats. *J. Appl. Physiol.* 59:1410–1415, 1985.
111. Marraccini, P., C. Palombo, S. Giaconi, et al. Reduced cardiovascular efficiency and increased reactivity during exercise in borderline and established hypertension. *Am. J. Hypertens.* 2:913–916, 1989.
112. McCarron, D.A. Is calcium more important than sodium in the pathogenesis of essential hypertension? *Hypertension* 7:607–627, 1985.
113. McCarron, D.A., C.D. Morris, H.J. Henry, and J.L. Stanton. Blood pressure and nutrient intake in the United States. *Science* 224:1392–1398, 1984.
114. McCarron, D.A., N. Nyung, B. Augoretz, and S. Krutzik. Disturbance of calcium metabolism in the spontaneously hypertensive rat. *Hypertension* 3(Suppl. I):I162–I167, 1981.
115. Melin, J.A., W. Wijns, H. Pouleur, et al. Ejection fraction response to upright exercise in hypertension: relation to loading condition and to contractility. *Int. J. Cardiol.* 17:37–49, 1987.
116. Molineux, D., and A. Steptoe. Exaggerated blood pressure responses to submaximal exercise in normotensive adolescents with a family history of hypertension. *J. Hypertens.* 6:361–365, 1988.
117. Montain, S.J., S.M. Jilka, A.A. Ehsani, and J.M. Hagberg. Altered hemodynamics during exercise in older essential hypertensive subjects. *Hypertension* 12:479–484, 1988.
118. Mondon, C.E., G.M. Reaven, S. Azhar, C.M. Lee, and R. Rabkin. Abnormal insulin metabolism by specific organs from rats with spontaneous hypertension. *Am. J. Physiol.* 257:E491–E498, 1989.
119. Mondon, C.E., and G.M. Reaven. Evidence of abnormalities of insulin metabolism in rats with spontaneous hypertension. *Metabolism* 37:303–305, 1988.
120. Mortensen, Luke H., C.M. Pawloski, N.L. Kanagy, and G.D. Fink. Chronic hypertension produced by infusion of endothelin in rats. *Hypertension* 15:729–733, 1990.
121. Noma, K., H. Rupp, and R. Jacob. Subacute and long term effect of swimming training on blood pressure in young and old spontaneously hypertensive rats. *Cardiovasc. Res.* 21:871–877, 1987.
122. Nomura, G., E. Kumagai, K. Midorikhwa, T. Kitano, H. Tashiro, and H. Toshima. Physical training in essential hypertension: alone and in combination with dietary salt restriction. *J. Cardiac. Rehab.* 4:469–475, 1984.

123. Oppliger, R.A., T. Hodgins, C.M. Tipton, A.C. Vailas, and K.D. Marcus. The influence of training on wall lumen ratio of WKY & SHR populations. *Med. Sci. Sports Exerc.* 12:130, 1980. (Abstract)

124. Overton, J.M., M.J. Joyner, and C.M. Tipton. Reductions in blood pressure after acute exercise by hypertensive rats. *J. Appl. Physiol.* 64:748–752, 1988.

125. Overton, J.M., C.M. Tipton, R.D. Matthes, and J.R. Leininger. Voluntary exercise and its effect on young SHR and stroke-prone hypertensive rats. *J. Appl. Physiol.* 61:318–324, 1986.

126. Paffenbarger, R.S., A.L. Wing, R.T. Hyde, and D.L. Jung. Physical activity and incidence of hypertension in college alumni. *Am. J. Epidemiol.* 117:245–257, 1983.

127. Painter, P.L., J.N. Nelson-Worel, M.M. Hill, et al. Effects of exercise training during hemodyalysis. *Nephron* 43:87–92, 1986.

128. Panico, S., E. Celentano, V. Krogh, et al. Physical activity and its relationship to blood pressure in children. *J. Chron. Dis.* 40:925–930, 1987.

129. Paulev, P-E., R. Jordal, O. Kristensen, and J. Ladefoged. Therapeutic effect of exercise on hypertension. *Eur. J. Appl. Physiol.* 53:180–185, 1984.

130. Perkins, K.A., P.M. Dubbert, J.E. Martin, M.E. Faulstich, and J.K. Harris. Cardio-vascular reactivity to psychological stress in aerobically trained versus untrained mild hypertensives and normotensives. *Health Psychol.* 5:407–421, 1986.

131. Petzl, D.H., E. Hartter, W. Osterode, H. Bohm, and W. Woloszcuk. Atrial natriuretic peptide release due to physical exercise in healthy persons and in cardiac patients. *Klin. Wochenschr.* 65:194–196, 1987.

132. Pfeffer, M.A., B.A. Ferrell, J.M. Pfeffer, A.K. Weiss, M.C. Fishbein, and E.D. Frohlich. Ventricular morphology and pumping ability of exercised spontaneously hypertensive rats. *Am. J. Physiol.* 235:H193–H199, 1978.

133. Podolsky, M.L. Don't rule out sports for hypertensive children. *The Physician Sports Med.* 17:(9)164–170, 1989.

134. Qualy, J.M., and T.C. Westfall. Release of norepinephrine from the paraventricular hypothalamic nucleus of hypertensive rats. *Am. J. Physiol.* 254:H993–H1003, 1988.

135. Rakusan, K., P. Wicker, M. Abdul-Samad, B. Healy, and Z. Turek. Failure of swimming exercise to improve capillarization in cardiac hypertrophy of renal hypertensive rats. *Circ. Res.* 61:641–647, 1987.

136. Raven, P.B., and G.H. Stevens. Endurance exercise training reduces orthostatic tolerance in humans. *Physiologist* 33:(Suppl. 1):S56–S58, 1990.

137. Reiling, M.J., L.A. Clayton-Bare, P.B. Chase, and D.R. Seals. Effects of low-level exercise training (ET) on resting and ambulatory blood pressure (BP) in older persons. *Physiologist* 31:A158, 1988 (Abstract).

138. Reiling, M.J., L.A. Bare, P.B. Chase, and D.R. Seals. Influence of regular exercise on 24-hour blood pressure (BP 24) in middle aged and older person with mild essential hypertension (EH). *Med. Sci. Sports Exerc.* 22:(2)S48, 1990 (Abstract).

139. Reis, D.J., S. Morrison, and D.A. Ruggiero. The C1 area of the brainstem in tonic and reflex control of blood pressure. *Hypertension* 11:(Suppl. I):I-8–I-13, 1988.

140. Ressel, J., J. Chrastek, and J. Jandova. Hemodynamic effects of physical training in essential hypertension. *Acta. Cardiol.* 32:121–133, 1977.

141. Robertson, J.S. Salt and hypertension—a dangerous myth? *Public Health* 102:513–517, 1988.

142. Rocchini, A.P., V. Katch, A. Schork, and R.P. Kelch. Insulin and blood pressure during weight loss in obese adolescents. *Hypertension* 10:267–273, 1987.

143. Rocchini, A.P., C.P. Moorehead, S. De Remer, and D. Bondie. Pathogenesis of weight-related changes in blood pressure in dogs. *Hypertension* 13:922–928, 1989.

144. Rogers, M.A., C. Yamamoto, J.M. Hagberg, W.H. Martin III, A.A. Ehsani, and J.O. Holloszy. Effect of 6d of exercise training on responses to maximal and submaximal exercise in middle-aged men. *Med. Sci. Sports Exerc.* 208:260–264, 1988.

145. Roman, O., A.L. Camuzzi, E. Villalon, and C. Klenner. Physical training program

in arterial hypertension: a long-term prospective follow-up. *Cardiology* 67:230–243, 1981.

146. Rupp, H. Differential effect of physical exercise volumes on ventricular myosin and peripheral catecholamine stores in normotensive and spontaneously hypertensive rats. *Cir. Res.* 65:370–377, 1989.

147. Saito, Y., K. Nakao, A. Sugawara, et al. Exaggerated secretion of atrial natriuretic polypeptide during dynamic exercise in patients with essential hypertension. *Am. Heart J.* 116:1052, 1988.

148. Sannerstedt, R., H. Wasir, R. Henning, and L. Werko. Systemic haemodynamics in mild atrial hypertension before and after physical training. *Clin. Sci. Molec. Med.* 45:S145–S149, 1973.

149. Savage, M.V., G.F. Mackie, and C.P. Bolter. Effect of exercise on the development of salt-induced hypertension in Dahl-S rats. *J. Hypertens.* 4:289–293, 1986.

150. Scheuer, J., and C.M. Tipton. Cardiovascular adaptations to physical training. *Annu. Rev. Physiol.* 39:221–251, 1977.

151. Schieken, R.M., W.R. Clarke, and R.M. Lauer. Left ventricular hypertrophy in children with blood pressures in the upper quintile of the distribution: the muscatine study. *Hypertension* 3:669–675, 1981.

152. Schneider, E.C., and P.V. Karpovich. *The Physiology of Muscular Activity*, 3rd ed. Philadelphia: W.B. Saunders, 1948, p. 197.

153. Seals, D.R., and J.M. Hagberg. The effect of exercise training on human hypertension: a review. *Med. Sci. Sports Exerc.* 16:207–215, 1984.

154. Secher, N.H., M. Kjaer, and H. Galbo. Arterial blood pressure at the onset of dynamic exercise in partially curarized man. *Acta Physiol. Scand.* 133:233–237, 1988.

155. Sharma, R.V., R.J. Tomanek, and R.C. Bhalla. Effect of swimming training on cardiac function and myosin ATPase activity in SHR. *J. Appl. Physiol.* 59:758–765, 1985.

156. Shen, Y-T, M.A. Young, J. Ohanian, R.M. Graham, and S.F. Vatner. Atrial natriuretic factor-induced systemic vasoconstriction in conscious dogs, rats and monkeys. *Circ. Res.* 66:647–661, 1990.

157. Shepherd, R.E., M.L. Kuehne, K.A. Kenno, J.L. Durstine, T.W. Balon, and J.P. Rapp. Attenuation of blood pressure increases in Dahl salt-sensitive rats by exercise. *J. Appl. Physiol.* 42:1608–1613, 1982.

158. Shindo, M., H. Tanaka, S. Ohara, and I. Tokuyama. Training of 50% $\dot{V}o_2$max on healthy middle aged men by bicycle ergometer. *Rep. Res. Cen. Phys. Ed.* 2:139–152, 1974 (In Japanese, see Kinoshita).

159. Shyu, B.C., and P. Thoren. Circulatory events following spontaneous muscle exercise in normotensive and hypertensive rats. *Acta. Physiol. Scand.* 128:515–524, 1986.

160. Simonson, M.S., and M.J. Dunn. Endothelin. Pathways of transmembrane signaling. *Hypertension* 15(2 Suppl.):I5–I12, 1990.

161. Sims, E.A.H. Mechanisms of hypertension in the overweight. *Hypertension* 4(Suppl. III):III43–III-40, 1982.

162. Skoog, K.M., and M.L. Mangiapane. Area postrema and cardiovascular regulation in rats. *Am. J. Physiol.* 254:H963–H969, 1988.

163. Sparling, P.B., and Cantwell, J.D. Strength training guidelines for cardiac patients. *The Physician Sportsmed.* 17(3):191–194, 1989.

164. Spence, D.W., L.H. Peterson, and V.E. Friedewald, Jr. Relation of blood pressure during exercise to anaerobic metabolism. *Am. J. Cardiol.* 59:1342–1344, 1987.

165. Stamler, R., J. Stamler, R. Grimm, et al. Nutritional therapy for high blood pressure: final report of a four-year randomized controlled trail—The hypertension control program. *J.A.M.A.* 257:1484–1491, 1987.

166. Stasch, J.P., S. Kazada, C. Hirth, and F. Morich. Role of nisoldipine on blood pressure cardiac hypertrophy and atrial natriuretic peptides in spontaneously hypertensive rats. *Hypertension* 10:303–307, 1987.

167. Steinhaus, A.H. Chronic effects of exercise. *Physiol. Rev.* 13:103–147, 1933.
168. Stewart, K.J. Resistive training effects on strength and cardiovascular endurance in cardiac and coronary prone patients. *Med. Sci. Sports Exerc.* 21:678–682, 1989.
169. Stokes, J., W.B. Kannel, P.A. Wolf, R.B. D'Agostino, and L.A. Cupples. Blood pressure as a risk factor for cardiovascular disease: the Framingham Study—30 years of follow-up. *Hypertension* 13(Suppl I):I13–I18, 1989.
170. Stoney, C.M., and K.A. Matthews. Parental history of hypertension and myocardial infarction predicts cardiovascular responses to behavioral stressor in middle-aged men and women. *Psychophysiology* 25:269–277, 1988.
171. Stump, C.S., S.M. Bealieu, J.M. Overton, L.A. Sebastian, Z. Rahman, and C.M. Tipton. The influence of anesthesia and exercise on plasma atrial natriuretic peptide (ANP) in trained and nontrained spontaneously hypertensive rats (SHR). *Physiologist,* 31:A128, 1988 (Abstract).
172. Sturek, M.L., T.G. Bedford, C.M. Tipton, and L. Newcomer. Acute cardiorespiratory responses of hypertensive rats to swimming and treadmill exercise. *J. Appl. Physiol.* 57:1328–1332, 1984.
173. Taguchi, J., and E.D. Fries. Partial versus complete control of blood pressure in the prevention of hypertensive complications. *Cir. Res.* 36(Suppl. I):I-257-I1260, 1975.
174. Takeshita, A., and A.L. Mark. Neurogenic contribution to hindquarters vasoconstriction during high sodium intake in Dadh-strain of genetically hypertensive rat. *Cir. Res.* 43(Suppl. I):I-86/I-91, 1978.
175. Tanabe, Y., J. Sasaki, H. Urata, et al. Effect of mild aerobic exercise in lipid and apolipo protein in patients with essential hypertension. *Jpn. Heart J.* 29:199–206, 1988.
176. Tanji, J.L., J.J. Champlin, G.Y. Wong, E.Y. Lew, T.C. Brown, and E.A. Amsterdam. Blood pressure recovery curves after submaximal exercise: a predictor of hypertension at ten year follow-up. *Am. J. Hypertens.* 2:135–138, 1989.
177. Terjung, R.L. Endocrine system. R.H. Straus (ed.). *Sports Medicine and Physiology.* Philadelphia: W.B. Saunders, 1979, pp. 147–165.
178. Terry, A.H. Obesity and hypertension. *J.A.M.A.* 31:1283–1284, 1923.
179. Tipton, C.M. Exercise, training and hypertension. *Exerc. Sports Sci. Revs.* 12:245–306, 1984.
180. Tipton, C.M., R.D. Matthes, K.D. Marcus, K.A. Rowlett, and J.R. Leininger. Influences of exercise intensity, age and medication on resting systolic blood pressure of SHR populations. *J. Appl. Physiol.* 55:1305–1310, 1983.
181. Tipton, C.M., R.D. Matthews, J.A. Wegner, and J.G. Edwards. A model for borderline hypertension: preliminary results. *Fed. Proc.* 44:818, 1985 (Abstract).
182. Tipton, C.M., S. McMahon, J.R. Leininger, E.L. Pauli, and C. Lauber. Exercise training and incidence of cerebrovascular lesions in stroke-prone spontaneously hypertensive rats. *J. Appl. Physiol.* 68:1080–1085, 1990.
183. Tipton, C.M., S. McMahon, E.M. Youmans, et al. Response of hypertensive rats to acute and chronic conditions of static exercise. *Am. J. Physiol.* 254:H592–H598, 1988.
184. Tipton, C.M., J.M. Overton, R.B. Pepin, J.G. Edwards, J. Wegner, and E.M. Youmans. Influence of exercise training on resting blood pressures of Dahl rats. *J. Appl. Physiol.* 63:342–346, 1987.
185. Tipton, C.M., L. Sebastian, J.M. Overton, S.B. Williams, and C.R. Woodman. Exercise training and resting hemodynamic measurements of hypertensive rats (SHR). *Abstracts of the Kuopio International Hypertension meeting.* Kuopio, Finland, 1989, p 10.
186. Tipton, C.M., M.S. Sturek, R.A. Oppliger, R.D. Matthes, J.M. Overton, and J.G. Edwards. Responses of SHR to combinations of chemical sympathectomy, adrenal demedullation and training. *Am. J. Physiol.* 247:H109–H118, 1984.
187. Tomanek, R.J., C.V. Gisolfi, C.A. Bauer, and P.J. Palmer. Coronary vasodilator

reserve, capillarity, and mitochondria in trained hypertensive rats. *J. Appl. Physiol.* 64:1179–1185, 1988.

188. Urata, H., Y. Tanabe, A. Kiyonaga, et al. Antihypertensive and volume-depleting effects of mild exercise on essential hypertension. *Hypertension* 9:245–252, 1987.

189. Van Hoof, R., P. Hespel, R. Fagard, P. Lijnen, J. Staessen, and A. Amery. Effect of endurance training on blood pressure at rest, during exercise and during 24 hours in sedentary men. *Am. J. Cardiol.* 63:945–949, 1989.

190. Wallin, B.G., C. Morlin, and P. Hjemdahl. Muscle sympathetic activity and venous plasma noradrenaline concentrations during static exercise in normotensive and hypertensive subjects. *Acta Physiol. Scand.* 129:489–497, 1987.

191. Walsh, K.P., T.D.M. Williams, S.E. Pitts, S.L. Lighman, and R. Sutton. Role of atrial pressure and rate in release of atrial natriuretic peptide. *Am. J. Physiol.* 254:R607–R610, 1988.

192. Weber, J.R. Left ventricular hypertrophy: its prime importance as a controllable risk factor. *Am. Heart J.* 116:272–279, 1988.

193. Weber, F., R.J. Barnard, and D. Roy. Effects of a high-complex-carbohydrate, low-fat diet and daily exercise on individuals 70 years of age and older. *J. Gerontology* 38:155–161, 1986.

194. Weinberger, M.H. Salt intake and blood pressures in humans. *Contemp. Nutr.* 13:(8)1–2, 1988.

195. Weinsier, R.L., D.J. Norris, R. Birch, et al. Serum insulin and blood pressure in an obese population. *Int. J. Obesity* 10:11–17, 1986.

196. Westheim, A., K. Simonsen, O. Schamaun, E.K. Qvigstad, P. Staff, and P. Teisberg. Effect of exercise training in patients with essential hypertension. The Soria Moria Hypertension Meeting. *Acta Medica Scand.*, Suppl. 714:99–103, 1986.

197. Widimsky, J., W. Debinski, O. Kuchel, and N.T. Buu. ANF disappearance and tissue distribution in rats. *Am. J. Physiol.* 258:H134–H139, 1990.

198. Wyatt, H.L., and J.H. Mitchell. Influences of physical training on the hearts of dogs. *Circ. Res.* 35:883–889, 1974.

199. Zambraski, E.J. Renal regulation of fluid homeostasis during exercise. C.V. Gisolfi and D.R. Lamb (eds.). *Fluid Homeostasis During Exercise. Perspectives in Exercise Science and Sports Medicine.* Indianapolis: Benchmark Press, 3:247–280, 1990.

14
Adenine Nucleotide Metabolism In Contracting Skeletal Muscle

PETER C. TULLSON, Ph.D
RONALD L. TERJUNG, Ph.D.

OVERVIEW

The proper management of adenine nucleotide metabolism in skeletal muscle is central to the role of muscle as a transducer of chemical energy into mechanical work. Adenine nucleotides are integrally important to nearly all energy transfer reactions within the cell, and the precise control of their concentrations and interconversions is essential during exercise when large, abrupt increases in the rate of energy transfer occur. This review concerns the interconversions, synthesis, and degradation of adenine nucleotides during and following muscle contraction. We have highlighted differences among skeletal muscle fiber types and included available information from human studies.

During steady-state exercise the rates of energy provision are carefully controlled to match the rates of energy expenditure (i.e., rates of adenosine 5′-triphosphate [ATP] hydrolysis [reaction 1]). The needed energy for steady state contractions comes primarily from

$$ATP \rightarrow ADP + HPO_4^{2-} \qquad [1]$$

aerobic metabolism through mitochondrial respiration. Over a wide range of sustainable exercise an excellent energy balance is maintained within muscle. This balance is reflected by the tight control of the muscle ATP concentration evident over a wide range of exercise intensities. However, the cell's phosphocreatine (PCr) concentration progressively declines as the exercise intensity increases. This decrease in PCr is related to the increase in free adenosine diphosphate (ADP_f) concentration, through the near-equilibrium creatine kinase reaction [reaction 2], and is in this way coupled

$$ADP + PCr + H^+ \leftrightarrow ATP + Cr \qquad [2]$$

to processes within the cell important for controlling energy metabolism (e.g., mitochondrial respiration and glycolysis). When the rate of ATP hydrolysis exceeds the rate of ADP phosphorylation, the ATP content of the muscle fiber can become depleted. The decrease in ATP content does not appear as a stoichiometric increase in ADP concentration, because the myokinase reaction [3] is operating. This reaction

$$ADP + ADP \leftrightarrow ATP + AMP \qquad [3]$$

leads to the restoration of ATP and the production of adenosine monophosphate (AMP). Thus, the net hydrolysis of ATP during high rates of energy expenditure leads to the formation of AMP within the muscle fiber. Because the muscle content of ATP is much greater than the available ADP_f and free AMP (AMP_f) (e.g., ATP: ≈ 8 μmol/g; ADP_f: ≈ 0.025 μmol/g; and AMP_f: ≈ 0.0001 μmol/g), a relatively small decrease in ATP would result in very large increases in ADP_f and AMP_f. However, skeletal muscle manages adenine nucleotide metabolism during and following conditions of high energy turnover in a unique way that involves alteration of the total adenine nucleotide content through a series of reactions termed the purine nucleotide cycle [70]. The functions of the purine nucleotide cycle are discussed in the following section.

In addition to deamination, increased concentrations of AMP and inosine 5′-monophosphate (IMP) can lead to net degradation of purine nucleotides from dephosphorylation catalyzed by 5′AMP (5′IMP) nucleotidase. Nucleosides, and their ensuing purine bases can be subsequently lost from the muscle cell. To maintain and restore the muscle adenine nucleotide content, those degradation products not recovered and recycled as purines must be replenished through the *de novo* synthesis pathway. Degradation of purines in skeletal muscle is discussed in the section Degradation of Adenine Nucleotides; *de novo* synthesis is discussed in the section De Novo Synthesis of Adenine Nucleotides.

PURINE NUCLEOTIDE CYCLE

The formation of AMP when ATP hydrolysis [reaction 1] exceeds rephosphorylation does not result in markedly elevated AMP concentrations owing to the enzymatic action of AMP deaminase [reaction 4], the first reaction of the purine nucleotide

$$AMP + H_2O \rightarrow IMP + NH_3 \qquad [4]$$

cycle (Fig. 14.1). This reaction leads to the depletion of the adenine nucleotide pool and the stoichiometric production of IMP and ammonia (NH_3). Restoration of adenine nucleotides by the reamination of IMP does not occur by simple fixation of ammonia, because the deamination reaction is irreversible. Instead, the reamination of IMP occurs through

FIGURE 14.1
Reactions of the purine nucleotide cycle. **AS** = *adenylosuccinate*

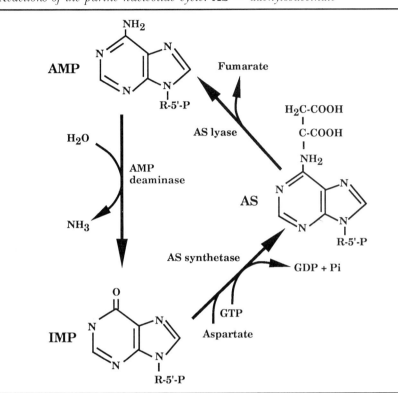

two reactions, the first catalyzed by adenylosuccinate synthetase [reaction 5] and the second by adenylosuccinate lyase [reaction 6], using the amine from aspartate with the energy obtained from guanosine 5'-triphosphate (GTP) [70].

$$\text{IMP + Aspartate + GTP} \rightarrow \text{Adenylosuccinate + GDP + P}_i \quad [5]$$

$$\text{Adenylosuccinate} \rightarrow \text{AMP + Fumarate} \quad [6]$$

Thus, one complete turn of the purine nucleotide cycle, in which there is no net loss of AMP, results in the deamination of aspartate to fumarate and ammonia and the consumption of energy. The AMP produced during reamination becomes part of the muscle ATP pool through the myokinase reaction [reaction 3].

As originally proposed by Lowenstein [70] and reviewed more recently [71, 110, 129], the purine nucleotide cycle has several possible functions, including the:

1. maintenance of a high ATP:ADP ratio by shifting the myokinase equilibrium [reaction 3] toward ATP by removing AMP through deamination to IMP;
2. regulation of phosphofructokinase activity by the ammonium ion (NH_4^+) concentration;
3. regulation of phosphorylase *b* activity by the IMP concentration;
4. replenishment of citric acid cycle intermediates by production of fumarate;
5. deamination of amino acids for oxidative metabolism.

The first three proposed functions are dependent on the initial reaction of the purine nucleotide cycle, because this reaction effects the ATP:ADP ratio and increases the cellular concentration of NH_4^+ and IMP. Proposed functions [4] and [5] would require the complete functioning of the purine nucleotide cycle because the reaminating limb of the purine nucleotide cycle is essential for fumarate production and deamination of aspartate. For this latter process to be useful during contractions, therefore, both the deamination and reamination reactions of the cycle would have to proceed concurrently. In addition, as discussed by Sabina et al. [105], deamination of AMP to IMP could serve to prevent massive adenine nucleotide degradation to purine bases and thereby favor recovery processes.

AMP Deamination to IMP and NH_3
The deamination of AMP within muscle occurs during relatively intense exercise when the rate of ATP hydrolysis is high relative to the rate of oxidative phosphorylation, and the concentration of AMP rises. In addition to the depletion of adenine nucleotides, it is apparent from reaction [4] that the process of AMP deamination leads to a stoichiometric production of NH_3. Ammonia readily leaves the active muscle and probably accounts for the increased concentration of blood NH_4^+ that occurs during intense exercise in humans [33, 50, 143] and animals [30, 31, 81, 120].

REGULATION OF AMP DEAMINASE. The activity of AMP deaminase is extremely low in resting muscle in part because of the low sarcoplasmic concentration of AMP_f, which is approximately four orders of magnitude below the Michaelis constant (K_m) for the enzyme (i.e., ≈ 0.1 vs. $\approx 1,000$ μM). Any elevation in AMP_f concentration within the fiber should directly increase IMP formation and is probably a major factor that contributes to AMP deamination during muscle contraction [35, 64, 140, 141].

A variety of energetically important muscle metabolites have been shown in in vitro experiments to exert allosteric control of AMP deaminase activity. The ADP_f, P_i, and H^+ are probably the most important modulators of AMP deaminase because the concentration of each is sensitive to the energetic status of muscle [71, 141]. Acidosis decreases the K_m of AMP deaminase toward AMP [90] and, along with increasing ADP_f, lessens the inhibition of deamination by P_i (K_i (inhibitor constant) $\approx$2 mmol/L) [141]. These modulators probably serve to increase the activity of AMP deaminase during severe exercise [35].

The binding of AMP deaminase to myosin may play a significant part in controlling deamination in addition to the well-studied mechanisms of substrate and allosteric control. The AMP deaminase was first recognized as a minor contaminant of myosin; this interaction was later shown to have considerable specificity in studies that demonstrated the exclusive tight binding of purified rabbit muscle AMP deaminase to subfragment 2 of heavy meromyosin, with a stoichiometry of two mol of enzyme per mol of myosin [6]. The addition of subfragment 2 to the purified enzyme activated deamination slightly and prevented inhibition by GTP [7]. Researchers using rat muscle AMP deaminase also have observed specific tight binding but have suggested that the enzyme binds to light meromyosin with a stoichiometry of 1 mol of enzyme per 3 mol of myosin [115], which results in an activation of $\approx$60% in AMP deamination rate [116]. The AMP deaminase binding was localized to the ends of the A-band in isolated chicken myofibrils and cultured chicken muscle fibers [8] and in isolated rabbit myofibrils [24] using immunofluorescent and histochemical techniques.

When deamination was activated by muscle contraction, the fraction of AMP deaminase in a soluble form decreased while the total activity of the muscle remained unchanged; this was interpreted as binding to myosin [117]. After muscle stimulation ceased, AMP deaminase reverted to the soluble form [117]. This reversible binding of AMP deaminase during exercise recently has been confirmed and extended by the demonstration that binding is associated with conditions in which energy utilization exceeds the aerobic capacity of specific fiber types [104]. This demonstrated importance of exercise intensity and duration in relation to the aerobic capacity of each fiber type may explain the lack of binding found with exercise by Westra et al. [140]. Recently, both the native 80 kilodalton (kDa) AMP deaminase subunit from rat skeletal muscle and the 66 kDa subunit formed by proteolysis were shown to bind to myosin heavy chain; binding of the 66 kDa species was reversed by 4–5 mmol/L ATP [77]. Thus, the interaction between myosin and AMP deaminase may play an integral part in the process of high rates of IMP and NH_3 production in contracting muscle.

The isoforms of AMP deaminase (discussed in the following section) present in skeletal muscle appear to have important differences in their regulatory properties. The heart-type isoform is less sensitive to changes in the adenylate energy charge [121] and to increases in H^+ [99] than the skeletal muscle isoform. Any potential regulation exerted by myosin binding would appear to be restricted to the skeletal muscle isoform, because the heart isoform from rat does not appear to bind to myosin [115]. As discussed below in the section Fiber Type Differences, fast- and slow-twitch muscle exhibit very different capacities for AMP deamination. IMP production in slow-twitch muscle is much less, even under severe conditions of energetic imbalance, such as intense contractions during ischemia [82, 134, 142]. It seems likely that regulatory differences between the isoforms present in skeletal muscle fiber types contribute to the control of AMP deamination.

Regardless of the precise basis of enzymatic control, it is apparent that AMP deaminase activity can effectively deplete up to approximately 50% of the adenine nucleotide pool within fast-twitch muscle in a brief period of time (e.g., less than 3 minutes of intense contractions). This occurs coincident with contraction failure reflected by the inability to sustain the same high rate of work output or tension development [64, 82].

ISOFORMS OF AMP DEAMINASE. AMP deaminase exists as distinct tissue-specific isoforms (e.g., skeletal muscle, heart, red blood cell) having unique chromatographic, electrophoretic, and immunologic characteristics [92]. All skeletal muscles, regardless of fiber type, have been shown to possess an isoform unique to this tissue. In addition, slow-twitch red skeletal muscle [41, 92, 98, 121] contains a second isoform which in rabbit [92, 98], rat [41, 98], and mouse [41] is similar to the isoform isolated from heart. In contrast, this second isoform in the cat slow-twitch red muscle (soleus) is reported to be immunologically similar to the enzyme isolated from erythrocytes [41]. AMP deaminase from human muscle was chromatographically resolved into either one [91] or two species [98] and immunologically characterized as being more than 90% of the skeletal muscle isoform [41]. The complementary DNA of the skeletal muscle isoform from rat has been recently cloned and sequenced, allowing the amino acid sequence of the enzyme to be deduced [107]. The skeletal muscle isoform is a tetramer with a native molecular weight of 320,000 composed of identical 80 kDa subunits [76, 77]. The 80 kDa peptide is prone to proteolytic cleavage [77, 102] which may explain the lower molecular weight found when muscle extracts have been prepared without protease inhibitors [91, 115, 121].

FIBER TYPE DIFFERENCES. The activity of AMP deaminase differs between fiber types. For example, in rat skeletal muscle the highest capacity for AMP deamination is found in fast-twitch muscle, with the fast-twitch white higher than the fast-twitch red muscle section. In contrast, the slow-twitch red muscle (i.e., soleus) of the rat has a relative low enzymatic capacity for AMP deamination, approximately 30–40% of fast-twitch muscle [97, 104, 145]. Similar differences were found in slow-twitch and fast-twitch rabbit [97] and cat [15] muscle. AMP deaminase activity in human mixed-fibered muscle [112] is similar to that measured in rats. Although these distinctions suggest that differences should be found in vivo, it is important to recognize that the highest rates of AMP deamination measured during intense contractions could easily be accomplished by using only a small fraction ($\approx 0.1-2\%$) of the cell's enzymatic capacity [35]. Nonetheless, marked differences in rates of AMP deamination are apparent among fiber types during brief, intense exercise. Although most of the information of fiber type responses comes from research with rats, information from human experiments shows that IMP accumulation is less in slow-twitch (type I), as compared to fast-twitch (type II) fibers [62, 64, 88, 89, 109].

Slow-twitch versus fast-twitch muscle. In contrast to the response in fast-twitch muscle, slow-twitch muscle of the rat does not show large decreases in adenine nucleotide content and corresponding increases in IMP during brief, intense exercise. Thus, the ATP content of the muscle is reasonably well maintained, even though the contractions were sufficiently intense to yield a significant loss of tension development [82]. Muscle contraction in this fiber type apparently does not readily produce cellular conditions sufficient to activate AMP deaminase. Even eliminating normal blood flow during brief, intense contractions does not succeed in activating deamination to an extent similar to that in fast-twitch muscle [35, 82], which emphasizes that fast- and slow-twitch fibers are distinctly different in some aspects of adenine nucleotide metabolism.

Slow-twitch muscle appears similar to heart muscle in demonstrating a dissociation between ATP depletion and failure of contraction [45]. Slow-twitch muscle appears to be very sensitive to oxygen delivery, failing during short-term ischemia and recovering rapidly following reflow, without deamination [82, 142]. Short-term ischemia coupled with intense contractions has been shown to cause an approximate 1 μmol/g depletion of adenine nucleotides with little deamination [82, 134, 142]. This observed loss of nucleotides could not be accounted for as nucleosides or bases, which has lead to the suggestion that some as yet unrecognized purine metabolite may be formed under these conditions [134].

Large differences in lactate content are found between slow-twitch and fast-twitch muscle rat during intense short-term ischemic contractions. A marked activation of AMP deaminase in rat fast-twitch muscle is coincident with a very high lactate content (e.g., 25–45 μmol/g). In contrast, the relatively low capacity for glycolysis in the rat slow-twitch red muscle apparently limits the rate of lactate production during the brief ischemic period, such that only 12–15 μmol/g lactate accumulated [82, 142], which leads to a lesser degree of acidosis under these conditions. When ischemic slow-twitch muscle contracts for a prolonged time (10 min), about 30% of the adenine nucleotide pool is depleted coincident with a high accumulation of lactate (21–30 μmol/g) [142]. This experimental condition further associates acidosis with deamination, but it is certainly extreme and not normally encountered, even during intense treadmill running in which lactate does not increase nearly as much [11, 81].

The differences in AMP deaminase activity normally observed between slow- and fast-twitch muscle of the rat may not be characteristic of fiber type differences in humans. The quantitatively large depletion in ATP content (up to $\approx 50\%$) of mixed-fibered muscle samples during intense exercise conditions [50, 123, 127] implies that both fast- and slow-twitch fibers are exhibiting AMP deamination. In vitro AMP deaminase activity of mixed-fibered muscle samples increased with the percentage of fast-twitch fibers, which indicates a 2.8-fold higher activity in fast- versus slow-twitch fibers [39]. Evidence obtained from individual human muscle fibers has demonstrated that slow-twitch fibers show significant increases in IMP following intense exercise, but only about half that found in fast-twitch fibers [62, 88, 89, 109]. The observation that adenine nucleotide depletion decreased as the percentage of slow-twitch fibers in mixed muscle biopsies increased further implies that slow-twitch fibers in human muscle possesses a lower capacity for AMP deamination [64]. In a similar fashion, Dudley et al. [33] found that the increase in plasma ammonia after maximal exercise decreased linearly as the proportion of slow-twitch fibers in their subjects increased. Nonetheless, differences in deamination evident between slow- and fast-twitch fibers in human are less than that seen in rat muscle. This may be reasonable if cellular acidosis is an important factor that enhances AMP deaminase activity, because the glycolytic capacity of human fast- and slow-twitch fibers is fairly similar and in contrast to the large difference between slow-twitch and fast-twitch muscle of the rat muscle. High lactate contents approaching $22–27$ $\mu mol/g$ have been measured in the slow-twitch red fibers of humans [130].

Fast-twitch red versus fast-twitch white muscle. Although both of these fiber types are capable of exhibiting extremely high rates of AMP deamination during very intense exercise [82], there can be marked differences between the low and high oxidative fibers [34, 35, 36]. Recall that the primary stimulus for AMP deamination is a sustained imbalance between the rates of ATP hydrolysis and ADP phosphorylation that lead to a rise in AMP_f. The potential for aerobic energy supply is much greater for fast-twitch red versus fast-twitch white fibers and results in a better energy balance over a wider range of exercise conditions. The 4- to 5-fold greater mitochondrial content [10, 32] and blood flow capacity [68, 72] of the rat fast-twitch red fibers versus the fast-twitch white fibers contribute to the excellent energy balance at higher rates of energy expenditure [34, 35]. During moderately intense exercise, the fast-twitch red accommodate the energy demand with only a modest decline in PCr content, whereas the low-oxidative, fast-twitch white muscle shows an extensive decline in ATP content and a stoichiometric accumulation of IMP [34, 35]. When the highly aerobic fast-twitch red muscle is made ischemic, approximately half of the ATP content is deaminated. Thus, the response among even the fast-twitch skeletal muscle fibers is heterogeneous and depends on the exercise severity, the inherent metabolic capabilities of the individual fibers, and the actual recruitment of fibers during exercise. This heterogeneity of muscle fiber type response makes interpretation of data obtained from mixed-fibered muscle samples difficult.

EFFECTS OF ENDURANCE TRAINING ON AMP DEAMINATION. In both rats [34] and humans [69] endurance training lessens the extent of AMP deamination at a given energy demand or work load. This is likely due to the increase in the sensitivity of respiratory control that occurs as muscle oxidative capacity increases. This results in lower concentrations of ADP_f and AMP_f with consequently lower rates of IMP formation over a wide range of oxygen consumption rates [36].

Metabolic Consequences of AMP Deamination

REGULATION OF THE ATP:ADP RATIO DURING CONTRACTION. With an imbalance between the rate of ATP hydrolysis (energy utilization) and ADP phosphorylation (energy provision), the concentration of ATP within the fiber must decrease. This decrease in ATP concentration per se probably would not alter muscle function, even if the concentration declined by 80–90% (i.e., to 1 mmol/L or less). Ferenczi et al. [37] found that maximal isometric tension and maximal shortening velocity of skinned muscle fibers were well maintained over a broad range of ATP concentrations, extending far below any ATP concentration ever measured in *intact* contracting mammalian skeletal muscle. It is possible, however, that the hydrolysis products of ATP breakdown could have an influence on muscle function. Dawson et al. [26] found a high correlation between the loss of tension development and the estimated increase in ADP_f. If the quantity of adenine nucleotide derived from a decrease of $\approx 50\%$ in ATP concentration were found as ADP_f and AMP_f, according to the myokinase equilibrium [78, 139], the increase in ADP_f concentration would be exceptionally high (cf. Fig. 14.2) and expected to produce marked changes in muscle function (i.e., reduced shortening velocity with a K_i of 0.2–0.03 mmol/L) [23]. Similarly, the AMP_f concentration would increase far in excess of that estimated to occur physiologically [78, 139].

Activation of AMP deaminase during conditions of net ATP hydrolysis serves to prevent the large increases in ADP_f and AMP_f concentrations within working muscle. In the situation described above, in which IMP formation does not occur, ADP_f and AMP_f would be ≈ 90-fold and $\approx 13,500$-fold elevated above rest, compared to ≈ 8-fold and ≈ 70-fold greater than when AMP deamination does occur [34]. Thus, it seems probable that AMP deaminase serves to prevent large increases in ADP_f

FIGURE 14.2

Expected increases in muscle ADP_f and AMP_f according to the myokinase re-action, as a function of the decrease in ATP, if the total adenine nucleotide content is kept constant (i.e., 7.50 µmol/g). These large increases in ADP_f and AMP_f are not typically found in skeletal muscle owing to deamination of AMP to IMP.

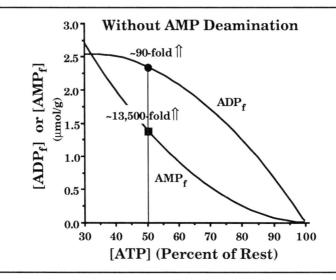

and AMP_f and the likely catastrophic consequences of such a decrease in energy state. It is conceivable that even a modest degree of deamination (≈ 0.25 µmol/g) could have important beneficial effects by attenuating the rise in ADP_f and, thus, enable the cell to continue ATP hydrolysis at a high rate [136].

REGULATION OF PHOSPHOFRUCTOKINASE BY AMMONIA. The higher rate of ATP utilization during exercise elicits an increase in the rate of glycolysis. Activation of phosphofructokinase (PFK), which catalyzes an important control reaction of glycolysis, is essential to meet an accelerated demand for ATP. Ammonium ion, the predominant form of ammonia within muscle, has been shown to activate phosphofructokinase by reducing the inhibition due to citrate and ATP [1]. Although the concentration-dependent effect of NH_4^+ [1] is within the range of 0.35 to 3.0 µmol NH_4^+ per gram of wet weight found within the muscle fiber [46, 82], it is unlikely to be physiologically relevant. First, as recently discussed by Katz et al. [64] the effect of ammonium ion appears to a specific cation effect with a response in common with K^+ [126]. With a normal high intracellular K^+ concentration, there should be no effect of NH_4^+. Second, even if NH_4^+ accumulation should influence phosphofructokinase per se, it would probably be of little effect in modulating glycolysis, because NH_4^+ accumulates only when the glycolytic rate is already high. Other factors that accelerate PFK activity must be effective in increasing the rate of glycolysis. The continued accumulation of lactate to high levels after acidosis develops within the cell [29, 35, 55, 123, 124] suggests that acidosis does not effectively inhibit PFK activity and argues that deamination is more likely facilitated by acidosis rather than a cause of it [35, 82].

REGULATION OF PHOSPHORYLASE *b* BY IMP. Early after the onset of contractions, the conversion of phosphorylase *b* to phosphorylase *a* probably accounts for the high rate of glycogenolysis. Shortly into the contraction period the activity of phosphorylase *a* declines by its conversion back to phosphorylase *b* [3, 22]. It has been proposed that the increase in IMP within muscle serves to sustain glycogenolysis in the face of phosphorylase *a* to *b* conversions [70, 71], because IMP activates phosphorylase *b* [3]. Evidence suggests that IMP stimulated glycogen breakdown in phosphorylase *b* kinase-deficient mice [101].

It is unlikely, however, that IMP plays a critical role in the control of glycogenolysis in normal muscle. First, glycogenolysis occurs in active muscle during conditions that do not involve any significant accumulation of IMP, and when IMP production does occur, antecedent glycogen breakdown already occurs at a high rate [34]. Thus, IMP can only be assigned a sustaining influence. Even in this role, its importance is questionable, because the need for glycogenolysis is waning at high IMP concentrations when fatigue has developed. Although a complete answer must await further research, it is now recognized that the greatly elevated PO_4^{2-} is an important factor that stimulates the continuation of glycogen breakdown during sustained exercise [21, 55].

SPARING ADENINE NUCLEOTIDES FROM DEGRADATION TO PURINE BASES. The production of IMP during intense exercise could act to conserve nucleotides within the cell [105]. If the metabolism of adenine nucleotides in skeletal muscle involved degradation to nucleosides and purine bases to the extent found in the heart [74], there could be a massive net loss of adenine nucleotides from the cell. Purine nucleosides and bases readily leave muscle tissue [63], resulting in depletion of important precursors necessary for adenine nucleotide recovery. Restoration of the ATP pool would then require the actions of the purine salvage and de novo purine nucleotide synthesis pathways. In contrast, IMP remains within the cell [82, 83] and is readily reaminated [47, 82]. Evidence that AMP deamination influences adenine nucleotide degradation has come from clinical studies with patients who lack muscle AMP deaminase where ischemic isometric forearm exercise causes a lesser increase in plasma inosine and hypoxanthine [95, 118, 147] and a greater increase plasma adenosine [118] than found in control subjects. Adenosine content increased 8-fold more in muscle biopsies from enzyme deficient as compared to normal subjects [106].

IMP Reamination to AMP

The three enzymes of the purine nucleotide cycle catalyze the following net reaction [7]. The reamination of IMP requires energy derived from GTP, an amine

$$\text{Aspartate } + \text{ GTP } + \text{ H}_2\text{O} \rightarrow \text{Fumarate } + \text{ GDP } + \text{ P}_i + \text{ NH}_3 \quad [7]$$

obtained from aspartate, and produces fumarate. These reactions could be an important means of supporting ancillary metabolic processes in muscle in addition to the obvious restoration of the adenine nucleotide pool.

ENZYMES OF REAMINATION. *Adenylosuccinate synthetase.* Adenylosuccinate synthetase exists as two isoforms, only one of which is found in muscle [125]. This isoform has been purified from rabbit and rat skeletal muscle [85, 93]. The active enzyme appears to exist as a dimer composed of two subunits of 52 kDa each [93], with a Km toward IMP of 0.2 mmol/L [46, 85, 125]. Because the content of IMP in resting muscle is only 5–10 nmol/g (wet wt), increases in IMP should increase adenylosuccinate synthetase activity. The enzyme is subject to both primary and secondary product inhibition by adenylosuccinate [93] and AMP [125], respectively. Further, adenylosuccinate synthetase activity is inhibited by high concentrations of IMP (i.e., >0.26 mM) [125].

An interesting feature of adenylosuccinate synthetase is that it binds to F-actin with a fairly high affinity, with a ratio of 1 mole of the synthetase per 4 moles of actin monomer [93]. In physiological buffers, adenylosuccinate synthetase also binds specifically to actin-tropomyosin complexes and myofibrils [75]. This observation has led to the proposal that the enzymes that produce and consume IMP are restricted to a functional intracellular "compartment" by binding to proteins of the contracile apparatus [75, 94].

Adenylosuccinate lyase. Adenylosuccinate lyase has been purified from rat skeletal muscle and found to have a subunit molecular weight of 52 kDa, with a native molecular weight of approximately 200 kDa, which suggests that it exists as a tetramer [20]. The Km of the enzyme toward adenylosuccinate was determined to be 1.5 μM [20]. Muscle adenylosuccinate content ranged from undetectable in resting muscle up to ≈4–5 nmol/g (wet wt) during mild stimulation conditions [46], which suggests that substrate concentration should be important in determining activity.

CONTROL OF IMP REAMINATION. It is technically difficult to evaluate the occurrence of IMP reamination in muscle in vivo. Even though the concurrent processing of the purine nucleotide reactions consumes energy and aspartate, and produces fumarate and NH3 (cf. Fig. 14.1) with little change in AMP concentration, measurement of the reamination rate from changes in muscle contents of these metabolites is not definitive, because each of the reactants and products are involved in other reactions or can easily leave the muscle (e.g., NH_3). Thus, metabolite concentration changes do not necessarily reflect the activity of the purine nucleotide cycle reactions.

In spite of this limitation some general features of the control of IMP reamination have been deduced. Goodman and Lowenstein [46] have provided evidence that IMP accumulation in skeletal muscle accelerates reamination to AMP at low IMP concentrations but not at high IMP concentrations. This can be explained by the substrate effect at low IMP concentrations (cf. section on enzymes of reamination) and the inhibition of adenylosuccinate synthetase by high concentrations of IMP [125]. Because reamination requires GTP, the process of IMP reamination should not be favored by the reduced energy state that occurs during intense exercise and results in a high rate of IMP formation. Further, adenylosuccinate synthetase is inhibited by elevated PO_4^{2-} [125], a condition that occurs during muscle contractions due to the hydrolysis of phosphocreatine. As IMP concentration increases above its normal resting value, the concentration of adenylosuccinate increases up to a limit and then decreases as IMP concentration increases further [46]. An increase in the substrate:product ratio is often typical of a reduced rate of reaction by an enzyme in a metabolic pathway relative to the preceding and following reactions [86].

TEMPORAL INTEGRATION OF THE PURINE NUCLEOTIDE CYCLE. *Control during high intensity exercise.* An indirect method to estimate IMP reamination has proved especially useful in assessing the response of different fiber types to a range of exercise intensities. Inhibition of IMP reamination produces a situation in which the accumulation of IMP is only a function of the deaminating limb of the purine nucleotide cycle. Because IMP does not leave the muscle, any extra accumulation within the cell should represent the amount of IMP that would have been reaminated without inhibiton. This experimental design was employed by Meyer and Terjung [83] and Aragón and Lowenstein [4] in contracting hindlimb muscle. The drug hadacidin at the doses employed was shown to be an effective (>80% inhibition), specific inhibitor of IMP reamination. A rate of IMP reamination of ≈ 7 nmol/min per gram of wet weight measured in the presence of hadacidin [83] established the lower limit of sensitivity with this experimental protocol.

During short-term intense exercise when there is a large depletion of adenine nucleotides, there is no evidence that reamination occurs at any significant rate [64, 82, 83]. Thus, the role of the purine nucleotide cycle during severe exercise appears solely related to the deamination of AMP to IMP and ammonia.

Control during low- to moderate-intensity exercise. Fast-twitch red muscle does not accumulate IMP except under relatively intense exercise conditions [34, 35, 36, 83]. Even with inhibition of adenylosuccinate synthetase activity with hadacidin, there was still no significant IMP accumulation in the fast-twitch red muscle section over a range of mild to moderate exercise conditions (1, 3 or 5 twitches/sec), a response indicating that this high-oxidative muscle could meet this range of energy demands without activating AMP deamination.

In contrast to the fast-twitch red muscle, the low-oxidative fast-twitch muscle section did accumulate excess IMP due to the presence of hadacidin. This became apparent at the higher contraction conditions (3 and 5 twitches/sec) after 30 minutes of stimulation. Thus, IMP was produced during contractions and retained in the muscle when the reamination pathway was inhibited, but was reaminated to ATP in the absence of hadacidin. These results provide strong evidence that the prime nucleotide reactions (Fig. 14.1) function as a complete cycle during contractions.

To better understand this process of purine nucleotide cycling, additional experiments were performed which demonstrated that IMP was produced early (within 5 min) during the 30-minute period of stimulation [83]. In the absence of hadacidin, IMP was subsequently reaminated to ATP during the remainder of the stimulation period, whereas in the hadacidin treated muscle a high IMP content was maintained. The activities of the deamination and reamination legs of the purine nucleotide cycle were out of phase, because IMP was produced early and reaminated later during the exercise period. Interestingly, the dissociation of deamination-reamination processes in fast-twitch muscle occurred even though the muscle was continually stimulated through the nerve for the 30-minute period. Thus, cellular conditions must have developed after the initial phase contractions which promoted the activities of adenylosuccinate synthatase and lyase. This would likely include a favorable energy balance for GTP utilization. The deamination/reamination sequence appears similar to the situation during intense short-term contraction conditions in which extensive ATP depletion to IMP occurs while restoration of the ATP pool proceeded by reamination of IMP during the subsequent recovery period [82]. One explanation, consistent with these observations, is that during intense exercise, the muscle fibers of the fast-twitch white section fatigued during the first few minutes of stimulation and were relatively unresponsive thereafter. Because tension development would be minimal, the fibers would then be able to exhibit a partial metabolic recovery during the remaining 25 minutes of the experiment. This interpretation is compatible with the well-characterized poor performance characteristics of this low-oxidatve, fast-twitch white fiber type (18). These experiments therefore suggest that the two limbs of the purine nucleotide cycle do not function simultaneously in the same fiber even though the whole muscle continues contracting.

The process of sequential AMP deamination/IMP reamination also could account for the recognized ammonia accumulation during submaximal exercise of moderate intensity in humans. Prolonged cycle exercise at 50–75% of maximal oxygen consumption could lead to IMP and NH_3 production in some fibers as fatigue ensues [16]; overall exercise performance could be sustained by the recruitment of other motor units, thereby permitting adenine nucleotide recovery in the originally recruited fibers. The accumulation of IMP in muscle during submaximal exercise [109], especially as fatigue develops [88] or when acclerated by prior glycogen depletion [16, 89] illustrates the need to appreciate the probable heterogeneity of muscle fiber response during submaximal exercise.

Two reports have suggested that inhibition of IMP reamination may be associated with accelerated fatigue. Swain et al [128] found that blocking the hydrolysis of adenylosuccinate to fumarate and AMP [reaction 6] with 5-amino-4-imidazolecarboxamide riboside (AICAr) caused a greater loss in tension development of mouse muscle during intense contraction conditions. An accelerated loss of muscle tension was also found in rat muscle [42] during more mild stimulation conditions. Recent evidence suggests that treatment with AICAr is not an appropriate means to inhibit IMP reamination because it lowers systemic blood pressure [43]. This could be related to excessive peripheral vasodilation, because AICAr inhibits adenosine deaminase [9]. Foley et al. [43] found normal twitch tension during mild stimulation conditions during AICAr treatment even though blood pressure was reduced by 20%. It is possible that the animals used in the study by Flanagan et al. [42] were hypotensive and suffered a large reduction in perfusion pressure to the muscle, a factor known to impair muscle performance [51].

Metabolic Consequences of AMP Reamination

REPLENISHMENT OF TCA CYCLE INTERMEDIATES DURING EXERCISE. The reamination limb of the purine nucleotide cycle could enhance mitochondrial respiration because the fumarate formed is readily oxidized to oxaloacetate and thereby available for condensation with acetyl-CoA to form citrate. Support for this hypothesis has come from Scislowski et al. [111] who demonstrated that the deamination of aspartate to fumarate through the purine nucleotide cycle served to enhance oxygen consumption in isolated mitochondria. Although a similar function may occur in skeletal muscle, some question exists over whether this process takes place to support metabolism during contractions.

The evidence that reamination is an important source of TCA cycle intermediates was obtained by a careful evaluation of critical metabolite contents during experiments with and without inhibition of the reaminating limb of the purine nucleotide cycle by hadacidin [4]. During moderately intense (5 Hz) contractions, approximately 70% of the increased levels of TCA cycle intermediates observed during 15 minutes of contractions could be accounted for by the reamination of IMP [4]. Unfortunately, the data cannot be interpreted plainly, because the muscles used in the experiments contained low- and high-oxidative muscle fibers. The rat hindlimb is composed of 60–70% fast-twitch, white fatigable fibers [2], which suggests that analyses of the mixed-fibered muscle would yield mass-averages of metabolites in fatigued and contracting fibers. The cellular response of fast-twitch white muscle is very different from that of the fast-twitch red during the 5 Hz twitch contraction condition [83] used in this study [4]. It is clear that reamination was occurring, but it is not possible to conclude from the data of Aragón and Lowenstein [4] that the purine nucleotide cycle served to enhance aerobic function by concurrent deamination/reamination reactions in *contracting* muscle. An alternative explanation can be offered. It is known that contraction failure of the low-oxidative, fast-twitch white fibers leads to a lower rate of muscle oxygen consumption [52]. Under these conditions, flux through the TCA cycle must decrease and may allow the transient accumulation of TCA cycle intermediates before a new steady-state rate is established. In perfused rat heart, a decrease in flux through the TCA cycle during a high work to low work transition is associated with increases in malate, oxaloacetate, and citrate [144]. After contraction failure, the production of fumarate by adenylosuccinate lyase during IMP reamination would be a likely source of the observed expansion of TCA cycle intermediates [4].

DEAMINATION OF AMINO ACIDS FOR OXIDATIVE METABOLISM. Another concomitant effect of the reamination leg of the purine nucleotide cycle is the potential deamination of amino acids. Amino acid metabolism is implicated because the reamination of IMP requires an amine from aspartate. The amount of aspartate required for full recovery of the adenine nucleotide content can be substantial. During intense stimulation conditions, in which 50% of the ATP pool is deaminated to IMP, approximately 10 times the normal tissue content of aspartate is required for full recovery of the ATP content. Thus, even though aspartate is the immediate substrate involved in the reamination of IMP, the amine must originate by transamination from other amino acids to aspartate (cf. Fig. 14.3).

One likely source is from the branched-chain amino acids (valine, isoleucine, and primarily leucine). The reasons are that, (a) these amino acids are taken up and oxidized by muscle [53, 54, 90], (b) muscle contains a high activity of the branched-chain, keto-acid transaminase enzyme [86], and (c) muscle is a major tissue in the body that oxidizes the branched-chain amino acids [48, 53, 54]. The amine nitrogen ultimately donated by aspartate to form AMP could originate through a sequence of transamination reactions [Fig. 14.3]. This pathway has

FIGURE 14.3

Deamination of branched-chain amino acids by means of the purine nucleotide cycle. Note that the amine transaminated from the branched-chain amino acids is used to reaminate IMP to AMP, whereas ammonia is produced in the deamination of AMP to IMP.

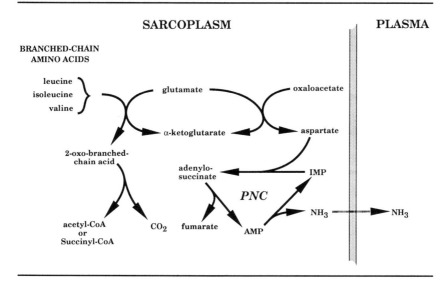

recently been shown to operate. Extracellularly derived leucine has been shown to account for a significant fraction of the amine used in the recovery of the adenine nucleotide pool following intense muscle stimulation [47]. If this occurred during contractions, the leucine-derived keto-acid (alpha-ketoisocaproate) would be available for oxidation [53]. The amine would appear as net ammonia production, originally cleaved during AMP deamination, because AMP is replaced by a complete turn of the purine nucleotide cycle. As discussed above, because high rates of AMP deamination/IMP reamination appear out of phase, it is unlikely that IMP reamination serves to enhance leucine oxidation in muscle during contractions. However, whether there may be a very low rate of amino acid deamination through the purine nucleotide cycle remains to be established experimentally.

Interestingly, the reamination of a large quantity of IMP would not necessarily produce an equivalent *net* increase in fumarate content within the cell. Any deamination of aspartate to fumarate would lead to oxaloacetate production, because fumarate is readily oxidized. The oxaloacetate, in turn, would be subject to reamination to aspartate via transamination with glutamate. This reformation of aspartate would maintain its tissue concentration while permitting a flux of amine to reaminate IMP.

Deficiencies of Enzymes of the Purine Nucleotide Cycle

AMP DEAMINASE DEFICIENCY. The most direct evidence for the importance of the purine nucleotide cycle comes from patients who exhibit a genetic deficiency in muscle AMP deaminase [38]. The inability to deaminate AMP coincides with altered muscle function in these patients who are typically intolerant of moderate to vigorous exercise though able to sustain mild work efforts [38, 65, 105]. Symptoms of easy fatigability, muscle pain, and cramps are consistent with muscle dysfunction that arises from an impaired ability to limit the increase in ADP_f and AMP_f expected in the absence of AMP deaminase [105, 106]. The association of symptoms and enzyme deficiency is controversial, however (80); performance during short-term ischemic isometric exercise is not necessarily impaired [118, 119].

Although nearly 90% of patients exhibit some degree of symptoms following exercise [108] the picture is not entirely clear. The age of onset and severity of symptoms vary widely with some persons who remain asymptomatic [40, 119]. Fishbein [40] has suggested that AMP deaminase deficiency may be present as a primary, inherited form with less than $\approx 1.5\%$ of normal activity, or alternatively, as an acquired deficiency secondary to other neuromuscular diseases, with considerably more (up to 10% of normal) activity present.

ADENYLOSUCCINATE LYASE DEFICIENCY. Deficiency of adenylosuccinate lyase recently has been identified in children who suffer from severe psychomotor retardation [60]. Muscle enzyme activity was deficient in three of six patients tested, with muscle wasting and growth retardation found [61]. Interestingly, adenylosuccinate was undetectable in adenylosuccinate lyase-deficient muscle, which suggests an effective dephosphorylation to succinyladenosine by 5'-nucleotidase [138]. This enzyme deficiency would have extensive consequences, because de novo adenine nucleotide synthesis and purine salvage from inosine and hypoxanthine would be impaired. Thus, disruption of the purine nucleotide cycle may be a minor issue compared to altered nucleic acid metabolism.

DEGRADATION OF ADENINE NUCLEOTIDES

Adenine nucleotide degradation in skeletal muscle was first studied during ischemia in which degradation products accumulate in the absence of oxidative phosphorylation [27, 56]. The potential activity of the degradative pathway is demonstrated by the 80–90% decrease in muscle adenine nucleotides during prolonged ischemia [27, 103]. Contraction of ischemic muscle further expands the difference between energy supply and utilization and accelerates degradation [28, 96, 103, 134]. With a prolonged energy imbalance, the concentration of ATP decreases and those of ADP and AMP rise, followed by the extensive accumulation of IMP. After the concentration of IMP has increased to high levels, inosine and subsequently hypoxanthine contents increase. This pattern of adenine nucleotide degradation is consistent with the high AMP deaminase activity present in skeletal muscle and also points to further degradation through the action of 5'-nucleotidase and nucleoside phosphorylase [136] (cf Fig. 14.4). Adenosine, in contrast, does not accumulate to a large extent in skeletal muscle. Although it is conceivable that AMP is dephosphorylated to adenosine and then deaminated to inosine by means of adenosine deaminase present in muscle [5, 59], the fact that inosine accumulates to a far greater extent than adenosine and that inosine rises only when the IMP concentration is already high [27, 28, 56, 96, 103, 106, 134], suggests that it is formed through the direct action of 5'-nucleotidase on IMP.

5'-Nucleotidase in Skeletal Muscle

The nucleotide monophosphates 5'-AMP or 5'-IMP may be dephosphorylated by 5'-nucleotidase [Reaction 8] to adenosine and inosine, respectively. Flux through

$$5'\text{-AMP } (5'\text{-IMP}) + H_2O \rightarrow \text{adenosine (inosine)} + PO_4^{2-} \quad [8]$$

this nonequilibrium reaction must be tightly controlled to prevent needless degradation and net loss of nucleotides which would require replacement by the energetically costly pathway of de novo synthesis.

Skeletal muscle 5'-nucleotidase activity is positively correlated with muscle oxidative capacity being highest in heart, intermediate in red skeletal muscle, and lower in fast-twitch white or predominantly low oxidative, mixed-fibered muscle [5, 59, 87, 112].

ENZYME LOCATION AND ISOFORMS. 5'-Nucleotidase was first studied in vitro using a semipurified enzyme extracted from rat and guinea pig skeletal muscle [25]. These authors found 5'-nucleotidase activity to be considerably higher in guinea pig than rat skeletal muscle; a somewhat higher maximal velocity was obtained with AMP as substrate as compared with IMP in the enzyme from both species. Camici et al [19] determined that about 85% of the 5'-nucleotidase activity was membrane bound and could be released by treatment with detergents. This finding is consistent with the cytochemical localization of the hydrolysis of AMP and IMP in rat skeletal muscle to endothelial cells and muscle fibers near blood vessels [103]. Moreover, Frick and Lowenstein [44] showed substantial accessibility of 5'-nucleotidase activity to the extracellular space by perfusing rat hindquarters with AMP and measuring the

FIGURE 14.4

Pathways of purine nucleotide synthesis and degradation.

1. *5-phosphoribosyl-1-pyrophosphate (PRPP) aminotransferase*
2. *AMP deaminase*
3. *adenylosuccinate synthetase*
4. *adenylosuccinate lyase*
5. *myokinase*
6. *adenosine kinase*
7. *5'-nucleotidase*
8. *5'-nucleotidase (probably cytoplasmic)*
9. *nucleosidase*
10. *purine nucleoside phosphorylase*
11. *adenine 5-phosphoribosyl 1-pyrophosphate transferase*
12. *hypoxanthine/guanine 5-phosphoribosyl 1-pyrophosphate transferase*
13. *adenosine deaminase*
14. *adenine deaminase*
15. *xanthine oxidase*
16. *S-adenosylhomocysteine hydrolase*

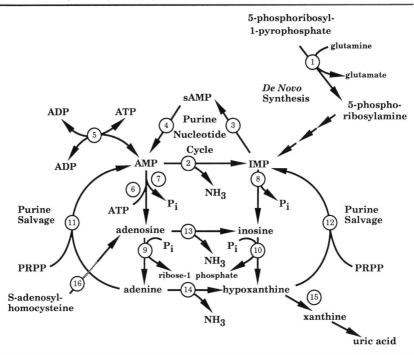

hydrolysis products. This observation provides good evidence to indicate that most 5'-nucleotidase is present as an ecto-enzyme.

Studies of 5'-nucleotidase in heart have revealed a membrane bound ecto-enzyme and a soluble, cytosolic 5'-nucleotidase; the membrane-bound 5'-nucleotidase is at least 10-fold more active than the soluble cytosolic enzyme in rat heart [79]. Recently, it has been reported that rat heart-soluble 5'-nucleotidase exists as two forms, favoring either AMP or IMP as substrate; the AMP-favoring isoform constitutes the majority of the total soluble 5'-nucleotidase activity [131]. Substantial evidence suggests that these cytosolic isoforms of 5'-nucleotidase are more important sources of adenosine formed from muscle AMP than the ecto-enzyme [58, 79, 131]. The ecto-enzyme has been postulated to be responsible for the production of adenosine from AMP that arises in the interstitial fluid by the action of pyrophosphatase on ATP released from sympathetic nerve endings [57].

Based on histochemical studies, it appears that a greater fraction of the 5'-nucleotidase activity might be located intracellularly in skeletal muscle as compared with heart [103]. Although isoforms of the soluble enzyme are likely to exist in skeletal muscle, to our knowledge, no direct information presently addresses this point.

REGULATION OF 5'NUCLEOTIDASE. The membrane-bound enzyme from guinea pig skeletal muscle exhibited half maximal velocities with 13 and 20 μM AMP and IMP, respectively, and was powerfully inhibited by μM concentrations of ATP [73]. A more highly purified 5'-nucleotidase showed even greater inhibition by ADP than ATP [19]; in contrast, the soluble form isolated from heart has a higher activity in the presence of ATP [59, 131]. The high substrate affinity of the ecto-enzyme would seem inconsistent with a primary role in degradation of intracellular adenine nucleotides because it would be highly active at physiological AMP_f concentrations. The fact that IMP (which is retained within the cell) can be extensively dephosphorylated in the presence of ATP suggests the possibility that skeletal muscle, like heart, also possesses soluble cytosolic 5'-nucleotidase(s). Alternatively, an ATP- and ADP-insensitive, membrane-bound ecto-enzyme with accessibility to the sarcoplasm also would be consistent with IMP dephosphorylation.

The heart-soluble 5'-nucleotidase has a K_m of 1–2 mmol/L for both the AMP- and IMP-favoring isoforms [131], much greater than that of the heart ecto-enzyme, in which half-saturation is about 14 μM [114]. The soluble 5'-nucleotidase from heart is activated by a decreasing energy charge [58]. If these regulatory features are applicable to skeletal muscle, an increase in AMP_f is probably important in the degradation of adenine nucleotides, whether degradation proceeds by AMP deamination to IMP with subsequent hydrolysis to inosine or by dephosphorylation to adenosine with ensuing deamination to inosine (cf. Fig. 14.4). Consistent with this view is the observation that hypoxanthine release from exercising muscle is increased at a lower exercise intensity in persons suffering arterial insufficiency, because AMP_f is likely to be higher owing to an impaired ability to meet the energy demands of exercise [122]. For a similar reason, exercise in patients with glycogen storage disease, in which muscle glycogenolysis and glycolysis are impaired, results in an exaggerated release of inosine and hypoxanthine [84].

Adenine Nucleotide Degradation During Exercise
With strenuous exercise in humans, the plasma concentrations of inosine [49] and hypoxanthine [49, 66, 122] increase, unlike adenosine which does not (49). This apparent net degradation of adenine nucleotides is reflected by the increased urinary excretion of inosine [49, 127] and hypoxanthine [49] after very intense exercise. Modest increases in muscle inosine and hypoxanthine [88, 106], along with the release of hypoxanthine by muscle (95, 122) after exhaustive exercise, suggest that skeletal muscle is the source of these degradation products.

Muscle nucleosides and bases do not accumulate to a measurable extent during exercise in which energy supply and utilization are well matched in either fast-twitch [96] or slow-twitch muscle [134]. In contrast, under fixed-flow conditions or frank ischemia, concentrations of adenosine [12, 14, 15, 28, 96, 134], inosine [14, 15, 27, 28, 56, 103, 118, 134] and hypoxanthine [14, 15, 27, 28, 56, 88, 103, 118] increase in proportion to the magnitude and duration of the apparent inequality between energy supply and demand.

Metabolic Consequences of Nucleoside Formation
Degradation of adenine nucleotides (Fig. 14.4) must be balanced by recovery through the salvage pathway or de novo synthesis if the adenine nucleotide pool size of skeletal muscle is to be maintained. The formation of adenosine also has been proposed to have important, local regulatory effects.

BLOOD FLOW REGULATION. Adenosine is a potent vasodilator [13] that accumulates during ischemia and during flow-restricted muscle contractions [12, 14, 15, 28, 96, 134]. During exercise in which oxygen delivery to the muscle is matched to the metabolic demand, adenosine does not measurably accumulate [12, 96], which suggests that adenosine's role in the regulation of skeletal muscle blood flow is probably restricted to oxygen-deficient conditions.

DE NOVO SYNTHESIS OF ADENINE NUCLEOTIDES

De novo synthesis of adenine nucleotides (Fig. 14.4) involves a series of 11 reactions that sequentially build on ribose-5-phosphate using the amino acids glutamine, glycine, and aspartate as well as formate and bicarbonate [86]. These reactions consume 6 high-energy phosphate bonds per IMP molecule synthesized. IMP thus formed is incorporated into the adenlyate pool by the purine nucleotide cycle as described previously. The capacity of skeletal muscle for de novo synthesis was first demonstrated in vivo [146], and later in isolated muscles incubated in vitro [113, 1137] and in cultured muscle cells [17, 148, 149, 150]. Nucleosides and bases lost from the cell and not restored by the salvage pathway therefore can be replenished by de novo synthesis. Under steady-state conditions (i.e., constant adenine nucleotide content) the de novo synthesis rate must equal the net loss of adenine nucleotides from the muscle adenine nucleotide pool.

Fiber Type Differences
Recent experiments using perfused rat skeletal muscle have shown that the rate of de novo synthesis differs among resting muscle fiber types. The red, high oxidative fast- and slow-twitch fibers show high rates of synthesis compared to low oxidative fast-twitch fibers. Activities in mixed-fibered muscles were found to be intermediate [132]. Muscle fibers experience different degrees of adenine nucleotide degradation during periods in which ATP hydrolysis exceeds rephosphorylation; red muscle produces more nucleosides and bases than white [15, 67]. This may explain why rates of de novo synthesis and adenine nucleotide pool turnover vary among fiber types according to the fibers' oxidative capacity [132].

Effect of Endurance Training and Exercise
The correlation between de novo synthesis rate and muscle oxidative capacity might imply that endurance training, which increases mito-chondrial content, may also increase the capacity for de novo synthesis. Recent evidence indicates that endurance training has little effect on de novo synthesis rates in resting skeletal muscle [135]; rather, the most important influence of training may be to improve the sensitivity of respiratory control such that energy turnover can be sustained with smaller increases in ADP_f and AMP_f [36] and thus reduce degradation. De novo synthesis of adenine nucleotides is lower in contracting muscle [133]; perhaps because of the first step of the de novo synthesis pathway, 5'phosphoribosyl pyrophosphate synthetase is inhibited by ADP [11b]. Synthesis in resting and fatigued muscle, however, are similar. There is no evidence that flux through the de novo synthesis pathway increases during muscle contraction to compensate for lost nucleosides and bases.

SUMMARY

During steady-state muscle contractions, ATP production and utilization are well matched. When the rate of ATP hydrolysis exceeds the capacity of a given muscle fiber to phosphorylate ADP, the ADP_f and AMP_f concentrations rise, first leading to the deamination of adenylates and subsequently to the dephosphorylation of AMP or IMP, or both, to their respective nucleosides and bases.

Several proposed roles for the purine nucleotide cycle in skeletal muscle have been reviewed and evaluated. The deaminating limb of the purine nucleotide cycle is most important; it maintains the ATP/ADP ratio and lessens adenine nucleotide degradation. Regulation of glycolytic pathway enzymes by the products of AMP deamination (IMP and NH_4^+) does not seem likely. During reamination there is a net production of fumarate, with the branch-chain amino acids potentially supplying a significant fraction of the amine; reamination, however, is probably not concurrent with a high rate of deamination. Evidence from some studies of AMP deaminase-deficient persons suggests that an intact purine nucleotide cycle is required for normal muscle function during intense exercise; the issue is clouded, however, by the occurrence of asymptomatic AMP deaminase deficiency.

Skeletal muscle is capable of extensive adenine nucleotide degradation during severe, energy-depleting conditions. Purine nucleosides and bases not reincorporated by the salvage pathway must be synthesized de novo. The capacity for de novo synthesis differs among fiber types, being highest in muscle with the highest oxidative capacity.

ACKNOWLEDGEMENT

Work cited from the authors' laboratory was supported by NIH Grant AR 21617.

REFERENCES

1. Abrahams, S.L., and E.S. Younathan. Modulation of the kinetic properties of phosphofructokinase by ammonium ions. *J. Biol. Chem.* 246:2464–2467, 1971.
2. Armstrong, R.B., and R.O. Phelps. Muscle fiber composition of the rat hindlimb. *Am. J. Anat.* 171:259–272, 1984.
3. Aragon, J.J., K. Tornheim, and J.M. Lowenstein. On a possible role of IMP in the regulation of phosphorylase activity in skeletal muscle, *FEBS Letts* 117 (Suppl.):K56–K64, 1980.
4. Aragón, J.J., and J.M. Lowenstein. The purine nucleotide cycle. Comparison of the levels of citric acid cycle intermediates with the operation of the purine nucleotide cycle in rat skeletal muscle during exercise and recovery from exercise. *Eur. J. Biochem.* 110:371–377, 1980.
5. Arch, J.R.S., and E.A. Newsholme. Activities and some properties of 5'-nucleotidase, adenosine kinase and adenosine deaminase in tissues from vertebrates and invertebrates in relation to the control of the concentration and the physiolgical role of adenosine. *Biochem. J.* 174:965:977, 1978.
6. Ashby, B., and C. Frieden. Interaction of AMP-aminohydrolase with myosin and its subfragments. *J. Biol. Chem.* 252:1869–1872, 1977.

7. Ashby, B., and C. Frieden. Adenylate deaminase. Kinetic and binding studies on the rabbit muscle enzyme. *J. Biol. Chem.* 253:8728–8735, 1978.

8. Ashby, B., C. Frieden, and R. Bischoff. Immunofluorescent and histochemical localization of AMP deaminase in skeletal muscle. *J. Cell Biol.* 81:361–373, 1979.

9. Baggot, J.E., W.H. Vaughn, and B.B. Hudson. Inhibition of 5-aminoimidazole-4-carboxamide ribotide transformylase, adenosine deaminase and 5'-adenylate deaminase by polyglutamates of methotrexate and oxidized folates and by 5-aminoimidazole-4-carboximide riboside and ribotide. *Biochem. J.* 236:193–200, 1986.

10. Baldwin, K.M., G.H. Klinkerfuss, R.L. Terjung, P.A. Mole, and J.O. Holloszy. Respiratory capacity of white, red and intermediate muscle: adaptive response to exercise. *Am. J. Physiol.* 222:373–378, 1972.

11. Baldwin, K.M., P.J. Campbell, and D.K. Cooke. Glycogen, lactate, and alanine changes in muscle fiber types during graded exercise. *J. Appl. Physiol.* 43:288–291, 1977.

11b.Becker, M.A., K.O. Raivio, and J.E. Seegmiller. Synthesis of phosphoribosylpyrophosphate in mammalian cells. *Adv. Enzymol.* 49:281–306, 1979.

12. Belloni, F.L., R.D. Phair, and H.V. Sparks. The role of adenosine in prolonged vasodilation following flow-restricted exercise of canine skeletal muscle. *Circ. Res.* 44:759–766, 1979.

13. Berne, R.M. The role of adenosine in the regulation of coronary blood flow. *Circ. Res.* 47:807–813, 1980.

14. Bockman, E.L., R.M. Berne, and R. Rubio. Adenosine and active hyperemia in dog skeletal muscle. *Am. J. Physiol.* 230:1531–1537, 1976.

15. Bockman, E.L., and J.E. McKenzie. Tissue adenosine content in active soleus and gracilis muscles of cats. *Am. J. Physiol.* 244:H552–H559, 1983.

16. Broberg, S., and K. Sahlin. Adenine nucleotide degradation in human skeletal muscle during prolonged exercise. *J. Appl. Physiol.* 67:116–122, 1989.

17. Brosh, S., P. Boer, E. Zoref-Shani, and O. Sperling. De novo purine synthesis in skeletal muscle. *Biochim. Biophys. Acta* 714:181–183, 1982.

18. Burke, R.E., D.N. Levine, F.E. Zajac, P. Tsairis, and W.K. Engel. Mammalian motorunits: physiological-histochemical correlation in three types of cat gastrocnemius. *Science* 174:709–712, 1971.

19. Camici, M., C. Fini, and P.L. Ipata. Isolation and kinetic properties of 5'-nucleotidase from guinea-pig skeletal muscle. *Biochem. Biophys. Acta* 840:6–12, 1985.

20. Casey, P.J., and J.M. Lowenstein. Purification of adenylosuccinate lyase from rat skeletal muscle by a novel affinity column. *Biochem. J.* 246:263–269, 1987.

21. Chasiotis, D., K. Sahlin, and E. Hultman. Regulation of glycogenolysis in human muscle at rest and during exercise. *J. Appl. Physiol.* 53:708–715, 1982.

22. Conlee, R.K., J.A. McLane, M.J. Rennie, W.W. Winder, and J.O. Holloszy. Reversal of phosphorylase activation in muscle despite continued contractile activity. *Am. J. Physiol.* 237:R291–R296, 1979.

23. Cooke, R., and E. Pate. The effects of ADP and Phosphate on the contraction of muscle fibers. *Biophys. J.* 48:789–798, 1985.

24. Cooper, J., and J. Trinick. Binding and location of AMP deaminase in rabbit psoas muscle myofibrils. *J. Mol. Biol.* 177:137–152, 1984.

25. Cozzani, I., P.L. Ipata, and M. Ranieri. Resolution of 5'-nucleotidase and nonspecific phosphatase activities from skeletal muscles. *FEBS Letts.* 2:189–92, 1969.

26. Dawson, M.J., D.G. Gadian, and D.R. Wilkie. Mechanical relaxation rate and metabolism studied in fatiguing muscle by phosphorous nuclear magnetic resonance. *J. Physiol.* (London) 299:465–484, 1980.

27. Deuticke, B., E. Gerlach, and R. Dierkesmann. Abbau freier nucleotide in herz, skeletmuskel, gehirn und leber der ratte bei sauerstoffmangel. *Pflügers Arch.* 292:239–254, 1966.

28. Dobson, J.G., Jr., R. Rubio, and R.M. Berne. Role of adenine nucleotides, adenosine,

and inorganic phosphate in the regulation of skeletal muscle blood flow. *Circ. Res.* 29:375–384, 1971.

29. Dobson, G.F., E. Yamamoto, and P.W. Hochachka. Phosphofructokinase control in muscle: nature and reversal of pH-dependent ATP inhibition. *Am. J. Physiol.* 250:R71–R76, 1986.

30. Dobson, G.P., W.S. Parkhouse, J.-M. Weber, E. Stuttard, J. Harman, D.H. Snow, and P.W. Hochachka. Metabolic changes in skeletal muscle and blood of greyhounds during 800-m track sprint. *Am. J. Physiol.* 255:R513–R519, 1988.

31. Driedzic, W.R., and P.W. Hochachka. Control of energy metabolism in fish white muscle. *Am. J. Physiol.* 230:579–582, 1976.

32. Dudley, G.A., W.M. Abraham, and R.L. Terjung. Influence of exercise intensity and duration on biochemical adaptations in skeletal muscle. *J. Appl. Physiol.* 53:844–850, 1982.

33. Dudley, G.A., R.S. Staron, T.F. Murray, R.C. Hagerman, and A. Luginbuhl. Muscle fiber composition and blood ammonia levels after intense exercise in humans. *J. Appl. Physiol.* 54:582–586, 1983.

34. Dudley, G.A., and R.L. Terjung. Influence of aerobic metabolism on IMP accumulation in fast-twitch muscle. *Am. J. Physiol.* 248:C37–C42, 1985.

35. Dudley, G.A., and R.L. Terjung. Influence of acidosis on AMP deaminase activity in contracting fast-twitch muscle. *Am. J. Physiol.* 248:C43–C50, 1985.

36. Dudley, G.A., P.C. Tullson, and R.L. Terjung. Influence of mitrochondrial content on the sensitivity of respiratory control. *J. Biol. Chem.* 262:9109–9114, 1987.

37. Ferenczi, M.A., Y.E. Goldman, and R.M. Simmons. The dependence of force and shortening velocity on substrate concentration in skinned muscle fibres from *Rana temporaria. J. Physiol.* 350:519–543, 1984.

38. Fishbein, W.N., V.W. Armbrustmacker, and J.L. Griffin. Myoadenylate deaminase deficiency: a new disease of muscle. *Science* 200:545–548, 1978.

39. Fishbein, W.N., V.W. Armbrustmacher, J.L. Griffin, J.I. Davis, and W.D. Foster. Level of adenylate deaminase, adenylate kinase, and creatine kinase in frozen human muscle biopsy specimens relative to type 1/type 2 fiber distribution: evidence for a carrier state of myoadenylate deaminase deficiency. *Ann. Neurol.* 15:271–277, 1984.

40. Fishbein, W.N. Myoadenylate deaminase deficiency: inherited and acquired forms. *Biochem. Med.* 33:158–169, 1985.

41. Fishbein, W.N., N. Ogasawara, R.L. Sabina, and E.W. Holmes. AMP deaminase isozymes in type 1 & type 1 muscles and in muscle biopsies with primary & secondary myoadenylate deaminase deficiency. *FASEB J.* 4:A1963, 1990.

42. Flanagan, W.F., E.W. Holmes, R.L. Sabina, and J.L. Swain. Importance of purine nucleotide cycle to energy production in skeletal muscle. *Am. J. Physiol.* 251:C795–C802, 1986.

43. Foley, J.M., G.R. Adams, and R.A. Meyer. Utility of AICAr for metabolic studies is diminished by systemic effects in situ. *Am. J. Physiol.* 257:C488–C494, 1989.

44. Frick, G.P., and J.M. Lowenstein. Studies of 5′-nucleotidase in the perfused rat heart including measurements of the enzyme in perfused skeletal muscle and liver. *J. Biol. Chem.* 251:6372–6378, 1976.

45. Gibbs, C.L. Cardiac energetics. *Physiol. Rev.* 58:174–254, 1978.

46. Goodman, M.N., and J.M. Lowenstein. The purine nucleotide cycle. Studies of ammonia production by skeletal muscle in situ and in perfused preparations. *J. Biol. Chem.* 252:5054–5060, 1977.

47. Gorski, J., D.A. Hood, O.M. Brown, and R.L. Terjung. Incorporation of ^{15}N-leucine amine into ATP of fast-twitch muscle following stimulation. *Biochem. Biophys. Res. Comm.* 128:1254–1260, 1985.

48. Harper, A.E., and C. Zapalowski. Metabolism of branched-chain amino acids. J.C. Waterlow and J.M.L. Stephen (eds.). *Nitrogen Metabolism in Man.* London: Applied Science Pub., 1981, pp. 97–116.

49. Harkness, R.A., R.J. Simmonds, and S.B. Coade. Purine transport and metabolism in man: the effect of exercise on concentrations of purine base, nucleosides and nucleotides in plasma, urine, leucocytes and erythrocytes. *Clin. Sci.* 64:333–340 1983.

50. Harris, R.C., and E. Hultman. Adenine nucleotide depletion in human muscle in response to intermittent stimulation in situ. *J. Physiol.* 365:78P, 1985.

51. Hobbs, S.F., and D.I. McCloskey. Effects of blood pressure on force production in cat and human muscle. *J. Appl. Physiol.* 63:834–839, 1987.

52. Hood, D.A., J. Gorski, and R.L. Terjung. Oxygen cost of twitch and tetanic contractions of rat skeletal muscle. *Am. J. Physiol.* 250:E449–E456, 1986.

53. Hood, D.A., and R.L. Terjung. Leucine metabolism in perfused rat skeletal muscle during contractions. *Am. J. Physiol.* 253:E636–E647, 1987.

54. Hood, D.A., and R.L. Terjung. Effect of endurance training on leucine metabolism in perfused rat skeletal muscle. *Am. J. Physiol.* 253:E648–E656, 1987.

55. Hultman, E., and L.L. Spriet. Skeletal muscle metabolism, contraction force and glycogen utilization during prolonged electrical stimulation in humans. *J. Physiol. Lond.* 374:493–501, 1986.

56. Imai, S., A.L. Riley, and R.M. Berne. Effect of ischemia on adenine nucleotides in cardiac and skeletal muscle. *Circulation Res.* 15:443–450, 1964.

57. Imai, S., W.-P. Chin, H. Jin, and M. Nakazawa. Production of AMP and adenosine in the interstitital fluid compartment of the isolated perfused normoxic guinea pig heart. *Pflügers Arch.* 414:443–449, 1989.

58. Itoh, R., J. Oka, and H. Ozasa. Regulation of rat heart cytosol 5'-nucleotidase by adenylate energy charge. *Biochem. J.* 235–847–851, 1986.

59. Jacobs, A.E.M., A. Oosterhof, and J.H. Veerkamp. Purine and pyrimidine metabolism in human muscle and cultured muscle cells. *Biochem. Biophys. Acta* 970:130–136, 1988.

60. Jaeken, J., and G. Van den Berghe. An infantile autistic syndrome characterized by the presence of succinylpurines in body fluids. *Lancet* 2:1058–1061, 1984.

61. Jaeken, J., S.K. Wadman, M. Duran, et al. Adenylosuccinase deficiency: an inborn error of purine nucleotide synthesis. *Eur. J. Pediatr.* 148:126–131, 1988.

62. Jansson, E., G. Dudley, B. Norman, and P. Tesch. ATP and IMP in single human muscle fibers after high intensity exercise. *Clin. Physiol.* 7:337–345, 1987.

63. Jennings, R.B., and C. Steenbergen Jr.. Nucleotide metabolism and cellular damage in myocardial ischemia. *Ann. Rev. Physiol.* 47:727–749, 1985.

64. Katz, A., K. Sahlin, and J. Henriksson. Muscle ammonia metabolism during isometric contract in humans. *Am. J. Physiol.* 250:C834–C840, 1986.

65. Keleman, J., D.R. Rice, W.G. Bradley, T.L. Munsat, S. DiMauro, and E.L. Hogan. Familial myoadenylate deaminase deficiency and exertional myalgia. *Neurology* 32:857–863, 1982.

66. Ketai, L.H., R.H. Simon, J.W. Kriet, and C.M. Grum. Plasma hypoxanthine and exercise. *Am. Rev. Respir. Dis.* 136:98–101, 1987.

67. Klabunde, R.E., and S.E. Mayer. Effects of ischemia on tissue metabolites in red (slow) and white (fast) skeletal muscle of the chicken. *Circ. Res.* 45:366–373, 1979.

68. Laughlin, M.H., and R.B. Armstrong. Muscle blood flow during locomotory exercise. *Exerc. Sport Sci. Rev.* 13:95–136, 1985.

69. Lo, P.-Y., and G.A. Dudley. Endurance training reduces the magnitude of exercise-induced hyperammonemia in humans. *J. Appl. Physiol.* 62:1227–1230, 1987.

70. Lowenstein, J.M. Ammonia production in muscle and other tissues: the purine nucleotide cycle. *Physiol. Rev.* 52:382–414, 1972.

71. Lowenstein, J.M. The purine nucleotide cycle revised. *Int. J. Sports Med.* 11(Suppl. 2):S37, 1990.

72. Mackie, B.G., and R.L. Terjung. Blood flow to the different skeletal muscle fiber types during contraction. *Am. J. Physiol.* 245:H265–H275, 1983.

73. Magni, G., E. Fioretti, F. Marmocchi, P. Natalini, and P.L. Ipata. Guinea pig skeletal muscle 5'-nucleotidase. *Life Sci.* 13:663–673, 1973.

74. Manfredi, J.P., and E.W. Holmes. Purine salvage pathways in myocardium. *Annu. Rev. Physiol.* 47:691–705, 1985.

75. Manfredi, J.P., R. Marquetant, A.D. Magid, and E.W. Holmes. Binding of adenylosuccinate synthetase to contractile proteins of muscle. *Am. J. Physiol.* 257:C29–C35, 1989.

76. Marquetant, R., N.M. Desai, R.L. Sabina, and E.W. Holmes. Evidence for sequential expression of multiple AMP deaminase isoforms during skeletal muscle development. *Proc. Natl. Acad. Sci.* 84:2345–2349, 1987.

77. Marquetant, R., R.L. Sabina, and E.W. Holmes. Identification of a noncatalytic domain in AMP deaminase that influences binding to myosin. *Biochem.* 28:8744–8749, 1989.

78. McGilvery, R.M., and T.W. Murray. Calculated equilibria of phosphocreatine and adenosine phosphates during utilization of high energy phosphate by muscle. *J. Biol. Chem.* 249:5845–5850, 1974.

79. Meghji, P., K.M. Middleton, and A.C. Newby. Absolute rates of adenosine formation during ischaemia in rat and pigeon hearts. *Biochem. J.* 249:695–703, 1988.

80. Mercelis, R., J-J. Martin, T. de Barsy, and G. Van den Berghe. Myoadenylate deaminase deficiency: absence of correlation with exercise intolerance in 452 muscle biopsies. *J. Neurol.* 234:385–389, 1987.

81. Meyer, R.A., G.A. Dudley, and R.L. Terjung. Ammonia and IMP in different skeletal muscle fibers after exercise in rats. *J. Appl. Physiol.* 49:1037–1041, 1980.

82. Meyer, R.A., and R.L. Terjung. Differences in ammonia and adenylate metabolism in contracting fast and slow muscle. *Am. J. Physiol.* 237:C111–C118, 1979.

83. Meyer, R.A., and R.L. Terjung. AMP deamination and IMP reamination in working skeletal muscle. *Am. J. Physiol.* 239:C32–C38, 1980.

84. Mineo, I., N. Kono, T. Shimizu, et al. Excess purine degradation in exercising muscles of patients with glycogen storage disease types V and VII. *J. Clin. Invest.* 76:556–560, 1985.

85. Muirhead, K.M., and S.H. Bishop. Purification of adenylosuccinate synthetase from rabbit skeletal muscle. *J. Biol. Chem.* 249:459–464, 1974.

86. Newsholme, E.A., and A.R. Leech. *Biochemistry for the Medical Sciences.* New York: John Wiley and Sons, 1983.

87. Newsholme, E.A., E. Blomstrand, J. Newell, and J. Pitcher. Maximal activities of enzymes involved in adenosine metabolism in muscle and adipose tissue of rats under conditions of variations in insulin sensitivity. *FEBS Letts.* 181:189–192, 1985.

88. Norman, B., A. Sollevi, L. Kaijser, and E. Jannson. ATP breakdown products in human skeletal muscle during prolonged exercise to exhaustion. *Clin. Physiol.* 7:503–509, 1987.

89. Norman, B., A. Sollevi, and E. Jannson. Increased IMP content in glycogen-depleted muscle fibers during submaximal exercise in man. *Acta Physiol. Scand.* 133:97–100, 1988.

90. Odessey, R., and A.L. Goldberg. Oxidation of leucine by rat skeletal muscle. *Am. J. Physiol.* 223:1376–1383, 1972.

91. Ogasawara, N., H. Goto, Y. Yamada, T. Watanabe, and T. Asano. AMP deaminase in human tissues. *Biochim. Biophys. Acta* 714:298–306, 1982.

92. Ogasawara, N., H. Goto, and Y. Yamada. AMP deaminase isozymes in rabbit red and white muscles and heart. *Comp. Biochem. Physiol.* 76B:471–473, 1983.

93. Ogawa, H., H. Shiraki, Y. Matsuda, K. Kakiuchi, and H. Nakagawa. Purification, crystallization, and properties of adenylosuccinate synthetase from rat skeletal muscle. *J. Biochem.* 81:859–869, 1977.

94. Ogawa, H., H. Shiraki, Y. Matsuda, and H. Nakagawa. Interaction of adenylosuccinate synthetase with F-actin. *Eur. J. Biochem.* 85:331–337, 1978.

95. Patterson, V.H., K.K. Kaiser, and M.H. Brooke. Exercising muscle does not produce hypoxanthine in adenylate deaminase deficiency. *Neurology* 33:784–786, 1983.
96. Phair, R.D., and H.V. Sparks. Adenosine content of skeletal muscle during active hyperemia and ischemic contraction. *Am. J. Physiol.* 237:H1–H9, 1979.
97. Raggi, A., S. Ronca-Testoni, and G. Ronca. Muscle AMP aminohydrolase. II. Distribution of AMP aminohydrolase, myokinase and creatine kinase activities in skeletal muscle. *Biochim. Biophys. Acta* 178:619–622, 1969.
98. Raggi, A., C. Bergamini, and G. Ronca. Isozymes of AMP deaminase in red and white skeletal muscles. *FEBS Letts.* 58:19–23, 1975.
99. Raggi, A., and M. Ranieri-Raggi. Regulatory properties of AMP deaminase isoenzymes from rabbit red muscle. *Biochem. J.* 242:875–879, 1987.
100. Rahim, Z.H.A., G. Lutaya, and J.R. Griffiths. Activation of AMP aminohydrolase during skeletal muscle contraction. *Biochem. J.* 184:173–176, 1979.
101. Rahim, Z.H.A., D. Perrett, G. Lutaya, and J.R. Griffiths. Metabolic adaptation in phosphorylase kinase deficiency. Changes in metabolite concentrations during tetani stimulation of mouse leg muscles. *Biochem. J.* 186:331–341, 1980.
102. Ranieri-Raggi, M., and A. Raggi. Effects of storage on activity and subunit structure of rabbit skeletal-muscle AMP deaminase. *Biochem. J.* 189:367–368, 1980.
103. Rubio, R., R.M. Berne, and J.G. Dobson, Jr.. Sites of adenosine production in cardiac and skeletal muscle. *Am. J. Physiol.* 225:938–953, 1973.
104. Rundell, K.W., P.C. Tullson, and R.L. Terjung. AMP deaminase binding in contracting rat skeletal muscle. *Med. Sci. Sports Exer.* 22:S7, 1990.
105. Sabina, R.L., J.L. Swain, B.M. Patten, T. Ashizawa, W.E. O'Brien, and E.W. Holmes. Disruption of the purine nucleotide cycle. A potential explanation for muscle dysfunction in myoadenylate deaminase deficiency. *J. Clin. Invest.* 66:1419–1423, 1980.
106. Sabina, R.L., J.L. Swain, C.W. Olanow, et al. Myoadenylate deaminase deficiency. Functional and metabolic abnormalities associated with disruption of the purine nucleotide cycle. *J. Clin. Invest.* 73:720–730, 1984.
107. Sabina, R.L., R. Marquetant, N.M. Desai, K. Kaletha, and E.W. Holmes. Cloning and sequence of rat myoadenylate deaminase cDNA. *J. Biol. Chem.* 262:12397–12400, 1987.
108. Sabina, R.L., J.L. Swain, and E.W. Holmes. Myoadenylate deaminase deficiency. J.B. Stanbury, J.B. Wyngaarden, D.S. Fredrickson, J.L. Goldstein, and M.S. Brown, (eds.) *Metabolic Basis of Inherited Disease*, 6th ed. New York: McGraw-Hill Information Services Co., Health Professions Division, 1989, pp. 1077–1084.
109. Sahlin, K., S. Broberg, and J.M. Ren. Formation of inosine monophosphate (IMP) in human skeletal muscle during incremental dynamic exercise. *Acta Physiol. Scand.* 136:193–198, 1989.
110. Sahlin, K., and A. Katz. Purine nucleotide metabolism. *Med. Sport Sci.* 27:120–139, 1988.
111. Scislowsi, P.W.D., Z. Aleksandrowica, and J. Swierczynski. Purine nucleotide cycle as a possible anapleurotic process in rat skeletal muscle. *Experientia* 38:1035–1037, 1982.
112. Schopf, G., M. Havel, R. Fasol, and M.M. Müller. Enzyme activities of purine catabolism and salvage in human muscle tissue. *Adv. Exp. Biol. Med.* 195B:507–509, 1986.
113. Sheehan T.G., and E.R. Tully. Purine biosynthesis de novo in rat skeletal muscle. *Biochem. J.* 216:605–610, 1983.
114. Shütz, W., J. Schrader, and E. Gerlach. Different sites of adenosine formation in the heart. *Am. J. Physiol.* 240:H963–H970, 1981.
115. Shiraki, H., H. Ogawa, Y. Matsuda, and H. Nakagawa. Interaction of rat muscle AMP deaminase with myosin. I. Biochemical study of the interaction of AMP deaminase and myosin in rat muscle. *Biochim. Biophys. Acta* 566:335–344, 1979.

116. Shiraki, H., H. Ogawa, Y. Matsuda, and H. Nakagawa. Interaction of rat muscle AMP deaminase with myosin. II. Modification of the kinetic and regulatory properties of rat muscle AMP deaminase by myosin. *Biochim. Biophys. Acta* 566:345–352, 1979.

117. Shiraki, H., S. Miyamoto, Y. Matsuda, E. Momose, H. Nakagawa. Possible correlation between binding of muscle type AMP deaminase to myofibrils and ammoniagenesis in rat skeletal muscle on electrical stimulation. *Biochem. Biophys. Res. Comm.* 100:1099–1103, 1981.

118. Sinkeler, S.P.T., E.M.G. Joosten, R.A. Wevers, et al. Ischaemic exercise test in myoadenylate deaminase deficiency and McArdle's disease: measurement of plasma adenosine, inosine and hypoxanthine. *Clin. Sci.* 70:399–401, 1986.

119. Sinkeler, S.P.T., R.A. Binkhorst, E.M.G. Joosten, R.A. Wevers, M.M. Coerwinkel, and T.L. Oei. AMP deaminase deficiency: study of the human skeletal muscle purine metabolism during ischaemic isometric exercise. *Clin. Sci.* 72:475–482, 1987.

120. Snow, D.H., R.C. Harris, and S.P. Gash. Metabolic response of equine muscle to intermittent maximal exercise. *J. Appl. Physiol.* 58:1689–1697, 1985.

121. Solano, C., and C.J. Coffee. Differential response of AMP deaminase isozymes to changes in the adenylate energy charge. *Biochem. Biophys. Res. Comm.* 85:564–571, 1978.

122. Sørlie, D., K. Myhre, O.D. Saugstad, and K.-E. Giercksky. Release of hypoxanthine and phosphate from exercising human legs with and without arterial insufficiency. *Acta Med. Scand.* 211:281–286, 1982.

123. Spriet, L.L., K. Soderlund, M. Bergstrom, and E. Hultman. Anaerobic energy release in skeletal muscle during electrical stimulation in men. *J. Appl. Physiol.* 62:611–615, 1987.

124. Spriet, L.L., K. Soderlund, M. Bergstom, and E. Hultman. Skeletal muscle glycogenolysis, glycolysis, and pH during electrical stimulation in men. *J. Appl. Physiol.* 62:616–621, 1987.

125. Stayton, M.M., F.B. Rudolph, and H.J. Fromm. Regulation, genetics, and properties of adenylosuccinate synthetase: a review. *Curr. Top. Cell. Regul.* 22:103–141, 1983.

126. Sugden, P.H., and E.A. Newsholme. Effects of ammonium, inorganic phosphate and potassium ions on the activity of phosphofructokinases from muscle and nervous tissue of vertebrates and invertebrates. *Biochem. J.* 150: 113–122, 1975.

127. Sutton, J.R., C.W. Toews, G.R. Ward, and I. Fox. Purine metabolism during strenuous muscular exercise in man. *Metabolism* 29:254–260, 1980.

128. Swain, J.L., J.J. Hines, R.L. Sabina, O.L. Harbury, and E.W. Holmes. Disruption of the purine nucleotide cycle by inhibition of adenylosuccinate lyase produces skeletal muscle disfunction. *J. Clin. Invest.* 74:1422–1427, 1984.

129. Terjung, R.L., G.A. Dudley, and R.A. Meyer. Metabolic and circulatory limitations to muscular performance at the organ level. *J. Exp. Biol.* 115:307–318, 1985.

130. Tesch, P., and J. Karlsson. Lactate in fast and slow twitch skeletal muscle fibers of man during isometric contraction. *Acta Physiol. Scand.* 99:230–236, 1977.

131. Truong, V.L., A.R. Collinson, and J.M. Lowenstein. 5'-Nucleotidases in rat heart. *Biochem. J.* 253:117–121, 1988.

132. Tullson, P.C., H. John-Alder, D.A. Hood, and R.L. Terjung. De novo synthesis of adenine nucleotides in different skeletal muscle fiber types. *Am. J. Physiol.* 255:C271–C277, 1988.

133. Tullson, P.C., and R.L. Terjung. De novo synthesis of adenine nucleotides in contracting skeletal muscle. *Med. Sci. Sports Exer.* 21:S17, 1989.

134. Tullson, P.C., D.M. Whitlock, and R.L. Terjung. Adenine nucleotide degradation in slow-twitch red muscle. *Am. J. Physiol.* 258:C258–C265, 1990.

135. Tullson, P.C., and R.L. Terjung. De novo synthesis of skeletal muscle adenine nucleotides following endurance training. *FASEB J.* 4:A541, 1990.

136. Tullson, P.C., and R.L. Terjung. Adenine nucleotide degradation in striated muscle. *Int. J. Sports Med.* 11:S47–S55, 1990.

137. Tully, E.R., and T.G. Sheehan. Purine metabolism in rat skeletal muscle. *Adv. Exp. Med. Biol.* 122B: 13–17, 1980.

138. Van den Berghe, G., and J. Jaeken. Adenylosuccinase deficiency. *Adv. Exp. Med. Biol.* 195A:27–33, 1986.

139. Vincent, A., and J.McD. Blair. The coupling of the adenylate kinase and creatine kinase equilibria. Calculation of substrate and feedback signal levels in muscle. *FEBS Letts.* 7:239–244, 1970.

140. Westra, H.G., A. De Haan, J.E. Van Doorn, and E.J. De Haan. IMP production and energy metabolism during exercise in rats in relation to age. *Biochem. J.* 239:751–755, 1986.

141. Wheeler, T.J., and J.M. Lowenstein. Adenylate deaminase from muscle. Regulation by purine nucleotides and orthphosphate in the presence of 150 mM KCl. *J. Biol. Chem.* 254:8994–8999, 1979.

142. Whitlock, D.M., and R.L. Terjung. ATP depletion in slow-twitch red muscle of the rat. *Am. J. Physiol.* 253:C426–C432, 1987.

143. Wilkerson, J.E., D.L. Batterton, S.M. Horvath. Exercise-induced changes in blood ammonia levels in humans. *Eur. J. Appl. Physiol.* 37:255–263, 1977.

144. Williamson, J.R., C. Ford, J. Illingworth, and B. Safer. Coordination of citric acid cycle activity with electron transport flux. *Circ. Res.* (Suppl. 1):I39–I48, 1976.

145. Winder, W.W., R.L. Terjung, K.M. Baldwin, and J.O. Holloszy. Effect of exercise on AMP deaminase and adenylosuccinase in rat skeletal muscle. *Am. J. Physiol.* 227:1411–1414, 1974.

146. Zimmer, H.-G., and E. Gerlach. Stimulation of myocardial adenine nucleotide biosynthesis by pentoses and pentitols. *Pflügers Arch.* 376:223–227, 1978.

147. Zöllner, N., S. Reiter, M. Gross, et al. Myoadenylate deaminase deficiency: successful symptomatic therapy by high dose oral administration of ribose. *Klin Wochenschr.* 64:1281–1290, 1986.

148. Zoref-Shani, E., A. Shainberg, and O. Sperling. Characterization of purine nucleotide metabolism in primary rat muscle cultures. *Biochim. Biophys. Acta* 716:324–330, 1982.

149. Zoef-Shani, E., A. Shainberg, and O. Sperling. Pathways of adenine nucleotide catabolism in primary rat muscle cultures. *Biochem. Biophys. Acta* 926:287–295, 1987.

150. Zoef-Shani, E., A. Shainberg, G. Kessler-Icekson, and O. Sperling. Production and degradation of AMP in cultured rat skeletal and heart muscle: a comparative study. *Adv. Exp. Med. Biol.* 195B:485–491, 1986.

15
Sport and Collective Violence

KEVIN YOUNG, Ph.D.

INTRODUCTION

Sports-related violence is considered to have become a critical social problem in many countries. Fans of European sport, particularly soccer, have gained notoriety for their violence inside and outside stadia. Violent disturbances at sport also have occurred with some frequency in Australia, Central and South America, Asia, and North America. In most of these places, sports-related violence has prompted solicitous responses from politicians, police, sports officials, and journalists. Scholars, however, have been relatively slow in turning their attention to the problem. Indeed, of the thousands of books and articles written on sport, little serious attention has been paid until recently to the disorderly behavior, roles, and rituals of athletes and spectators. Early attempts by sociologists and social psychologists to apply mainstream theories of collective behavior to the analysis of sports-related violence often have been considered incomplete and unhelpful and are gradually being replaced by more sophisticated, issue-specific theoretical frameworks based on careful empirical research.

Despite lay and official perceptions to the contrary, it is clear that disorderly incidents at sport have occurred in almost all international contexts in which sports have established consistent spectator followings. A wide range of sports are involved, including baseball [39], golf [180], cricket [36, 57], Australian rules football [100], wrestling [81], ice hockey [50, 77], boxing [85], horseracing [85, 176], basketball [64], motorcycle racing [37], cockfighting [7], lacrosse [49, 115], American and Canadian football [197], rugby [170], and soccer [191] (for examples see Table 15.1). It is equally clear that such incidents are not recent phenomena, as the historical accounts of Cameron [21] and Guttman [65, 66] attest. Most of the work conducted to date and reviewed here, however, refers to soccer-related violence, and specifically to what is known broadly as British soccer "hooliganism." This no doubt reflects both a bias in research selection on the part of scholars working in this area, and a commonly made assumption that collective violence is more prevalent in soccer in the United Kingdom than elsewhere or in other sports. Reasons for this assumption also are addressed.

This review has three central objectives. The first is to briefly review

539

TABLE 15.1
Noteworthy Incidents of Sports-Related Collective Violence

Date	Sport	Location	Description
March, 1955	Ice Hockey	Montreal, Quebec, Canada	After home-team player had been ejected from play-offs for on-ice violence, hundreds of Montreal fans rioted inside and outside of Montreal Forum. Fifteen blocks of stores looted, cars overturned, and windows smashed. Over 100 rioters arrested.
May, 1964	Soccer	Lima, Peru	Over 300 dead, 500 injured when riot broke out following disallowed last minute goal during Olympic qualifying game between Argentina and Peru.
March, 1969	Ice Hockey	Prague, Czechoslovakia	Following a victory by the Czechoslovakian team over USSR in Sweden, thousands of Czechs celebrated in Prague's Wenceslas Square. Police brought in as celebrating gangs broke window of Soviet airline office, vandalizing property and building bonfires.
Jan., 1969	Soccer	Glasgow, Scotland	66 fans trampled to death, over 150 injured following stadium collapse at game between Glasgow Celtic and Rangers.
June, 1969	Soccer	El Salvador and Honduras	Following World Cup qualifying game between El Salvador and Honduras played in Mexico hundreds of Hondurans attacked Salvadoran nationals in Honduras. El Salvador retaliated with arms. Diplomatic relations between two countries severed. Seven days of violence subsequently dubbed "soccer war."
June, 1974	Baseball	Cleveland, Ohio, USA	Cleveland Indians' "Nickle Beer Night" idea backfired as hundreds of fans rioted on playing field, bombarding players and officials with bricks, cans, bottles, and firecrackers.
Nov., 1976	American Football	Foxboro, Massachusetts, USA	60 fans arrested, 35 hospitalized, and one stabbed at riot after National Football League game.
July, 1979	Baseball	Chicago, USA	Chicago White Sox's "Disco Demolition Night" backfired as 7000 fans rioted on the field. Bases, turf, and batting cage destroyed . 39 fans arrested.
Jan., 1980	Cricket	Sydney, Australia	80 fans arrested and jailed during fighting between Australian and New Zealand fans at World Cup series match.
Aug., 1981	Rugby	Wellington, New Zealand	Police in riot gear fought with anti-apartheid demonstrators at game between New Zealand and visiting South Africa. 18 arrested and 12 demonstrators injured.
May, 1985	Soccer	Brussels, Belgium	39 fans crushed to death, hundreds injured following a charge by fans of Liverpool, England into section housing fans of Juventus, Italy, at European Cup Championship game.
Nov., 1986	Canadian Football	Hamilton, Ontario, Canada	Following Hamilton's Grey Cup victory, over 3000 fans "celebrated" in downtown area. Over $55,000 worth of damage to vehicles, stores, and public property. 13 arrests.
April, 1989	Soccer	Sheffield, England	94 fans of Liverpool soccer club crushed to death as fans arriving late attempted to force way into game.

traditional or mainstream theories of collective behavior. The second is to comprehensively examine various explanations of sport and collective violence proposed by sociologists and social psychologists of sport. The third objective is to review research in which the relationship between collective violence in sport and the media process has been considered. The review concludes with brief comments on three important additional issues: methodological problems in research sport and collective violence, feminist concerns with extant research in the area, and future research on sport and collective violence.

MAINSTREAM THEORIES OF COLLECTIVE BEHAVIOR

Traditional perspectives on collective behavior provide the general foundation on which more sophisticated, issue-specific theories of collective action in political and popular culture, and sport, have been constructed. One of the earliest treatments of collective behavior, *The Crowd*, was first published nearly a century ago by Le Bon [88] and it is no surprise that since then social science has amassed a great wealth of theoretical commentary on the subject. Although Le Bon is widely considered the founder of theories of crowd psychology [146], it was in fact Robert Park, one of the central figures of the Chicago school of sociology, who introduced the term "collective behavior" to the discipline. Park [127, p. 42] actually defined sociology as "the science of collective behavior."

Scholars have disagreed, however, as Quarantelli and Weller [134] note, on formal definitions of collective behavior. This can be explained at least in part by the fact that no social phenomenon can be viewed intrinsically as "collective behavior." The potential scope of behaviors that can be considered under this label is diverse, ranging from interpersonal action in relatively small groups, to action between hundreds of thousands of individuals brought together by a common interest or cause. Hence, collective behavior can include action at bus stops and at weddings, in subways, shopping malls, and parks, on beaches and concert stages, as well as action during riots, stampedes, panics, revolution, war, and, of course, sports events. It is, however, forms of relatively disorganized collective action in which a group responds in an apparently spontaneous, unexpected manner to a given stimulus that seem to be the fundamental concern of theorists of collective behavior to date. Much of this research was conducted during the late 1960s and included assessments of infamous cases of American collective violence such as the Kent State shootings, or inner-city race riots.

Generally, theoretical perspectives on collective behavior have attempted to locate causal factors either in the person or in his or her social situation [8]. Most frequently, however, the emphasis is on deindividualization (loss of personal identity) and anonymity in the crowd. Widely employed in the literature are at least six major theoretical paradigms, all of which can be applied very loosely to collective violence in sport. These are briefly outlined in Table 15.2.

Most of the theories noted in Table 15.2 (particularly those aligned with the contagion and convergence paradigms) focus on the essential spontaneity of collective behavior as if, as Blumer [14, p. 68] puts it, there were no "pre-established understandings or traditions" in crowds [see also 86, pp. 11–14; 175, pp. 4–5]. Indeed, a number of authors have adopted such a view on the sports crowd as collective behavior [15, 101, 152]. In many contexts, such a view is simply incomplete. In the subsequent review of contemporary theories of sports crowd disorder, it becomes clear that it is quite possible for members of crowds to bring to an event an intricate collection of rational pre-understandings and expectations based on notions of social structure, class culture, relationship to other crowd members, and so forth. As Gerth and Mills [58] have argued, it is important to realize that in any given situation, the complex sequence of small-group relations at work is probably molded as much by the influence of larger social structural factors as by spontaneously emerging order. Moreover, behaviors arising from such pre-understandings need to be seen as being performed normatively in their own context. For example, rival gangs of English soccer "hooligans" have been in conflict with each other for so long that most informed sources consider their unique form of collective behavior normative and highly structured. Thus, assertions such as Lang and Lang's [87, p. 556] that collective behavior is typically behavior that displays a "derailment . . . from its normatively structured course" cannot be considered universally accurate or indeed helpful.

When applied to specific sports milieux, all of the theories outlined above offer little more than superficial theoretical frameworks. Collective crowd disorders at sports events are extremely complex, varied, and often highly organized rather than spontaneous phenomena, and attempts to explain their occurrence must be based on historically-grounded interpretations of, among other factors, social structure, class, politics, and gender. That is, there should be an understanding of both form and context. Although the mainstream theories can be used to explain certain aspects and phases of collective violence in sport, it is naive to expect that a perfect analytical fit can be achieved between forms of sports violence and any one of these theories. Consequently, the presumption implicit in much of the literature that all crowd processes are alike is incorrect. It is argued in this paper that because crowds can differ enormously by context (e.g., time, place, culture, history), and form (e.g., class, gender composition) causal explanations for crowd behavior must be grounded in contextual rather than broad,

TABLE 15.2
Summary of Mainstream Theories of Collective Behavior

Theory	Proposed Cause (References)	Possible Application to Sports Violence (References)	Major Weaknesses
Contagion	Behavior of self-elected leaders in crowds becomes contagious. Members copy each other. Result is completely homogeneous action [34,88,111,145,162].	Chanting rituals and fighting by British soccer hooligans as an example of contagious behavior [150]. Roman chariot race crowds acting as homogeneous organism [16].	Ignores differences in crowd members (class, definition of situation, etc.). Fails to explain why some crowds become violent and others remain passive. Fails to understand that violent crowd behavior may be rational and systematic.
Convergence	Persons sharing common values and goals come together to form crowds [3,116,175].	Persons exploit protection of crowd to engage in normally repressed behavior (profanity, aggression, etc.).	Fails to explain why persons with similar values and goals behave differently in crowds.
Decision/ Gaming	Crowd members engage in a rational decision-making process regarding estimated rewards of action versus potential costs [13].	Persons willing to engage in unruly action (e.g., field invasion, fighting) only in large groups. Individual disorder increases possibility of apprehension and sanction.	Overlooks contagious, spontaneous effect of crowds. Assumes all crowd action is rational.
Emergent norm	Governing norms in crowds emerge spontaneously. Actors respond to behavioral cues from each other, especially in moments of ambiguity [6,134,151,175].	Sports events characterized by suspended norms. Temporary norms arise and act as behavioral guides in fan celebrations at and around events [84].	Fails to explain how and why violence may be ordered and preconceived, not spontaneous.
Value-added	Crowd action determined by a sequence of incremental steps (e.g., structural conduciveness, strain, hostile beliefs) [153].	Hostile outbursts at British soccer as examples of "structural strain" [95,156,187].	"Necessary" precipitants for violence to occur may not be incremental and may not exist at all.
Catharsis	Human frustration accumulated in daily activity can be diffused by behaving aggressively or by observing violent action [97,120,129].	Violence on the playing field provides outlet for frustrations that arise for both athletes and fans. Violence in sport keeps other forms of social violence at acceptable levels [10,17,19,61,109].	More evidence for "disinhibition" effect than catharsis, i.e., participating in violence actually enhances further violence.

nonspecific analyses. Such culturally specific explanations for sports-related collective violence are now considered.

EXPLANATIONS OF COLLECTIVE VIOLENCE IN SPORT

Undoubtedly, the sports crowd is as significant a force in sport as the athletes and the events themselves. When large crowds gather at emotionally charged public events such as sport, many of the preconditions for collective behavior exist [116]. Although various factors of sociological and social psychological importance have been considered (e.g., cultural history, social organization, class experience, gender), there has been no widespread agreement among sociologists and social psychologists about the behavioral tendencies of sports crowds or the disorder perpetrated by them. Because the proposed explanations have tended to be geographically specific, the following discussion is organized according to North American, British, and "Other" explanations for sports crowd disorder.

North America

SOCIAL PSYCHOLOGICAL PERSPECTIVES. A number of early studies into sports-related violence in North America adopted social psychological perspectives. For the most part, attention has been paid in these studies to ways in which certain sports affect the mood and aggression levels of spectators and to how some sports attract certain personality types. The following is a brief review of such studies which fall into *Catharsis* and *Other* camps.

Catharsis. Several sport psychologists have attempted to show how the work of Lorenz [97] and others can be used to throw light on violent behavior in sport. Using original or revised versions of drive-discharge theory, noted in Table 15.2, which assumes stored aggressiveness within the human body, studies by Kingsmore [81], Moore [117], Roberts [143], and Johnson and Hutton [76] have attempted to provide empirical support for the catharsis hypothesis. Moore has summarized the general thrust of this work: ". . . sports are particularly valuable as a means or partial outlet of aggressive and sexual impulses whether we are participant or observer" [p. 74]. Kingsmore's study of the aggressive effects on male spectators of watching wrestling and a basketball game is especially interesting here because it provides what the author views as evidence in support of the catharsis position—notably, wrestling fans displayed a decrease in postevent aggression.

However, other studies measuring hostility or aggression levels of sports spectators, such as Russell's [147] analysis of spectator moods at aggressive sports events, Goldstein and Arms' [60] study of male spectators' responses to Army-Navy football and gymnastics events, and their follow-up investigation of female spectators' responses to swimming and ice hockey events [5] lend only limited support to the catharsis or drive-discharge hypotheses or indeed none at all. As Arms et al. write, their research endeavors "provide ... support for a general disinhibition position" [p. 140].

Other. Of course, such tests of pre- and postevent hostility levels constitute only one direction of sports violence research conducted by social psychologists. Others have examined, for example, stimuli and cues occurring in the sports crowd which, when combined with other factors such as "emotional readiness," ultimately give way to aggression [89], as well as variations in personality types of participants in sport and nonsport groups. In the latter case, Bennet [12] claims that sport spectators (specifically of tennis, boxing, and basketball) display a greater need for power and prestige (and therefore presumably higher violence levels?) than members of nonsport groups.

A sociological critique of these and similar studies quickly indicates some serious weaknesses. For the most part, they are ahistorical, astructural, and apolitical. Because they follow earlier theorists such as Lorenz, these researchers inevitably assume that causes of sports violence can be located within the individual rather than the social structure. This is a premise that sociologists find myopic and unpersuasive. The dubious technique of deriving meanings and relationships from limited, nonrepresentative samples is certainly a criticism that one could justifiably apply to much of this work. Moreover, one of the major findings of psychological studies, the disinhibition effect, is entirely amenable to sociological interpretation.

SOCIOLOGICAL PERSPECTIVES. Sociological research on sport and collective violence in North America has attempted to place individual behavior at sport in a wider social framework. It tends to fall into three thematic categories: conflicts taking place in the wider society, the carnival or celebratory nature of sport, and precipitating factors occurring at the sport event itself.

Conflicts taking place in the wider society. Fimrite's well-known "Take Me Out to the Brawl Game" [55] attributes the apparent increase in spectator violence in North America to certain socioeconomic "dis-affections" emerging between the fan, the athlete, and society. According to Fimrite, a growing alienation between these three is resulting in widespread social frustration which is being vented in sports stadia. Fontana's [56] thesis is similar: he proposes that increasing loss of individuality and excessive bureaucratic practices are central causes of social frustration. Life in contemporary society is becoming overly structured and predictable for the individual which, says Fontana, is undermining each person's sense of distinctness. Violence and inordinate participation in the sports crowd are seen, therefore, in this argument as an attempt to reassert individualism "... by resurrecting the primitive feelings of simulation and vertigo" [p. 225].

A popular perspective, found in the work of both scholars and laypersons (including journalists), follows from Fimrite's and Fontana's work, and this is what may be called the "reintegration" thesis. Some sociologists [e.g., 10, 130] have suggested that life in modern cities is essentially anonymous and mundane. With the disintegration of the extended family network, and the steady drive of people towards the large cities, modern man and woman, it is argued, are losing membership with valued groups and, concomitantly, the necessary sense of belonging derived from association with such groups. Violence in sports stadia is thus understood in terms of spectators' needs to reestablish forms of group identification. As Petryszak [130, p. 1] writes:

> Incidents of violence and aggression that occur in the stadium are understood as overt displays of competition. It is ... suggested that sports violence as an overt and visible index of group competition is the means by which the spectator is able to temporarily satisfy the basic human need for group membership. The spectators' joy in sports violence represents in fact his enthusiasm in the realization of this essential need.

Goldaber, founder of the Centre for the Study of Crowd and Spectator Behavior in Miami, Florida, agrees with Petryszak. He sees problems in sport as linked to problems in mainstream society. To illustrate, Goldaber argues [cited in 59, p. 1]:

> ... more people aren't making it. You work hard, you exist, but you haven't got much to show for it. There are increasing numbers of people who are deeply frustrated because they feel they have very little power over their lives. They come to sporting events to experience, vicariously, a sense of power.

Like broader convergence theories, Goldaber's thesis is one of vicarious power-seeking: sports violence is an attempt to distinguish oneself in a milieu that, unlike the workplace, provides the person with the possibility for so doing.

Of course, it is possible to claim, as several British and North American scholars have done, a relationship between sports violence and socio-demographic factors such as race, religion, and ethnicity as an indication of social conflict affecting sport. At times such claims have been supported by convincing empirical evidence. Edwards [52], for example, argues that blacks take great pride in defeating white teams or teams from predominantly white areas, and that racially driven rivalry often leads to violence. His arguments proceed from the assumption that racial tension often directly affects the hostility of rioters. Of course, American history is replete with examples of collective violence so caused outside sport. In American sport, numerous high school and college riots at football and basketball games in the 1960s and 1970s were clearly motivated along these lines. Similarly, Levitt and Shaffir [94] show how the Christie Pits softball riots in Toronto in 1933 were actually the result of a series of anti-Semitic incidents perpetrated by English Canadians.

Possibly the most notorious and well-documented [50, 77, 197] incident that contained racial or ethnic overtones occurred in Canada in March, 1955. The Montreal/Rocket Richard Riot remains one of the largest single crowd riots in the history of North American sport. All commentators of the Montreal riot have pointed to ethnic hostility between anglophones and francophones as a principal cause. The riot stands as such a classic example of sports violence prompted by social conflict that a brief description of its antecedents is in order.

In the early part of this century, the Montreal Canadiens established a reputation as one of Canada's (and particularly French Canada's) most avidly followed sports teams. In an era of growing political strife between anglophone and francophone Canadians, *Les Canadiens* became almost synonymous with the political plight and cultural experience of French Canadians as a whole. In the 1950s, their French Canadian hockey idol was Maurice "Rocket" Richard, a highly talented but volatile player whose career had been punctuated by a number of widely publicized violent incidents.

During a home game against Boston on March 13, 1955, an altercation took place between Richard and Boston's Hal Laycoe. With only 6 minutes left in the game, Laycoe retaliated against the persistent high-sticking of Richard by hitting the Canadien and opening a gash above his eye. Although the referee signalled for a penalty, Richard, bent on revenge, circled his opponent and attacked him twice with his stick, actually breaking it on the second occasion. Undeterred, Richard proceeded to punch a linesman in the face as the latter attempted to restrain him.

Richard was ejected from the game and fined by the National Hockey League, whose anglophone President, Clarence Campbell, decided to levy further sanctions (in the face of Richard's violent history) in the form of a suspension for the remainder of the season including the play-offs—an unprecedented penalty. The implication of the suspension for Richard himself was that his once imminent goal-scoring record was now out of reach, and the team's chances of going on to win the Stanley Cup had been greatly diminished. The subsequent crowd reaction has been described by Mark et al. [103, p. 84].

. . . fifty-five Montreal Canadiens' fans made threats on the life of National Hockey League Commissioner, Clarence Campbell. When the commissioner appeared at the Montreal Forum at a Canadiens–Detroit Red Wings game, he was pelted with fruit, programs, galoshes, and other missiles. A smoke bomb was exploded and many spectators fled to the exits. Because of the fans' disruptive behavior, the Montreal Fire Chief evacuated the Forum (resulting in a Canadiens' forfeit). When the fans from inside the Forum mixed with people mingling outside, a major riot ensued. Fifteen blocks of stores were looted, windows were smashed, cars were over-turned, and corner newsstands and street kiosks were burned down. Over 100 people were arrested.

On the international sporting scene, social, racial, or ethnic hostility and xenophobia have in fact been pointed to frequently to explain numerous soccer riots involving fans in Brazil [93], Israel [149], Scotland [123], and England [167, 179].

The celebratory nature of sport. A second set of explanations for collective violence at North American sport has been based on the notion that the whole organization and structure of sport encourages expressive, if not blatantly aggressive, behavior by players and fans alike, normally in a carnival-like atmosphere. Because most sport spectators have an informed knowledge of "their" game (owing to the cultural relevance of sport in contemporary society), they can immediately identify the significance of an event either in terms of seasonal goals (e.g., making the play-offs, winning championships) or in terms of the relations ("rivalries") that have developed historically between the contestants, and, indeed in the case of some sports, between the fans. For these reasons, sports crowds, unlike crowds in many other contexts, have a vested interest—a fanaticism—in the outcome of the event at hand. Combined with factors caused by aggregation (e.g., physical proximity, tension, noise, competition), it is therefore rather unsurprising that sporting contests are characterized by highly emotionally charged behavior on the part of participants and spectators alike, in which proceedings can, under the appropriate conditions, "get out of hand."

The carnival and celebratory aspects of sport, then, have frequently been addressed in research. Both Listiak [96] and Manning [102] demonstrate how sport is a setting for scheduled revelry. Listiak, for example, uses the context of Grey Cup celebrations in Canada to show how widespread public revelry and in some cases violence is ignored or condoned by bar owners, uninvolved passers-by, and even by agents of social control. Making a case for the utility of emergent-norm theory, Kutcher [84] argues that under conditions of suspended conventional norms, such as this, temporary norms take over and act as behavioral guides in a setting conducive to deviance. Kutcher writes:

> . . . those who refuse to accept the definition of revelry are the deviants. It is a huge party that does not tolerate easily the party-

pooper, who may be the unfortunate policeman whose job it is to curb excess. In many stadia, the most frequent problem is the inebriated fan who . . . feels this is a carnival, and he has a right to behave any way he wishes . . . Other fans observing the arrest will often see the police as the deviant, violating the spirit of carnival [p. 39].

For the purposes of this discussion, what becomes pertinent is the sports-related celebration that becomes excessive even by its own expectations and turns criminal or violent, or both.

In a study of the structural aspects of sports crowd disorder in North America, Young [197] explains that, for North American spectators, destruction and vandalism as well as the now infamous victory riot are consistently manifested forms of such excess. Although the former often include ripping up parts of the field, dismantling goalposts (common in amateur and professional football), and theft at the site of the game itself, the latter typically includes postevent revelry which becomes disruptive. In brief, celebration rioting is characterized by inebriation, brawling, looting, and vandalism. Young [197, p. 182] notes:

> Over the last two decades, celebration rioting in a large number of cities has left a long trail of violence and vandalism. Locations include: New York (Mets—World Series, 1969); Pittsburgh (Pirates—World Series, 1971); Pittsburgh (Steelers—Superbowl, 1975); Philadelphia (Phillies–World Series, 1980); Toronto (Argonauts—Grey Cup, 1983); Detroit (Tigers—World Series, 1984); San Francisco (49'ers—Superbowl, 1985); Montreal (Canadiens—Stanley Cup, 1986); Hamilton (Tiger-Cats—Grey Cup, 1986).

According to the official police report [197, p. 183] of the last victory riot on the list:

> Following the Hamilton Tiger-Cat Grey Cup victory on November 30, 1986, 3,000 to 5,000 fans converged in the downtown core to celebrate. Most had been drinking and some were clearly intoxicated. During the course of the evening, the exuberance of some fans was transformed into spontaneous acts of destruction. It is estimated that just over $55,000 worth of damages to passing automobiles, public utility vehicles and commercial premises was caused and 13 charges were laid by the early morning hours of December 1st.

Hoch [72], Klapp [82], and Dunstan [49] provide similar accounts of postevent celebrations turning violent at United States college football,

World Series baseball, and international rubgy games, respectively. Importantly, all these studies emphasize the implicit approval given to destructive and violent fans by police, politicians, and sports authorities. Apparently the cultural significance of sport is such that it often represents a site for tolerated crime and violence closed off to participants of other cultural pursuits. Interestingly, Kutcher [84] argues that sports owners have consciously encouraged the carnival-like nature of sport to attract people who may lead very tedious, routinized lives.

Precipitating factors at sports events. A third category of explanations for collective violence at North American sport focuses on aspects of the event itself—usually action on the field of play—as the site of a number of 'precipitating factors.' Several sociologists have applied a structural-functionalist perspective to the analysis of spectator disorder. Smith's [156] early work, for example, examined crowd violence at a number of soccer riots using Smelser's [153] value-added theory of collective behavior. Focusing on Smelser's notions of structural conduciveness and precipitating factors, Smith found the most common determinants of crowd hostility to be unpopular decisions by officials and player violence. These findings led Smith [156, p. 205] to conclude that: "Sport probably often exacerbates the very strains that initially give rise to collective hostility." More recently, Smith [159] went on to further validate what he calls the "violence-precipitates-violence hypothesis" for which he used examples from hockey, baseball, and basketball games. Elsewhere, White [187], Edwards and Rackages [53], and Lewis [95] also have used Smelser's value-added theory to examine hostile outbursts in sport, and their findings regarding the violence-precipitates-violence hypothesis support those of Smith.

Cheffers and Meehan have conducted work similar to Smith's in which they investigated how fans respond to player violence, or what they call "unwarranted actions" on the part of athletes. Gilbert and Twyman [59, p. 66] cite their findings:

> In soccer, fights among the players have triggered violence in the stands in 57% of the cases the researchers have observed. For football and baseball, the percentages are 49 and 34 respectively.

According to Gilbert and Twyman, Cheffers and Meehan's data revealed that only 8.5% of hockey fights prompted fan violence. The latter two researchers account for this by asserting that hockey, like roller-derby and professional wrestling, has become normatively grounded in violence, and that fans witness on-ice violence so frequently that they are becoming blasé about it and hence rarely react aggressively.

In general, this category of explanations views sports crowd disorder as a response to game-related phenomena only. What occurs in fans' lives before and following games is apparently unimportant. Further examples of such "ecological" explanations are Dewar's [39] study which attempts to establish correlations between spectator fights at baseball and such factors as the day of the week, starting time, seat location, temperature, and inning of the game, as well as Green and O'Neal's [63] account of how crowd size affects fan violence.

Sociological research into North American sports violence has so far examined a number of important aspects of the phenomenon. Specifically, sociologists have attempted to trace links between violent behavior at and around sport stadia and broader conflicts in society, and to locate features of sport as a cultural form and organizational structure that may actually encourage unruly behavior. some important steps have been taken in these directions. These initial attempts, however, have not yet been developed into more sophisticated, insightful theoretical frameworks. In general, North American research in this area appears to be rather individualistic, functionalist, and static (this is especially evident in social psychological and "precipitating factor" explanations). These are problems that several researchers of soccer hooliganism in the United Kingdom have attempted to overcome.

United Kingdom

Generally speaking, the vast majority of research into sports violence in the United Kingdom has examined causes and forms of soccer hooliganism from a sociological perspective, but there are exceptions. For instance, Pearton and Gaskell [128] have explained soccer hooliganism using frustration-aggression theory, but their account suffers from the same weaknesses addressed earlier vis-á-vis social psychological work in North America (notably, it is largely ahistorical and apolitical). At least four major sociological research programs on the British hooliganism issue can be identified. Each has been cited widely in the literature, and each has its own strengths and weaknesses.

THE RITUAL OF SOCCER VIOLENCE THESIS. Peter Marsh and his colleagues [105–109] are the principle exponents of the ritual violence thesis following their observational work at Oxford United Football Club. Marsh et al. [109] have employed what they call the "ethogenic method" in their research programs to detail the career structure of hooligan fans, as well as the norms (or rules) intrinsic to that structure. They start from the premise that one has to view disorder ". . . through the eyes of the people who take part in it" [p. 2]. The ethogenic method, as Marsh et al. see it, is thus a means of empathizing with subjects of sociological investigation, and it was established as a research method in response to ". . . middle-class investigators who enter the social world of working-class children from the outside and without credentials valid in that world" [p. 6].

Building on Tiger's [171] study of the aggressive behavior of *Men in Groups*, and on notions of male bonding, Marsh and his colleagues offer a type of "psychology of action," conceptualizing aggression as a constructive and rule-governed means of controlling the social world, in the process of achieving certain goals. They argue that it is the culture of specific groups that determines their expression of aggression. Hence, soccer crowd disorder is viewed as a specific cultural adaptation to the lower working-class environment, which manifests itself in aggressive (but largely symbolic and harmless) rituals in soccer stadia, and thereby facilitates the cathartic release of aggressive impulses for young working-class adolescents, i.e., it is a "ritual of teenage aggro" (aggression). Moreover, Marsh et al. [109, p. 134] caution authorities that the catharsis offered by soccer aggression is an indispensable cultural requisite, and that if they:

> . . . take away the opportunities for boys and young men to engage in structured aggro, then we might very well be faced with a set of problems that are far more serious and much more difficult to control.

Ironically, then, as Marsh et al. see it, authorities are faced with having to tolerate ritualized soccer aggression to avert more serious violence at soccer and elsewhere.

It is evident that the work of Marsh et al. also has ties with the ethological and catharsis theories of Lorenz [97], discussed above, in addition to other writers who emphasize the ritualistic and even tribal aspects of soccer fan behavior [e.g., 51, 70, 121]. Edgell and Jary [51, p. 226], for example, posit the notion of the relatively non-violent soccer crowd, and focus on the predictability of its behavior which ". . . tends to be highly ritualized rather than 'undefined'." For empirical support, they draw our attention to two points: first, the manner in which officials or authority figures can be verbally insulted by fans with a near immunity from retaliation; and second, the profane, threatening nature of regular songs and chants, reciprocally used by rival fan groups, which are viewed as aggressive rituals rather than precipitants per se of violent interchanges.

To minimize the frequency and form of soccer "aggro" in these ways, however, and to suggest that the phenomenon is only a ritualistic "fantasy" of violence, fails to provide a fully adequate account and leaves several questions unanswered. What advocates have failed to recognize is the regularity with which serious (and sometimes fatal) injury is caused at soccer. Marsh et al. [109] in particular make no reference to the pre- or postmatch context, in which undoubtedly violence is particularly prevalent. Rather, the main focus of their analysis is on "hand to hand" combat during games. This completely overlooks several significant aspects of hooligan transaction, not the least of which are extra-stadia incidents of organized violence between rival fighting groups, and aerial confrontations through the use of missiles, both well-established characteristics of contemporary hooligan deportment. Moreover, theories that focus on the ritual of soccer "aggro" entirely omit any notion of structural differentiation and political backdrop of fans involved, so fundamental to adequately explaining the phenomenon sociologically.

There is no denying some ritualistic flavor to soccer violence—many of the songs, chants, profanities, and even aspects of inter-group fighting are clearly ritualistic—but to argue that the very essence of hooliganism is ritualistic, and that actual violence plays no more than a peripheral role, raises serious doubts as to the validity of all these hypotheses, particularly in the wake of several recent, but already infamous, hooligan incidents that occurred in the 1970s and 1980s. Many of these incidents actually started out as relatively harmless rituals and escalated into destructive, violent exchanges. Moreover, one wonders how responsible such theses are in an era in which soccer-related disorders show no sign of abatement. Actual violence is as central to the problem as its ritualistic counterpart. Finally, in addition to these weaknesses, we already have seen that any argument based on the catharsis view remains, at the least, unsubstantiated and unpersuasive.

SOCIAL DEPRIVATION AND THE "LITTLE ENGLAND" PERSPECTIVE. Sports crowd disorder, as noted previously, has been explained by some North American writers in terms of the effects of spectators' experiences of social deprivation. With respect to disorder that has occurred at soccer matches over the last few decades in the United Kingdom, several sociologists [e.g., 33, 163–166] have posed similar deprivation hypotheses. The work of Taylor [163–166] is foremost in this category.

In an explanation of soccer hooliganism that is centrally concerned with class differentiation, Taylor argues that contemporary changes in the (English) game have combined to bring about important alterations in the behavior of traditional fans. Central to Taylor's analysis are notions of a 'soccer subculture' and 'soccer consciousness'. For him, the subculture of soccer in a working-class community comprises groups of working men socially and culturally bound together in a general concern for the game—soccer consciousness—and for the local team in particular. He writes [164, p. 143]:

> During the last quarter of the nineteenth century and throughout the Depression, the evidence is that players were very much subject to control by such soccer subcultures: expected to receive advice and "tips," expected to conform to certain standards of behavior (as the subculture's public representative) and (in return) given a wage for so long as they fulfilled these expectations.

According to Taylor, the rank-and-file supporter could thus view himself as a member of a ". . . collective and democratically structured enterprise" [p. 145] in which players, managers, owners, and fans were all engaged in a kind of working-class "participatory democracy."

Taylor argues, however, that certain postwar changes in the British game have threatened this state of affairs. Soccer clubs now enter international competitions and have introduced new domestic competitions. Moreover, clubs have recently set out to "bourgeoisify" the game in becoming more oriented towards profit maximization, and the player has:

> . . . been incorporated into the bourgeois world, his self-image and his behaviour have become increasingly managerial and entrepreneurial, and soccer has become . . . a means to personal (rather than subcultural) success. [164, p. 146].

For the members of the working-class soccer subculture, Taylor argues, these changes have had a traumatic effect. Their relatively deprived socio-economic status is allegedly exacerbated by a feeling that they are now being cast off by the clubs that have traditionally provided their cultural raison d'être. Taylor suggests that these people constitute a "subcultural-rump," and argues that it is principally they who engage in the sorts of behavior that authorities usually designate as hooliganism. Hence, the invasion of pitches, destruction of property in and around stadia, the pillaging of soccer buses and trains returning from games, and the like are all, according to this view, attempts by the remnants of a working-class subculture to reclaim a game that has become increasingly removed from their control. Disorder represents, as Edgell and Jary [51, p. 227] have written elsewhere, ". . . a highly specific protest against football's loss of class exclusivity."

Taylor [165–168] has comprehensively revised portions of his earlier thesis and now argues that contemporary soccer hooliganism can only be understood if placed against the ongoing crises of the British state and the economy [167]. The latter would include dislocations (industrial and residential) in working-class experience that have given way to differentiation within the working-class itself. For instance, Taylor [167] believes that an increased upper working-class jingoism or "Little Englanderism" developing during the Thatcher period has exacerbated Britain's hooligan problem:

> The general point to be made is that the violence of working-class soccer supporters in the 1980s occurs within a different conjuncture in the development of class relationships in Britain to the violence of the 1960s: the form and content of contemporary soccer violence is a product of a generalized anxiety which is obviously affecting both the bourgeois and the traditional worker, *but in different ways*. The older traditional worker, experiencing the reality or the threat

of unemployment, at least has the familiar framework of neighborhood, kinship group, and class institutions as some kind of personal cultural, and even economic support. But the new bourgeois worker, and of course also the mass of unemployed young brought up increasingly in the desperate bourgeois ethic of competitive market individualism and jingoism that is a *necessary* accompaniment of the economic radicalism of the Thatcher "experiment," has no such set of cultural, economic or, of course, political alternatives. In the absence of a political and economic program from the social democratic opposition that gives meaning and hope to the experience of decline and collapse in working-class life, the only possible development is toward a more intense, nihilistic form of racist, sexist, and nationalist paranoia. The alternative to socialism, especially in periods of fundamental crisis in capitalist society, is indeed, barbarism. [p. 179]

Such arguments clearly show that Taylor's most recent contributions to the hooligan issue locate many of the participants themselves in an altogether different segment of the working class than his earlier work. It is precisely this point of interpretation in the revised Taylor thesis that has been criticized most by other researchers, particularly the Leicester group (discussed subsequently).

In locating soccer hooliganism in the context of certain changes that have occurred recently in the structure and form of the British game, and the effects of Thatcherism on working-class experience and values as a whole (and on soccer support specifically), Taylor [167, p. 179] has succeeded in demonstrating, crucially, that ". . . no sensible discussion" of this phenomenon can proceed unless developed against a cultural and political backdrop. His incisive responses [167, 168] to the Brussels and Sheffield tragedies (see Table 15.1) represent attempts to place concrete events against this backdrop. Nevertheless, several flaws in Taylor's (particularly early) work require identification.

First, Taylor nowhere provides convincing evidence to support the notion of a participatory democracy in the 1920s and 1930s, i.e., that fans ever believed they were in a position to exert control over the game or its players. In fact, as Carroll [22] points out in another account of hooliganism in England, it is extremely doubtful whether current soccer hooligans are cognizant of any participatory democracy or 'illusion of control' as Taylor puts it, or, moreover, are concerned with regaining it. Taylor's view of a golden age of soccer in the United Kingdom when clubs and fans shared identical backgrounds and experiences is probably more a romanticized image of British sporting history than one grounded in evidence. Second, if as Taylor suggests, fans have only recently turned to hooliganism through feelings of estrangement from the participatory democracy of the club-fan relationship, how do we account for the regular soccer crowd disturbances of the late 19th century and early 20th century [47, 195] when this relationship allegedly reached a peak. Although he mentions pre-1960 forms of violence sporadically in his work, Taylor continues to refute (without empirical testimony) the possibility of extended phases of crowd disorder at soccer before the 1960s. His failure to examine the span of the phenomenon surely results in an overall lack of historical clarity in his argument. Finally, (and linked to this point), because they are not based on any (acknowledged) empirical work, many of Taylor's insights regarding soccer hooliganism must remain speculative and impressionistic. Taylor's work forces us, however, to consider social context in a far more sophisticated way than that implied by North American deprivation theses.

THEORIES OF WORKING-CLASS SUBCULTURES. Several writers at the Centre for Contemporary Cultural Studies at Birmingham University, England [e.g., 27, 28, 35, 68], have been similarly concerned to position soccer hooliganism in the class and cultural experiences of certain groups of fans. As Clarke [28, pp. 49–50] writes:

> Hooliganism comes out of the way in which the traditional forms of football watching encounter the professionalization and spectacularization of the game. It is one of the consequences of the changing relationship of the audience to the game.

In this way, soccer hooliganism is once again seen (in part) as a reaction by working-class men to commercializing processes, such as the increasing presentation of soccer as spectacle, appearing in what has traditionally been construed as "the people's game" [182].

However, Clarke and others have modified Taylor's thesis slightly with a new focus on adolescent subcultural characteristics that have emerged out of post-World War II changes in British working-class culture. These changes include breakdown in family ties, decline in the heavy industries, loss of communal space, dislocations in relations between generations, and the emergence of a range of youth styles (e.g., teddy boys, mods, rockers, skinheads). Clarke believes that the changing relationship between adults and youths in working-class communities has facilitated greater freedom and independence for youths, and thus provided fewer (social and physical) constraints on them at soccer and elsewhere in their lives. Hence, traditional forms of crowd behavior at soccer, including such things as profanity, pushing, and 'controlled aggression', are now seen as escalating into new styles of spectatorship—specifically, forms of aggressiveness and violence that the authorities have designated as hooliganism. These are processes that White [186] also has recognized.

In arguing that hooliganism is integrally related to dislocations in working-class life in the postwar period—"Into the hiatus between the traditional supporter and the modern consumer stepped the football hooligan"—Critcher's [35, p. 171] thesis is compatible with Clarke's. Like Clarke, Critcher is concerned to rework Taylor's (early) thesis which locates soccer-related crowd disorders entirely within the context of the game itself. Critcher prefers instead to view them as representative of changes occurring in working-class culture, i.e., in the social position of the working-class as a whole.

There can be no doubt that relating soccer hooliganism to the context of a culture in flux is a very helpful framework of analysis. Equally, there can be no doubt that the sociohistorical approaches of Taylor, Clarke, and others offer considerably more explanatory insight into a complex social problem than the ethological and rather microsociological ventures of Marsh and his colleagues. In combining understandings of transformations in social relations and in the composition of the soccer crowd, Clarke and others seem in many ways to have transcended Taylor's [164] narrow early focus on the latter account alone, although it must be emphasized once again that Taylor has very recently rectified this position in his work on soccer hooliganism as related to the effects of structural differentiation within the British working-class [165–168].

As was previously noted about Taylor's early work, however, Clarke, Critcher, and others unfortunately produce little concrete evidence to support the argument that hooliganism is a response to the establishment's challenge to working-class traditions and values. Stability of working-class social relations in the past, i.e., in the pre-1960 era, is a view that both parties tend to assume rather too uncritically and, because both assume that soccer hooliganism began on a widespread basis for the first time during the early 1960s, is a view they are unlikely to relinquish in the foreseeable future.

THE SOCIAL ROOTS OF SOCCER VIOLENCE THESIS. A group of sociologists at the Universities of Leicester and Loughborough, England (Eric Dunning, John Williams, Joe Maguire, and Patrick Murphy), have been interested, like Taylor and the working-class subculture theorists, to place the sociogenesis of British soccer hooliganism in historical and class perspectives, although, unlike these other writers, their work is grounded in extensive, empirically-tested comparisons of this phenomenon in its past and present contexts.

Theoretically, this group's now extensive body of work [40–47, 188–193] has been influenced in diverse ways. Most fundamentally, their work is predicated on Norbert Elias's [54] evolutionary theories of the civilizing process, although supplementary impetus has clearly been provided by Suttles's [161] socioanthropological work on the social order of American slums, and by several histories of British soccer and rugby [e.g., 48, 74, 75, 104, 110, 176, 182, 200].

Dunning and his colleagues argue that certain standards of behavior displayed by soccer hooligans are directly influenced by social conditions and characteristics inherent in the class-cultural background of those involved. A predominant theme of their work, and one that represents a direct conflict with Taylor's recent "Little England" thesis, is that hooligan groups largely comprise persons from the roughest sector of the working-classes. Aligning themselves with notions of deprivation, they argue that the hooligan's deprived social condition is instrumental in the production and reproduction of normative modes of behavior, including strong emphases on ties of kinship and territory, loyalty to peers and family, conjugal role separation, male dominance, and a need to express masculinity through physical means such as fighting. In a recent television documentary [*Holligan*, 73] developed around the Leicester researchers' work, Williams says:

> They spend a lot of time in the same areas, they do the same kinds of jobs, they have the same sorts of interests, they have relatively narrow social horizons given the kinds of opportunities they have for status and expressing themselves. They have very strong bonds of loyalty and group solidarity. They prize many of the things that are more generally prized and accepted in our society ... they prize pride in their own area and their community ... you also find in communities of this kind ... a much stronger division between the sexes ... and the males tend to dominate ... there tend to be dominance hierarchies built up between males and one way you can gain status is through the ability to fight.

It is precisely the reproduction of this social condition that is presumed to lead to the development of a specific violent masculine style manifested regularly on the soccer terraces. The context is soccer because:

> The match on the field of play itself is a match as they (hooligans) see it on behalf of their community, not just the wider city but in particular the working-class sections of their city, because they see the game as part and parcel of their working-class culture ... they're also involved in a competition with the fans of the opposing side because they're battling on behalf of their community. [Dunning, in Hooligan].

This is the thrust of the Leicester school's "social roots' explanation of soccer hooliganism in Britain. To explain fan violence at international soccer matches, we are introduced to what Paul Harrison [70, p. 604] has called the "Bedouin Syndrome." Simply stated, this means that in the same way that usually hostile neighborhood groups come together to define their "home territory" against visiting fans, so, too, is social solidarity of this type manifested on a regional scale (e.g., northern fans fighting against southern fans) and even on a national scale (e.g., English fans fighting against Italian fans). Harrison's concept of the Bedouin Syndrome is thus usually explained in terms such as ". . . the enemy of your enemy is your friend" [p. 604]. *Hooligans Abroad* [191], the first book-length study produced by the Leicester group was, in fact, an attempt to substantiate such a scenario empirically in the context of international soccer competition (World Cup, Spain, 1982).

Most explanations of soccer hooliganism in Britain [e.g., 35, 109, 164, 166] have postulated that the phenomenon began on a broad scale for the first time in the early 1960s, and is therefore quite recent. The Leicester research, by contrast, is based on a very different assumption, i.e., that patterns of soccer crowd disorder (although varied in their manifestations) can be traced as far back as the last quarter of the 19th century. Moreover, Dunning et al. [42, p. 342] argue that ". . . every phase of the Association game in Britain . . . has been accompanied by episodes of spectator disorder," although the pre-World War I and post-1960 periods are seen as most prolific in this regard. For example, the *Hooligan* documentary shows that the English Football Association was so concerned with increasing crowd disorder prior to World War II that military personnel were regularly allowed into matches free of charge to help informally police unruly crowd members.

The argument that hooliganism has prevaded the entire history of British soccer requires discussion, however, and possibly represents a principal weakness in the "social roots" explanation. Because their work is theoretically grounded in Eliasan evolutionary notions of the civilizing process, the Leicester scholars are led to view the current hooligan problem as no more pressing than during other periods of British soccer history. This is, at the very least, a contentious position (particularly in the wake of several recent incidents that have involved British soccer fans, such as the Heysel Stadium riot and the Hillsborough tragedy), and it must be said that the empirical evidence, at least as we have seen it to date, may be a little selective in its support of the Eliasan model of behavior. This is an aspect of the research that has also concerned Curtis [38].

The work of Dunning and others provides, however, one of the most sophisticated, informed analyses of the complex issues and meanings behind soccer hooliganism. Despite the limitations noted above, these writers have gone far in mapping the sociogenesis of the phenomenon and linking it to the broader culture in which it emerges. It should be pointed out that unlike other approaches reviewed earlier, the perspective of the Leicester school is grounded in comprehensive, longitudinal empirical research (using methods such as content analysis, historical methods, participant observation, and interviewing), not only of soccer hooligan action, but also of the lifestyles, behaviors, and attitudes of young men normally involved in hooligan action away from soccer. Such a sound empirical background has led them to make a number of recommendations vis-á-vis conflict resolution in this area [e.g., 191]. This is a compelling aspect of their work that others have been reluctant or unable to emulate. Additional features of the soccer-collective violence nexus have been researched by other sociologists, although this research is not normally aligned with the four widely cited approaches discussed above.

ADDITIONAL STUDIES. Like Taylor, Dunning, and others, a number of other authors consider the meaning of local community, national honor, and pride to be integrally linked with hooligan action. Observations at and around soccer matches have led Murray [124], for instance, to agree with the now well-established argument of Dunning and others that at the root of domestic hooligan action is pride in and defense of local working-class community reputation, which in a sense becomes magnified at regional, national, and international levels. As one of Murray's hooligan respondents puts it: "Good supporters don't like a team getting beat, so we wait for the other supporters to come out and give it to them. Show them who's boss" [p. 9]. Although he never states his case unequivocally, Murray's argument implies that team defeat and hooligan action are necessarily correlated. But this is only partly correct, because fans defend their local and national pride against opposing fans whether victory or defeat is the outcome, and, indeed, long before and after games have been played, as Dunning et al. [47] have shown convincingly. Murray's argument is thus a relatively unsophisticated explanation for a set of practices that are altogether more complex in their genesis and meaning.

Arguments concerning hooligan honor and pride have been developed into more compelling theses by Vulliamy [179] and Weir [184]. Like Taylor, both authors point crucially to a number of contradictions in dominant ideologies in the United Kingdom that ultimately contribute to collective violence at British soccer. Asserting that "hooligans are closer to Mrs. Thatcher than she thinks," Weir argues:

> . . . it is plain to see that, apart from their rampant anti-authoritarianism, the football hooligans are anything but aliens from the rest of British society. Their well-documented chauvinism, racist and sexist attitudes, hostility towards intellectuals and homosexuals, physical aggression, drunkenness, are quite evident in the culture and values of the dominant society in which Mrs. Thatcher and the rest are so at home. Enough people by now have drawn attention to the striking parallels with the Falklands. When the whole nation was invited to glory in "our boys" aptitude for what Major Keeble of the parachute Regiment called "gutter fighting" at Goose Green, our hypocritical press called Brussels a "massacre;" Goose Green really was. [p. 21]

In an equally sociopolitically astute account of the Heysel Stadium riot of May, 1985, Vulliamy [179, p. 8] points to what he sees as the inevitability of sports-related violence in a cultural setting that actively encourages physical defense of masculinity and national honor:

> The English supporters came less to win the cup for football or even "their club" than to assert their collective English manhood, free from the ties of job or poverty, of "normality," of women and girls of whom there were almost none to be seen. They bellowed tireless songs about "wops" and "spiks" and drank themselves into a state where nothing was real but their mass violence . . . it was a matter for their drunken, blood-thirsty and racist English "honor" that the terraces be cleared of "spiks" and the Union Jack flown unchallenged. I saw one Liverpool fan with a t-shirt: "Keep the Falklands British" as though he and his mates were the task force. Perhaps, as he kicked and punched, he thought, in the *Sun's* infamous screech of violent chauvinism, "GOTCHA!" . . . The behavior of English fans was, and is, sickening. It is hypocritical to belabor them for besmirching British values when in so many other areas of national life violence is made heroic, narrow chauvinism is appealed to and the need of the whole community for sports they can enjoy and take part in is ignored.

Along with Taylor's most recent work, then, Weir and Vulliamy are careful to position soccer hooliganism and the working-class males who perpetrate it in a unique, contemporary cultural and political context currently experiencing crisis, in which aspects of a radical right-wing world view pervade both the upper and lower echelons of the social strata and becomes expressed aggressively in diverse ways.

Also noteworthy here are studies of the relationship between soccer hooliganism and religion. Murray's *The Old Firm* [123], probably the best known of these, richly details the history of religious dogmatism and its effects with two well-known Glasgow teams, Rangers and Celtic. Murray shows how the sectarian, bigoted attitudes and practices of these clubs towards persons (including players and fans) of alternative religious faith has in fact enhanced the antagonisms of their respective fan groups towards each other and helped create a long tradition of hostility and violence between them. In a much earlier piece, McIlvanney [112] also gave a simplified account of these processes.

A number of other studies in this area make important contributions to our understanding of soccer hooliganism in the United Kingdom. Briefly, these include Wagg's [181] Marxist-critical appraisal of the cultural transformations taking place in soccer which have left cultural "spaces" currently filled by the destructive activities of young working-class supporters; Redhead and McLaughlin's [136] and Robins's [144] fascinating accounts of the popular cultural and stylistic elements of hooligans and their action; as well as Clarke and Madden's [25, 26] trenchant socioeconomic analyses of soccer's fiscal problems and how sports authorities in Britain have misunderstood shifts in leisure interests in that context. Other studies provide evidence of Scottish hooliganism [30] and compare hooligan rates and practices in England and Scotland [118, 119]; still others offer demographic and arrest data on hooliganism [47, 172]; Redhead [135] incisively examines the cultural meaning of soccer to its officials, players, and followers; and O'Brien [125] briefly describes how soccer affects the lives of committed fans.

Although recognizing the diverse theoretical origins of the four major perspectives examined above, as well as the impracticality of marrying ethological, cultural, Marxist, and Eliasan positions, the most adequate explanation of hooliganism could perhaps best be achieved by combining all of the strengths of these perspectives. Indeed, they demonstrate a number of recognizable parallel interests. These include concerns with class background, youth culture, postwar changes in the dynamics of violence itself, and the role played by the media in sensationalizing soccer hooliganism. As a result of such research in the United Kingdom, we are now quite well informed about how and why hooliganism occurs. This body of research shows, for example, that since the 19th century, soccer has come to represent pride in local, regional, and national community for many millions of British people, that much of the aggressive action in and around soccer stadia is both ritualistic and potentially injurious, that hooliganism is linked closely with broader ideologies of "manliness" embraced by large numbers of British men, and that as a historically grounded practice, hooliganism is unlikely to disappear in the near future. As the work of Dunning and his colleagues [40–48] has shown, in this regard we also know that recommendations for solutions based on punishment alone are incapable of resolving a complex social problem. (See the subsequent section on Recommendations.) To complete this review of explanations of collective violence in sport it is necessary to examine research on sports violence outside North America and the United Kingdom.

Other International Contexts

In the introduction it was noted that collective violence at sport can be found in almost all national contexts. Indeed, most countries where organized sport is played have recorded problems of crowd disturbance at one time or another. This includes locations with diverse cultures and political systems. Sadly, however, despite a growing body of literature on collective violence in various international settings, at the time of this writing such literature remains limited, particularly the portion of it written in or translated into English. Although there are no clear international schools of theory, this section provides a series of examples of explanations for sports-related violence where they have been offered. Once again, most research addresses the issue of soccer-related violence.

Perhaps best known of the work on sports crowd disorder outside North America and the United Kingdom is Lever's research on soccer in Brazil [91–93]. Implementing a structural-functionalist framework of analysis, Lever shows how in South America, sport (sport here almost always means soccer) paradoxically demonstrates both unifying and divisive elements: unifying in the sense that it enhances inter- and intracommunity relations, but divisive because it magnifies the realization that in Brazil only athletes and the very affluent can be socially mobile. For the purposes of this paper, Lever raises at least two crucial issues. First, she shows how the way the Brazilian government organizes and markets the game is consistent with the crude Marxist "opiate of the masses" argument. For example, she writes that informal Brazilian policy "seems to include the notion that soccer can be used to distract workers from their serious grievances" [93, p. 61]. Second, and again paradoxically, this unofficial attempt to mask proletarian social deprivation apparently fails as frequently as it succeeds, because we are at once told that soccer games consistently attract huge paying audiences and that there are a number of ways that class conflict is acted out inside stadia. The latter includes the throwing of urine bags by working-class fans into the middle-class sections of fans below them. Lever's work is theoretically unsophisticated (for example, structural-functionalism cannot easily account for these lived contradictions), but her data are rich and her research constitutes the most comprehensive sociological appraisal of the cultural meanings of sport in South America currently available.

By now, most students of sport and violence recognize the spurious nature of the common official and lay claim that soccer hooliganism is a "British disease." Scholars in continental Europe are increasingly turning to their own continent's collective violence at soccer games as can be witnessed by an expanding literature.

In a critique of dominant messages of sports crowd disorder constructed in the popular media, Young [197] notes the following European examples. French hooligan groups have prompted closure of sections of stadia, escalations in policing at games, and in some cases games being played behind closed doors. Following violence and destruction in Holland (where clubs such as Ajax and Feyenoord are known to have disruptive followers), the state-owned railway system recently banned alcohol on all soccer excursions, and West German police have assigned special investigation units to detect neo-Nazi hooligans who attack immigrant workers at soccer games. Robins [144, p. 89] informs us that certain Italian clubs have amassed gangs of fighting followers similar to those of British clubs, which also adopt their own suggestive nicknames (e.g., the Commandos of A.C. Milan and the Ulras of Torino). Finally, following the Heysel Stadium riot in 1985 in which 39 fans lost their lives when Liverpool fans attacked their Juventus rivals, supporters of other Italian and French clubs were reported to have sprayed graffiti in their local towns congratulating the Liverpool contingent for their "triumph" [*Hamilton Spectator*, June 1, 1985; *Daily Telegraph*, June 19, 1985].

Throughout Europe, there is currently much concern that soccer fans are consolidating connections with extreme right-wing groups. Taylor [167] and Young [197] have argued that British neo-Nazi groups such as the British Movement and the National Front use soccer for recruitment purposes, distributing fascist propaganda and flaunting Nazi symbols. Williams et al. [193] note that fans of several northern Italian clubs such as Bergano, Brescia, Milan, and Verona have neo-Nazi connections, and Bell [11] has pointed to similar social problems in France and Austria.

One needs to exercise caution here. It is clear that problems of collective violence at European soccer matches have been exacerbated by expressions of fascism, but there is little evidence that the problem of soccer hooliganism per se is caused by fascism. This would be too quick and simple an explanation, though it has certainly been adopted, curiously in both right- and left-wing quarters (for example, following the Heysel stadium riot, the National Front was blamed both by the chairman of the Liverpool club itself, Mr. John Smith, and by the communist newspaper *Workers Vangard*, June 14, 1985). A much broader historical and sociological framework is needed to explain these issues in which relations of politics, class, and gender are seen to translate into violent action at sport.

In February, 1989, the Greek Ministry of Culture hosted a special conference on sport and collective violence entitled European Congress on Violence Control in the World of Sports. Papers presented at the conference represented, at the time, an important sample of European research in this area. Papers included sociological explanations of hooliganism, its manifestations and policies created around it, in Denmark [131], the Netherlands [177], Belgium [178], Germany [113], Greece [126], and England and Wales [154]. Outside the British context, most work on soccer-related violence has probably been conducted by German scholars [e.g., 67, 132, 133]. Indeed, as an indication of Germans' perceptions of their own problems, Hahn et al. [67, p. 7] cite August Kirsch, Director of the Federal Institute of Sports Science in the Federal Republic of Germany, who recently argued: "Spectator riots at big sports events are the negative accompaniment of modern sport."

Despite common references to a "British disease," in terms of total numbers of fatalities, some of the most serious cases of soccer crowd disorder in the history of the sport have not involved British supporters at all. In May, 1964, for example, over 300 fans were killed in a riot that broke out at the National Stadium in Lima, Peru [*New York Times*, May 25, 1964], and in perhaps the most notorious case of soccer-related violence, a one week "soccer war" was waged between Honduras and El Salvador in the summer of 1969 following a game played between the two countries on neutral ground in Mexico. To end the conflict, the Organization of American States had to intervene [*Newsweek*, July 28, 1969, p. 54].

Contrary to the popular myth of soccer hooliganism as a phenomenon exclusive to the United Kingdom, then, soccer-related violence appears to be endemic wherever the game is played. Young [197] provides a long list of examples from settings as diverse as Uruguay, Chile, the United Arab Emirates, China, Libya, Turkey, the Soviet Union and Bangladesh. Semyonov and Farbstein's [149] recent work on the ecology of soccer riots in Israel is worthy of note here also.

Finally, despite clear evidence that world soccer has more problems with violence off the field than other sports, it should not be perceived as the only sport around which regular forms of collective violence have developed. The very few studies indicating that violence also accompanies other sports have unfortunately been theoretically unso-phisticated and empirically limited but do include Adedeji's [2] study of violence in Nigerian school sports, Main's [100] brief commentary on Australian rules football and cricket fans, Crot's [36] illustration of crowd violence at one-day cricket events in Australia, and Gammon's [57, p. 37] account of "unseemly behavior, on the pitch and off" in West Indies cricket. And finally, at least one crowd riot following a European ice hockey game can be interpreted in terms of symbolic responses to oppression through sport. Following a victory by the Czechoslovakian national team over Russia in 1969, thousands of Czechoslovakian fans in Prague shouted anti-Soviet slogans and van-dalized offices of Aeroflot, the Soviet national airline [*Life*, April 11, 1969, pp. 93–94]. Like other politically driven sports protests noted above, this example shows how sport can be and has been used in symbolic ways to challenge forms of oppression. In this specific case, public disruption was clearly less about sport than the Russian invasion of Czechoslovakia that had occurred in the previous year.

Recommendations

Increasing recognition of sports-related violence that occurs in a number of international contexts has prompted numerous recommendations for dealing with such violence. Measures that have been proposed emanate from groups representing various interests, although in most countries they have been initiated almost exclusively by police, sports officials, and politicians. Scholarly evaluations of suggested solutions are scarce, and what is available once again relates mostly to British hooliganism. The following is a brief analysis of measures discussed and introduced in North America and the United Kingdom to challenge sports crowd disorder and those who take part in it.

So many recommendations for solutions have been made in the United Kingdom at so many levels that space is available here to review only the most common among them. During the 1980s, the Thatcher government perceived hooliganism as a national social problem that required remedial attention. The British government's concern has been amply demonstrated by a number of what can only be called "hit and miss" policies, which include increases in strict security and policing procedures at soccer games and the spiraling of sentences imposed upon offenders. For example, the 1984–1985 soccer season in England witnessed the first life jail-term given to a soccer hooligan (subsequently rescinded by the courts). Prime Minister Thatcher's now notorious "War Cabinet," a special committee established in the post-Heysel era to combat hooliganism, demanded that soccer "get its own house in order," basically refusing to acknowledge that hooliganism as a problem was in any way indicative of larger social, political, or economic conflict.

The number of government-sponsored investigations into hooliganism and its surrounding issues [137–141] also has risen. Reports resulting from these investigations have elicited critical responses from scholars such as Taylor and Dunning. Most interesting here is the report *Committee of Inquiry into Crowd Safety and Control at Soccer Grounds* supervised by Mr. Justice Popplewell following the now infamous Bradford fire and Heysel Stadium riot of 1985. Taylor's [167, p. 174] description of the report's content is an accurate one and is broadly applicable to other official reports written to date:

> The Report is . . . notable for the general support it gives to the theory, held to so fruitlessly by authority in Britain since the mid-1960s, that there is some kind of solution to the problem of soccer hooliganism in the extension of police powers of search and arrest and in the general revision of the criminal law.

Both Popplewell's report and Taylor's response are undoubtedly imbued with their own political biases. But such official assessments of soccer's problems with violence are crucial in illuminating ways in which various British politicians and sports authorities have traditionally viewed possibilities for resolving hooliganism. As Taylor shows, this has typically included some call for increasing sanctions and punitive procedures, for increases in law and order. The usefulness of such measure has been strongly challenged by a number of scholars mentioned previously [especially 47, 191].

Similar criticisms have been made of measures taken by British soccer clubs themselves. A number of these attempts to combat hooliganism have been radical and desperate, as was the case with Chelsea Football Club in 1985 when the chairman of the club installed an electrified fence around the playing field and was intent on making it operational until the Greater London Council pressured the club into removing it. Not surprisingly, however, most other measures taken or discussed by clubs have been more thoughtful, if not more successful. Possibly the most widely publicized suggestion has been to introduce a national identity card scheme which would principally be aimed at removing the protection of anonymous membership in the soccer crowd normally enjoyed by hooligan fans. The long-term effects of the scheme remain speculative. One wonders at the feasibility of implementing this presumably expensive identity card program when many British soccer clubs are experiencing financial crises. Its potential costliness is underlined when one considers that many of the larger First and Second Division clubs have a cumulative regular and occasional spectator following of over 80,000. Moreover, several of the clubs themselves have hinted at the futility of introducing a widespread identity card program when those with hooligan proclivities represent a very small minority of the overall fan support.

Believing that violence inside stadia has been caused or exacerbated by the traditional arrangement of standing to watch the games, many British clubs have dramatically increased the numbers of seats and some have even changed entirely to all-seat stadia. This policy also appears to have been entirely unsuccessful, because hooligan groups are now known to vandalize these new sections and have been captured on film several times using seats as missiles in aerial confrontations with police.

In contrast to measures of this type, academics such as Taylor and Dunning have generally been critical of all sources who look solely to game-centered explanations and solutions for soccer hooliganism and who advise short-term and punitive measures only. Events over the last two decades in the United Kingdom show that the incidence of hooliganism does not decrease as more draconian policies are imposed. Rather, such scholars have emphasized that practical short-term solutions must be combined with more considered long-term ones.

Despite their theoretical differences, both Taylor and Dunning would agree that because hooliganism is symptomatic of broader social crises, nothing less than a major revision of the British social and political structure itself will help dissolve the hooligan issue entirely. Recognizing the unlikelihood of such a suggestion in the immediate or long-term, Dunning and his colleagues have made several practical recommendations for tackling hooliganism domestically and abroad. These include more efficient ticket distribution, comprehensive travel schedules that enable specially appointed stewards to supervise groups of travelling fans, and adequate segregation by host clubs. Although the government and the Football Association in the United Kingdom appear to be paying some attention to the work of the Leicester group, at the time of this writing government officials, soccer officials, and scholars unfortunately concur on only a handful of possible explanations for hooliganism, its causes, and its resolution. In such a situation, it is inevitable that recommendations that are taken seriously remain almost entirely police and politician initiated.

Although North Americans generally believe that sports crowd disorder is minimal and unworthy of serious attention, evidence suggests that a large number of clubs have become sufficiently concerned with a perceived crowd disorder problem to have introduced policy changes. Generally, these changes have taken the form of revisions in security procedures and efforts to decrease the abusive, destructive, and violent behavior of fans. Young [197] discovered that these recent changes often have included stiff increases in fines for trespassing on the field of play; increases in numbers of security personnel, and reductions in the level of police tolerance of profane, abusive, and violent fan conduct; the construction of special family enclosures and protective tunnels for players to enter and exit from the playing area safely; the closing of bleacher sections known to contain consistently disorderly fans; and increases in frisking and searches at stadium entrances.

North American clubs also have expressed concern with increasing numbers of alcohol-related offences, but even though recommendations are regularly made by fans, officials, and police to restrict the sale of alcohol, the vast majority of North American stadia continue to sell alcohol. Although many of these now sell only low (or lower) alcohol beer and frequently terminate sales long before the end of games, Young [197] has argued that these attempts represent only a token effort by clubs to appease frustrated orderly fans and security personnel. His study notes that clubs experiencing security problems with inebriated fans frequently underplay the seriousness and number of offences taking place. This, he argues, may be explained by the fact that many North American clubs are actually sponsored or owned by breweries.

Of course, as Williams [189] indicates, a similarly embarrassing scenario exists for British soccer clubs. The Control of Alcohol Bill, introduced in 1985, has now banned the possession or consumption of alcohol inside soccer stadia. This rests uneasily with many clubs who are once again sponsored by breweries. One might note here that recommendations to reduce or ban the sale of alcohol at sports events, a popular position with politicians, as well as legal and sports authorities, may in fact be meaningless. It is clear that in the United Kingdom anti-alcohol policies have had only limited results because hooligans are quick to discover alternative ways of drinking. And in North America, where alcohol restrictions amount to little more than tokenism so far, it seems that fans who want to drink will also find a way to do so.

Crucially, what many of these recommendations for curbing aspects of sports crowd disorder in the United Kingdom and North America demonstrate is the apparent persuasiveness in popular and legal discourse of explanations for disorder that focus on the ecology of the sport stadium, i.e., on how disorder is linked to game-related phenomena alone (such as alcohol consumption). Some ecological explanations (such as lack of seats) were discussed previously as "precipitating factors" [53, 59, 95, 156]. Understanding alcohol as a main cause of fan violence is a classic example of such an ecological explanation. Although excessive alcohol consumption may be a partial explanation for fan violence, and although such a popular explanation has apparently been legitimated by concrete policies and sanctions introduced in both the United Kingdom and North America, sociologists argue that the alcohol and other ecological explanations necessarily entail leaving out the social, historical, and political context.

As Young [197] has argued, if sports violence is representative of contested ideological terrain where favored explanations reflect political interests, such an imbroglio is likely to endure. Governments will continue to blame crowd violence on poorly organized and policed sport, sports officials will continue to blame society, and sociologists will continue to argue that neither explanation is helpful when used alone. Of course, recommendations will continue to reflect these assumed causes.

SPORT, VIOLENCE AND THE MASS MEDIA

The vast majority of people have neither seen nor participated in sport crowd disorder. Thus, our perceptions of such behavior are likely to be mediated, and the media must take a great deal of responsibility for our perceptions and misperceptions of the form and meaning of spectator violence in sport. As Young and Smith [199, p. 298] have noted:

> The effect of mass media portrayals of violence on violence itself in society has for decades generated heated public debate and a huge volume of research and writing . . . while this outpouring of energy has not resulted in the conclusive establishment of a direct cause-and-effect relationship between media and real-life violence, the bulk of the evidence, especially that pertaining to television, points strongly in this direction.

Young and Smith's comments allude to how crowd violence in sport is affected as much by media coverage as by participant violence. The role played by the media in developing and confirming popular images of sport, its players, its followers, and its violence, has prompted some research. This is particularly true of research concerned with contextualizing sports crowd disorder in a broad sociological framework that includes not just microsociological inquiries into how problems of violence are manifested but also macrosociological examinations of how those manifestations may be linked to official and unofficial responses to violence, class structure, and political ideology.

Hall's [68, p. 267] early description of the treatment of soccer hooliganism in the British popular press since the 1960s is in a sense indicative of the manner in which sports violence is reported in the press more generally:

> ... graphic headlines, bold type-faces, warlike imagery and epithets, vivid photographs cropped to the edges to create a strong impression of physical menace, and the stories have been decorated with black lines and exclamation marks.

Hall speaks of the process of "editing for impact," a process in which hooligan action comes to be marketed by a newspaper industry concerned largely with profit maximization. A cluster of issues including lurid news values, distorted reporting, and conservative world views combine to "excite" the phenomenon, argues Hall, an effect that tends to be heightened public and official sensitization to soccer-related violence, increased policing at and around games, and ultimately more arrests and violence.

Adams [1], Walvin [183], Murphy et al. [122], Whannel [185], and Young [196] also have pointed to the cyclical nature of this process. In an analysis of television coverage of soccer in the United Kingdom, Walvin [183, p. 88] is careful to argue that "television violence may be less significant in stimulating acts of violence than it is in encouraging a stiffening of the law and order lobby." But his thesis arguably fails to reach its logical conclusion. Walvin is certainly correct to underline how, especially during the Thatcher years, draconian measures have become the norm in England, but this is where his argument wanes and research by the Leicester group gathers pace.

In a much more historically grounded fashion, Murphy et al. [122] illustrate the connection between soccer violence, media, and politics in terms of long-term social processes and trends. They show how at various phases of British history, official responses to and press coverage of hooliganism have played both amplifying or indeed deamplifying roles in very contrived ways. In the years immediately following the Brussels riot, for instance, and despite a number of serious incidents of disorder outside soccer grounds, media treatment of hooliganism was, if anything, underplayed. In fact, the press particularly, we are told, took it upon themselves to broadly celebrate decreases in overall arrest figures, which did occur, but also to ignore a number of violent interchanges.

Clearly, the Leicester group understands political backdrop as a key determinant of the nature of news in the context of soccer hooliganism. In this specific case, in the post-Heysel era, authorities and the media in Britain have frequently made statements that suggest that hooliganism has now been controlled. Such statements, contrived as they are, serve to send out a plethora of messages to a national and international audience, notably that the British government and sports authorities are concerned and responsible, and that stringent law and order measures have been effective. Because English soccer clubs are still banned by the ruling bodies of soccer from involvement in European competitions, and are attempting to have the ban lifted, such a message has very serious practical and political connotations.

Whannel [185], Young [196, 197], and Taylor [166, 167] concur that the media play an active role in collective violence at British soccer, and that the hooliganism-media nexus can best be understood using a framework that is historically and politically informed. Using critical theory approaches, Whannel and Young provide models of normative media discourses on hooliganism (including themes of war talk, dehumanized quantities, mindless behavior, and blame) and view them broadly as representative of right-wing ideologies and practices at work in contemporary Britain. Taylor [166, 167], Vulliamy [179], and Keen [78] have elaborated on these issues and have tied ongoing media discourses on sports violence in Britain, which are paradoxically as aggressive, jingoistic, and sexist as the activities and groups they depict, to the emergence of a widely accepted radical right-wing philosophy in the Thatcher era. Crucially, all these authors underline fundamental lived contradictions in dominant ideology in Britain, and collectively make the trenchant argument that hooliganism (and male violence more generally) is inevitable in a cultural setting that actively encourages physical displays and defense of masculinity and national honor on a number of levels.

Several in-depth examinations of media coverage of collective violence at North American sport have been conducted. Bryant and Zillman [20], Smith [159], and Young and Smith [199] have examined ways in which the media exploit (mostly) participant violence in sport. For example, Smith and Young concentrate on the messages that accompany violence and show at least three common patterns in sports commentary, including the melodramatic headline, commendations of violent players, and graphic depictions of violence in photographs. The net result of such common procedures, they insist, is at least to condone violent athletic conduct and perhaps to help reproduce it.

It appears that critical appraisals of the social genesis of violence in sport are conspicuous by their absence in North American media discourses [197]. There tends to be an assumption that participant violence is part of the natural and unchangeable ordering of a world in which men compete together [198]. Theberge [169] has conducted a case study of media coverage of a bench-clearing brawl between the Canadian and Soviet teams at the 1987 World Junior Hockey Championships in Piestany, Czechoslovakia, to make a similar argument. Her incisive study shows how North American hockey officials and the media invariably rationalize incidents of violence (if indeed incidents are so perceived) as the inefficiency of officials on the ice or technical failures (in this case the stadium lights were extinguished), and never as the cultural and social basis of a sport fundamentally orchestrated around traditional notions of masculinity and aggressive role requirements.

Young's [197] comparative study of media treatment of sports crowd disorder in North America and the United Kingdom is an in-depth cross-cultural analysis of dominant images and ideologies of sports crowd disorder. He demonstrates how soccer fans in the United Kingdom have for decades been viewed in both the British media and the public as "internal enemies" against whom the state is forced to use extreme sanctions. But he also introduces evidence to indicate that hooligans (and perhaps British youth in general) have been considered "external enemies" by the North American media. The notion of hooliganism as a "British disease" has been disseminated widely in North America.

Despite a number of indications of increases in sports crowd disorder at North American sports events (although nothing as pronounced, violent, or collective as its British counterpart), and despite reports of and responses to British soccer hooliganism that have displayed all the classic symptoms of moral panic, any presence or threat of sports crowd disorder in North America appears to be consistently downplayed by clubs, officials, and the media, if not denied in more explicit terms.

To interpret this, Young uses a cultural studies framework, specifically the notion of hegemony. Dominant ideologies of sports crowd disorder, he argues, are representative of hegemonic processes in North American sport. Powerful groups (e.g., sports organizations, media, breweries) have contributed towards the masking or distorting of a social issue which in actuality is more pronounced and perhaps more insidious than they are willing to acknowledge. He shows, for instance, that stadia security personnel and police often discuss the sports crowd disorder issue in far more serious tones than do clubs, owners, and the media. (The alcohol issue raised earlier is an example.) Political and business interests are being protected here, argues Young. Elements of critical media theory also are used to show how the content and format of news normally depends on its proximity to its subject. With this in mind, Young [83, p. 243] interprets dominant approaches on the part of the North American media to the "British disease" as an attempt by that media ". . .to exploit its relative distance from its object, and insert a critical stance." The axiom that what one does not say is as important as what one does say is now brought into sharper relief. This ongoing process of denial of sports crowd violence in North America by those inside sports and those whose job it is to bring sports to the public (the media) not only represents a striking example of what Taylor [165, p. 165] calls a "significant silence," but a clear indication that by pointing to serious social problems elsewhere, one's own problems inevitably appear less important and menacing.

Studies by Coakley [29] and Young and Smith [199] are careful to emphasize that a direct cause-and-effect relationship between media coverage of sports violence and spill-over violence in society is yet to be empirically validated, and both address the attendant problem of generalizing vis-á-vis media effects on the basis of limited studies and data. Because audience readings of texts and discourses are differentially linked to factors such as social experience, ideology, and gender, caution should be exercised in assuming that media reports affect all sports audiences in the same fashion or indeed at all. Nevertheless, several writers have argued persuasively that there may be certain discourse effects of media treatment of sports violence [78, 165], and Young's [197] study attempts to provide evidence for both discourse and (some limited) behavioral effects. Considerable evidence certainly shows that media coverage of sports violence by fans or players is linked to practice and performance itself, at least indirectly. Media discourses contribute to a social climate that is conducive to violent behavior. Once again, as Young and Smith [199] point out, most people are not exposed to sports violence directly but indirectly through the media.

CONCLUSIONS

In general, research into sports-related violence has paid insufficient attention to methodological problems and issues, and almost none of it has critically evaluated the phenomenon from a feminist perspective. This review concludes with a brief discussion of these important issues, and some suggestions for future research.

A Methodological Critique

A diversity of procedures have been employed in studies of sport and collective violence. These include observation [60, 109], historical methods [66, 98, 99, 110, 176], qualitative content analysis [185, 196, 197], quantitative content analysis [62, 157, 159], questionnaire [24, 90, 197], experimental design studies [4, 148, 197], secondary data analysis of criminal offence categories [172, 173], ethnography [191], and review of literature [15, 23, 101, 155, 159]. However, although the literature on violent collective processes taking place in sport continues to expand, this advance has not, for the most part, been accompanied by improvements in the types of research procedures employed or by reflexive uses of them. Most notably, it is still true that methods often are adopted singly. One can only assume from this that like the early perspectives of those working from a social facts or social definitions paradigm [142], methods continue to be viewed by sports scholars as mutually exclusive. Such an outdated and indeed insidious perspective has correctly been criticized by methodologists in mainstream sociology for inevitably producing studies that tend to be one-sided and incomplete.

Very recently, a handful of studies have been conducted that demonstrate not only that multiple methods can be used in integrated and coherent ways, but also that research based on such an approach ultimately produces deeper sociological interpretations and understandings.

Smith's [159] study is a review of much that has been written in the area of sport and violence which pays considerable attention to the methodological and conceptual problems in defining violence. It combines statistically recorded results from Smith's own original research into violence in ice hockey [158] with other approaches, which include subcultural analyses of violent sports groups and the development of a typology of sports violence built on data from numerous extant sources, to produce a thorough examination of sports violence in international perspective. The research produced on soccer hooliganism in Britain by the Leicester group, notably Williams's ethnography of the conduct of hooligans at the 1980 World Cup in Spain [191], Maguire's content analysis of nineteenth and twentieth century newspaper reports [98], and Dunning et al.'s analysis of the sociogenesis of hooliganism [47] surely stands as the most comprehensive, empirically grounded set of studies of the violent associations of any one sport conducted by sociologists to date. Crucially, Dunning and his colleagues provide a thorough examination of the demographic characteristics of participants and of actual violent crowd processes, which are relatively rare in the literature and are components of violence studies that have long been required [see 13, 155]. This group, now internationally renowned for its work, has been careful to use a number of methods to illuminate what is a highly complex issue. Although their methods are principally historical, they also have included such sources as content analysis, ethnography, interviews, and official data on arrest figures to show how contemporary hooliganism and responses to it compare with earlier times. Finally, Young's [197] comparative study of dominant images of sports crowd disorder in North America and the United Kingdom shows how semiotic content analysis, interviewing and observation, and questionnaires can be used in a complementary fashion. Each method contributes to the overall sociological picture painted by the study. Questionnaires distributed to sports organizations in North America and interviews with stadium security and police provide official commentaries on the issue, interviews with fans and media personnel demonstrate how sports-related violence is respectively understood and broadcast by members of the public and the media, and an in-depth semiological component discloses the nature of signs transmitted to mass audiences.

All three studies use very different theoretical perspectives. Smith's eclectic sociological analysis proceeds from a completely different premise than the figurational perspective of Dunning and his colleagues and Young's cultural studies approach. What all three studies share is a consensus on the significance of historical analysis in sociological research. As Beamish [9, p. 59] has argued, "because sport is a dialectical form it is always in a state of change and must be reviewed and studied historically." Combining historical and other methods, then, these three studies attempt to avoid the static, confining results inevitably produced by single-method approaches.

Unfortunately, studies such as these that advocate the advantages of multiple-method approaches represent the exception rather than the rule in research on sport and collective violence. Despite this, Trow's [174, p. 33] early argument that "most sociological problems are so complex that they require the use of multiple methods" is still pertinent to the study of sport structures and processes in society. As Trow puts it:

> Every cobbler thinks leather is the only thing. Most social scientists . . . have their favorite research methods with which they are familiar and have some skill in using. And I suspect we mostly choose to investigate problems that seem vulnerable to attack through these methods. But we should at least try to be less parochial than cobblers. Let us be done with the arguments of "participant observation" versus interviewing . . . and get on with the business of attacking our problems with the widest array of conceptual and methodological tools that we possess and they demand. This does not preclude discussion and debate regarding the relative usefulness of different methods for the study of specific problems or types of problems. But that is very different from the assertion of the general and inherent superiority of one method over another on the basis of some intrinsic qualities it presumably possesses. [pp. 33–35]

Given that the study of sports crowd disorder, a phenomenon that is unpredictable, spontaneous and often lacks a permanent institutional base, is an extremely complicated task, and one that usually renders direct techniques of data gathering difficult and time consuming, it is surprising that few researchers have so far explored syntheses between direct and indirect methodological procedures. The adoption of a multiple-method approach undoubtedly would increase the chances of obtaining reliable empirical data and, importantly, would contribute toward more complete sociological research.

A Feminist Critique

Given the considerable attention that has been paid to the phenomenon of collective violence in sport to date, remarkably few studies have provided a feminist interpretation of the behaviors, processes, and structures they address. I suspect that this has much to do with the assumption that because sports violence appears to be predominantly expressed and participated in by men (Smith [160] shows that there are exceptions to this norm), an analysis of women's roles or a feminist perspective is superfluous. Such a view is neither accurate nor indicative of an appropriate sociological imagination. Violence, like much that occurs in sport, is certainly gendered, but like all practices that appear gender exclusive, it is not only amenable to interpretation from a feminist perspective, but in fact best proceeds from one. What women and men do in sport tells us much about larger structures of ostracism, power, and cultural legitimacy in any given context. Connell makes these arguments in convincing ways in both a theoretically sophisticated study of sexual politics [31], and in a case study of an Australian Iron Man triathlon event [32].

With regard to accounts of British soccer hooliganism, only Taylor [167] has recognized the importance of a feminist critique of soccer's violence and broader social problems in Britain in anything other than a fleeting manner. Indeed, a feminist critique is integral to Taylor's entire argument of cultural and political crisis in a bigoted society in which sport is at once a breeding ground for chauvinism and male dominance and comfortably provides its own justifications for sexist attitudes and practices. Specifically, Taylor, like Weir [184] and Vulliamy [179], shows how for thousands of working-class males in Britain the weekend only makes sense away from women. He cites Brown's [18, p. 14] sociologically insightful commentary on this weekend regimen:

> Saturday steeped in soccer, *Football Focus* with Bob Wilson, off to the match, back home for the results and a prepared tea. Post match analysis, out to the pub, *Match of the Day* dictating sexual behavior. Sunday morning, on with the boots for ninety minutes in the mud. Drinks with the lads and then back for a bath and Sunday lunch. Play with the kids and *Match of the Week*. In the evening a special treat for the wife—drink in the pub or perhaps

a visit to the mother-in-law. All over the country this is the pattern of life every weekend, week in, week out, August to May.

Taylor underlines a plethora of traditionally prized but deeply sexist rituals of British soccer clubs, including the hosting of female beauty pageants, the use of bathing beauties on cars during half-time sales pitches, sexist pin-ups in soccer newspapers and magazines, and links them all to what he calls the "failure of orthodox social democracy" [167, p. 187] in Britain. Redhead [135, p. 51] similarly describes how seminude women in soccer equipment frequently adorn the pages of the soccer press. Given all this, it is again remarkable that so little interest has been shown in women's experiences of soccer, at or away from the game. This has been given only passing and implicit attention by Hazelton [71], who demonstrates how the experience of soccer spectatorship in Britain, replete with its macho, sexist, and militaristic trappings, can be uncomfortable and intimidating for both men and women, especially those new to the culture. As noted earlier, immediately following the Heysel stadium riot, two brief but powerfully insightful pieces were written which, like Taylor's thesis, drew connections between traditional notions of Britishness on the one hand and values at work in soccer hooliganism on the other. Weir's [184] and Vulliamy's [179] commentaries highlight the meanings of events taking place at Heysel which include repressive attitudes to women.

Of course, the Leicester group also has noted the importance of gender in British soccer hooliganism, although in a less direct manner than Taylor (they nowhere explicitly advocate a feminist critique). The video *Hooligan* [73] showed clearly how in rough working-class communities traditional gender structures can be found. These include radical conjugal role separation, expressions of pride in the local community, and physical displays of manliness. Moreover, the Leicester group points to ways in which women from such class backgrounds actually approve of their male partners validating their masculinity through hooligan endeavors. Unfortunately, what the researchers do not tell us is what happens when such approval is not offered (presumably some women are critical of violence), or indeed whether these gender structures and values are more broadly representative of other class groupings or in fact British society as a whole. At least in part, one suspects that the latter is the case, and that a sole focus on "rough" sections of the working class results in a limited and incomplete thesis.

In general, in all contexts more detailed and theoretically informed critiques of gender ideologies at work in sport are required. Contributions by Hargreaves [69] in England, Kidd [79, 80] and Theberge [169] in Canada, and Messner [114] in the United States have made important strides in this direction, but more is needed. All five studies use critical and cultural studies approaches to show how women are relatively disempowered through sport, and how notions of aggressive masculinity are produced and reproduced. As Theberge [169, p. 253] puts it:

> Sport is a cultural practice that embodies qualities of toughness, aggression, and physical dominance. Not only is it a setting wherein individual males learn these traits; in sport the cultural meaning and social reality of masculinity are continually reinforced and reproduced. Moreover, the apparent "naturalness" of gendered experiences of sport, based upon their assumed basis in physical differences between the sexes, makes sport a particularly powerful setting for the reproduction of hegemonic masculinity.

Following these studies, to ignore social and political context, which includes issues of gender, in accounting for sports violence is to provide only an incomplete sociological explanation of the phenomenon under scrutiny.

Future Research

Since the 1960s, sport's relation to collective violence has prompted much research and writing. What is noticeable in North American work [e.g., 23, 53, 95, 194] is that a considerable portion of the total research conducted has proceeded from the assumption that sports-related violence on and off the field is spiralling alarmingly. This is a position embraced less readily by British researchers with the conspicuous exception of Marsh [106], whose work builds on a premise similar to the North American one. Curiously few attempts have been made to empirically substantiate this rather striking and, if validated, important claim. What is missing in these and many other studies is an appreciation of an historical perspective, as Dunning's [41] work in particular is quick to point out. Only the latter can provide appropriate sociological tools in the explanation of behavior that occurs today at and around sport.

If anything is clear from the collective behavior literature, it is that mainstream theories adopted so broadly in the 1960s and 1970s to account for counter-cultural movements, riots, protests, and so forth, although able to cast some light on aspects of collective violence at sport, for the most part are simultaneously limited and limiting. This can be witnessed in the way they aspire only to explain isolated moments and phases of collective action. No doubt, complex sociological issues are at work in sports violence, and a helpful framework of analysis must be capable of illuminating these issues on both microsociological and macrosociological levels. As argued above, because sports violence is normally manifested in widely different ways by form and context, what also is required is a contextualized perspective, atuned to the specific history, culture, and politics of the setting in which the violence occurs. For this reason, attempts to use a uniform theory to account for all forms and expressions of sports violence are likely to meet with as much success as the mainstream collective behavior perspectives. One might note here that these approaches, discussed at the beginning of the paper, are adopted less and less in research, and when they are, it is usually to rehash now familiar and belabored moments of American cultural and political crisis (e.g., counter-cultural and protest movements of the 1960s).

Future research in this area must proceed, as has the respected work of Taylor and the Leicester school in England, from a perspective that is as complex as the issue on which it seeks to throw light. It must recognize history and social structure, the latter comprising factors such as political backdrop, class experience, and gender. Of course, the work of Taylor and Dunning is far from complete in these respects. Although Taylor's recent work resonates uneasily with his early soccer subculture thesis and thus stumbles at the historical or developmental level used so seductively by the Leicester group, the latter's account of the effects of modern British political crisis in sport is at times cursory. But what is impressive about these studies is their respective levels of appreciation for the unique culture in which one particular aspect of collective violence at sport has become an institutionalized feature of sport in that context. This is borne of approaches, different as they are, that recognize that history, social structure, and politics all play a crucial role in both passive and violent sports-related practices. Future research must proceed from such an understanding.

REFERENCES

1. Adams, R. Soccer hooliganism and the mass media: fictions and reality. *Youth and Society* 30:13–16, 1978.
2. Adedeji, J.A. Sport, violence and collective behavior in Nigerian post-primary and secondary school games. Paper presented at the Tenth World Congress of Sociology, Mexico City, 1982.
3. Allport, G.W. *Social Psychology*. Boston: Houghton Mifflin, 1924.
4. Arms, R.L., G.W. Russell, and M.L. Sandilands. Effects on the hostility of spectators of viewing aggressive sports. *Rev. of Sport and Leisure* 4:115–127, 1979.
5. Arms, R.L, G.W. Russell, and M.L. Sandilands. Effects of viewing aggressive sports on the hostility of spectators. R.M. Suinn (ed.). *Psychology in Sports: Methods and Applications*. Minneapolis: Burgess, 1980, pp. 133–142.
6. Asch, S.E. Effects of group pressure upon modification and distortion of judgements. E. Macoby (ed.). *Readings in Social Psychology*. New York: Holt, 1958, pp. 174–183.
7. Atyeo, D. *Violence in Sports*. Toronto: Van Nostrand Reinhold, 1979.
8. Aveni, A.F. The not-so-lonely crowd: friendship groups in collective behavior. *Sociometry* 40:96–99, 1977.
9. Beamish, R. The materialist approach to sport study: an alternative prescription to the discipline's methodological malaise. *Quest* 33:55–71, 1981.
10. Beisser, A.R. *The Madness in Sports*. New York: Appleton Century Crofts, 1967.

11. Bell, A. *Against Racism and Fascism in Europe*. Socialist Group, European Parliament, 1986.

12. Bennet, M.J. Sport Fans and Others. Ph.D. Dissertation, Ohio State University, 1975.

13. Berk, R.A. *Collective Behavior*. Chicago: William Brown, 1974.

14. Blumer, H. Collective behavior. A.M. Lee (ed.). *Principles of Sociology*. New York: Barnes and Noble, 1951, pp. 167–222.

15. Boire, J.A. Collective behavior in sport. *Rev. of Sport and Leisure* 5:2–45, 1980.

16. Breaux, J. Factors Affecting Social Contagion in Crowds. Ph.D. Dissertation, Oxford University, 1975.

17. Brill, A.A. The way of the fan. *North Am. Rev.* 226:400–434, 1929.

18. Brown, L. Men on home ground. *The Leveller*, 16–29 Oct.:14–16, 1981.

19. Browne, J. The sociological aspects of the sports audience. *Aust. J. Phys. Ed.* 58:15–24, 1972.

20. Bryant, J., and D. Zillmann. Sports violence and the media. J.H. Goldstein (ed.). *Sports Violence*. New York: Springer-Verlag, 1983, pp. 195–208.

21. Cameron, A. *Circus Factions: Blues and Greens at Tome and Byzantium*. Oxford: Clarendon, 1976.

22. Carroll, R. Football hooliganism in England. *Int. Rev. Sport Sociol.* 15:77–92, 1980.

23. Case, R.W., and R.L. Boucher. Spectator violence in sport: A selected review. *J. Sport and Social Issues* 5:1–15, 1981.

24. Cavanaugh, B.M., and J.M. Silva. Spectator perceptions of fan misbehavior: an attitudinal inquiry. C.H. Nadeau (ed.). *Psychology of Motor Behavior and Sport*. Champaign, IL: Human Kinetics, 1980, pp. 189–198.

25. Clarke, A., and L. Madden. Professional football: the limits of economic analysis. *Leis. Management*: 36–38, October, 1986.

26. Clarke, A., and L. Madden. Sportacular: the club, the community and the common cause. *Leis. Management*: 16–17, Feb., 1987.

27. Clarke, J. Football Hooliganism and the Skinheads. Occasional Paper, University of Birmingham, 1973.

28. Clarke, J. Football and working-class fans: tradition and change. R. Ingham (ed.). *Football Hooliganism: The Wider Context*. London: Inter-Action Inprint, 1978.

29. Coakley, J. Media coverage of sports and violent behavior: an elusive connection. *Curr. Psych: Res. and Reviews* 7:322–330, 1988–1989.

30. Coalter, F. Crowd behavior at football matches: a study in Scotland. *Leis. Studies* 4:111–117, 1985.

31. Connell, R.W. *Gender and Power*. Stanford, CA: Stanford University Press, 1987.

32. Connell, R.W. An iron man. M.A. Messner and D.F. Sabo (eds.). *Sport, Men and the Gender Order: Critical Feminist Perspectives*. Champaign, IL: Human Kinetics, 1989.

33. Corrigan, P. *Schooling the Smash Street Kids*. London: MacMillan, 1979.

34. Couch, C.J. Dimensions of association in collective behavior episodes. *Sociometry* 33:457–471, 1970.

35. Critcher, C. Football since the war. J. Clarke (ed.). *Working Class Culture*. London: Hutchinson, 1979, pp. 161–184.

36. Crofts, M. Crowd behavior: Bay 13 at the World Series one day internationals. *Pelops* 5:17–21, 1984.

37. Cunneen, C., and R. Lynch. The social meanings of conflict in riots at the Australian grand prix motorcycle races. *Leis. Studies* 7:1–18, 1988.

38. Curtis, J. Isn't it difficult to support some of the notions of "The Civilizing Process"?: a response to Dunning. C.R. Rees and A.W. Miracle (eds.). *Sport and Social Theory*. Champaign, IL: Human Kinetics, 1986, pp. 57–65.

39. Dewar, C.K. Spectator fights at professional baseball games. *Rev. Sport and Leis.* 4:12–26, 1979.

40. Dunning, E. Soccer: The Social Origins of the Sport and its Development as a Spectacle and a Profession. Leicester: University of Leicester Press, 1979.
41. Dunning, E. Sociological reflections on sport and civilization. *Int. Rev. Sport Sociol.* 25:65–81, 1990.
42. Dunning, E., J. Maguire, P. Murphy, and J. Williams. If you think you're hard enough. *New Society:* 342–344, Aug. 27, 1981.
43. Dunning, E., J. Maguire, P. Murphy, and J. Williams. The social roots of football violence. *Leis. Studies* 1:139–156, 1982.
44. Dunning, E., J. Maguire, P. Murphy, and J. Williams. Football hooliganism in Britain before the first World War. *Int. Rev. Sport Sociol.* 19:215–239, 1984.
45. Dunning, E., P. Murphy, and J. Williams. Working Class Social Bonding and the Sociogenesis of Football Hooliganism: A Report to the Social Science Council. Leicester: University of Leicester, 1982.
46. Dunning, E., P. Murphy, and J. Williams. Football hooliganism. *Research Council Newsletter* 51:91–21, 1984.
47. Dunning, E., P. Murphy, and J. Williams. *The Roots of Football Hooliganism: An Historical and Sociological Study.* London: Routledge and Kegan Paul, 1988.
48. Dunning, E., and K. Sheard. *Barbarians, Gentlemen and Players: A Sociological Study of the Development of Rugby Football.* New York: New York University Press, 1979.
49. Dunstan, K. *Sports.* Melbourne: Cassell, 1973.
50. Duperault, J.R. L'Affaire Richard: a situational analysis of the Montreal hockey riot. *Can. J. Hist. Sport* XII:66–83, 1981.
51. Edgell, S., and D. Jary. Football: a sociological eulogy. M.A. Smith, S. Parker, and C.S. Smith (eds.). *Leisure and Society in Britain.* London: Allen Lane, 1973, pp. 214–229.
52. Edwards, H. *The Sociology of Sport.* Homewood, IL: Dorsey Press, 1973.
53. Edwards, H., and V. Rackages. The dynamics of violence in sport. *J. Sport and Social Issues* 1:3–31, 1977.
54. Elias, N. *The Civilizing Process.* London: Basil Blackwell, 1978.
55. Fimrite, R. Take me out to the brawl game. A. Yiannakis (ed.). *Sport Sociology: Contemporary Themes.* Dubuque, IA: Kendall/Hunt, 1976, pp. 200–203.
56. Fontana, A. Over the edge: a return to primitive sensation in play and games. *Urban Life* 7:213–229, 1978.
57. Gammon, C. This isn't cricket . . . but it is. *Sports Illust.:* 37–42, Apr. 6, 1981.
58. Gerth, H., and C.W. Mills. *Character and Social Structure.* New York: Harcourt Brace and World, 1953.
59. Gilbert, B., and L. Twyman. Violence: out of hand in the stands. *Sports Illust.:* 62–74, Jan. 31, 1983.
60. Goldstein, J.H., and R.L. Arms. Effects of observing athletic contests on hostility. *Sociometry* 34:83–90, 1971.
61. Goodhart, P., and C. Chataway. *War Without Weapons.* London: W.H. Allen, 1968.
62. Goranson, R.E. The Impact of Television Hockey Violence. La Marsh Research Program Reports on Violence and Conflict Resolution. Toronto: York University Press, 1982.
63. Green, R.G., and E.C. O'Neal. *Perspectives on Aggression.* New York: Academic Press, 1976.
64. Greer, D.L. Spectator booing and the home advantage: a study of influence in the basketball arena. *Social Psych. Qt.* 46:252–261, 1983.
65. Guttmann, A. Sports spectators from antiquity to renaissance. *J Sports Hist.* 8:5–27, 1981.
66. Guttmann, A. *Sports Spectators.* New York: Columbia University Press, 1986.
67. Hahn, E., G. Pilz, H.J. Stollenwerk, and K. Weis. *Fanverhalten, Massenmedien und Gewalt im Sport.* Schorndorf: Verlag Karl Hofmann, 1988.

68. Hall, S. The treatment of football hooliganism in the press. R. Ingham (ed.). *Football Hooliganism: The Wider Context.* London: Inter-Action Inprint, 1978, pp. 15–37.

69. Hargreaves, J. Where's the virtue? Where's the grace? A discussion of the social production of gender relations in and through sport. *Theory, Culture and Society* 3:109–121, 1986.

70. Harrison, P. Soccer's tribal wars. *New Society*: 602–604, Sept. 5, 1974.

71. Hazleton, L. British soccer. *New York Times*: 40–41, May 7, 1989.

72. Hoch, P. *Rip Off the Big Game: The Exploitation of Sport by the Power Elite.* Garden City, NY: Anchor, 1972.

73. *Hooligan.* Thames Television, England. Produced by Ian Stuttard, 1985.

74. Hopcraft, A. *The Football Man.* London: Penguin, 1968.

75. Hutchinson, J. Some Aspects of Football Crowds Before 1914. Proceedings from Conference for the Study of Labour History, University of Sussex, Paper 13, 1975.

76. Johnson, W., and D. Hutton. Effects of Boxing Upon Spectators as Measured by a Projective Test. Unpublished paper, University of Maryland, 1953.

77. Katz, S. Strange forces behind the Richard hockey riot. *Macleans* 17:11–110, 1955.

78. Keen, D. Exterminate them. *New Statesman*: 16, Jan. 31, 1986.

79. Kidd, B. Of ice and men. *Integral: The Magazine for Changing Men* 1:16, 1987.

80. Kidd, B. Sports and masculinity. M. Kaufmann (ed.). *Beyond Patriarchy: Essays by Men on Pleasure, Power and Change.* New York: Oxford, 1987, pp. 250–265.

81. Kingsmore, J. The Effect of Professional Wrestling and Professional Basketball Contests Upon the Aggressive Tendencies of Male Spectators. Ph.D. Dissertation, University of Maryland, 1968.

82. Klapp, O.E. *Currents of Unrest.* New York: Holt, Rinehart and Winston, 1972.

83. Knight, G., and I. Taylor. News and political censensus: CBC television and the 1983 British election. *Can. Rev. Soc. and Anthro.* 23:230–246, 1986.

84. Kutcher, L. The American sport event as carnival: an emergent norm approach to crowd behavior. *J. Pop. Cult.* 16:34–42, 1983.

85. Lang, G.E. Riotous outbursts at sports events. G.R. Luscher and G.H. Sage (eds.). *Handbook of Social Sciences of Sport.* Champaign, IL: Stipes, 1981, pp. 415–439.

86. Lang, K., and G.E. Lang. *Collective Dynamics.* New York: Crowell, 1961.

87. Lang, K., and G.E. Lang. Collective behavior. D. Sills (ed.). *Int. Encycl. Soc. Sciences* 2:556–564, 1968.

88. Le Bon, G. *The Crowd.* New York: Viking, 1960. (First published 1895).

89. Lennon, J.X., and F.C. Hatfield. The effects of crowding and observation of athletic events on spectator tendency toward aggressive behavior. *J. Sports Behav.* 3:61–68, 1980.

90. Leuck, M.R., G.S. Krahenbohl, and J.E. Odenkiuk. Assessment of spectator aggression at intercollegiate basketball contests. *Rev. Sport and Leis.* 4:40–53, 1979.

91. Lever, J. Soccer: opium of the Brazilian people. *Trans-action* 7:36–43, 1969.

92. Lever, J. Soccer as a Brazilian way of life. G.P. Stone (ed.). *Games, Sport and Power.* New Brunswick, NJ: Transaction Inc., 1972, pp. 138–159.

93. Lever, J. *Soccer Madness.* Chicago: University of Chicago Press, 1983.

94. Levitt, C., and W. Shaffir. *The Riot at Christie Pits.* Toronto: Lester and Orpen Dennys, 1987.

95. Lewis, J.M. Fan violence: an American social problem. *Res. in Soc. Probs. and Pub. Policy* 12:175–206, 1982.

96. Listiak, A. "Legitimate deviance" and social class: bar behavior during Grey Cup week. M. Hart and S. Birrell (eds.). *Sport in the Sociocultural Process.* Dubuque, IA: Wm. C. Brown, 1981, pp. 532–563.

97. Lorenz, K. *On Aggression.* Toronto: Bantam, 1966.

98. Maguire, J. The emergence of football spectating as a social problem 1880–1985: a figurational and developmental perspective. *Sociol. of Sport J.* 3:217–244, 1986.

99. Maguire, J. Violence of soccer matches in Victorian England: issues in the study of

sports violence, popular culture and deviance. *Curr. Psych.: Res. and Review* 7:285–297, 1988–1989.

100. Main, J. Sport cops a bloody nose. *Your Sport: Australia's Monthly Sport Magazine* 1:8–11, 1985.

101. Mann, L. Sports crowds from the perspective of collective behavior. J.H. Goldstein (ed.). *Sports, Games, and Play: Social and Psychological Viewpoints.* Hillsdale, NJ: Laurence Erlbaum Associates, 1979, pp. 337–371.

102. Manning, F. (ed.). *The Celebration of Society: Perspectives on Contemporary Cultural Performance.* Bowling Green, OH: Bowling Green State University Press, 1983.

103. Mark, M., F.B. Bryant, and D.R. Lehman. Perceived lifestyle and sports violence. J.H. Goldstein (ed.). *Sport Violence.* New York: Springer-Verlag, 1983, pp. 83–105.

104. Marples, M. *A History of Football.* London: Secker and Warburg, 1954.

105. Marsh, P. Understanding aggro. *New Society*: 7–9, Apr. 3, 1975.

106. Marsh, P. *Aggro: The Illusion of Violence.* Oxford: Basil Blackwell, 1982.

107. Marsh, P., and A. Campbell (eds.). *Aggression and Violence.* Oxford: Basil Blackwell, 1982.

108. Marsh, P., and R. Harré. The world of football hooligans. M. Hart and S. Birrell (eds.). *Sport in the Sociocultural Process.* Dubuque, IA: Wm. C. Brown, 1981, pp. 609–623.

109. Marsh, P., E. Rosser, and R. Harré. *The Rules of Disorder.* London: Routledge and Kegan Paul, 1978.

110. Mason, A. *Association Football and English Society, 1863–1915.* Brighton, England: Harvester, 1980.

111. McDougall, W. *The Group Mind.* New York: G.P. Putnam, 1920.

112. McIlvaney, H. Fierce holy war in a violent city. *Sports. Illust.*:40–43, Jan. 15, 1968.

113. Meijs, J., and H. Van Der Burg. Dutch supporters at the European championship in Germany. Paper presented at the European Congress on Violence Control in the World of Sports, Athens, Greece, Feb. 17–19, 1989.

114. Messner, M. Sports and male domination: the female athlete as contested ideological terrain. *Sociol. of Sport J.* 5:197–211, 1988.

115. Metcalfe, A. Working Class Physical Recreation in Montreal, 1860–1895. H. Cantelon and R. Gruneau (eds.). Working Papers in the Sociological Study of Sport and Leisure (Monograph 1). Kingston, Ontario: Queen's University Press, 1978.

116. Milgram, S., and H. Toch. Collective behavior: crowds and social movements. G. Lindsey and E. Aronson (eds.). *Handbook of Social Psychology.* Reading, MA: Addison-Wesley, 1969, pp. 507–610.

117. Moore, R. *Sport and Mental Health.* Springfield, IL: Charles C. Thomas, 1966.

118. Moorhouse, H.F. Professional football and working class culture: English theories and Scottish evidence. *Sociol. Rev.* 32:285–316, 1984.

119. Moorhouse, H.F. Scotland against England: football and popular culture. *Br. J. Sports Hist.* 1:4, 1987.

120. Morris, D. *The Naked Ape.* New York: McGraw Hill, 1967.

121. Morris, D. *The Soccer Tribe.* London: Jonathon Cape, 1981.

122. Murphy, P., E. Dunning, and J. Williams. Soccer crowd disorder and the press: processes of amplification and de-amplification in historical perspective. *Theory, Cult. and Society* 5:645–693, 1988.

123. Murray, B. *The Old Firm: Sectarianism, Sport and Society in Scotland.* Edinburgh: John Donald, 1984.

124. Murray, C. The soccer hooligan's honour system. *New Society*: 9–1, Oct. 6, 1977.

125. O'Brien, T. The fans' beliefs. *Curr. Psych.: Res. and Reviews* 7:347–359, 1988–1989.

126. Panayiotopoulos, D. Violence as a Crime in the Athletic Field and Greek Law. Paper presented at the European Congress on Violence Control in the World of Sports, Athens, Greece, Feb. 17–19, 1989.

127. Park, R.E. *Introduction to the Science of Sociology*. Chicago: University of Chicago Press, 1924.
128. Pearton, R.E., and G. Gaskell. Youth and social conflict: sport and spectator violence. *Int. Rev. Sport Sociol.* 2, 57–69, 1981.
129. Perls, F.S. *Ego, Hunter, and Aggression*. New York: Random House, 1969.
130. Petryszak, N. The bio-sociology of joy in violence. *Rev. Sports and Leis.* 2:1–16, 1977.
131. Pietersen, B. The Emergence of the Roligan—A Danish Aspect of Fan Behavior. Paper presented at the European Congress on Violence Control in the World of Sports, Athens, Greece, Feb. 17–19, 1989.
132. Pilz, G. Report on "Sport and Violence." Committee for the Development of Sport, Council of Europe, Strasbourg, Sept. 1981.
133. Pitz, G. Violence in West German Sport—Some Theoretical and Empirical Remarks. Paper presented at the third annual meeting of the North American Society for the Sociology of Sport, Toronto, Ontario, Nov. 3–7, 1982.
134. Quarantelli, E.L., and J. Weller. The structural problem of a sociological speciality: collective behavior's lack of a critical mass. *The Am. Sociol.* 9:59–68, 1974.
135. Redhead, S. *Sing When You're Winning*. London: Pluto, 1986.
136. Redhead, S., and E. McLaughlin. Soccer's style wars. *New Society*: 225–228, Aug. 16, 1985.
137. Report on Football Hooliganism to the Minister of Sport (The Harrington Report). Unpublished, 1968.
138. Report of the Working Party on Crowd Behavior at Football Matches (The Lang Report). London: HMSO, 1969.
139. Report of the Inquiry into Crowd Safety at Sports Grounds (The Wheatley Report). London: HMSO, 1972.
140. Report of a Joint Sports Council/Social Science Research Council Panel, *Public Disorder and Sporting Events*. London: Social Sciences Research Council, 1978.
141. Report of Committee of Inquiry into Crowd Safety and Control at Soccer Grounds (The Popplewell Report). London: HMSO, 1985.
142. Ritzer, G. *Sociological Theory*. New York: Alfred A. Knopf, 1983.
143. Roberts, J. The Effects of Degree of Involvement Upon the Level of Aggression of Spectators Before and After a University Basketball Game. Ph.D. Dissertation, University of Maryland, 1972.
144. Robins, D. *We Hate Humans*. Markham, Ontario: Penguin, 1984.
145. Ross. E.A. *Foundations of Sociology*. New York: MacMillan, 1905.
146. Rude, G. *The Crowd in History: A Study of Popular Disturbances in France and England 1730–1848*. New York: John Wiley, 1964.
147. Russell, G.W. Spectator moods at an aggressive sports event. *J. Sports Psych.* 3:217–227, 1981.
148. Russell, G.W., S.L. Di Lullo, and D. Di Lullo. Effects of observing competitive and violent versions of a sport. *Curr. Psych.: Res. and Reviews* 7:312–321, 1988–1989.
149. Semyonov, M., and M. Farbstein. Ecology of sports violence: the case of Israeli soccer. *Sociol. of Sport J.* 6:50–59, 1989.
150. Sheed, W. This riotous isle. *Sports, Illust.*: 78–95, Apr. 12, 1969.
151. Sherif, M. *The Psychology of Social Norms*. New York: Harper and Row, 1936.
152. Sloan, L.R. The function and impact of sports for fans: a review of theory and contemporary research. J.H. Goldstein (ed.). *Sports, Games and Play: Social and Psychological Viewpoints*. Hillsdale, NJ: Laurence Erlbaum Associates, 1979, pp. 219–263.
153. Smelser, N.J. *The Theory of Collective Behavior*. New York: Free Press, 1962.
154. Smith, F. New legislation on football hooliganism—England and Wales. Paper presented at the European Congress on Violence Control in the World of Sports, Athens, Greece, Feb. 17–19, 1989.
155. Smith, M.D. Sport and collective violence. D.W. Ball and J.W. Loy (eds.). *Sport and*

Social Order: Contributions to the Sociology of Sport. Reading, MA: Addison-Wesley, 1975, pp. 277–333.

156. Smith, M.D. Hostile outbursts in sport. A Yiannakis (ed.). *Sport Sociology: Contemporary Themes.* Dubuque, IA: Kendal/Hunt, 1976, pp. 203–205.
157. Smith, M.D. Precipitants of crowd violence. *Sociol. Inquiry* 48:121–131, 1978.
158. Smith, M.D. Hockey violence: A test of the violent subculture hypothesis. *Soc. Probs.* 27:234–247, 1979.
159. Smith, M.D. *Violence and Sport.* Torono: Butterworths, 1983.
160. Smith, M.D. Violence in Canadian Amateur Sport: A Review of Literature. Report for Commission for Fair Play, Government of Canada, 1987.
161. Suttles, G. *The Social Order of the Slum.* Chicago: University of Chicago Press, 1968.
162. Tarde, G. *The Laws of Imitation.* New York: Holt, 1903.
163. Taylor, I. Hooligans: soccer's resistance movement. *New Society,* Aug. 7, 1969.
164. Taylor, I. Soccer consciousness and soccer hooliganism. S. Cohen (ed.). *Images of Deviance.* New York: Penguin, 1971, pp. 134–165.
165. Taylor, I. On the sports violence question: soccer hooliganism revisited. J. Hargreaves (ed.). *Sport, Culture and Ideology.* Boston: Routledge and Kegan Paul, 1982, pp. 152–197.
166. Taylor, I. Class, violence and sport: the case of soccer hooliganism in Britian. H. Cantelon and R. Gruneau (eds.). *Sport, Culture and the Modern State.* Toronto: University of Toronto Press, 1982, pp. 39–97.
167. Taylor, I. Putting the boot into a working-class sport: British soccer after Bradford and Brussels. *Soc. of Sport J.* 4:171–191, 1987.
168. Taylor, I. Hillsborough, 15 April 1989: Some Personal Contemplations. Unpublished paper, 1989.
169. Theberge, N. A feminist analysis of responses to sports violence: Media coverage of the 1987 World Junior Hockey Championship. *Sociol. of Sport J.* 6:247–256, 1989.
170. Thompson, R. Sport and Deviance: A Subcultural Analysis. Ph.D. Dissertation, University of Alberta, 1977.
171. Tiger, L. *Men in Groups.* London: Thomas Nelson and Son, 1969.
172. Trivizaz, E. Offences and offenders in football crowd disorders. *Br. J. Criminol.* 20:276–289, 1980.
173. Trivizaz, E. Sentencing the football hooligan. *Br. J. Criminol.* 21:342–347, 1981.
174. Trow, M. Comment on participant observation and interviewing. *Human Organization* 16, 1957.
175. Turner, R.H., and L.M. Killian. *Collective Behavior.* Englewood Cliffs, NJ: Prentice-Hall, 1972.
176. Vamplew, W. Sports crowd disorder in Britain, 1870–1914: causes and controls. *J. Sport Hist.* 7:5–21, 1980.
177. Van Der Brug, H. Football Hooliganism in the Netherlands. Paper presented at the European Congress on Violence Control in the World of Sports, Athens, Greece, Feb. 17–19, 1989.
178. Van Limbergen, K. The Societal Backgrounds of Hooliganism in Belgium. Paper presented at the European Congress on Violence Control in the World of Sports, Athens, Greece, Feb. 17–19, 1989.
179. Vulliamy, E. Live by aggro, die by aggro. *New Statesman*: 8–10, June 7, 1985.
180. Wade, D. Are golf's galleries getting out of hand? *Gold Digest*: 60–61, Nov. 1978.
181. Wagg, S. *The Football World: A Contemporary Social History.* Brighton, England: Harvester, 1984.
182. Walvin, J. *The People's Game: The Social History of British Football.* Harmondsworth, England: Allen Lane, 1975.
183. Walvin, J. *Football and the Decline of Britain.* Basingstoke, England: MacMillan, 1986.
184. Weir, S. Oi for England, *New Socialist*:20–21, July, 1985.

185. Whannel, G. Football crowd behavior and the press. *Med. Cult. and Society* 1:327–342, 1979.
186. White, A. Soccer hooliganism in Britain. *Quest* 34:154–164, 1982.
187. White, C. Analysis of hostile outbursts in spectator sports. *Dissertation Abstracts Int.* 31:6390A, 1970.
188. Williams, J. Football hooliganism: offences, arrests and violence—a critical note. *Br. J. Law Society.* 7:104–111, 1980.
189. Williams, J. In search of the hooligan solution. *Social Studies Rev.* 1:3–5, 1985.
190. Williams, J. "C,mon, la! We'll get in!" *New Statesman and Society*: 14–15, 21 April, 1989.
191. Williams, J., E. Dunning, and P. Murphy. *Hooligans Abroad: The Behavior and Control of English Fans in Continental Europe.* London: Routledge and Kegan Paul, 1984.
192. Williams, J., E. Dunning, and P. Murphy. The rise of the English soccer hooligan. *Youth and Society* 17:362–380, 1986.
193. Williams, J., E. Dunning, and P. Murphy. *Hooliganism After Heysel: Crowd Behavior in England and Europe, 1985–1988.* Leicester: University of Leicester Press, 1988.
194. Yeager, R.C. *Seasons of Shame: The New Violence in Sports.* Toronto: McGraw-Hill, 1979.
195. Young, K.M. A sociological study of football crowd disorder, 1863–1980. Unpublished paper, University of Leicester, 1980.
196. Young, K.M. The killing field: themes in mass media responses to the Heysel stadium riot. *Int. Rev. Sport Sociol.* 21:253–264, 1986.
197. Young, K.M. Sports Crowd Disorder, Mass Media and Ideology. Ph.D. Dissertation, McMaster University, Ontario, 1988.
198. Young, J.M. Violence in the workplace of professional sport from victimological and cultural studies perspectives. *Int. Rev. Sport Sociol.* 1, 1991 (forthcoming).
199. Young, K.M., and M.D. Smith. Mass media treatment of violence in sports and its effects. *Curr. Psych: Res. and Reviews* 7:298–312, 1988–1989.
200. Young, P.M. *A History of British Football.* London: Stanley Paul, 1968.

Index

Page numbers followed by "t" denote tables; those followed by "f" denote figures.